HORSEOWNER'S GUIDE
TO LAMENESS

Horseowner's Guide to Lameness

TED S. STASHAK, DVM, MS

Diplomate American College of Veterinary Surgeons;
Professor of Surgery, Department of Clinical Sciences,
College of Veterinary Medicine and Biomedical Sciences,
Colorado State University, Fort Collins, Colorado

IN COLLABORATION WITH CHERRY HILL

A Lea & Febiger Book

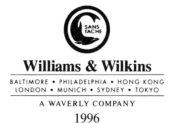

Williams & Wilkins

BALTIMORE • PHILADELPHIA • HONG KONG
LONDON • MUNICH • SYDNEY • TOKYO

A WAVERLY COMPANY

1996

Executive Editor: Carroll C. Cann
Developmental Editor: Susan Hunsberger
Production Coordinator: Peter J. Carley
Project Editor: Robert D. Magee

Copyright © 1995
Williams & Wilkins
Rose Tree Corporate Center
1400 North Providence Road
Building II, Suite 5025
Media, PA 19063-2043 USA

Accurate indications, adverse reactions, and dosage schedules for drugs are provided in this book, but it is possible they may change. The reader is urged to review the package information data of the manufacturers of the medications mentioned.

Printed in the United States of America

Library of Congress Cataloging-in-Publication Data

Stashak, Ted S.
    Horseowner's guide to lameness / Ted S. Stashak; in collaboration with Cherry Hill
        p.   cm.
    "A Lea & Febiger book."
    Includes index.
    ISBN 0-683-07985-9
    1. Lameness in horses.   I. Hill, Cherry, 1947–   .   II. Title.
SF959.L25S73   1995
636.1'089758—dc20
                                                        94-30066
                                                              CIP

The Publishers have made every effort to trace the copyright holders for borrowed material. If they have inadvertently overlooked any, they will be pleased to make the necessary arrangements at the first opportunity.

95 96 97 98 99
1 2 3 4 5 6 7 8 9 10

Reprints of chapters may be purchased from Williams & Wilkins in quantities of 100 or more. Call Isabella Wise, Special Sales Department, (800) 358-3583.

Dedication

To conscientious horse owners, trainers, veterinarians,
equine science students, and farriers everywhere
so that together
we might make our horses more comfortable.

Acknowledgments

- Peggy Judy for her much-appreciated assistance with the drawings throughout the book and especially for Chapters 2 and 6.

- Richard Klimesh for his technical assistance, drawings, and photos for Chapter 6, Shoeing for Soundness.

- Macmillan Publishing, New York, NY, for use of materials from *Maximum Hoof Power*, 1994, by Cherry Hill and Richard Klimesh, AFA CJF.

- Breakthrough Publications, Ossining, NY, for use of materials from *Making Not Breaking*, 1992 by Cherry Hill.

- Storey Communications, Pownal, VT, for use of materials from *From the Center of the Ring*, 1988 by Cherry Hill.

Preface

When lameness strikes, it is often painful for the horse and can be frustrating, disappointing, heart-breaking, and costly. Because *Adam's Lameness in Horses*, Fourth Edition, is generally considered too technical for horse owners, trainers, and students in equine science and farrier programs, we elected to develop a comprehensive text that was user friendly. We extracted some of the information from the Fourth Edition and updated every topic. We heavily revised the Conformation and Shoeing chapters.

We hope that this information, coupled with conscientious management, will result in fewer horses suffering from lameness. When a lameness does occur, and you seek professional assistance, we suggest you stay informed and actively involved in the case yourself. It will be most helpful for the horse if you are knowledgeable about the lameness that is being treated. Toward that end, we have provided detailed information about all equine lamenesses: description, causes, signs, treatment, and prognosis. For the horse's sake, we strongly encourage you to develop a cooperative team involving yourself, your veterinarian, and your farrier. This is the key to your horse's recovery and comfort.

Ted S. Stashak and Cherry Hill

Contents

CHAPTER ONE

Functional Anatomy*

Anatomy, by nature, is a complex, technical subject. Rather than simplify it too much, we have retained the detail for your future reference.

Anatomic Nomenclature

In Figure 1–1, note that the positional adjectives "proximal" and "distal" refer to the limbs and "dorsal" and "ventral" refer to the upper body, head, and neck. "Rostral" is used to indicate the direction toward the nose. With the exception of the eye, the terms "anterior" and "posterior" are not applicable to quadrupeds. "Cranial" and "caudal" apply to the limbs proximal to the knee (antebrachiocarpal radiocarpal) joint and the hock (tarsocrural tibiotarsal) joint. Distal to these joints, "dorsal" and "palmar" (on the forelimb) or "plantar" (on the hindlimb) are the correct terms. The adjective "solar," is used to designate structures on the palmar (plantar) surface of the coffin bone (distal phalanx) and the ground surface of the hoof.

Thoracic Limb (Fig. 1–2)

Digit and Fetlock

The foot and pastern comprise the equine digit. The bones of this region include the coffin bone (also known as [a.k.a.] the distal phalanx, third phalanx, or P_{III}), the navicular bone (a.k.a. the distal sesamoid), the short pastern bone (a.k.a. the middle phalanx, the second phalanx, or P_{II}), and the long pastern bone (a.k.a. the proximal phalanx, the first phalanx, or P_I). The fetlock is the region where the long pastern bone articulates with the cannon bone and the two proximal sesamoid bones.

Foot

The foot consists of the hoof (epidermis) and all it encloses: the corium (dermis), digital cushion, coffin bone, lateral cartilages, coffin joint, distal extremity of the short pastern bone, navicular bone, navicular bursa, several ligaments, tendons of insertion of the common digital extensor and deep digital flexor muscles, blood vessels, and nerves.

* A large portion of this material is extracted from Karner RA, Functional Anatomy of Equine Locomotor Organs, In Adam's Lameness in Horses, edited by Ted Stashak, 4th Edition, Philadelphia, PA, Lea & Febiger, 1987.

The hoof is continuous with the epidermis (outer skin) at the coronet. Here the dermis (inner layer) of the skin is continuous with the dermis (corium) of the hoof. Regions of the corium correspond to the parts of the hoof under which they are located: perioplic corium, coronary corium, laminar corium, corium of the frog, and corium of the sole (Fig. 1–3).

The exterior parts of the hoof protect underlying structures of the foot and dissipate concussive forces when the hoof strikes the ground. Figure 1–4 illustrates the sole, frog, heels, bars, and ground surface of the wall. The ground surface of the forefoot is wider than that of the hindfoot, corresponding to the rounder coffin bone of the forefoot.

The hoof wall extends from the ground surface to the coronary border, where the soft white horn of the periople joins the epidermis of the skin at the coronet. Regions of the wall are the dorsal toe, the medial and lateral quarters, and the heels. From the thick toe, the wall becomes progressively thinner and more elastic toward the heels, where it thickens again at the junction of the bars (the "buttress" of the hoof). The medial wall is usually steeper (more upright) than the lateral wall.

The horn's tubules are sometimes visible as fine lines on the hoof wall, running from the coronet to the ground (Fig. 1–5). Differential growth rates of the wall from the coronary border toward the ground account for the smooth ridges parallel to the coronary border.

Most of the epidermis is devoid of nerve endings; it is the "insensitive" part of the foot.

Three layers comprise the hoof wall: the stratum tectorium, stratum medium, and stratum internum (see Fig. 1–5). The superficial stratum tectorium is a thin layer of horn extending distally from the periople a variable distance that decreases with age. The bulk of the wall is a stratum medium consisting of horn tubules and intertubular horn. The horn tubules are generated by the germinal layer of the coronary epidermis covering the long papillae of the coronary corium. Intertubular horn is formed in between the projections.

Distal to the coronary groove, approximately 600 primary insensitive (epidermal) laminae interlock with the primary sensitive (dermal) laminae of the laminar corium (Figs. 1–4 and 1–5). Approximately 100 microscopic secondary laminae branch at an angle from each primary lamina, further binding the hoof and corium together (Fig. 1–6).

Some confusion exists concerning the terms "insensitive" and "sensitive" laminae. In the strictest sense, the keratinized parts of the primary epidermal

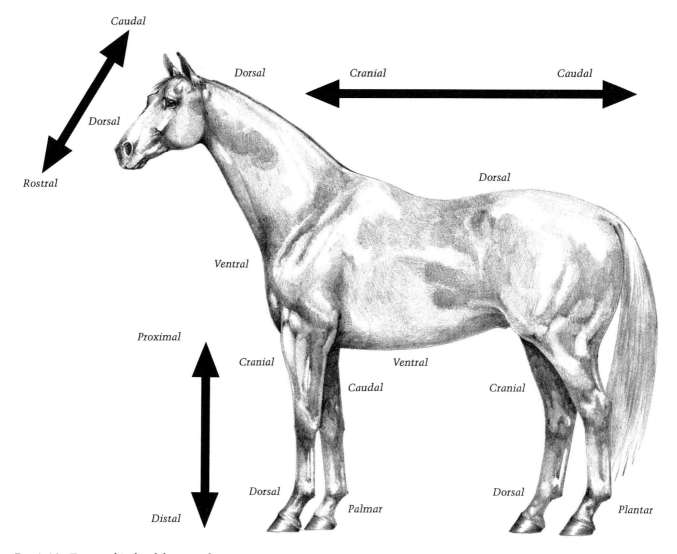

FIG. 1–1A. Topographical and directional terms.

laminae are insensitive; the stratum germinativum, which includes all of the secondary epidermal laminae, and the laminar corium are "sensitive." Although the terms "epidermal" and "dermal" are far more accurate adjectives, the terms "sensitive" and "insensitive" are still in common use.

Submicroscopic, peglike dermal projections increase the surface of attachment of the sensitive and insensitive structures (dermis and epidermis) of the hoof. This configuration and the blending of the laminar corium with the periosteum of the coffin bone suspend and support the bone, aiding in the dissipation of concussion and the movement of blood.

The wall grows approximately 0.25 inch (6 mm) per month, taking from 9 to 12 months for the toe to grow out. Growth tends to be slower in cold or dry environments.

Stratum medium may be pigmented or nonpigmented. Contrary to popular belief, pigmented hooves are not stronger than nonpigmented hooves.

The slightly concave sole should not bear weight on its ground surface, except near its junction with the white line, but it bears internal weight transmitted from the solar surface of the coffin bone through the solar corium. That portion of the sole at the angle formed by the wall and the bars is the angle of the sole (seat of corn). When the wall is trimmed, the white line is visible where the wall joins the sole. The sensitive corium is immediately internal to the white line that serves as a landmark for determining the position and angle for driving horseshoe nails.

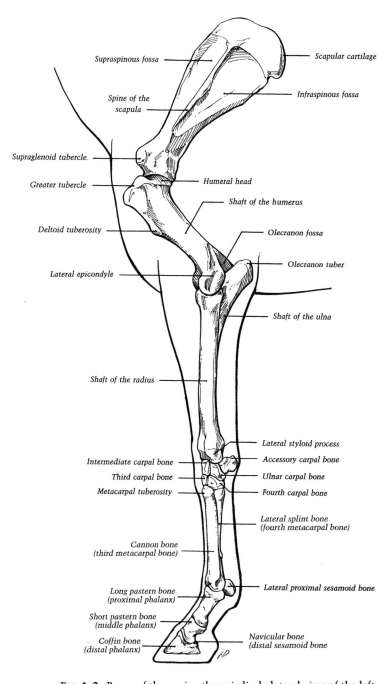

Supraspinous fossa

Scapular cartilage

Spine of the scapula

Infraspinous fossa

Supraglenoid tubercle

Greater tubercle

Humeral head

Shaft of the humerus

Deltoid tuberosity

Olecranon fossa

Olecranon tuber

Lateral epicondyle

Shaft of the ulna

Shaft of the radius

Lateral styloid process

Accessory carpal bone

Intermediate carpal bone

Ulnar carpal bone

Third carpal bone

Fourth carpal bone

Metacarpal tuberosity

Lateral splint bone
(fourth metacarpal bone)

Cannon bone
(third metacarpal bone)

Long pastern bone
(proximal phalanx)

Lateral proximal sesamoid bone

Short pastern bone
(middle phalanx)

Coffin bone
(distal phalanx)

Navicular bone
(distal sesamoid bone)

FIG. 1–1B (continued). Topographical and directional terms.

FIG. 1–2. Bones of the equine thoracic limb; lateral view of the left limb.

The sole's horn tubules are oriented vertically, conforming to the direction of the papillae of the solar corium. Intertubular horn binds the tubules together. The relationship of the solar epithelium to the solar corium is responsible for this configuration (Fig. 1–7). Near the ground, the horn tubules curl, accounting for the self-limiting growth of the sole, and cause shedding from the superficial part. Approximately one-third of the sole is water.

The frog (Fig. 1–4) is a wedge-shaped mass of keratinized epithelium rendered softer than other parts of the hoof by a 50% water content. Merocrine glands deliver their secretions onto the surface superficial to the frog stay (Fig. 1–3). The proximally projecting frog stay contacts the digital cushion.

The corium is rich in elastic fibers, highly vascular, and well supplied with nerves. The arterial supply is from numerous branches radiating outward from the

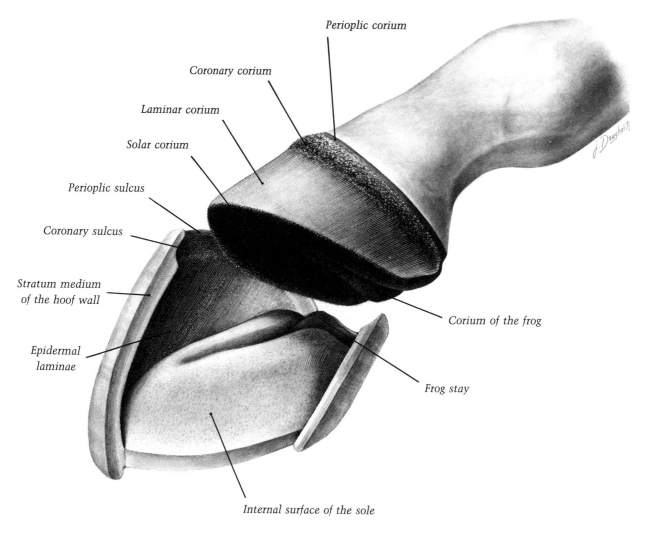

FIG. 1–3. Dissected view of the relationships of the hoof to the underlying regions of the corium.

terminal arch in small canals extending from the solar (semilunar) canal in the coffin bone and from the dorsal and palmar branches of the coffin bone from the digital arteries (Fig. 1–8).

Deep to the coronary band is the highly elastic coronary cushion. The coronary band and cushion form the bulging mass that fits into the coronary groove of the hoof. Part of the coronary venous plexus (network) is within the coronary cushion. The plexus receives blood from the dorsal venous plexus in the laminar corium.

Where the corium is adjacent to the coffin bone, it blends with the bone's periosteum, serving (particularly in the laminar region) to connect the hoof to the bone.

The medial and lateral (collateral) cartilages of the coffin bone lie under the corium of the hoof and the skin, covered by the coronary venous plexus. Roughly rhomboid in shape, they extend above the coronary border of the hoof, where they may be palpated.

Four ligaments stabilize each cartilage of the coffin bone (Fig. 1–9). The cartilages of the coffin bone are hyaline cartilage in young horses and fibrocartilage in middle-aged animals. In older horses, the cartilages tend to ossify (calcify), forming "sidebones."

Between the cartilages is the digital cushion, a highly modified meshwork of collagenous and elastic fibers, depots of adipose (fat) tissue, and small masses of fibrocartilage. It contacts the corium of the frog and thus encloses the frog stay (Fig. 1–10). The apex of the wedge-shaped digital cushion is attached to the deep digital flexor tendon as the latter expands to its insertion on the solar surface of the coffin bone. The base of the digital cushion bulges into the bulbs of the heels, which are separated superficially by a central shallow groove. The structure and relationships of the digital cushion indicate its anticoncussive function.

As the deep digital flexor tendon courses to its insertion on the coffin bone, it is bound in place by the distal digital anular ligament, a sheet of deep fascia supporting the terminal part of the tendon and sweeping proximally to attach on each side of the long pastern bone (Fig. 1–11). The tendon passes deeply over

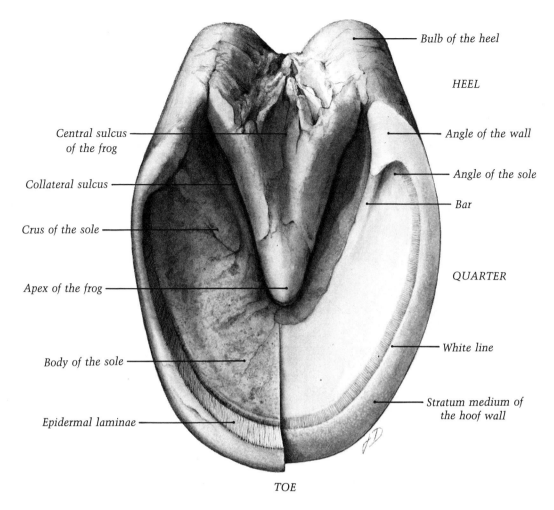

Central sulcus
of the frog

Collateral sulcus

Crus of the sole

Apex of the frog

Body of the sole

Epidermal laminae

Bulb of the heel

HEEL

Angle of the wall

Angle of the sole

Bar

QUARTER

White line

Stratum medium of
the hoof wall

TOE

FIG. 1–4. Ground (solar) surface of a right hind hoof. The left half has the epidermal laminar growth extending past the sole to illustrate its contribution to the formation of the white line. The right half has been trimmed to emphasize the formation of the white line by the epidermal laminae.

the navicular bone. The navicular bone is a sesamoid bone that changes the direction of the tendon as it goes to its attachment on the coffin bone. The navicular bursa is interposed between the tendon and the navicular bone, cushioning the movement of the tendon against the bone (see Fig. 1–10). From the exterior, the location of the navicular bursa and bone may be approximated deep to the middle third of the frog.

The proximal border of the navicular bone has a groove containing openings for the passage of small vessels. The distal border of the bone has a small, elongated facet for articulation with the coffin bone. Two concave areas on the main articular surface of the navicular bone contact the distal articular surface of the short pastern bone, resulting in the formation of the coffin joint. The navicular bone is supported in this position by three ligaments. Paired collateral sesamoidean (suspensory navicular) ligaments arise from the distal end of the long pastern bone on each side

dorsal to the collateral ligaments of the pastern joint. (Figs. 1–11 and 1–12). They sweep on each side of the short pastern bone and attach to the extremities and proximal border of the navicular bone. Distally, the navicular bone is stabilized by the impar ligament, which attachs it to the flexor surface of the coffin bone palmar to the insertion of the deep digital flexor tendon (see Fig. 1–12).

The distal articular surface of the short pastern bone, the articular surface of the coffin bone, and the two articular surfaces of the navicular bone form the coffin joint. Short collateral ligaments arise from the distal end of the short pastern bone, pass distally deep to the cartilages of the coffin bone and terminate on either side of the extensor process and the dorsal part of each cartilage (Fig. 1–9).

A small dorsal pouch of the joint capsule of the coffin joint blends with the common digital extensor tendon (Fig. 1–10). On either side, the joint capsule blends

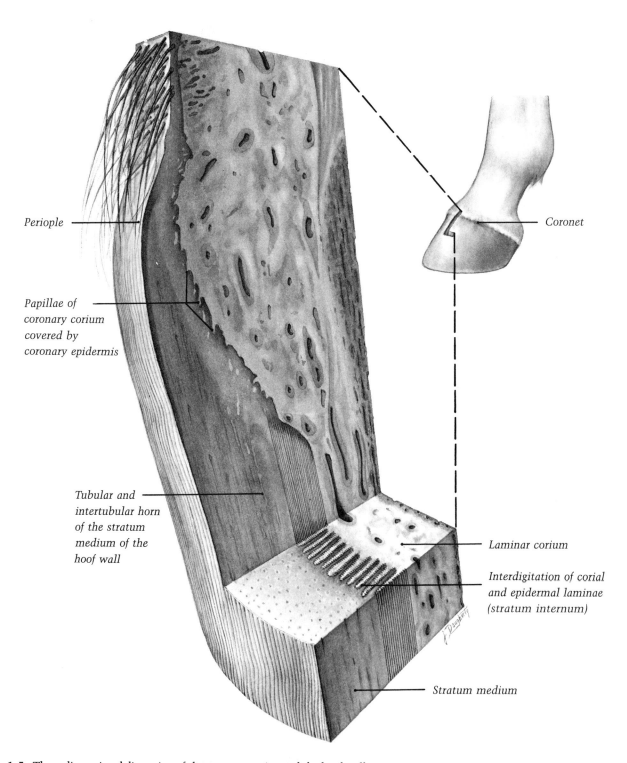

Periople

*Papillae of
coronary corium
covered by
coronary epidermis*

*Tubular and
intertubular horn
of the stratum
medium of the
hoof wall*

Coronet

Laminar corium

*Interdigitation of corial
and epidermal laminae
(stratum internum)*

Stratum medium

Fig. 1–5. Three-dimensional dissection of the coronary region and the hoof wall.

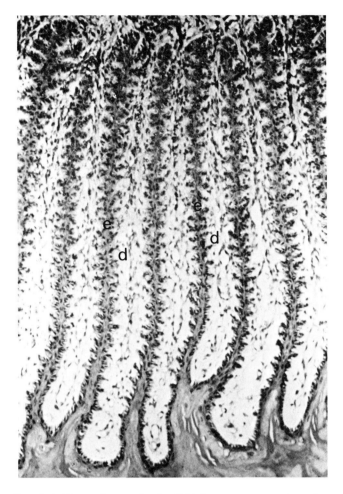

FIG. 1–6. Photomicrograph of a field from a cross section of an equine fetal hoof (×40). Interdigitations of epidermal laminae (e) and dermal (corial) laminae (d). Note the small secondary laminae.

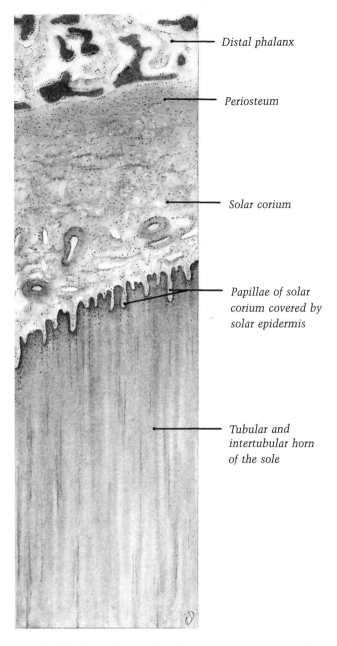

— *Distal phalanx*

— *Periosteum*

— *Solar corium*

— *Papillae of solar corium covered by solar epidermis*

— *Tubular and intertubular horn of the sole*

FIG. 1–7. Histologic relationships of periosteum, corium, and horn of the sole.

with the collateral ligaments. The palmar pouch is more extensive, extending proximally midway on the short pastern bone to a transverse fibrous band, the so-called "T ligament" separating the joint capsule from the digital synovial sheath of the flexor tendons (see Fig. 1–10). Medially and laterally protruding pouches of the joint capsule lie against the cartilages of the coffin bone palmar to the collateral ligaments, especially during flexion.

The tendon of insertion of the common digital extensor muscle terminates on the extensor process of the coffin bone, receiving a ligament from each cartilage as it inserts (Fig. 1–9).

Pastern

Deep to the skin and superficial fascia on the palmar aspect of the pastern, the proximal digital anular ligament adheres to the superficial digital flexor tendon and extends to the medial and lateral borders of the long pastern bone (Fig. 1–13). This fibrous band of deep fascia covers the superficial digital flexor as it bifurcates (splits) and aids in binding the deep digital flexor tendon as well.

Two ligaments of the ergot diverge from beneath the horny ergot on the palmar skin of the fetlock. Each ligament descends obliquely just under the skin

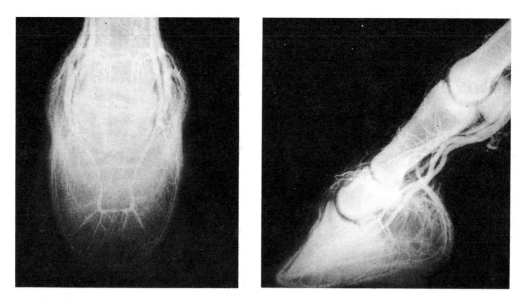

FIG. 1–8. Angiograms of the foot following intra-arterial injection of radiopaque medium.

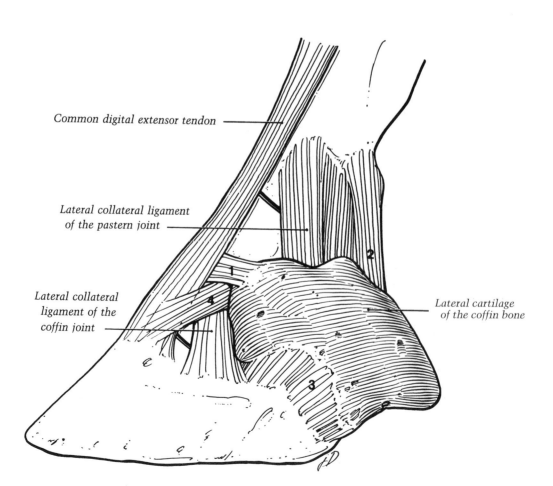

Common digital extensor tendon

Lateral collateral ligament
of the pastern joint

Lateral collateral
ligament of the
coffin joint

Lateral cartilage
of the coffin bone

FIG. 1–9. Four ligaments (1, 2, 3, and 4) stabilizing each cartilage of the coffin bone.

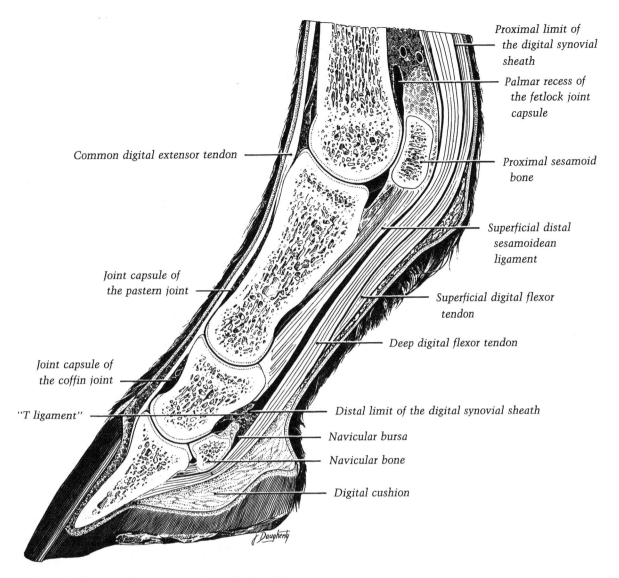

Common digital extensor tendon

Joint capsule of
the pastern joint

Joint capsule of
the coffin joint

"T ligament"

*Proximal limit of
the digital synovial
sheath*

*Palmar recess of
the fetlock joint
capsule*

*Proximal sesamoid
bone*

*Superficial distal
sesamoidean
ligament*

*Superficial digital flexor
tendon*

Deep digital flexor tendon

Distal limit of the digital synovial sheath

Navicular bursa

Navicular bone

Digital cushion

FIG. 1–10. Parasagittal section through the equine fetlock and digit.

superficial to the proximal digital anular ligament, the terminal branch of the superficial digital flexor tendon, and the palmar digital artery and nerve, finally widening and connecting with the distal digital anular ligament (Fig. 1–13).

The tendon of insertion of the superficial digital flexor muscle terminates by bifurcating into two branches that insert on the distal extremity of the long pastern bone and the proximal extremity of the short pastern bone just palmar to the collateral ligaments of the pastern joint (see Fig. 1–11). The tendon of insertion of the deep digital flexor muscle descends between the two branches of the superficial flexor tendon. A digital synovial sheath enfolds both tendons,

including both branches of the superficial flexor tendon and continuing around the deep flexor tendon as far as the T ligament (see Fig. 1–10). The latter is a fibrous partition attaching to the middle of the palmar surface of the short pastern bone.

Deep to the flexor tendons, three distal sesamoidean ligaments extend distally from the bases of the two proximal sesamoid bones (Fig. 1–11). The superficial straight sesamoidean ligament attaches distally on the proximal extremity of the palmar surface of the short pastern bone; the triangular middle sesamoidean ligament attaches distally to a rough area on the palmar surface of the long pastern bone; and the pair of deep sesamoidean ligaments cross, each attaching to

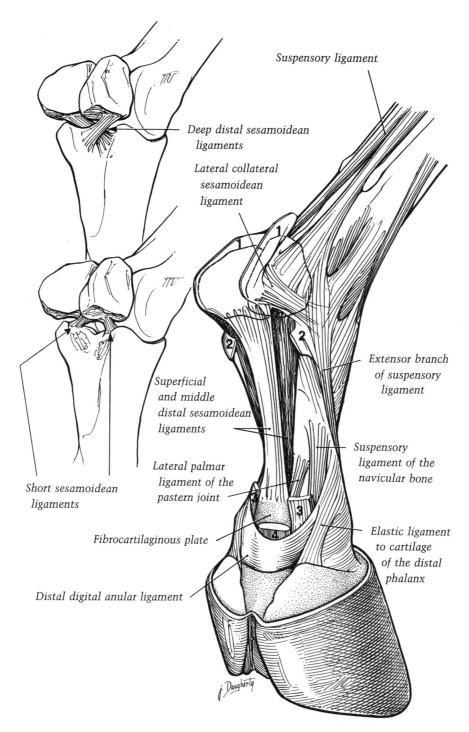

Suspensory ligament

Deep distal sesamoidean
ligaments

Lateral collateral
sesamoidean
ligament

Extensor branch
of suspensory
ligament

Superficial
and middle
distal sesamoidean
ligaments

Suspensory
ligament of the
navicular bone

Lateral palmar
ligament of the
pastern joint

Short sesamoidean
ligaments

Fibrocartilaginous plate

Elastic ligament
to cartilage
of the distal
phalanx

Distal digital anular ligament

j. Daugherty

Fig. 1–11. Dissections of the sesamoidean ligaments. Dashed lines indicate the positions of the proximal sesamoid bones embedded in the metacarpointersesamoidean ligament. Numbers indicate the cut stumps of the palmar anular ligament of the fetlock (1), proximal digital anular ligament (2), superficial digital flexor tendon (3), and deep digital flexor tendon (4).

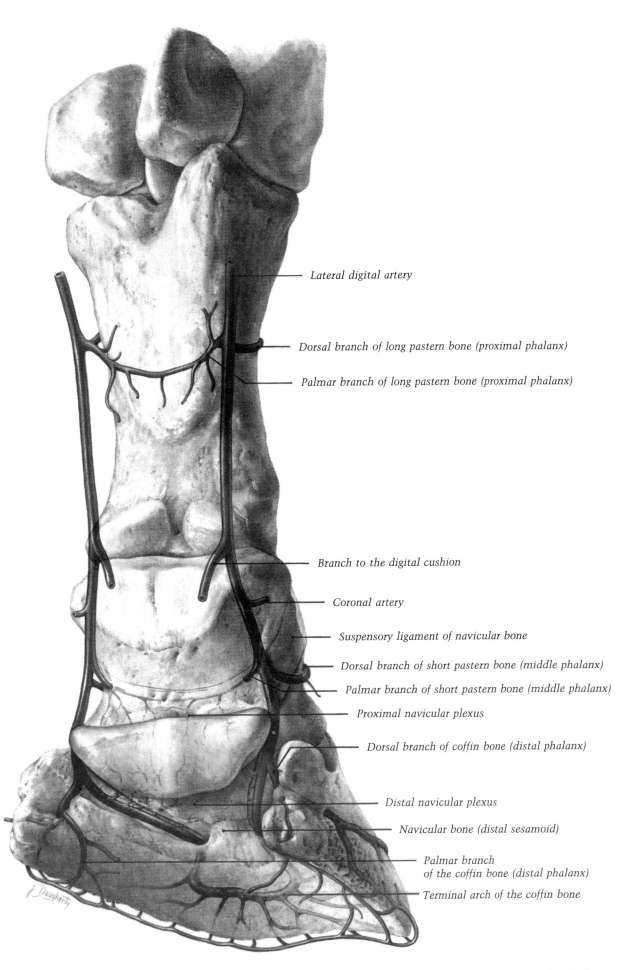

Lateral digital artery

Dorsal branch of long pastern bone (proximal phalanx)

Palmar branch of long pastern bone (proximal phalanx)

Branch to the digital cushion

Coronal artery

Suspensory ligament of navicular bone

Dorsal branch of short pastern bone (middle phalanx)

Palmar branch of short pastern bone (middle phalanx)

Proximal navicular plexus

Dorsal branch of coffin bone (distal phalanx)

Distal navicular plexus

Navicular bone (distal sesamoid)

Palmar branch
of the coffin bone (distal phalanx)

Terminal arch of the coffin bone

FIG. 1–12. Arterial supply to the digit of the forelimb with emphasis on branches supplying the navicular bone and coffin bone.

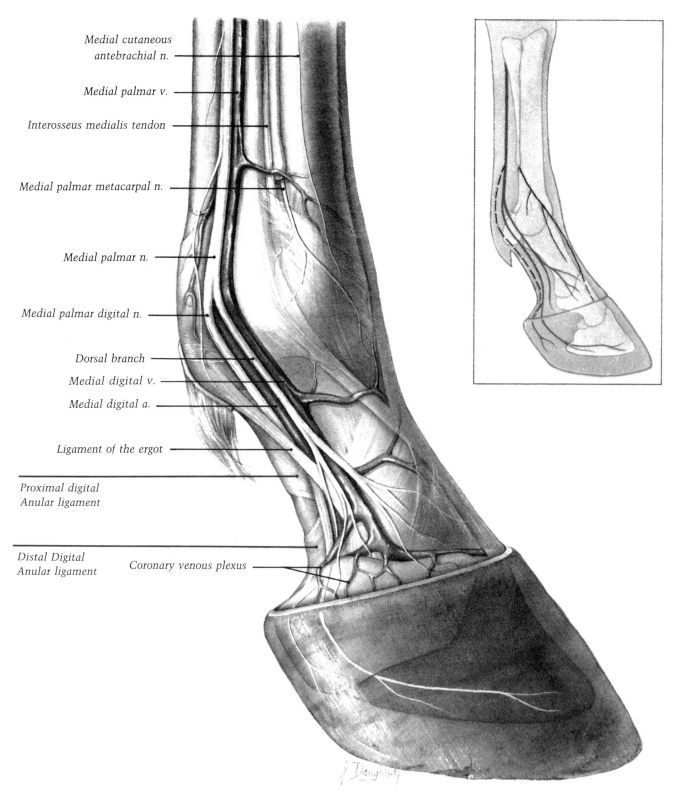

Medial cutaneous
antebrachial n.

Medial palmar v.

Interosseus medialis tendon

Medial palmar metacarpal n.

Medial palmar n.

Medial palmar digital n.

Dorsal branch

Medial digital v.

Medial digital a.

Ligament of the ergot

Proximal digital
Anular ligament

Distal Digital
Anular ligament

Coronary venous plexus

FIG. 1–13. Medial aspect of the distal cannon, the fetlock, and digit. Skin and superficial fascia removed. n., nerve; v., vein; a., artery. Inset: schematic of the distribution of major nerves indicating variant branches (dashed lines).

a prominence on the opposite side of the long pastern bone (see Fig. 1–11).

In addition, each sesamoid bone is further attached to the long pastern bone by a short sesamoidean ligament (Fig. 1–11).

A ligamentous extensor branch of the suspensory ligament (Figs. 1–11 and 1–12) passes from the respective proximal sesamoid bone obliquely across each side of the long pastern bone to the dorsal surface where each branch joins the tendon of insertion of the common digital extensor muscle near the distal extremity of the long pastern bone.

The tendon of the common digital extensor muscle inserts partially on the proximal extremities of the long and short pastern bones on its way to a final insertion on the extensor process of the coffin bone.

The pastern joint is formed by two convex areas on the distal extremity of the long pastern bone and two shallow concave areas on the proximal extremity of the short pastern bone. Bones of the pastern joint are held together by two short collateral ligaments and four palmar ligaments.

The joint capsule of the pastern joint blends with the deep surface of the common digital extensor tendon (see Fig. 1–10).

Fetlock (Metacarpophalangeal Joint)

The fetlock of the thoracic limb is the region around the fetlock joint. The horny ergot gives origin to the two distally diverging ligaments of the ergot.

Deep to the skin and superficial fascia, the palmar anular ligament of the fetlock binds the digital flexor tendons and their enclosing digital synovial sheath in the sesamoid groove.

The sesamoid groove contains the deep digital flexor tendon. Immediately proximal to the canal formed by the palmar anular ligament of the fetlock and the sesamoid groove, the deep digital flexor tendon perforates through a circular opening in the superficial digital flexor tendon.

The common and lateral digital extensor tendons pass over the dorsal aspect of the fetlock joint.

The distal extremity of the cannon bone, the proximal extremity of the long pastern bone, the two proximal sesamoid bones, and the extensive ligament in which the proximal sesamoids are embedded form the fetlock joint.

A pouch of the fetlock joint capsule extends proximally between the cannon bone and the suspensory ligament. This pouch is palpable and even visible when the joint is inflamed, distending the palmar recess with synovial fluid.

Support for the fetlock and stabilization during locomotion is provided by its suspensory apparatus, a part of the stay apparatus. The suspensory apparatus of the fetlock includes the suspensory ligament (interosseus medius muscle) and its extensor branches to the common digital extensor tendon and the distal sesamoidean ligaments extending from the bases of

the proximal sesamoid bones distal to the long or short pastern bones.

The blood vessels and nerves of the digit and fetlock are illustrated in Figures 1–12, 1–13, and 1–14.

Functions of the Digit and Fetlock

In the standing position, essentially in extension, the fetlock and digit are supported by the suspensory apparatus of the fetlock (interosseus muscle, intersesamoidean ligament, and distal sesamoidean ligaments), the digital flexor and extensor tendons, and the collateral ligaments of the joints. The forelimbs support more weight than the hindlimbs. On the forelimb, the angle of the toe (with the ground) varies from 53 to 58°.

The locomotor functions of the digit and fetlock include the flexion essential to movement, extension when the foot is off the ground, the dissipation of concussion when the hoof contacts the ground, and the recovery from extension.

During flexion of the fetlock and digit, most of the movement is in the fetlock; the least amount of movement is in the pastern joint; and movement in the coffin joint is intermediate.

Contraction of the common and lateral digital extensor muscles brings the bones and joints of the digit into alignment just before the hoof strikes the ground.

Normally, when the unshod hoof contacts the ground, the heels strike first. Most of the impact is sustained by the hoof wall, and compression of the wall creates tension on the interlocking insensitive and sensitive laminae and to the periosteum of the coffin bone. The domed sole is depressed slightly by the pressure of the coffin bone, causing expansion of the quarters. Descent of the coffin joint occurs and the navicular bone is compressed between the deep digital flexor tendon and the coffin joint. Concussion is dissipated by the digital cushion and the cartilages of the coffin bone.

Compression of the venous plexus between the laterally expanding digital cushion and the nonyielding hoof wall forces blood out of the hoof capsule. The hydraulic shock-absorption by the blood within the vessels augments the direct cushioning by the frog and digital cushion and the resiliency of the hoof wall.

During concussion, the four palmar ligaments of the pastern joint, the straight sesamoidean ligament, and the tendon of the deep digital flexor provide the tension necessary to prevent overextension of the joint. Tension of the contracting superficial digital flexor muscle tightens against its tendon's insertions on the distal end of the long pastern bone and proximal end of the short pastern bone, preventing the pastern joint from buckling.

The suspensory apparatus of the fetlock and the digital flexor tendons ensure that overextension of the fetlock joint, i.e., decreasing the dorsal articular angle, is minimal when the hoof strikes the ground. Yet at the gallop, when all of the horse's weight is on one

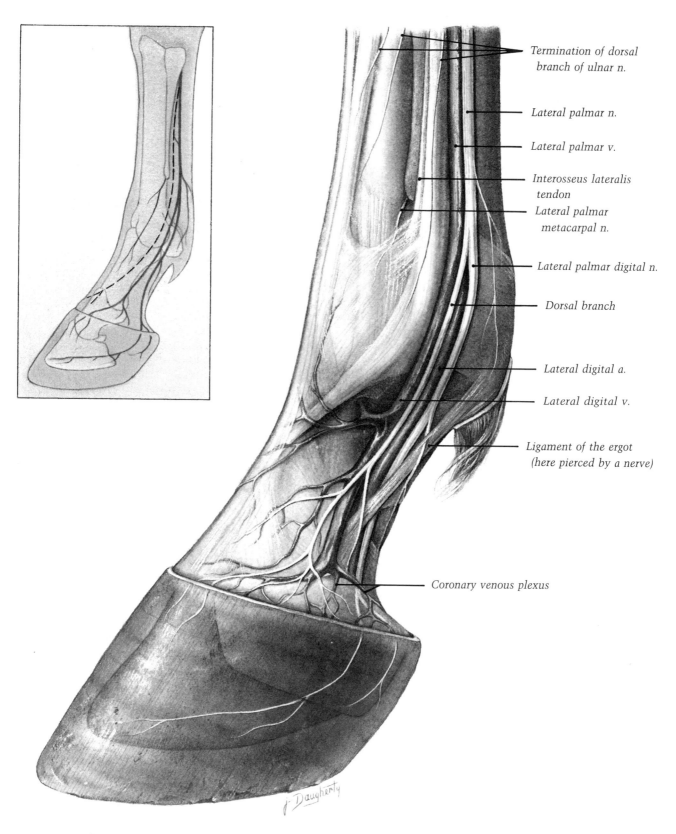

Termination of dorsal
branch of ulnar n.

Lateral palmar n.

Lateral palmar v.

Interosseus lateralis
tendon

Lateral palmar
metacarpal n.

Lateral palmar digital n.

Dorsal branch

Lateral digital a.

Lateral digital v.

Ligament of the ergot
(here pierced by a nerve)

Coronary venous plexus

FIG. 1–14. Lateral aspect of the distal cannon, the fetlock, and digit. Skin and superficial fascia have been removed. n., nerve; v., vein; a.,
artery. Inset: schematic of the distribution of major nerves indicating variant branches (dashed lines).

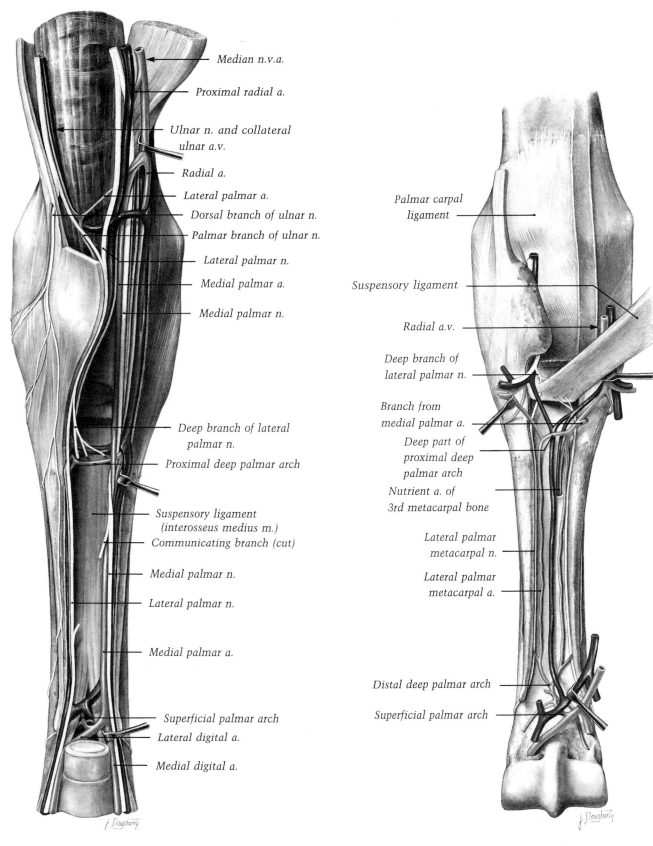

Median n.v.a.

Proximal radial a.

Ulnar n. and collateral ulnar a.v.

Radial a.

Lateral palmar a.

Dorsal branch of ulnar n.

Palmar branch of ulnar n.

Lateral palmar n.

Medial palmar a.

Medial palmar n.

Deep branch of lateral palmar n.

Proximal deep palmar arch

Suspensory ligament (interosseus medius m.)

Communicating branch (cut)

Medial palmar n.

Lateral palmar n.

Medial palmar a.

Superficial palmar arch

Lateral digital a.

Medial digital a.

Palmar carpal ligament

Suspensory ligament

Radial a.v.

Deep branch of lateral palmar n.

Branch from medial palmar a.

Deep part of proximal deep palmar arch

Nutrient a. of 3rd metacarpal bone

Lateral palmar metacarpal n.

Lateral palmar metacarpal a.

Distal deep palmar arch

Superficial palmar arch

FIG. 1–15. Caudal view of the left carpus and cannon; most of the digital flexor tendons have been removed. n., nerve; v., vein; a., artery.

FIG. 1–16. Deep dissection of the caudal aspect of left carpus and cannon, with the medial palmar artery removed. n., nerve; v., vein; a., artery.

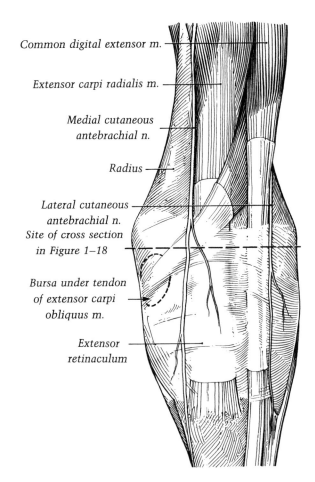

Common digital extensor m.

Extensor carpi radialis m.

Medial cutaneous antebrachial n.

Radius

Lateral cutaneous antebrachial n.
Site of cross section in Figure 1–18

Bursa under tendon of extensor carpi obliquus m.

Extensor retinaculum

FIG. 1–17. Dorsal view of the left carpus. m., muscle; n., nerve.

forelimb momentarily, the palmar aspect of the fetlock comes very close to the ground.

Cannon Bone Region (Metacarpus)

The equine metacarpus consists of the cannon bone and the medial and lateral splint bones and the structures associated with them. Each splint bone is united by an interosseous ligament to the cannon bone. Length and curvature of the shafts and the prominence of the free distal extremities ("buttons") of the splint bones are variable. The proximal extremities of the metacarpal bones articulate with the distal row of carpal bones.

Deep to the skin, the common digital extensor tendon is located on the dorsal surface of the cannon bone (Fig. 1–15).

The superficial digital flexor tendon is deep to the skin and subcutaneous fascia throughout the length of the cannon. The deep digital flexor tendon lies against the superficial surface of the suspensory liga-

ment. The carpal synovial sheath extends distally to enclose both digital flexor tendons as far as the middle of the cannon. At this level, the deep digital flexor tendon is joined by its accessory ligament (carpal check ligament or "inferior" check ligament) (see Fig. 1–22). The digital synovial sheath around the flexor tendons extends proximally into the distal fourth of the cannon (see Fig. 1–10).

The metacarpal groove, formed by the palmar surface of the cannon bone and the axial surfaces of the splint bones contains the suspensory ligament (interosseus medius muscle) and the diminutive interosseus medialis and lateralis muscles. The suspensory ligament arises from the distal row of carpal bones and the proximal end of the cannon bone (Fig. 1–16). In the distal fourth of the cannon, the suspensory ligament splits into two branches (see Fig. 1–15). Each branch extends to a sesamoid bone with an extensor branch and extends to the distal third of the pastern region continuing on to join the common digital extensor tendon.

Knee (Carpus)

The carpal region includes the carpal bones (radial, intermediate, ulnar, and accessory in the proximal row; first, second, third, and fourth in the distal row), the distal extremity of the radius (and fused ulna), the proximal extremities of the cannon and splint bones, and the structures adjacent to these bones.

Under the skin on the dorsal aspect of the carpus are the tendon sheaths of the extensor carpi radialis, extensor carpi obliquus, and the common digital extensor tendons, which are enclosed in fibrous extensor retinaculum. The tendon sheaths of the common digital and oblique carpal extensor tendons extend from the carpometacarpal articulation proximally to 6 to 8 cm proximal to the carpus (see Figs. 1–17 and 1–18).

The tendon sheath of the extensor carpi radialis muscle terminates at the middle of the carpus, and then the tendon becomes adherent to the retinaculum as it extends to its insertion on the metacarpal tuberosity. Deeply, the extensor retinaculum serves as the dorsal part of the common fibrous joint capsule of the carpal joints. Blood vessels and nerves of the carpus are illustrated in Figs. 1–17, 1–18, and 1–19.

The lateral collateral carpal ligament extends distally from its attachment on the styloid process of the radius (Fig. 1–20). The superficial part of the ligament attaches distally on the lateral splint bone and partly on the cannon bone. A canal between the superficial part and the deep part of the ligament provides passage for the tendon of the lateral digital extensor muscle and its synovial sheath. The deep part of the ligament attaches on the ulnar carpal bone.

Palmar to the lateral collateral carpal ligament, four ligaments support the accessory carpal bone (Fig. 1–20). Tendons of two muscles are associated with the accessory carpal bone. The short tendon of the ulnaris

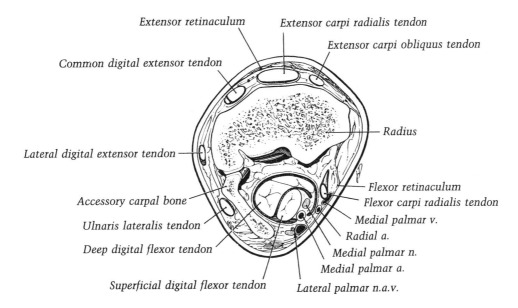

FIG. 1–18. Cross section of left forearm immediately proximal to the antebrachiocarpal joint. n., nerve; v., vein; a., artery.

lateralis muscle attaches to the proximal border and lateral surface of the bone; the muscle's long tendon passes through a groove on the bone's lateral surface and then continues distally to insert on the proximal extremity of the lateral splint bone (see Fig. 1–17). The single tendon of the flexor carpi ulnaris muscle attaches to the proximal border of the accessory carpal bone.

On the medial side of the carpus, the medial collateral carpal ligament extends from the medial styloid process of the radius and widens distally to attach to the proximal ends of the medial splint and cannon bones. Bundles of fibers also attach to the radial, second, and third carpal bones (Fig. 1–21). The inconstant first carpal bone may be embedded in the palmar part of the medial collateral carpal ligament adjacent to the second carpal bone.

The flexor retinaculum is a broad fibrous band extending from the medial collateral carpal ligament to the accessory carpal bone, bridging the carpal groove and forming the carpal canal (see Fig. 1–18). Fibrous connective tissue fills the carpal canal, supporting several structures that pass through the canal. The superficial and deep digital flexor tendons are enclosed in the carpal synovial sheath extending from a level 8 to 10 cm proximal to the carpus distally to the middle of the metacarpus (see Fig. 1–19).

The palmar carpal ligament forms the dorsal wall of the carpal canal, its deep face serving as the palmar part of the common fibrous capsule of the carpal joints. It attaches to the three palmar radiocarpal ligaments, three palmar intercarpal ligaments, four palmar carpometacarpal ligaments, and the palmar surfaces of the carpal bones. Distally, the palmar carpal ligament gives origin to the accessory ligament (carpal check ligament) of the deep digital flexor tendon, which joins the tendon at the middle of the metacarpus.

The antebrachiocarpal joint is located between the radius and ulna and the proximal row of carpal bones. The midcarpal joint is located between the proximal and distal rows of carpal bones (these are hinge joints). The carpometacarpal joint is located between the distal row of carpal bones and the cannon and splint bones form a plane joint with minimal movement. An extensive antebrachiocarpal synovial sac is deep to the fibrous joint capsule. A palmarolateral pouch extends from this sac. The midcarpal synovial sac communicates with the small carpometacarpal sac between the third and fourth carpal bones.

The antebrachiocarpal and midcarpal joints are flexed by the combined action of the flexor carpi radialis, flexor carpi ulnaris, and ulnaris lateralis muscles; the joints are extended by the extensor carpi radialis and extensor carpi obliquus (abductor digiti I longus) muscles. The flattened dorsal articular areas of the carpal joints and the palmar carpal ligament uniting the palmar aspect of the carpal bones all serve to prevent overextension of the antebrachiocarpal and midcarpal joints.

Further stability is given to the extended carpus dorsally by the tendon of the extensor carpi radialis tendon and palmarly by the tendoligamentous support of the "check ligaments" and the digital flexor tendons. The accessory (radial check) ligament (really the radial head) of the superficial digital flexor is a flat fibrous band originating on a ridge on the caudomedial aspect of the distal part of the radius and joining the tendon

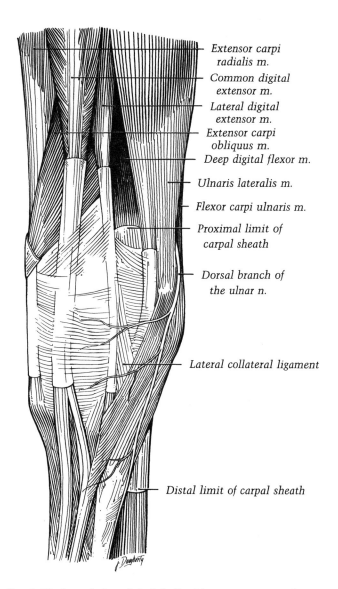

Extensor carpi
radialis m.

Common digital
extensor m.

Lateral digital
extensor m.

Extensor carpi
obliquus m.

Deep digital flexor m.

Ulnaris lateralis m.

Flexor carpi ulnaris m.

Proximal limit of
carpal sheath

Dorsal branch of
the ulnar n.

Lateral collateral ligament

Distal limit of carpal sheath

FIG. 1–19. Lateral view of the left distal forearm, carpus, and proximal metacarpus. m., muscle; n., nerve.

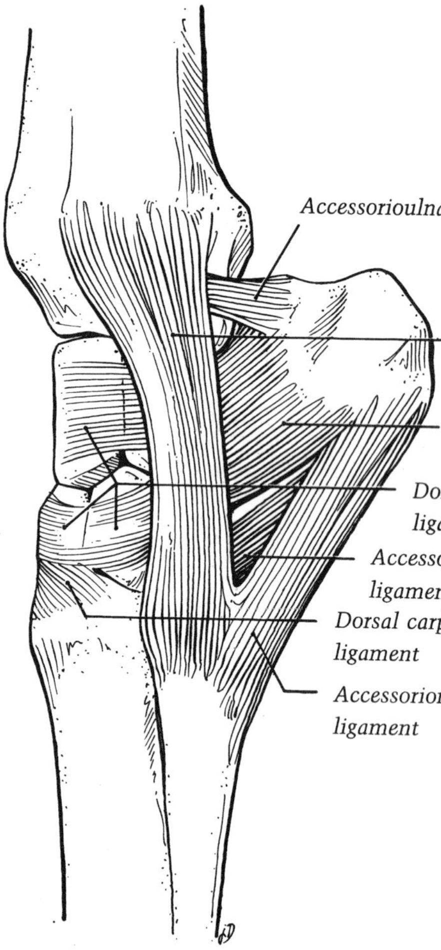

Accessorioulnar ligament

Lateral
collateral
ligament

Accessoriocarpo-
ulnar ligament

Dorsal intercarpal
ligaments

Accessorioquartal
ligament

Dorsal carpometacarpal
ligament

Accessoriometacarpal
ligament

FIG. 1–20. Dissection of carpal ligaments; lateral view.

of the humeral head under the proximal part of the flexor retinaculum (Fig. 1–22). The accessory (carpal check) ligament of the deep digital flexor continues distally from the palmar carpal ligament to join the main tendon near the middle of the metacarpus.

Forearm (Antebrachium)

The forearm includes the radius and ulna and the muscles (Fig. 1–22), vessels, nerves (Fig. 1–23), and skin surrounding the bones. The prominent muscle belly of the extensor carpi radialis muscle bulges under the skin on the cranial aspect (Fig. 1–24). A horny cutaneous structure, the chestnut, is present on the medial skin of the distal one-third of the forearm. The chestnut is considered to be a vestige of the first digit.

Four muscles comprise the extensor group of the antebrachium. The lateral digital extensor muscle, the common digital extensor muscle, the extensor carpi radialis muscle, and the smallest muscle of the extensor group, the extensor carpi obliquus muscle (Figs. 1–19 and 1–24).

The flexor carpi radialis, the flexor carpi ulnaris, and the ulnaris lateralis muscles flex the carpal joint and extend the elbow joint (Fig. 1–25).

The superficial digital flexor muscle and the deep digital flexor muscle flex the digit and fetlock. The accessory ligament (radial or "superior" check ligament) attaches the mediocaudal surface of the distal half of the radius to the superficial flexor tendon (see Fig. 1–22).

Some nerves and blood vessels are illustrated in Figure 1–23.

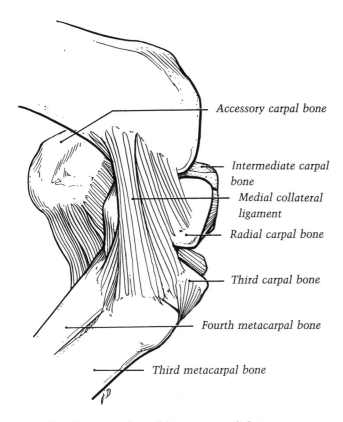

Accessory carpal bone

Intermediate carpal bone

Medial collateral ligament

Radial carpal bone

Third carpal bone

Fourth metacarpal bone

Third metacarpal bone

FIG. 1–21. Dissection of carpal ligaments; medial view.

An interosseous ligament attaches the shaft of a foal's ulna to the radius. Ossification of the ligament occurs in the young horse, but the proximal part of the ligament persists until it becomes ossified in very old horses.

Elbow Joint (Humeroradiol Joint and Olecranon)

Muscles associated with the elbow joint include two principal flexors, the biceps brachii and the brachialis (aided by the extensor carpi radialis and common digital extensor muscles), and three principal extensors, the tensor fasciae antebrachii, the triceps brachii, and the anconeus (assisted by the flexors of the carpus and digit) (Figs. 1–26 and 1–27).

A medial collateral ligament (Fig. 1–27) and a lateral collateral ligament add stability to this joint.

Arm and Shoulder (Humerus and Scapula)

The arm is the region around the humerus. The shoulder includes the shoulder joint (scapulohumeral joint), the region around the scapula (which blends dorsally into the withers) (Figs. 1–22 and 1–25) and the muscles of the shoulder (see Figs. 1–22, 1–25, and 1–26).

The articular configuration of the ball-and-socket shoulder joint and the support of the surrounding muscles give great stability to the joint. Major movements are flexion and extension. While standing, the angle of the shoulder joint is 50 to 60°.

The equine shoulder girdle is muscular and ligamentous. Component parts of the shoulder girdle connect the shoulder, arm, and forearm to the trunk, neck, and head.

The medial aspect of the arm and shoulder contains the large vessels and nerves supplying the thoracic limb (Fig. 1–27).

Stay Apparatus of the Thoracic Limb

The stay apparatus consists of the ligaments, tendons, and muscles serving to stabilize the joints of the thoracic limb in the standing position. This permits the horse to sleep while standing with a minimum of muscular activity (see Fig. 1–22).

The four palmar ligaments stretched tightly across the pastern joint, the straight distal sesamoidean ligament attached to the short pastern bone, and the deep digital flexor tendon stabilize the pastern joint and prevent its overextension. Under tension in the standing position, the superficial digital flexor tendon forestalls flexion of the pastern joint by exerting palmar force on the joint.

The suspensory apparatus of the fetlock consists of the suspensory ligament (interosseus medius muscle), the metacarpointersesamoidean ligament and embedded proximal sesamoid bones, and the three distal sesamoidean ligaments. The suspensory apparatus prevents extreme overextension of the fetlock joint. Reinforcing support is provided by the digital flexor tendons, the superficial digital flexor tendon as it extends from the accessory (radial check) ligament on the radius to the long and short pastern bones, and the deep digital flexor tendon as it extends from the accessory (carpal check) ligament off the palmar carpal ligament to the coffin bone.

The carpus is stabilized by the palmar carpal ligament and the configuration of the articular surfaces of the carpal bones. The digital flexor tendons in the carpal canal and the extensor tendons dorsally, especially the extensor carpi radialis tendon, lend further stability to the carpus.

Although a certain amount of muscle tone is present in all "resting" muscles of the limb, the tension exerted by the long head of the triceps brachii muscle is essential to prevention of flexion of the elbow joint and collapse of the forelimb. The elbow joint is stabilized further by its collateral ligaments and surrounding muscles originating from the humerus.

A tendinous continuum extending from the supraglenoid tubercle to the metacarpal tuberosity is

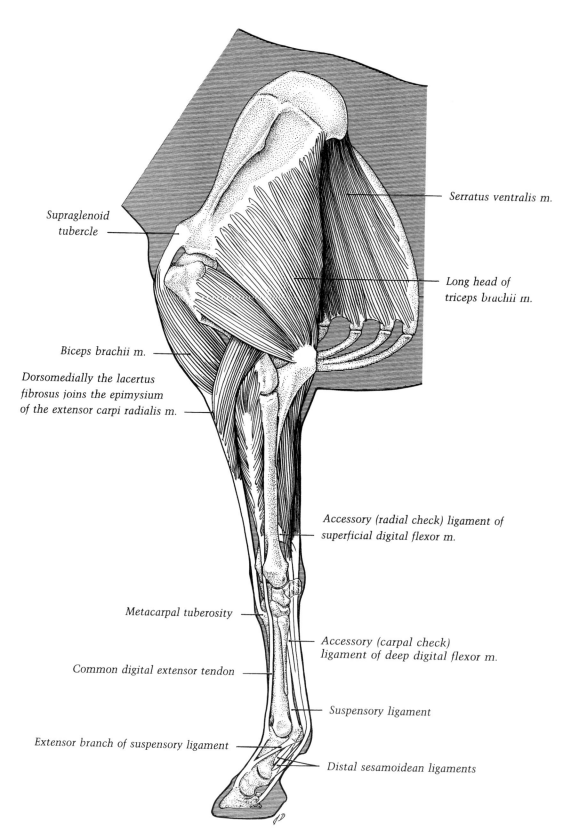

Supraglenoid
tubercle

Biceps brachii m.

Dorsomedially the lacertus
fibrosus joins the epimysium
of the extensor carpi radialis m.

Metacarpal tuberosity

Common digital extensor tendon

Extensor branch of suspensory ligament

Serratus ventralis m.

Long head of
triceps brachii m.

Accessory (radial check) ligament of
superficial digital flexor m.

Accessory (carpal check)
ligament of deep digital flexor m.

Suspensory ligament

Distal sesamoidean ligaments

FIG. 1–22. Stay apparatus of the thoracic limb. m., muscle.

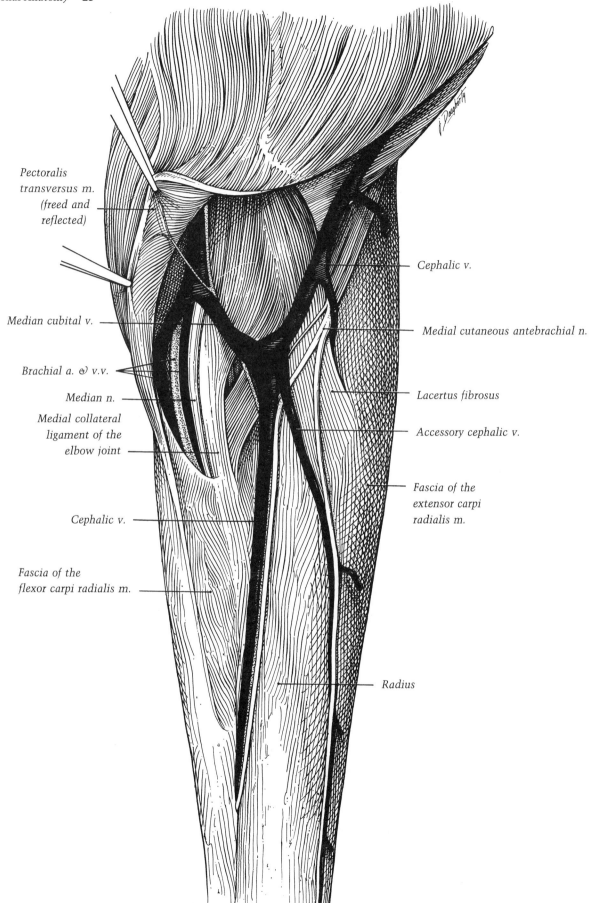

Pectoralis
transversus m.
(freed and
reflected)

Cephalic v.

Median cubital v.

Medial cutaneous antebrachial n.

Brachial a. & v.v.

Median n.

Lacertus fibrosus

Medial collateral
ligament of the
elbow joint

Accessory cephalic v.

Fascia of the
extensor carpi
radialis m.

Cephalic v.

Fascia of the
flexor carpi radialis m.

Radius

FIG. 1–23. Caudomedial view of a superficial dissection of the left elbow and forearm. m., muscle; n., nerve; v., vein; a., artery.

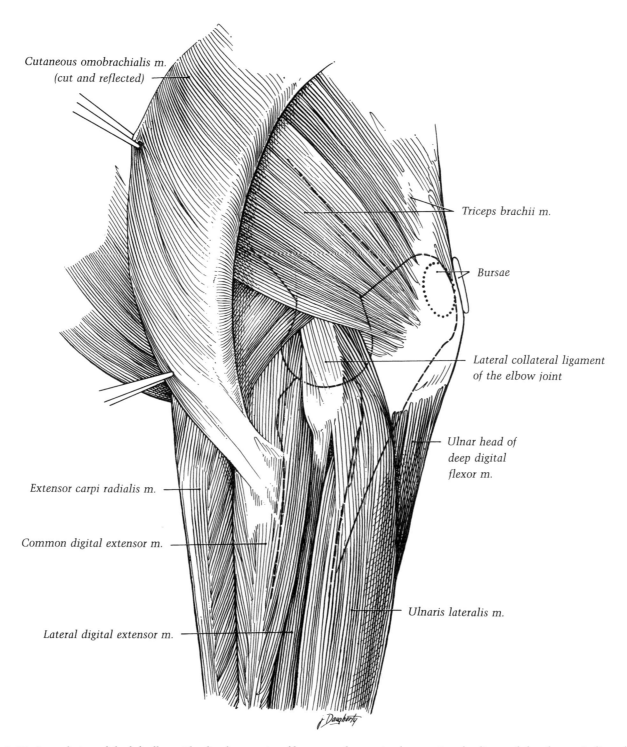

Cutaneous omobrachialis m.
(cut and reflected)

Triceps brachii m.

Bursae

Lateral collateral ligament
of the elbow joint

Ulnar head of
deep digital
flexor m.

Extensor carpi radialis m.

Common digital extensor m.

Ulnaris lateralis m.

Lateral digital extensor m.

Fig. 1–24. Lateral view of the left elbow. The distal extremity of humerus, the proximal extremity of radius, and the ulna are indicated by dashed lines. m., muscle.

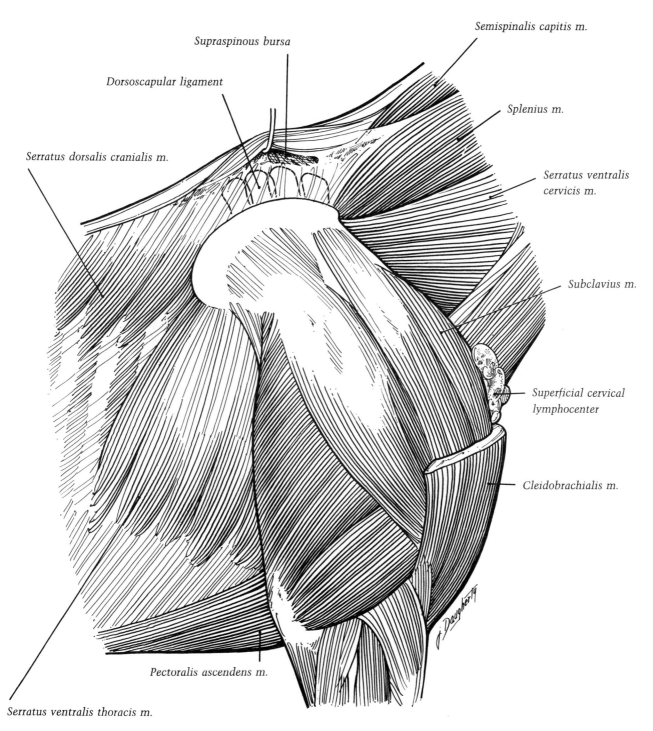

FIG. 1–25. Dissection of the right shoulder and dorsoscapular ligament. Spines of thoracic vertebrae 2 to 5 are outlined by dashed lines. m., muscle.

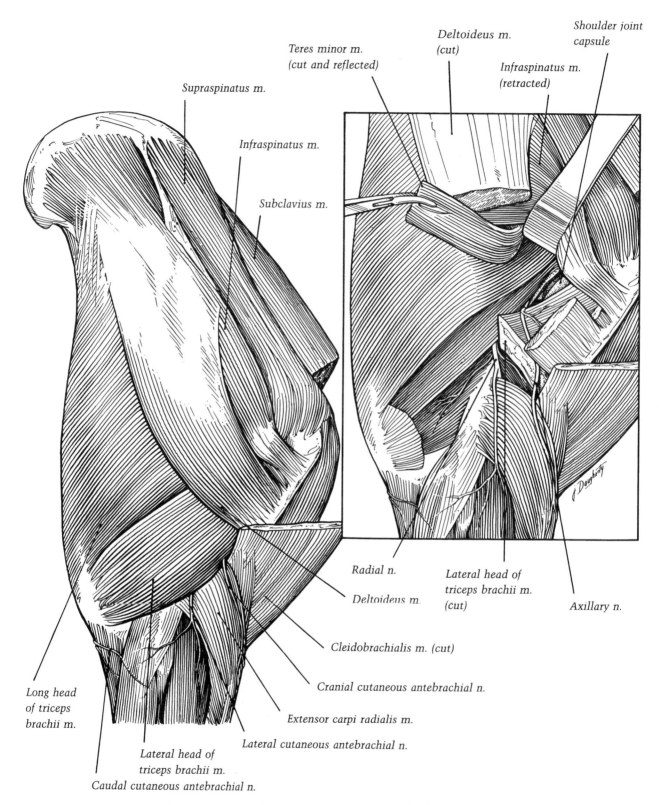

Supraspinatus m.

Teres minor m. (cut and reflected)

Deltoideus m. (cut)

Shoulder joint capsule

Infraspinatus m. (retracted)

Infraspinatus m.

Subclavius m.

Radial n.

Deltoideus m.

Lateral head of triceps brachii m. (cut)

Axillary n.

Cleidobrachialis m. (cut)

Cranial cutaneous antebrachial n.

Extensor carpi radialis m.

Lateral cutaneous antebrachial n.

Long head of triceps brachii m.

Lateral head of triceps brachii m.

Caudal cutaneous antebrachial n.

FIG. 1–26. Lateral aspect of the right shoulder. Inset: deeper dissection exposing the shoulder joint. m., muscle; n., nerve.

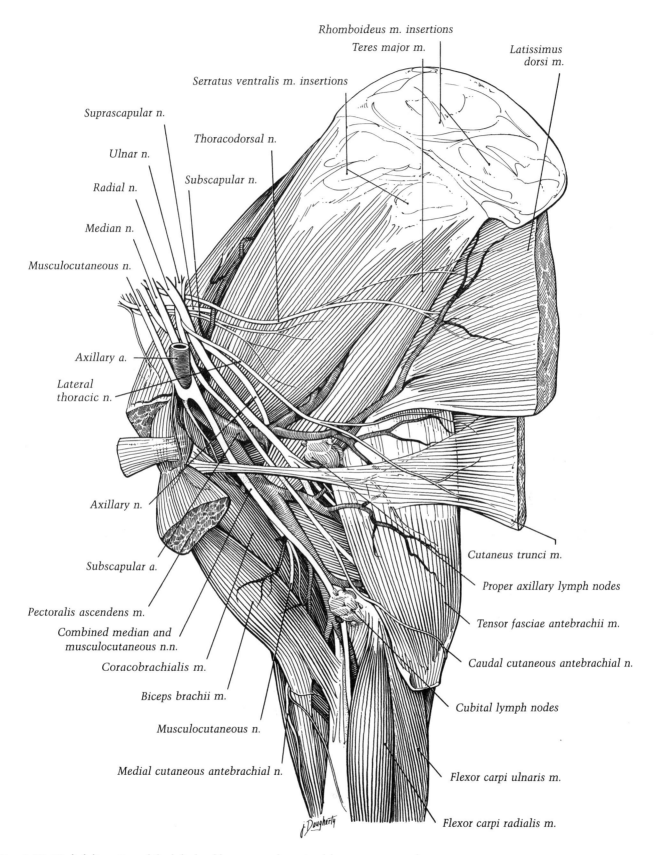

FIG. 1–27. Medial dissection of the left shoulder, arm, and proximal forearm. m., muscle; n., nerve; a., artery.

formed by the main tendon of the biceps brachii muscle and its distal superficial tendon joining the tendon of the extensor carpi radialis muscle. This complex prevents flexion of the shoulder joint caused by the weight of the trunk. Additionally, the deep radial tendon of the biceps brachii helps stabilize the elbow joint, and the tendon of the extensor carpi radialis opposes flexion of the carpus.

Growth Plate Closure

Several investigators have reported on closure times for the growth plates (epiphyseal cartilages) of the bones in equine limbs. Tables 1–1 and 1–2 (see p. 40) summarize the ranges of reported closure times based on examination of x-rays and gross and microscopic specimens.

Pelvic Limb (Fig. 1–28)

Digit and Fetlock

The hindfoot is narrower than the forefoot, corresponding to the shape of the coffin bone. Compared to the forefoot, the angle of the toe of the hindfoot is slightly greater, varying from 55 to 60°.

The long digital extensor muscle's tendon attaches to the dorsal surfaces of the long and short pastern bones and the extensor process of the coffin bone.

The hind cannon is about 16% longer than the corresponding front cannon, and the hind cannon bone is more rounded than the front cannon bone. The hind's lateral splint bone, particularly its proximal extremity, is larger than the hind's medial splint bone.

The nerves, arteries, veins, and muscles of the cannon bone region are portrayed in Figures 1–29 and 1–30.

Hock (Tarsus)

The bones of the hock include the talus, calcaneus, and the central, first and second fused, third and fourth tarsal bones (Fig. 1–28). Proximally, the trochlea of the talus articulates with the tibia in the tarsocrural (tibiotarsal) joint; distally, the distal row of tarsal bones and the cannon and two splint bones articulate in the tarsometatarsal joint. The nerves and vessels of the hock region are illustrated in Figures 1–29, 1–30, and 1–31. The long and lateral digital extensor tendons and their sheaths are illustrated in Figure 1–29.

The tendon of the peroneus tertius muscle is superficial to the tendon of the tibilias cranialis muscle (see Figs. 1–31, 1–32, and 1–33). The tendon of the peroneus tertius forms a sleevelike cleft through which the tendon of the tibialis cranialis and its synovial sheath pass. The latter tendon then bifurcates into a dorsal tendon, which inserts on the large metatarsal bone, and a medial (cunean) tendon, which inserts on the first tarsal bone.

A horny chestnut, the presumed vestige of the first digit, is located in the skin on the medial aspect of the hock.

A palpable feature of the medial aspect of the hock is the medial (cunean) tendon of the tibialis cranialis muscle as it goes to its insertion on the first tarsal bone (see Fig. 1–32).

The principal component of the composite hock joint is the tarsocrural joint, a hinge based on the shape of the articular surfaces or a snap joint based on

TABLE 1–1. *Ranges of Growth Plate Closure Times in Equine Thoracic Limbs*

Scapula Proximal* 36+ mo. Distal 9–18 mos.	Cannon Bone Proximal Before Birth Distal 6–18 mos.
Humerus Proximal 26–42 mos. Distal 11–34 mos.	Long Pastern Bone Proximal 6–15 mos. Distal Before Birth to 1 mo.
Radius Proximal 11–25 mos. Distal 22–42 mos.	Short Pastern Bone Proximal 6–15 mos. Distal Before Birth to 1 wk.
Ulna Proximal 27–42 mos. Distal 2–12 mos. (some up to 4 yrs.)	Coffin Bone Proximal Before Birth

*Ossification center

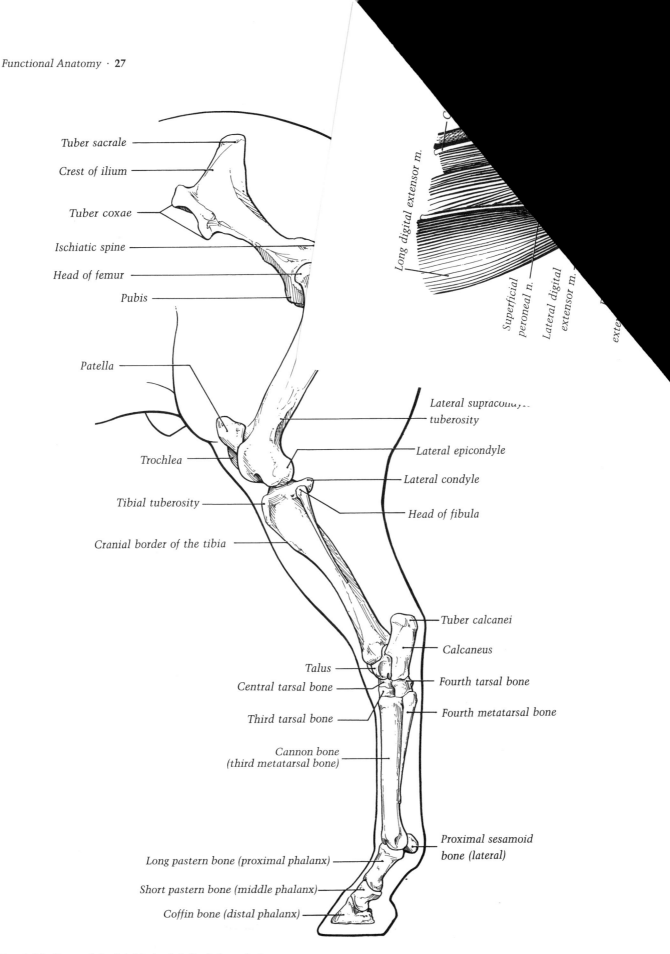

Tuber sacrale

Crest of ilium

Tuber coxae

Ischiatic spine

Head of femur

Pubis

Patella

Trochlea

Tibial tuberosity

Cranial border of the tibia

Long digital extensor m.

Superficial peroneal n.

Lateral digital extensor m.

Lateral supracondylar tuberosity

Lateral epicondyle

Lateral condyle

Head of fibula

Tuber calcanei

Calcaneus

Talus

Central tarsal bone

Third tarsal bone

Fourth tarsal bone

Fourth metatarsal bone

Cannon bone (third metatarsal bone)

Proximal sesamoid bone (lateral)

Long pastern bone (proximal phalanx)

Short pastern bone (middle phalanx)

Coffin bone (distal phalanx)

FIG. 1–28. Bones of the left hind pelvic limb; lateral view.

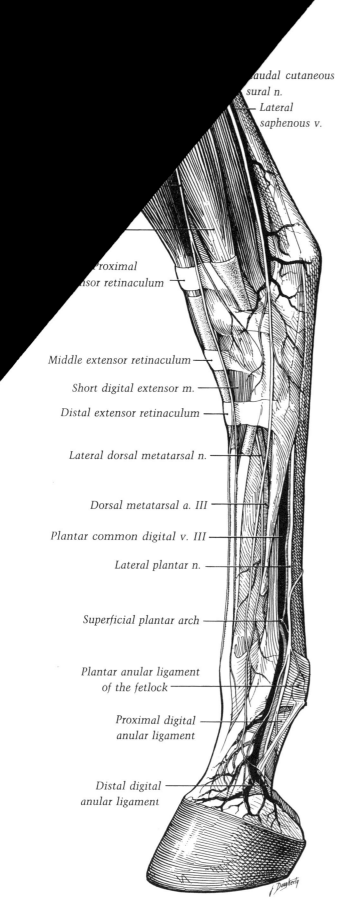

Caudal cutaneous
sural n.

Lateral
saphenous v.

Proximal
extensor retinaculum

Middle extensor retinaculum

Short digital extensor m.

Distal extensor retinaculum

Lateral dorsal metatarsal n.

Dorsal metatarsal a. III

Plantar common digital v. III

Lateral plantar n.

Superficial plantar arch

Plantar anular ligament
of the fetlock

Proximal digital
anular ligament

Distal digital
anular ligament

FIG. 1–29. Lateral view of the left distal hind limb. Skin and some of the fascia have been removed. m., muscle; n., nerve; v., vein; a., artery.

the snapping movement of the joint into or out of extension. The interarticular and tarsometatarsal joints are plane joints capable of only a small amount of gliding movement.

A long collateral ligament and three short collateral ligaments bind each side of the equine hock (Figs. 1–34 and 1–35).

Three pouches can protrude from the large tarsocrural synovial sac where it is not bound down by ligaments.

The tarsocrural joint is flexed by contraction of the tibialis cranialis muscle and the passive pull of the tendinous peroneus tertius muscle. Contraction of the gastrocnemius, biceps femoris, and semitendinosus muscles and the passive pull of the tendinous superficial digital flexor muscle extends the joint. By virtue of its attachments in the extensor fossa of the femur proximally, and on the lateral aspect of the hock and dorsal surface of the cannon bone distally, the peroneus tertius passively flexes the joint when the stifle joint is flexed. The superficial digital flexor muscle originates in the supracondyloid fossa of the femur and inserts first on the calcaneal tuber. This part of the superficial digital flexor serves to passively extend the hock joint when the stifle joint is extended. The two tendinous, passively functioning muscles constitute the reciprocal apparatus (see Fig. 1–36).

During flexion of the hock joint, the lower leg limb moves slightly outward due to the configuration of the joint. As the hock articulates, approximately one-third of the distance from the point of maximum extension to the point of maximum flexion, a snapping motion occurs influenced through tension exerted by the three short medial collateral ligaments (Fig. 1–37).

Gaskin (Crus)

The gaskin is the region of the hind limb containing the tibia and fibula. Thus, it extends from the hock joint to the stifle joint.

Stifle (Femorotibial and Femoropatellar Joint)

The stifle is the region including the stifle joint and surrounding structures. Deep to the skin, three patellar ligaments descend from the patella, converging to their attachments on the tibial tuberosity.

Overall, the two joints of the stifle, the femoropatellar and femorotibial joints, form a hinge.

The patella is essentially a sesamoid bone interposed in the termination of the quadriceps femoris muscle with the three patellar ligaments comprising the tendon of insertion.

The femorotibial joint is complex, the cranial and caudal cruciate ligaments lie between the joint capsule's medial and lateral synovial sacs.

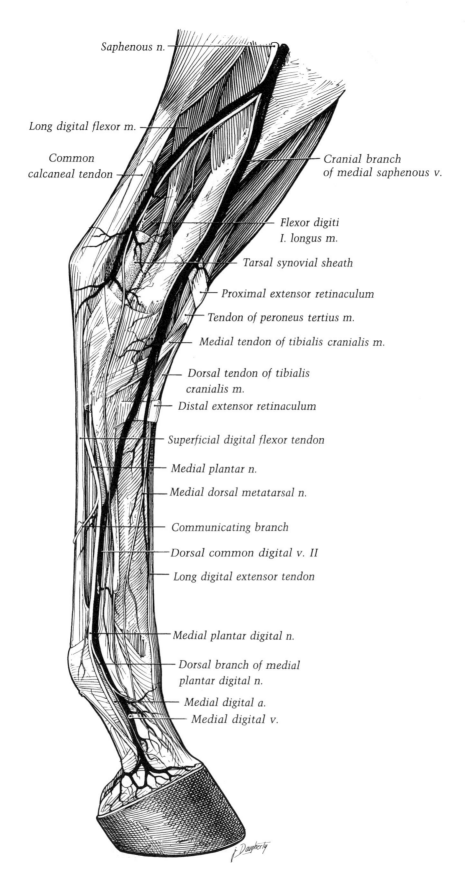

Saphenous n.

Long digital flexor m.

Common calcaneal tendon

Cranial branch of medial saphenous v.

Flexor digiti I. longus m.

Tarsal synovial sheath

Proximal extensor retinaculum

Tendon of peroneus tertius m.

Medial tendon of tibialis cranialis m.

Dorsal tendon of tibialis cranialis m.

Distal extensor retinaculum

Superficial digital flexor tendon

Medial plantar n.

Medial dorsal metatarsal n.

Communicating branch

Dorsal common digital v. II

Long digital extensor tendon

Medial plantar digital n.

Dorsal branch of medial plantar digital n.

Medial digital a.

Medial digital v.

FIG. 1–30. Medial view of the left distal hind limb. Skin and some of the fascia have been removed. m., muscle; n., nerve; v., vein; a., artery.

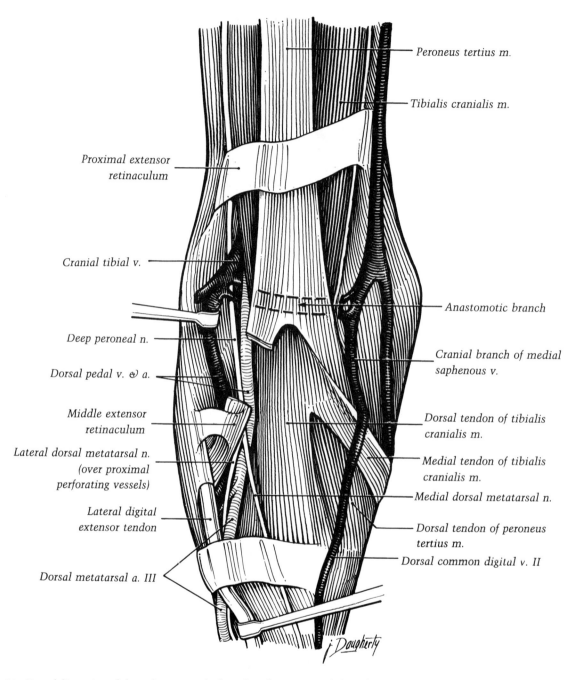

Peroneus tertius m.

Tibialis cranialis m.

Proximal extensor retinaculum

Cranial tibial v.

Anastomotic branch

Deep peroneal n.

Cranial branch of medial saphenous v.

Dorsal pedal v. & a.

Middle extensor retinaculum

Dorsal tendon of tibialis cranialis m.

Lateral dorsal metatarsal n. (over proximal perforating vessels)

Medial tendon of tibialis cranialis m.

Medial dorsal metatarsal n.

Lateral digital extensor tendon

Dorsal tendon of peroneus tertius m.

Dorsal common digital v. II

Dorsal metatarsal a. III

j. Daugherty

FIG. 1–31. Dorsal dissection of the right tarsus. The long digital extensor and short digital extensor muscles have been removed. The lateral tendon of the peroneus tertius is sectioned. Note its junction with the middle extensor retinaculum. m., muscle; n., nerve; a., artery; v., vein.

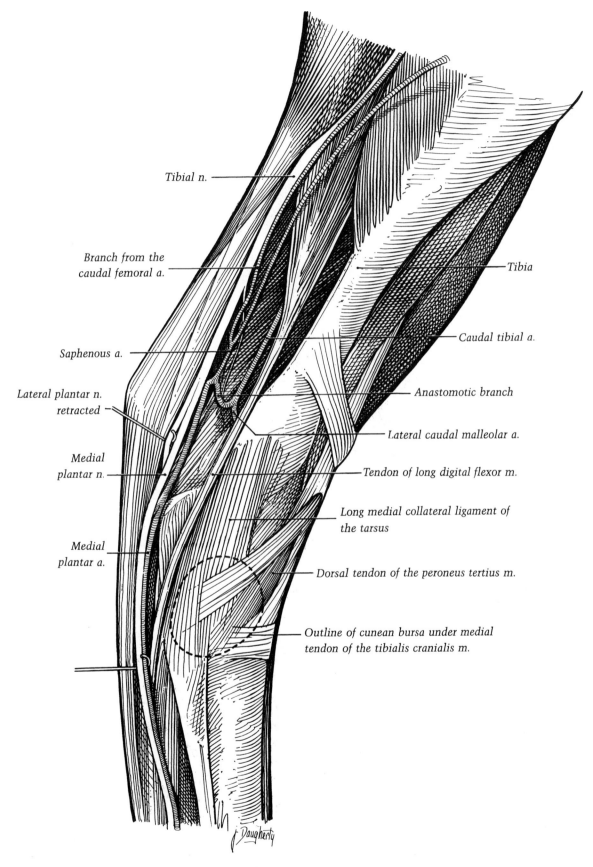

Tibial n.

Branch from the
caudal femoral a.

Saphenous a.

Lateral plantar n.
retracted

Medial
plantar n.

Medial
plantar a.

Tibia

Caudal tibial a.

Anastomotic branch

Lateral caudal malleolar a.

Tendon of long digital flexor m.

Long medial collateral ligament of
the tarsus

Dorsal tendon of the peroneus tertius m.

Outline of cunean bursa under medial
tendon of the tibialis cranialis m.

FIG. 1–32. Medial view of the left hock region. m., muscle; n., nerve; a., artery.

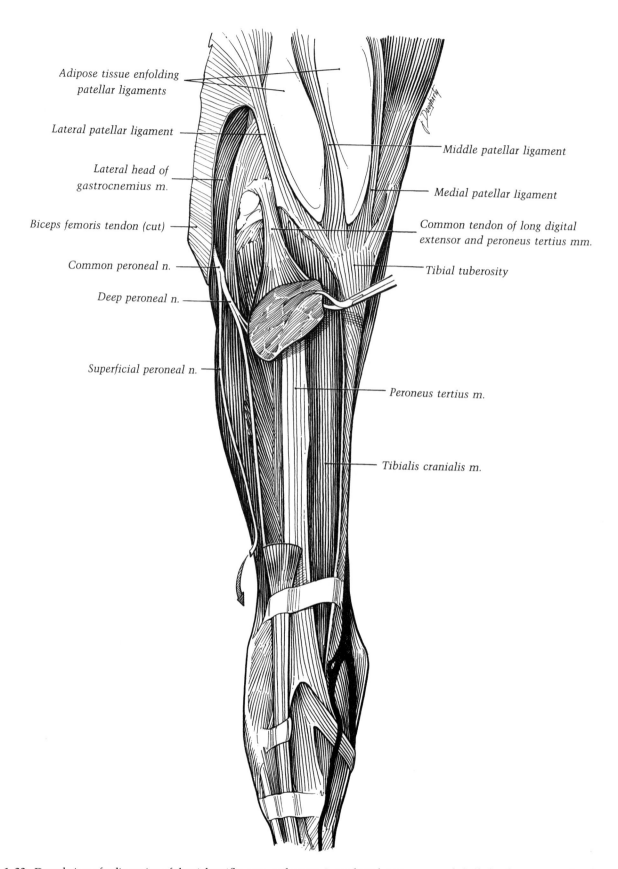

Adipose tissue enfolding
patellar ligaments

Lateral patellar ligament

Lateral head of
gastrocnemius m.

Biceps femoris tendon (cut)

Common peroneal n.

Deep peroneal n.

Superficial peroneal n.

Middle patellar ligament

Medial patellar ligament

Common tendon of long digital
extensor and peroneus tertius mm.

Tibial tuberosity

Peroneus tertius m.

Tibialis cranialis m.

Fig. 1–33. Dorsal view of a dissection of the right stifle, crus, and tarsus. Long digital extensor muscle belly has been removed and a portion of the superficial peroneal nerve has been removed with the fascia (arrow). m., muscle; n., nerve.

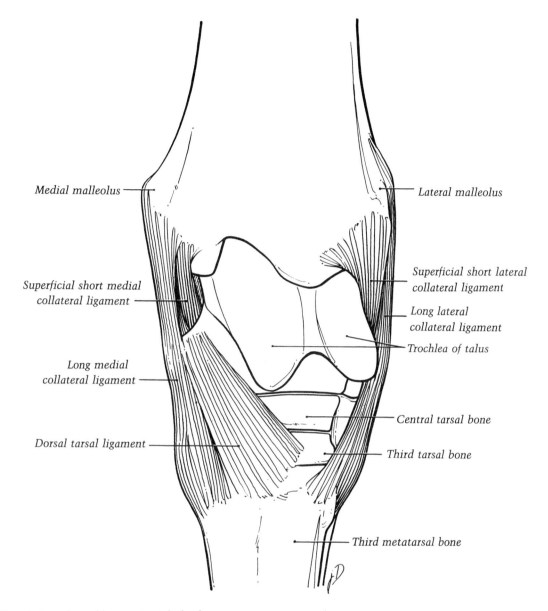

Medial malleolus

Lateral malleolus

Superficial short medial
collateral ligament

Superficial short lateral
collateral ligament

Long lateral
collateral ligament

Long medial
collateral ligament

Trochlea of talus

Central tarsal bone

Dorsal tarsal ligament

Third tarsal bone

Third metatarsal bone

FIG. 1–34. Dorsal view of tarsal ligaments; right hock.

Movements of the Stifle Joint

In the standing position, the quadriceps femoris muscle is relatively relaxed. Extension of the stifle joint through action of the quadriceps femoris, tensor fasciae latae, and cranial division of the biceps femoris muscles plus passive traction exerted by the peroneus tertius is limited by tension from the collateral and cruciate ligaments. There is minimal lateral rotation of the gaskin during full extension. During flexion, the gaskin is rotated slightly medially.

When a horse shifts its weight more to one hind limb, the relaxing limb flexes slightly and rests on the toe. The pelvis is tilted so that the hip of the supporting limb is higher. The stifle on the supporting limb is locked in position due to a slight medial rotation of the patella as the medial patellar ligament and parapatellar cartilage slip farther caudally on the proximal part of the medial trochlear ridge. The locked position achieved by this configuration together with the support rendered by the other components of the stay apparatus minimizes muscular activity in the supporting limb while the relaxed hind limb is resting. When the position is shifted, the patella snaps off the proximal part of the medial trochlear ridge.

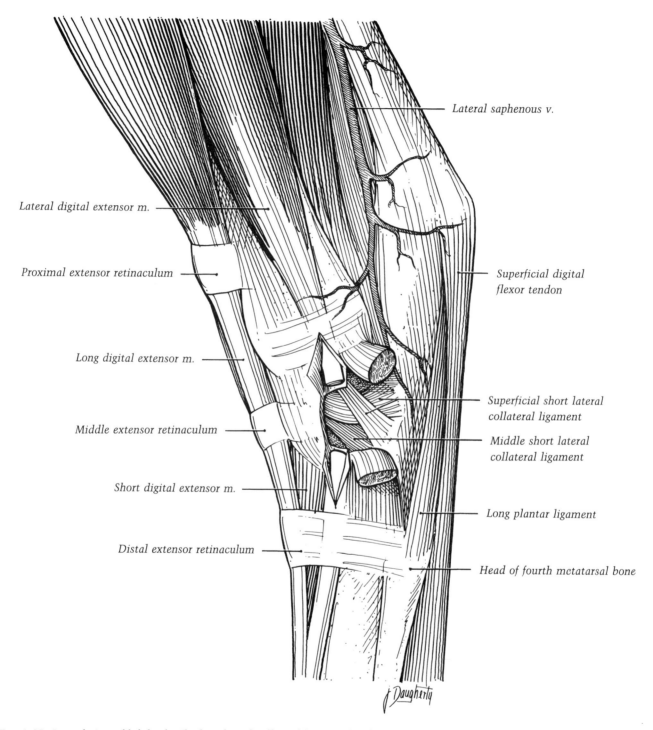

Lateral saphenous v.

Lateral digital extensor m.

Proximal extensor retinaculum

Superficial digital flexor tendon

Long digital extensor m.

Middle extensor retinaculum

Superficial short lateral collateral ligament

Middle short lateral collateral ligament

Short digital extensor m.

Long plantar ligament

Distal extensor retinaculum

Head of fourth metatarsal bone

FIG. 1–35. Lateral view of left hock. The long lateral collateral ligament has been cut and reflected. To the left of it, a section of lateral digital extensor tendon has been removed. m., muscle; v., vein.

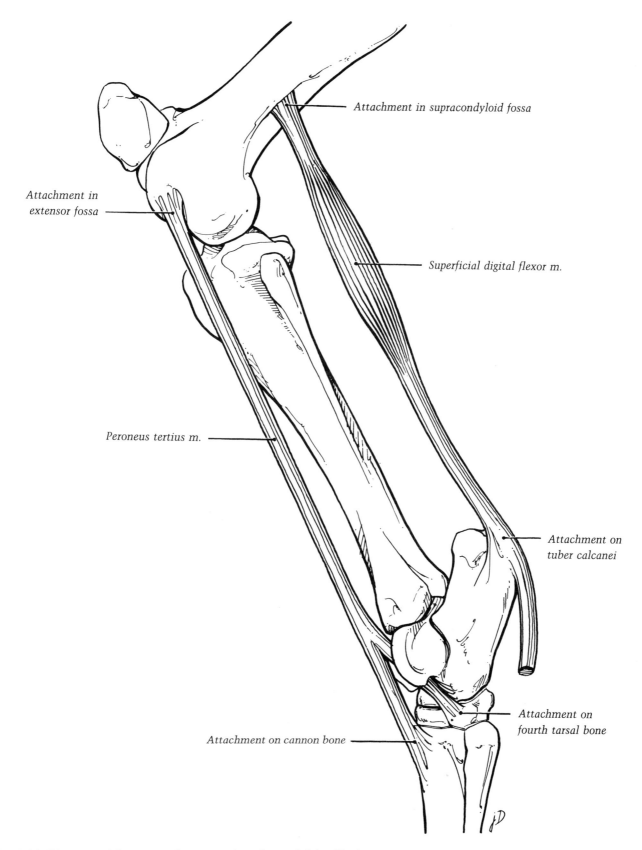

Attachment in supracondyloid fossa

Attachment in extensor fossa

Superficial digital flexor m.

Peroneus tertius m.

Attachment on tuber calcanei

Attachment on fourth tarsal bone

Attachment on cannon bone

FIG. 1–36. Dissection of the reciprocal apparatus; lateral view, left hind limb.

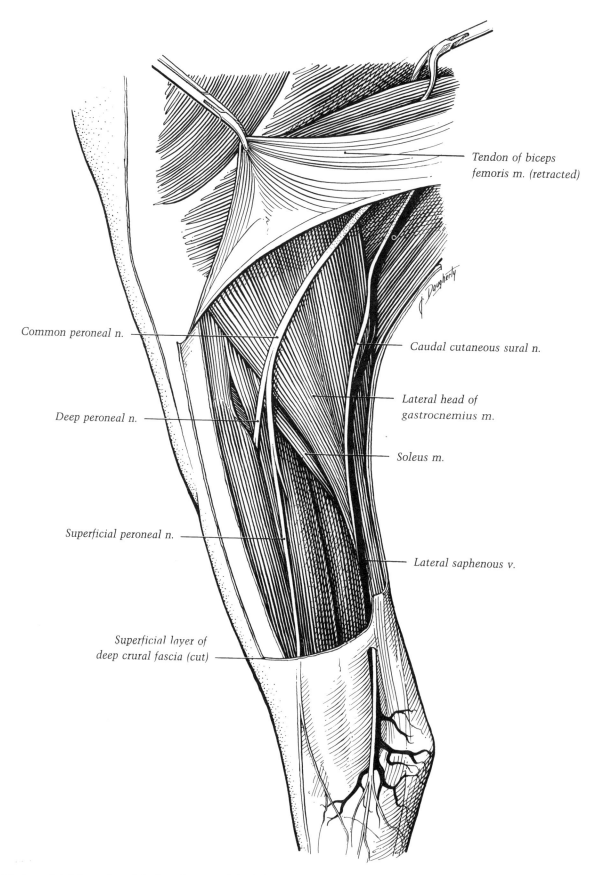

Tendon of biceps
femoris m. (retracted)

Common peroneal n.

Deep peroneal n.

Superficial peroneal n.

Superficial layer of
deep crural fascia (cut)

Caudal cutaneous sural n.

Lateral head of
gastrocnemius m.

Soleus m.

Lateral saphenous v.

FIG. 1–37. Superficial dissection of the lateral aspect of the left stifle, gaskin, and hock. m., muscle; n., nerve; v., vein.

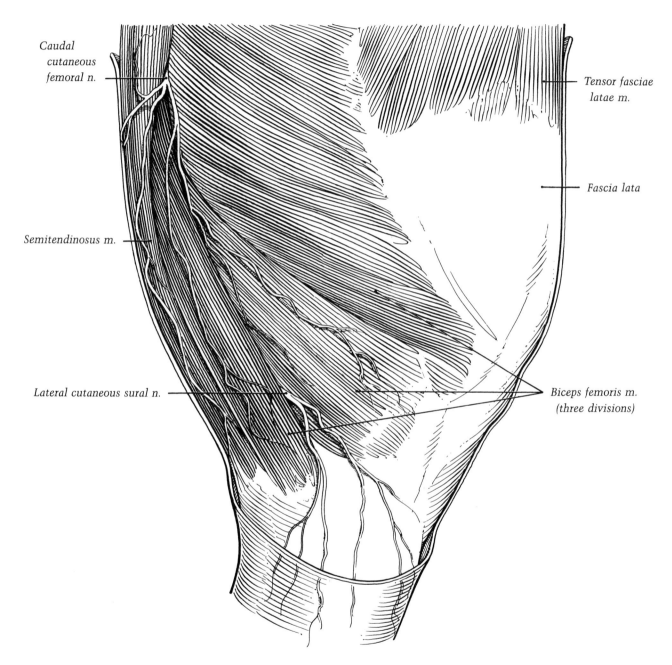

Caudal cutaneous femoral n.

Tensor fasciae latae m.

Fascia lata

Semitendinosus m.

Lateral cutaneous sural n.

Biceps femoris m. (three divisions)

Fig. 1–38. Lateral view of the right stifle and thigh, deep to the skin. m., muscle; n., nerve.

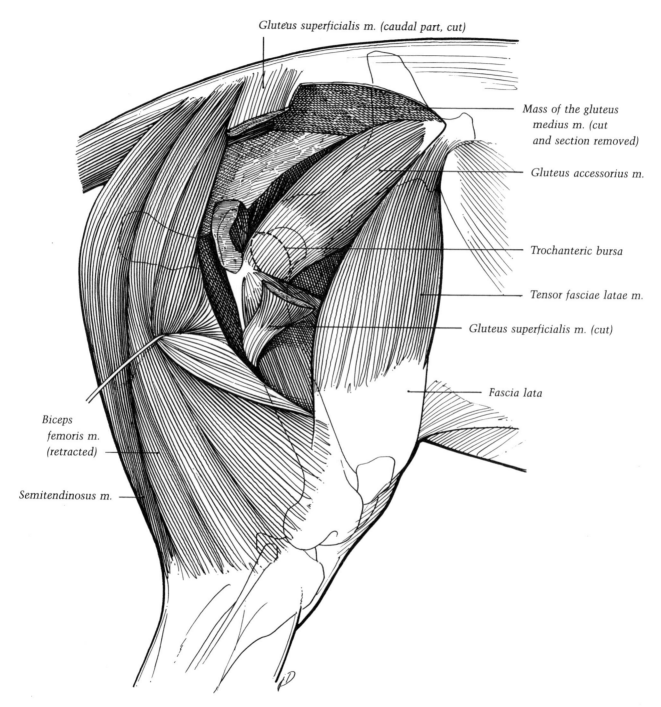

Gluteus superficialis m. (caudal part, cut)

Mass of the gluteus
medius m. (cut
and section removed)

Gluteus accessorius m.

Trochanteric bursa

Tensor fasciae latae m.

Gluteus superficialis m. (cut)

Fascia lata

*Biceps
femoris m.
(retracted)*

Semitendinosus m.

FIG. 1–39. Dissection of the right thigh and hip. Most of the gluteus superficialis and gluteus medius have been removed; lateral view. m., muscle.

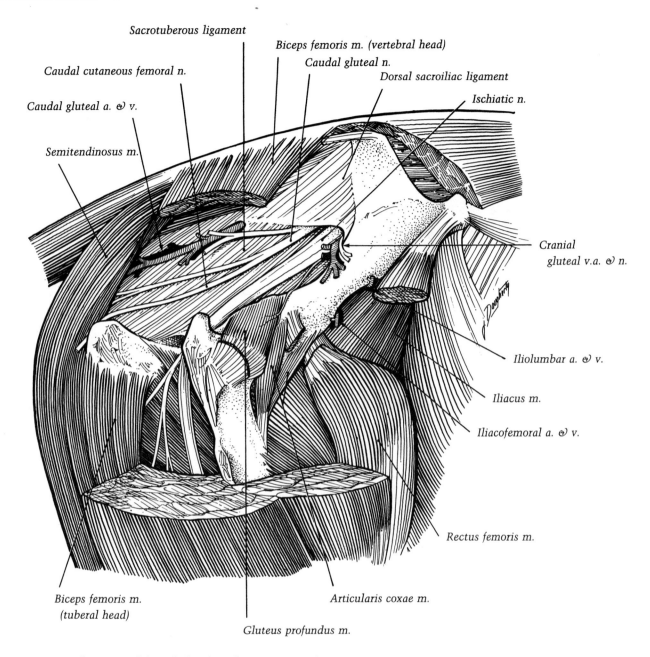

Caudal cutaneous femoral n.

Sacrotuberous ligament

Biceps femoris m. (vertebral head)

Caudal gluteal n.

Dorsal sacroiliac ligament

Ischiatic n.

Caudal gluteal a. & v.

Semitendinosus m.

Cranial
gluteal v.a. & n.

Iliolumbar a. & v.

Iliacus m.

Iliacofemoral a. & v.

Rectus femoris m.

Biceps femoris m.
(tuberal head)

Articularis coxae m.

Gluteus profundus m.

FIG. 1–40. Deep dissection of the right hip; lateral view. m., muscle; n., nerve; v., vein; a., artery.

Thigh and Hip (Femur and Coxal Joint)

Extending from the hip to the stifle, the thigh includes the femur and the structures around it. The region adjacent to and the muscles acting upon the coxal joint comprise the hip (Figs. 1–38, 1–39, and 1–40).

A prominent longitudinal groove evident when viewing a horse from the rear marks the site of the intermuscular septum between the semitendinosus and the biceps femoris muscles.

The hip joint is formed at the junction of the ilium, ischium, and pubis. The acetabulum articulates with the head of the femur. (Fig. 1–28).

Whereas the hip joint is a ball-and-socket joint capable of very limited rotation, the principal movements are flexion and extension. The range of motion between extreme flexion and extension is only 60°.

Flexor muscles of the hip joint are the gluteus superficialis, tensor fasciae latae, rectus femoris, iliopsoas, sartorius, and pectineus. Extensor muscles of the hip joint are the gluteus medius, biceps femoris,

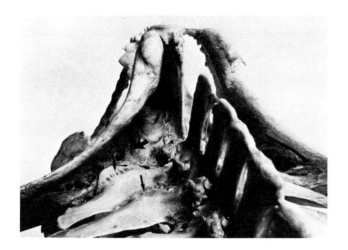

FIG. 1–41. Photograph of the sacroiliac joint (large arrow) and intertransverse joints (small arrows). Dorsocranial view.

semitendinosus, semimembranosus, adductor, and quadratus femoris.

Pelvis

Sacroiliac Joint

Because it is provided with a joint capsule and because the roughened articular surfaces of the sacrum and ilium are covered with a minimal layer of hyaline cartilage, the nearly immovable sacroiliac joint is classified as a synovial joint (Fig. 1–41). However, the joint cavity is just a slit, and it may be crossed by bands of dense white fibrous connective tissue. As the animal ages, the apposed surfaces become even rougher. The joint is stabilized by the surrounding strong fibrous bands of the ventral sacroiliac ligament.

Symphysis Pelvis

The medial borders of pubis and ischium from each side meet ventrally at the symphysis pelvis. In the young animal, fibrocartilage joins the bones. Later in life, the cartilage ossifies.

Stay Apparatus of the Pelvic Limb (see Fig. 1–42)

The quadriceps femoris muscle and the tensor fasciae latae act to pull the patella, parapatellar cartilage, and medial patellar ligament proximally to the locked position over the medial trochlear ridge of the femur when the limb is positioned to bear the weight of the

caudal part of the trunk and the hip. Through the restraint of the components of the reciprocal apparatus, the hock is locked correspondingly. Minimal muscular activity assures continuation of this locked configuration, preventing flexion of the stifle and hock joints. Distal to the hock, the digital flexor tendons support the lower limb. Prevention of overextension of the fetlock joint during the fixed, resting position is accomplished through the support rendered by the digital flexor tendons on the way to their digital attachments, the two extensor branches of the suspensory ligament extending from the proximal sesamoid bones to the long digital extensor tendon, and the sesamoidean ligaments, particularly the three distal sesamoidean ligaments.

Growth Plate Closure

Table 1–2 summarizes the ranges of reported closure times for the growth plates of bones in the pelvic limb.

Axial Contributors to Locomotion

Certain muscles of the trunk (the psoas minor, quadratus lumborum, and the four abdominal muscles on each side) act to flex the vertebral column during the gallop. Other muscles of the trunk and neck (from lateral to medial, the iliocostalis system, the longissimus system, and the transversospinalis system) are extensors of the vertebral column. Acting unilaterally, muscles from both of these groups are responsible for lateral movement of the trunk and neck.

TABLE 1–2. *Ranges of Growth Plate Closure Times in Equine Pelvic Limbs*

Ilium, ischium, pubis	10–12 mos.
Secondary centers for crest, tuber coxae, ischiatic tuber and acetabular part of pubis	$4\frac{1}{2}$–5 yrs.
Femur	
Proximal	36–42 mos.
Distal	22–42 mos.
Tibia	
Proximal	36–42 mos.
Distal	17–24 mos.
Fibula	
Proximal	$3\frac{1}{2}$ yrs.
Distal (lateral malleolus of tibia)	3–24 mos.
Calcaneus	19–36 mos.

Growth plate closure times for bones distal to the tarsus are similar to those distal to the carpus.

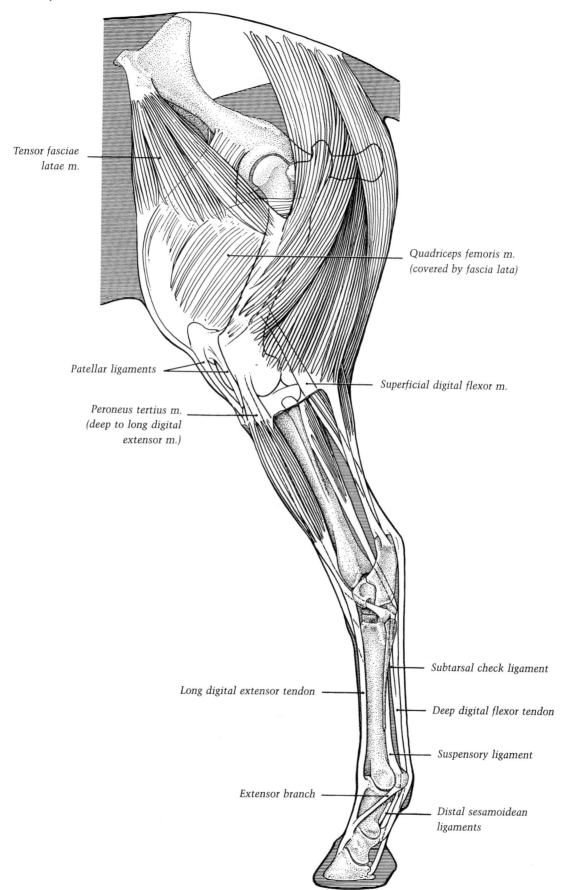

Tensor fasciae latae m.

Quadriceps femoris m. (covered by fascia lata)

Patellar ligaments

Superficial digital flexor m.

Peroneus tertius m. (deep to long digital extensor m.)

Subtarsal check ligament

Long digital extensor tendon

Deep digital flexor tendon

Suspensory ligament

Extensor branch

Distal sesamoidean ligaments

Fig. 1–42. Stay apparatus of the left pelvic limb. m., muscle.

Excluding the joint between the atlas and axis, the joints of the vertebral column all permit flexion, extension, lateral flexion, and even limited rotation. Whereas these movements are limited at each joint, taken as a whole, the movement is fairly extensive. Intervertebral discs of fibrocartilage are interposed between adjacent vertebrae. These are termed "symphysial joints." Joint cavities exist between the last cervical and first thoracic vertebral bodies and between the last lumbar and first sacral vertebral bodies. Articulations between articular processes on vertebral arches are true joints—arthrodial in the cervical and thoracic regions, and trochoid in the lumbar region. True joints also exist between the transverse processes of the fifth and sixth lumbar vertebrae and between the transverse processes of the sixth lumbar vertebra and the wings of the sacrum (see Fig. 1–41).

CHAPTER TWO

Conformation and Movement

TED S. STASHAK and CHERRY HILL

To develop a clearer understanding of lameness and gait defects, it is important to have a knowledge of conformation and movement. While many lamenesses occur in the lower limbs, the causative factors may be located in the upper limbs or body; therefore, overall conformation must be considered. Certain conformation traits may predispose to lameness and these should be eliminated through responsible breeding. Understanding the relationship between conformation, movement, and lameness is essential for making wise breeding decisions and devising sound management and training programs.

Conformation

Conformation refers to the physical appearance and outline of a horse as dictated primarily by bone and muscle structures. It is impractical to set a single standard of perfection or to specifically define *ideal* or *normal* conformation because the guidelines would depend on the classification, type, breed, and intended use of the horse. Therefore, a conformation evaluation must relate to function.

When discrepancies are discovered, it is important to differentiate between "blemishes" and "unsoundnesses." Blemishes are scars and irregularities that do not affect the serviceability of the horse. Unsoundnesses cause a horse to be lame or otherwise unserviceable. Old wire cuts, small focal muscle atrophies, and white spots from old injuries are considered blemishes if they do not affect the horse's soundness. Unsoundnesses include but are not limited to blindness, parrot mouth, defective hearing, heaves, roaring, cryptorchidism, sterility, and lameness caused from such conditions as navicular syndrome, wounds, ring bone, spavin, curb, and bowed tendons.

Types and Breeds

Horses are classified as draft horses, light horses, or ponies. Classifications are further divided by type (Fig. 2–1) according to overall body style and conformation and the work for which the horse is best suited. Light (riding and driving) horses can be described as one of six types: pleasure horse, hunter, stock horse, sport horse, animated (show) horse, and race horse.

Pleasure horses have comfortable gaits, are well designed for ease of riding, and are typified by smooth movement in any breed. Hunters move with a long, low (horizontal) stride, are suited to cross-country riding and negotiating hunter fences, and are typified by the American Thoroughbred. Stock horses are well-muscled, agile, and quick, are suited to working cattle, and are typified by the American Quarter Horse. The sport horse can be one of two types: a large, athletic horse suited for one or all of the disciplines of eventing (dressage, cross-country, and jumping) and typified by the European warm bloods, or a small, lean, tough horse suited for endurance events and typified by the Arabian. The animated (show) horse is one with highly cadenced, flashy gaits (usually with a high degree of flexion), is suited mainly for the show ring, and is typified by the American Saddlebred. The race horse is lean in relation to height with a deep but not round barrel and is typified by the racing Thoroughbred.

A "breed" is a group of horses with common ancestry and usually strong conformational similarities. In most cases, a horse must come from approved breeding stock to be registered with a particular breed. If a horse is not eligible for registration, it is considered to be a "grade" or "crossbred" horse.

Several breeds can have similar makeup and be of the same type. For example, most Quarter Horses, Paint Horses, and Appaloosas are considered to be stock horse types. Some breeds contain individuals of different types within the breed. American Thoroughbreds can be of the race, hunter, or sport horse type.

Method of Evaluation

Although breed characteristics vary greatly, the process of evaluating any horse is similar. First, a general assessment of the horse's four functional sections is made, giving each section approximately equal importance. (Wildly colored horses and those with dramatic limb markings can result in visual distortions and inaccurate conclusions.) The horse's conformational components are then evaluated in detail. The horse is viewed in a systematic fashion and the observations are summarized.

Systematic Conformation Evaluation

Evaluation begins by viewing the horse from the near side in profile and assessing balance by compar-

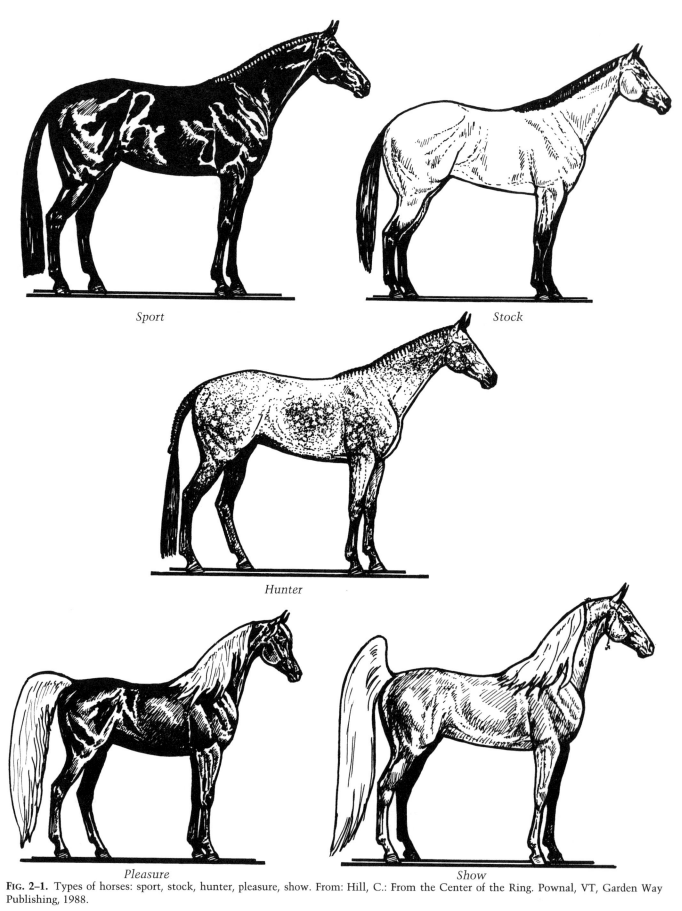

Sport

Stock

Hunter

Pleasure

Show

FIG. 2–1. Types of horses: sport, stock, hunter, pleasure, show. From: Hill, C.: From the Center of the Ring. Pownal, VT, Garden Way Publishing, 1988.

ing the forehand to the hindquarters. When viewing the horse in profile, attention must be paid to the curvature and proportions of the top line. The horse should be observed from poll to tail and down to the gaskin. Then, the attachment of the appendicular skeleton (limbs) to the axial skeleton (head and trunk) is observed. Angles are evaluated.

From the front of the horse, the limbs and hooves are evaluated for straightness and symmetry. The depth and length of the muscles in the forearm and chest are observed. The head, eyes, nostrils, ears are evaluated and the teeth are examined.

Then, from the off side, the evaluation of the balance, top line, and limb angles is confirmed or modified.

From the hindquarter and directly behind the tail, the straightness and symmetry of the back, croup, point of hip and buttock, and the limbs are evaluated. Observation should be made slowly from the poll to the tail because this is the best vantage point for evaluating back muscling, alignment of the vertebral column, and (provided the horse is standing square) left-to-right symmetry. The observer's position may need to be elevated if the horse is tall. The spring (width) of rib is also best observed from the rear view.

The observer then makes another entire circle around the horse, this time stopping at each quadrant to look diagonally across the center of the horse. From the rear of the horse, the observer steps to the left hind and looks toward the right front. This angle will often reveal abnormalities in the limbs and hooves that were missed during the side, front, and rear examinations. The horse is then viewed from the left front toward the right hind and from the right front toward the left hind. The revolution is completed at the right hind looking toward the left front. Finally, from the near side, the whole horse in profile once again is viewed.

While looking at a horse, it is helpful to obtain an overall sense of the correctness of each of the four functional sections: the head/neck, the forehand, the barrel, and the hindquarter.

Head and neck. The vital senses are located in the head, so it should be correct and functional. The neck acts as a lever to help regulate the horse's balance while moving; therefore, it should be long and flexible with a slight convex curve to its top line.

Forehand. The front limbs support approximately 65% of the horse's body weight, so they must be strong and sound. Most lameness is associated with the front limbs.

Barrel. The midsection houses the vital organs; therefore, the horse must be adequate in the heart girth and must have good spring to the ribs. The back should be well muscled and strong so that the horse is able to carry the weight of its intestines and the rider and saddle.

Hindquarters. The rear hand is the source of power for propulsion and stopping. The hindquarter muscling should be appropriate for the type, breed, and use. The croup and points of the hip and buttock

should be symmetric, and the limbs should be straight and sound.

CONFORMATION COMPONENTS

Balance. A well-balanced horse has a better chance of moving efficiently, thereby experiencing less stress. Balance refers to the relationship between the forehand and hindquarters, between the limbs and the body, and between the right and the left sides of the body (Figs. 2–2 through 2–4).

The center of gravity is a theoretical point in the horse's body around which the mass of the horse is equally distributed. At a standstill, the center of gravity is the point of intersection of a vertical line dropped from the highest point of the withers and a line from the point of the shoulder to the point of the buttock. This usually is a spot just behind the elbow and two-thirds the distance down from the top line of the back (Fig. 2–4).

Although the center of gravity remains relatively constant when a well-balanced horse moves, most horses must learn to rebalance their weight (and that of the rider and tack) when ridden. To simply pick up a front foot to step forward, the horse must shift his weight toward the rear. How much the weight must shift to the hindquarters depends on the horse's conformation, the position of the rider, the gait, the degree of collection, and the style of the performance. The higher the degree of collection, the more the horse steps under the center of gravity with the hindlimbs.

If the forehand is proportionately larger than the hindquarters, especially if it is associated with a downhill top line, the horse's center of gravity tends to be forward. This causes the horse to travel heavy on his front feet, setting the stage for increased concussion, stress, and lameness. When the forehand and hindquarters are balanced and the withers are level with or higher than the level of the croup, the horse's center of gravity is located more toward the rear. Such a horse can carry more weight with his hindquarters, thus moving in balance and exhibiting a lighter, freer motion with the forehand than the horse with withers lower than the croup.

When evaluating young horses, the growth spurts that result in a temporarily uneven top line should be taken into consideration. However, 2-year-olds that show an extremely downhill configuration should be suspect. Even if a horse's top line is level, if the forehand is excessively heavily muscled in comparison to the hindquarters, the horse is probably going to travel heavy on the forehand and have difficulty flowing forward freely.

A balanced horse has approximately equal lower limb length and depth of body. The lower limb length (chest floor to the ground) should be equal to the distance from the chest floor to the top of the withers (Fig. 2–4). Proportionately shorter lower limbs are associated with a choppy stride.

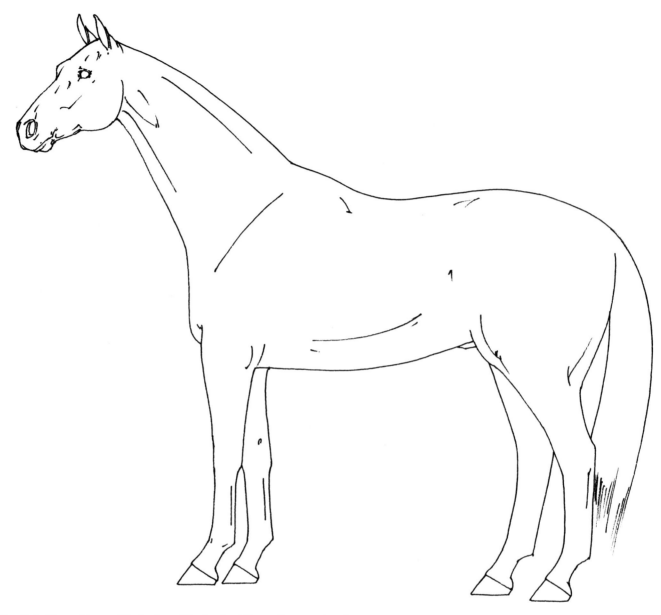

FIG. 2–2. Normal horse. The body and limbs should be well proportioned.

The horse's height or overall limb length (point of withers to ground) should approximate the length of the horse's body (the point of the shoulder to the point of buttock) (Fig. 2–4). A horse with a body that is a great deal longer than its height often experiences difficulty in synchronization and coordination of movement. A horse with limbs proportionately longer than the body may be predisposed to forging, over-reaching, and other gait defects.

Overall, the right side of the horse should be symmetric to the left side.

Proportions and curvature of the top line. The ratio of the top line's components, the curvature of the top line, the strength of loin, the sharpness of withers, the slope to the croup, and the length of the underline in relation to the length of back all affect a horse's movement.

The neck is measured from the poll to the highest point of the withers (Fig. 2–4). The back measurement is taken from the withers to the area of the loin located above the last rib and in front of the pelvis. The hip length is measured from the loin to the point of buttock (Figs. 2–4 and 2–5).

A neck that is shorter than the back tends to decrease a horse's overall flexibility and balance. A back that is very much longer than the neck tends to hollow. A very short hip, in relation to the neck or back, is associated with lack of propulsion and often a downhill configuration. A rule of thumb is that the neck should be greater than or equal to the back and

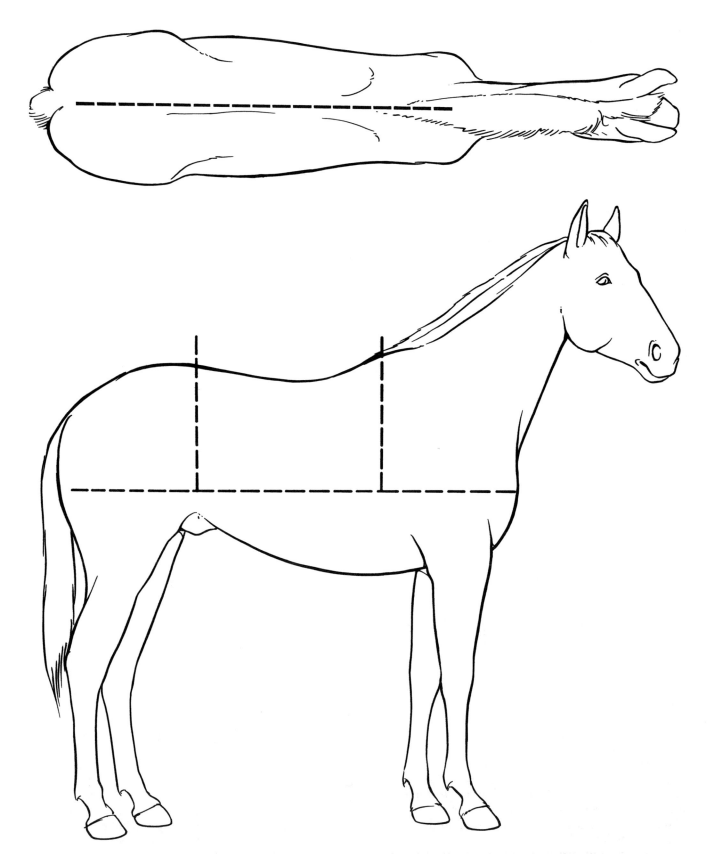

FIG. 2–3. Axial alignment is evaluated. A line drawn from the center of the withers through the center of the back roughly divides the body into two equal halves.

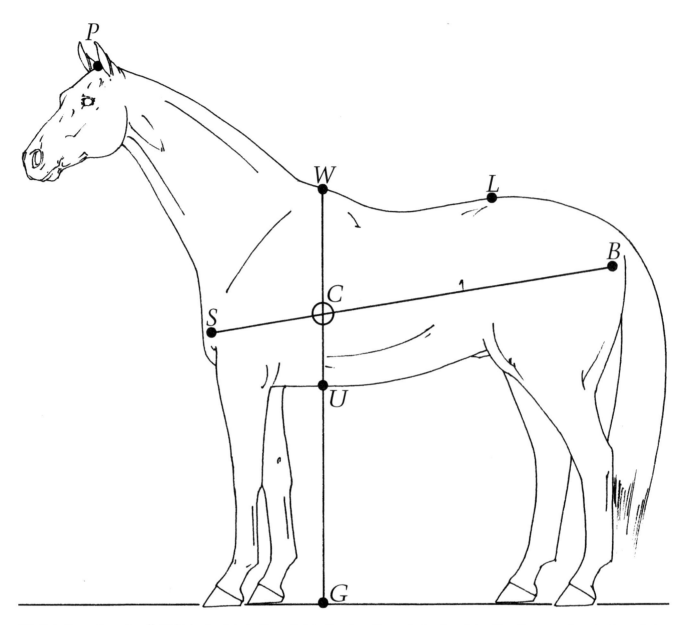

Fig. 2–4. Proportions. P, poll; W, highest point of withers; L, loin; B, point of buttock; S, point of shoulder; C, center of gravity; U, underline; G, ground; WU, depth of body; UG, lower limb length; WG, height and overall limb length; SB, length of body; PW, length of neck; WL, length of back; LB, length of hip. From: Hill, C., Klimesh, R.: Maximum Hoof Power. New York, Macmillan, Publishing, 1994.

that the hip should be at least two-thirds the length of the back (Fig. 2–4).

The neck should have a graceful shape that rises up out of the withers, not dipping downward in front of the withers. The shape of the neck is determined by the "S" shape formed by the seven cervical vertebrae. A longer, flatter (more horizontal) curve to the upper vertebrae results in a smoother attachment at the poll behind the skull and results in a cleaner, more flexible throat latch. If the upper cervical vertebrae form a short, straight line to the skull, it is associated with an abrupt attachment to the skull, resulting in a thick throat latch and a hammerhead appearance. The curve to the lower neck vertebrae should be short and shal-

low and should attach relatively high on the horse's chest. The thickest point in the neck is at the base of the lower curve. Ewe-necked horses often have necks that have a long, deep lower curve that appear to attach low on the chest. The attachment of the neck muscles to the shoulders should be smooth. Prominent depressions in the muscles in front of the shoulder blade are undesirable.

The upper neck length (poll to withers) should be twice the lower neck length (throat latch to chest). This is dictated to a large degree by the slope of the shoulder. A horse with a steep shoulder has an undesirable ratio (approaching 1 : 1) between the upper neck length and lower neck length.

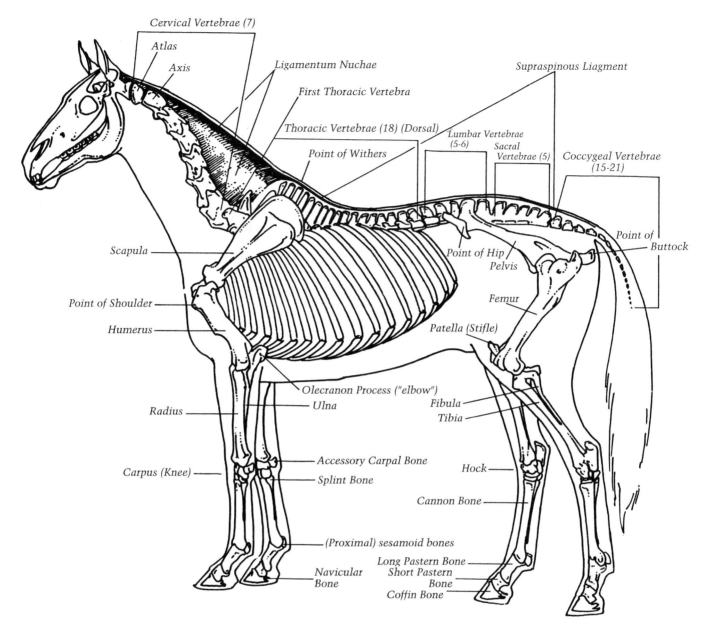

FIG. 2–5. Equine skeleton. From: Hill, C.: Making Not Breaking. Ossining, N.Y., Breakthrough Publications, 1992

The back should look like it has a natural place for a saddle, beginning with prominent withers located above or behind the heart girth. The withers should blend gradually into the back, ending ideally at about the midpoint of the back. The withers provide a place for the neck and forearm muscles and the ligamentum nuchae to anchor; the neck muscles should attach at the highest point of the withers. There should not be a prominent dip in the muscles in front of or behind the withers.

The withers also act as a fulcrum. As a horse lowers and extends its neck, the back rises. Low, mutton withers limit a horse's ability to raise his back. A horse with a well-sloped shoulder usually has correctly placed withers. The heart girth should be deep, which indicates adequate room for the heart and lungs.

The longissimus muscles that run along the spine should be flat and strong rather than sloped and weak. The back muscles aid in counteracting the gravitational pull from the weight of the horse's intestines as well as to supporting the rider's weight.

The loin is located along the lumbar vertebrae from the last rib-bearing (dorsal) vertebrae to the lumbosacral joint (Fig. 2–5). The loin should be well muscled and relatively short. Horses termed "long-backed" often have an acceptable back length but a long, weak loin. A horse with a weak and/or long loin and loose coupling tends to have a hollow back. (The coupling is the area behind the ribs and in front of a vertical line dropped from the point of hip.) A horse that chronically hollows its back may be predisposed to focal myofacial pain, pinched nerves, or vertebrae damage.

The loin and the coupling transfer the motion of the hindquarters up through the back and forward to the forehand; therefore, they must be strong and well connected. A short, heavily muscled loin has great potential strength, power, and durability but may lack the flexibility of a more moderately muscled loin. A lumpy appearance in the loin may indicate abnormal alignment (subluxations) of the vertebrae.

The croup is measured from the lumbosacral joint (approximately indicated by the peak above and slightly behind the points of hip) to the tail head (Fig. 2–5). The croup should be fairly long, as this is associated with a good length to the hip and a desirable forward-placement of lumbosacral joints.

The top line should be short in relation to the underline. Such a combination indicates strength plus desirable length of stride.

Head. The head should be functionally sound. The brain coordinates the horse's movements; therefore, adequate cranial space is necessary. The length from the ear to the eye should be at least one-third the distance from the ear to the nostril. The width between the eyes should be a similar distance as that from the ear to the eye. A wide-open throat latch allows proper breathing during flexion; a narrow throat latch is often associated with a ewe-neck attachment. Eyes set off to the side of the head allow the horse to have a panoramic view. The eye should be prominent without bulging. Prominence refers to the bony eye socket, not a protruding eyeball. The expression of the eye should indicate a quiet, tractable temperament.

The muzzle can be trim, but if it is too small, the nostrils may be pinched and there may be inadequate space for the incisors, resulting in dental misalignments. The width of the cheek bones indicates the space for molar teeth; adequate room is required for sideways grinding of food. The shape of the nasal bone and forehead is largely a matter of breed and personal preference.

Quality. Quality is depicted by "flat" cannon bones, clean joints, sharply defined (refined) features, smooth muscling, overall blending of parts, and a fine, smooth hair coat. "Flat" bone is a misnomer because the cannon bone is round. "Flat" refers to well-defined tendons that stand out cleanly behind the cannon bone and give the impression, when viewed from the side, that the cannon bone is flat.

Substance. Thickness, depth, and breadth of bone, muscle, and other tissues are described as "substance." Muscle substance is described by type of muscle, thickness of muscle, length of muscles, and position of attachment. Other substance factors include weight of the horse, height of the horse, size of the hoofs, depth of the heart girth and flank, and spring of rib.

"Spring of rib," which is best viewed from the rear, refers to the curve of the ribs. In addition to providing room for the heart, lungs, and digestive tract, a well-sprung rib cage provides a natural, comfortable place for a rider's legs. A slab-sided horse with a shallow heart girth is difficult to sit upon properly; an extremely wide-barreled horse can be stressful to the rider's legs.

"Substance of bone" refers to adequacy of the bone to weight ratio. Traditionally, the circumference around the cannon bone just below the knee serves as the measurement for substance of bone. For riding horses, an adequate ratio is approximately 0.7 inches of bone for every 100 lb. of body weight. Using that rule, a 1200-lb. horse should have an 8.4-inch cannon bone.

Correctness of angles and structures. The correct alignment of the skeletal components provides the framework for muscular attachments. The length and slope to the shoulder, arm, forearm, croup, hip, stifle, and pasterns should be moderate and should work well together. There should be a straight alignment of bones when viewed from the front and rear, large clean joints, high-quality hoof horn, adequate height and width of heel, concave sole, and adequate size hoof.

Forelimbs

Both forelimbs should appear to be of equal length and size and should appear to bear equal weight. A line dropped from the point of the shoulder to the ground should bisect the limb. The toes should point forward and the feet should be as far apart on the ground as the limbs are at their origin in the chest (Fig. 2–6). The shoulder should be well muscled without being heavy and coarse.

The muscles running along the inside and outside of the forearm should go all the way to the knee, ending in a gradual taper rather than ending abruptly a few inches above the knee. It is generally believed that this will allow the horse to use its front limbs in a smooth sweeping, forward motion. The pectoral muscles at the horse's chest floor (an inverted "V") should also reach far down onto the limb. The pectoral and the forearm muscles help a horse to move its limbs laterally and medially as well as to elevate the forehand.

Limbs, when viewed from the side, should exhibit a composite of moderate angles so that shock absorption is efficient (Fig. 2–7). The shoulder angle is measured along the spine of the scapula, from the point of the shoulder to the point of the withers. The shorter and straighter the shoulder, the shorter and quicker the stride and the more stress and concussion is transmitted to the limb. Also important is the angle the shoulder makes with the arm, which should be at least 90°, and the angle of the pastern.

The length of the humerus, the point of the shoulder to the point of elbows, affects stride length. A long humerus is associated with a long, reaching stride and

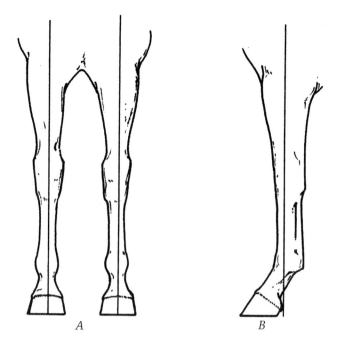

FIG. 2–6. Cranial and lateral views of normal forelimbs. *A*, Line dropped from the point of the shoulder joint bisects the limb. *B*, Line from the tuber spinae of the scapula bisects the limb as far as the fetlock and drops at the heel.

good lateral ability; a short humerus is related to a short, choppy stride and poor lateral ability. The steeper the angle of the humerus, generally, the higher the action; the closer the angle is to horizontal, the lower the action.

The medial-lateral slope of the humerus is evaluated from the front by finding the left point of shoulder and a spot in front of the left point of elbow, the same is done on the right side. The four points are then connected. If the resulting box is square, the humerus lies in an ideal position for straight lower limbs and straight travel. If the bottom of the box is wider, the horse may toe in and travel with loose elbows and paddle. If the bottom of the box is narrower, the horse will probably toe out, have tight elbows, and wing in.

The manner in which the shoulder blade and arm (humerus) are conformed and attach to the chest dictates, to a large degree, the alignment of the lower limbs. Whether the toes point in or out is often a result of upper limb structures, which is the reason why it is dangerous, in many cases, to attempt to alter a limb's structure and alignment through radical hoof adjustments. It is important to be sure the horse is standing square when assessing the lower limbs.

The knees should be large and clean, not small and puffy. The bone column should be functionally straight and sound, not buck-kneed or calf-kneed (Fig. 2–8).

Normal front pastern angles range from 53 to 58°. Exceptionally long, sloping pasterns can result in tendon strain, bowed tendon, and damaged proximal sesamoids. Short, upright pasterns deliver greater concussive stresses to the fetlock, pastern joints, and foot, which may result in osselets (fetlock arthritis), ring bone, and possibly navicular syndrome. Fetlock joints should be large enough to allow free movement, but they should be devoid of puffiness. The hoof should be appropriate for the size of the horse, well shaped, and symmetric with high-quality hoof horn, adequate height and width of heel, concave sole, and adequately sized hoof.

Faults in Conformation of the Forelimbs

Base-Narrow (Fig. 2–9)

In base-narrow conformation, the distance between the center lines of the feet at their placement on the ground is less than the distance between the center lines of the limbs at their origin in the chest when viewed from the front. This is found most often in horses having large chests and well-developed pectoral muscles, such as the Quarter Horse. This conformation may be accompanied by a toe-in (pigeon-toed) or toe-out (splay-footed) conformation.

Base-narrow conformation inherently causes the horse to bear more weight on the outside of the foot than on the inside. The base-narrow condition makes it impossible for the weight to be borne in any other way. Consequently, whether the foot toes-in or toes-out, the outside of the foot will land first, and most of the weight will be taken on this area. Because of this, the outside of the foot and limb is subjected to more strain. Articular windpuffs of the fetlock joint, lateral ringbone, lateral sidebone, and heel bruising may develop from this conformation.

Base-Wide (Fig. 2–10)

In base-wide conformation, the distance between the center lines of the feet on the ground is greater than the distance between the center lines of the limbs at their origin in the chest when viewed from the front. This condition is found most commonly in narrow-chested horses such as the American Saddlebred and the Tennessee Walking Horse. In base-wide conformation, the horse is often affected with a toe-out (splay-footed) position of the feet. Base-wide, toe-out conformation usually causes winging to the inside (Figs. 2–11*B* and 2–12).

Base-wide conformation forces the horse to bear more weight on the inside of the foot than the outside of the foot. Because the weight is distributed in this fashion, the horse will usually land on the inside of the foot, a situation opposite to that seen in base-narrow conformation. Consequently, the inside of the limb takes the most stress in base-wide conformation. Articular windpuffs (idiopathic synovitis/capsulitis) of the fetlock joint, medial ringbone, and medial sidebone may develop as a result of this conformation.

FIG. 2–7. The angle of the shoulder joint usually influences the angle of the pastern.

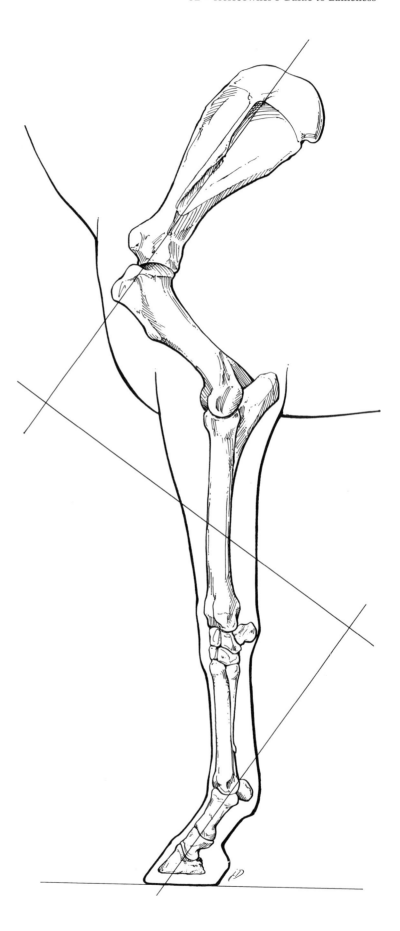

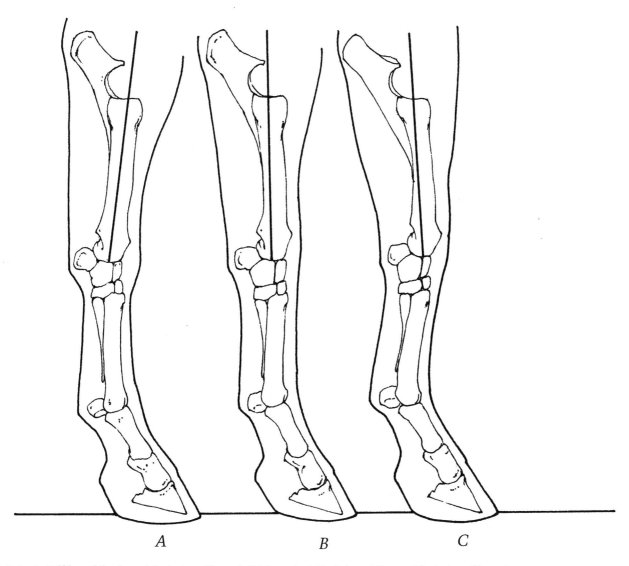

FIG. 2–8. *A*, Calf-kneed (backward deviation of knees). *B*, Normal. *C*, Buck-kneed (forward deviation of knees).

Toe-In or Pigeon-Toed (Figs. 2–13 and 2–14)

Toe-in is the position of the feet in which the toes point toward one another when viewed from the front. It is congenital, and the limb may be crooked as high as its origin at the chest or as low as the fetlock down. It is usually accompanied by a base-narrow conformation but rarely is present when the horse is base-wide. In the young foal, the condition may be partially corrected by proper trimming of the feet, and young horses may be correctively shod to prevent a worsening of the condition (see Chapter 6, Shoeing for Soundness). If an angular limb deformity is contributing to the problem, surgery may be helpful. When the affected horse moves, there is a tendency to paddle with the feet (Figs. 2–11*C* and 2–15). This is an outward deviation of the foot during flight. The foot breaks over the outside toe and lands on the outside wall. If a horse toes-in, it will usually paddle whether it is base-narrow or base-wide. If there is inward de-

viation of the pastern and foot from the fetlock down (varus deformity), the horse may carry the foot to the inside instead of the outside. This complication of base-narrow, toe-in conformation can cause interference, especially at the fetlock joint, causing damage to the medial sesamoid bone.

Toe-Out or Splay-Footed (Figs. 2–16 and 2–17)

In toe-out or splay-footed position, when viewed from the front, the toes point away from one another. The condition is usually congenital and is usually due to limbs that are crooked from their origin down. In some cases, however, the condition is aggravated by a twisting at the fetlock. It may be accompanied by either base-wide or base-narrow conformation. As with a toe-in conformation, it may be controlled or partially corrected by corrective trimming or corrective

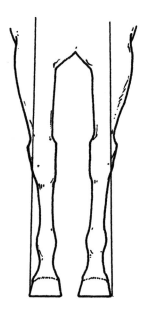

FIG. 2–9. Base-narrow. Note that the distance between the center lines of the limbs at their origin is greater than the distance between the center lines of the feet on the ground.

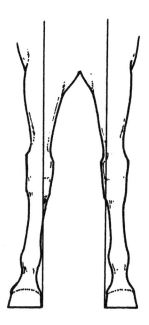

FIG. 2–10. Base-wide conformation. Note that the distance between the center lines of the feet is wider than the distance between the center lines of the limbs at the chest.

shoeing in the foal. If an angular limb deformity is contributing to the problem, surgery may be helpful. The flight of the foot goes through an inner arc when advancing and may cause interference with the opposite forelimb (Figs. 2–11B and 2–12). A horse that toes-out will usually wing to the inside, whether it is base-narrow or base-wide. When a toe-out attitude of the feet occurs with base-narrow conformation, there

is a greater likelihood of limb interference and plaiting (Fig. 2–18A).

Base-Narrow, Toe-In Conformation (Fig. 2–13)

Base-narrow, toe-in conformation causes excessive strain on the lateral collateral ligaments of the fetlock and pastern joints. Articular windpuffs, lateral ringbone, and lateral sidebone are common conditions with this conformation; they result from the mechanical strains caused by the base-narrow conformation and an excess of body weight on the outside hoof wall. Base-narrow, toe-in conformation usually causes paddling (Figs. 2–11C and 2–15). This is a common type of conformational abnormality.

Base-Narrow, Toe-Out Conformation (Fig. 2–16)

Base-narrow, toe-out conformation is one of the worst types of conformation in the forelimb. Horses having this conformation can seldom shoulder the strain of heavy work. The closely placed feet, combined with a tendency to wing inwardly from the toe-out position, commonly cause limb interference. The base-narrow attitude of the limb places the weight on the outside wall, as with base-narrow, toe-in conformation. The hoof breaks over the inside toe, swings inward, and lands on the outside wall. This causes great strain on the limb below the fetlock. Plaiting (Fig. 2–18A) may be evident. One should study the foot closely in flight before making any corrections (Fig. 2–18B).

Lesions on the medial aspect of the cannon bone, fractures of the medial splint bone, and an occasional fracture of the medial sesamoid may result from the interference. Diagnosis of interference is discussed later in this chapter. Corrective shoeing is discussed in Chapter 6.

Base-Wide, Toe-Out Conformation (Fig. 2–17)

When a horse is base-wide, the usual attitude of the feet is to toe-out. The base-wide conformation places the greatest stress on the inside of the limb. This means that there is greater stress on the medial collateral ligament of the fetlock and pastern joints. In addition, medial sidebone and ringbone may develop. With this conformation, the foot usually breaks over the inside toe, deviates (wings) to the inside, and lands on the inside hoof wall. Blemishes on the medial aspect of the cannon bone, medial splints, and fracture of the medial splint bone occur with this conformation because of interference.

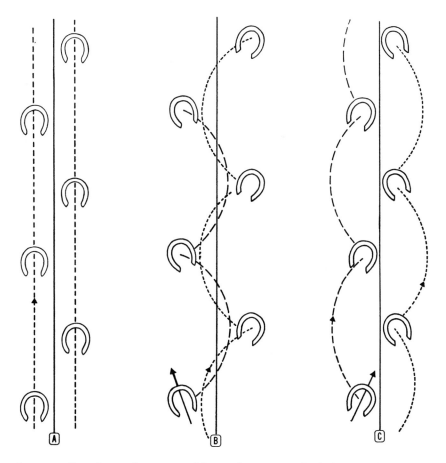

FIG. 2–11. How toe-in and toe-out affects foot path. *A,* Normal foot path. *B,* Foot path of a horse with toe-out conformation. *C,* Foot path of a horse with toe-in conformation.

Base-Wide, Toe-In Conformation (Fig. 2–14)

This type of conformation is unusual, but it does occur. The base-wide attitude of the limbs throws the greatest stress on the inside of the limb, with the same resulting pathologic changes as for base-wide, toe-out conformation. In most cases, a horse affected with base-wide, toe-in conformation will paddle to the outside even though it breaks over the inside toe and lands on the inside wall.

There is always the possibility that other conformational abnormalities of the limb, especially from the fetlock down, may change the path of the foot so it does not correspond to the above descriptions. These abnormalities include twisting of the fetlock so that the base-narrow, toe-in horse actually wings to the inside. These variations are rare and because they all cannot be listed, there will be no discussion of them here.

Plaiting (Fig. 2–18A)

Some horses, especially those with base-narrow, toe-out conformation, tend to place one forefoot directly in front of the other. This is an undesirable characteristic, because it can produce interference and stumbling resulting from an advancing forelimb hitting the one placed in front of it.

Backward (Palmar) Deviation of the Carpal Joints (Calf Knees or Sheep Knees) (Fig. 2–19)

Backward deviation of the carpus or carpal joints is a weak conformation, and the limbs seldom remain sound under heavy work. The weight of the horse descends through the misaligned limb to end behind the hoof. This conformation places stress on the carpal and radial check ligaments, the proximal middle and distal accessory carpal ligaments, the palmar carpal ligament, and the palmar reflection of the antebrachiocarpal joint capsule, and increases compression on the dorsal aspect of the carpal bones. Chip fractures from the third, radial, and intermediate carpal bones are common with horses working at speed and especially those with calf knees (Figs. 2–20 and 2–21). Small chip fractures from the radius may also occur.

Forward (Dorsal) Deviation of the Carpal Joints (Bucked Knees or Knee Sprung) (Fig. 2–19)

This condition may also be called "goat knees" or "over in the knees." It is a forward deviation of the

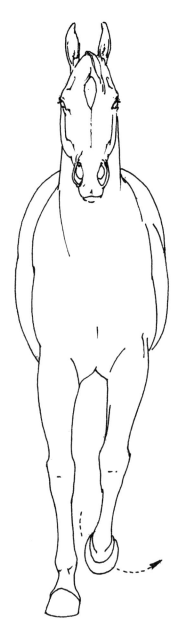

FIG. 2–12. Winging, which may cause interference, is caused by a toe out position of the feet.

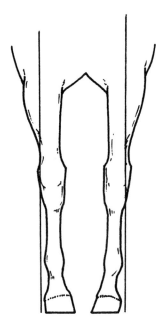

FIG. 2–13. Base-narrow, toe-in conformation.

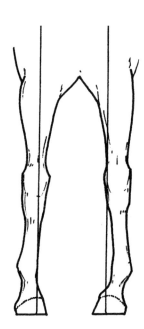

FIG. 2–14. Base-wide, toe-in position of feet.

carpus. Although it causes less damage to the horse than the calf-knee condition described above, it is more dangerous for the rider because the horse's knees are on the verge of buckling forward. Forward deviation of the carpus may be caused by contraction of the carpal flexors, i.e., ulnaris lateralis, flexor carpi ulnaris, and flexor carpi radialis. Extra strain is placed on the sesamoid bones, the superficial flexor tendon, the extensor carpi radialis, and the suspensory ligament. The condition is often present at birth, but if it is not severe, it usually disappears by 3 months of age. Congenital forms are nearly always bilateral and may be accompanied by a knuckling of the fetlocks. For-

ward deviation of the carpal joints may be accompanied by an enlarged epiphysis and distal metaphysis of the radius.

Medial Deviation of the Carpal Joints (Knock Knees, Carpus Valgus, or Knee-Narrow Conformation) (Fig. 2–22*B*)

Medial angular deviation of the knees can result from abnormalities of the distal physis (growth plate) and epiphysis of the radius, from abnormal development and alignment of the carpal bones and small metacarpal bones, or from joint laxity. As a result of this deviation, an increased tensional strain is placed on the medial collateral ligaments of the carpus with increased compression on the lateral (concave) surface of the carpus. Varying degrees of stresses are also transmitted to the joints proximal and distal to the carpus. Usually, varying degrees of outward rotation of the cannon bone, fetlock, and foot accompany this entity.

Lateral Deviation of the Carpal Joints (Bow Legs, Carpus Varus, or Bandy-Legged Conformation) (Fig. 2–22A)

Carpus varus is an outward deviation of the carpal joints when viewed from the front of the horse. It may be accompanied by a base-narrow, toe-in conformation. This condition causes increased tension on the lateral surface of the limb, particularly the lateral collateral ligament of the carpus. An increased compression is distributed to the medial surface of all joints, and an increased compression is brought to bear on the medial carpal bones.

Open Knees

The term "open knees" refers to an irregular profile of the carpal joints when viewed from the side (Fig. 2–23). This irregularity gives the impression that the carpal joints are not fully closed. This conformation is usually found in young horses (1 to 3 years of age) before full maturity and is often accompanied by epiphysitis. As the horse matures, the joints usually become more pleasing in appearance. Most people regard this as a weak conformation subject to carpal injury. On the basis of experience, this is probably so. Radiographically, this irregularity in the carpal joints does not show outstanding changes.

Lateral Deviation of the Metacarpal Bones (Offset or Bench Knees) (Fig. 2–24)

Offset knee is a conformation in which the cannon bone is offset to the lateral side and does not follow a straight line from the radius. It is evident when the limbs are viewed from the front. It is congenital in origin and should be considered a weak conformation. The medial splint bone is under greater stress than normal, and medial splints are common. The medial splint bone normally carries more weight than the lateral splint bone, because the medial splint bone has a flat articulation and the lateral splint bone has an oblique articulation. In offset knees, there is even more direct weight bearing on the medial splint bone, which in turn carries more weight to the interosseous ligament, increasing the possibility of splints.

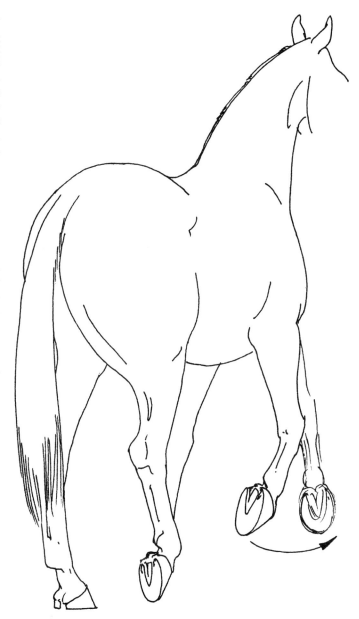

FIG. 2–15. Paddling at the pace. This accompanies toe-in conformation.

Tied-In Knees (Fig. 2–25B)

Viewed from the side, the flexor tendons appear to be too close to the cannon bone just below the carpus. This is poor conformation and it appears to inhibit free movement. A heavy fetlock may give the appearance of tied-in knees, even though the condition is not actually present.

Cut Out Under the Knees (Fig. 2–25A)

Viewed from the side, this condition causes a "cut out" appearance just below the carpus on the dorsal surface of the cannon bone. It is a fundamentally weak

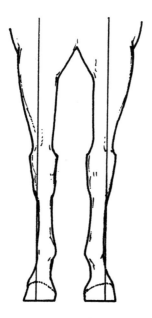

FIG. 2–16. Base-narrow, toe-out conformation.

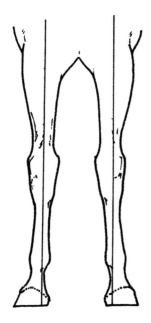

FIG. 2–17. Base-wide, toe-out position of the feet.

conformation because the cannon bone does not line up with the carpal bones dorsally.

Standing Under in Front (Fig. 2–26A)

This is a deviation in which the entire forelimb from the elbow down is placed in back of the perpendicular and too far under the body when the animal is viewed from the side. This may be brought about by disease and may not be caused by conformation.

With this conformation, the base of support is shortened, overloading the forelimbs and limiting the cranial phase of the stride by overburdening the forelimb left on the ground. The limb in motion must come down sooner and therefore has a low arc of foot flight. The steps are more frequent, the arc of foot flight is low, and the foot is carried too close to the ground, predisposing the horse to stumbling. Overall, it is believed to cause excessive wear and fatigue of bones, ligaments, and tendons. There is a reduction of speed, and the horse is predisposed to falling.

Camped in Front (Fig. 2–26B)

This is a condition opposite to that described above. The entire forelimb, from the body to the ground, is too far forward when viewed from the side. This limb attitude may be present in certain conditions, such as bilateral navicular syndrome and laminitis.

Short Upright Pastern (Fig. 2–27B)

A short upright pastern increases concussion on the fetlock joint, the pastern joint, and the navicular bone. A horse with this conformation has increased predisposition to osselets (traumatic arthritis of the fetlock joint), ringbone of the pastern joint, and navicular syndrome. This type of conformation is often associated with a base-narrow, toe-in conformation and is most often present in the horse with short limbs and powerful body and limb musculature. A straight shoulder usually accompanies this type of conformation.

Long Sloping Pastern (Fig. 2–28)

A long sloping pastern is one characterized by a normal or subnormal angulation of the forefoot (45° or under) with a pastern that is too long for the length of the limb. This type of conformation predisposes the horse to injury of the flexor tendons (tendosynovitis), sesamoid bones (sesamoiditis and fractures), and the suspensory ligament (desmitis).

Long Upright Pastern (Fig. 2–27C)

A long upright pastern predisposes the fetlock joint and the navicular bone to injury. Concussion to these regions is increased because the anticoncussion mechanism of a normally sloping pastern is not present. Osselets (traumatic arthritis) and navicular syndrome may be seen with this type of conformation, and both types of lameness may be present at the same time. The stresses are very similar to those found in the short upright pastern (Fig. 2–27B), but pathology of the pastern joint is not so common.

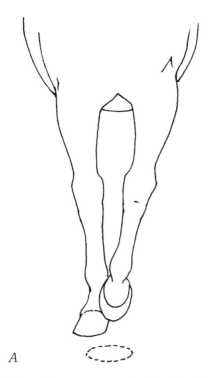

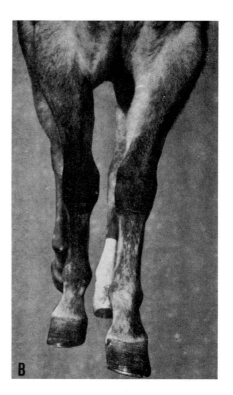

Fig. 2–18. *A,* Plaiting. Plaiting is most often found in a horse with base-narrow, toe-out conformation. After the foot travels an inward arc, it lands more or less directly in front of the opposite forefoot. In some cases, this leads to stumbling as a result of interference. *B,* Base-narrow, toe-out conformation. Note left forefoot landing on the outside wall, typical of this type of conformation. There is also a degree of plaiting.

The Hindlimbs

The bone structure and muscling of the hindlimb should be appropriate for the intended use. Endurance horses are characterized by longer, flatter muscles; stock horses are characterized by shorter, thicker muscles. All-around horses have moderate muscles.

Limbs, when viewed from the side, should exhibit a composite of moderate angles, so that shock absorption will be efficient (Fig. 2–29). A line from the point of buttock to the ground should touch the hock and end slightly behind the bulbs of the heels. A hindlimb in front of this line is often standing under (Fig. 2–30) or sickle-hocked (Fig. 2–31); a hindlimb behind this line is often post-legged (Fig. 2–32) or camped out (Fig. 2–33).

The hindquarter should be symmetric and well connected to the barrel and the lower limb. The gluteals should tie well forward into the back. The hamstrings should tie down low into the Achilles tendon of the hock.

The relationship of the length of the bones, the angles of the joints, and the overall height of the hindlimb will dictate the type of action and the amount of power produced. The length and slope to the pelvis (croup) are measured from the point of hip to the point of buttock. A flat, level croup is associated with hindlimb action that occurs *behind* the hindquarters rather than underneath it. A goose rump is a very steep croup that places the hindlimbs so far under the horse's belly that structural problems may occur due to the over-angulation.

A short femur is associated with the short, rapid stride characteristic of a sprinter. A long femur results in a stride with more reach. High hocks are associated with snappy hock action and a difficulty getting the hocks under the body. Low hocks tend to have a smoother hock action and the horse usually has an easier time getting the hocks under the body. The gaskin length (stifle to hock) should be shorter than the femur length (buttock to stifle). A gaskin longer than the femur tends to be associated with cow hocks and sickle hocks.

Hindlimbs with open angles (straighter hindlimbs when viewed from the side) have a shorter overall limb length and produce efficient movement suitable for hunters or race horses. Hindlimbs with more closed joints (more angulation to the hindlimb) have a longer overall limb length and produce a more vertical, folding action necessary for the collection characteristic of a high-level dressage horse. If the overall limb length is too long, it can be associated with either camped-out or sickle-hocked conformation. No matter what the hindlimb conformation is at rest, however, the connection to the loin and operation in motion is most important.

From the rear, both hindlimbs should appear to be symmetric, to be of the same length, and to bear equal

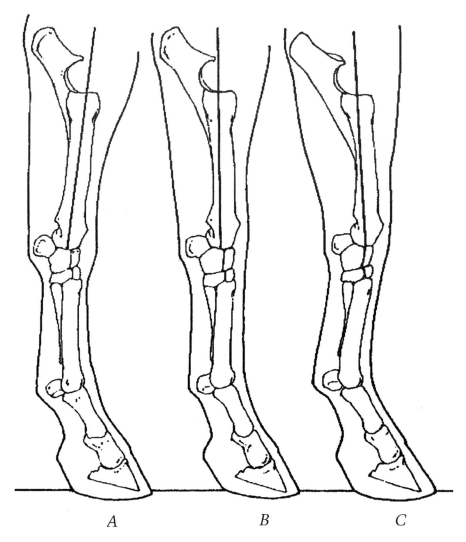

FIG. 2–19. *A*, Calf-kneed. *B*, Normal. *C*, Buck-kneed.

weight (Fig. 2–34). A left-to-right symmetry should be evident between the peaks of the croup, the points of the hip, the points of the buttock, and the midline position of the tail (Fig. 2–35). The widest point of the hindquarters should be the width between the stifles. A line dropped from the point of the buttock to the ground will essentially bisect the limb, but hindlimbs are not designed to point absolutely straight forward. It is necessary and normal for the stifles to point slightly outward in order to clear the horse's belly. This causes the points of the hocks to face slightly inward and the toes to point outward to the same degree. The rounder the belly and/or the shorter the loin and coupling, the more the stifles must point out and the points of the hocks will appear to point inward. The more the horse is slab-sided and/or longer coupled, the more straight ahead the stifles and hocks can point. When the cannon bone faces outward, the horse is often cow-hocked (Fig. 2–36); when cannons face inward the horse is bow-legged (Fig. 2–37).

Soundness problems can occur when the hocks point absolutely straight ahead and the hooves toe-out; in this situation, there is stress on the hock and fetlock joints. The hindfeet should be as far apart on the ground as the limbs are at their origin in the hip. Normal pastern angles for the hind range from 55 to 60°.

Faults in Conformation of the Hindlimbs

Standing Under Behind (Fig. 2–30)

Viewed from the side, the entire limb is placed too far forward or sickle hocks are present. A perpendicular line drawn from the point of buttock (tuber ischii) would strike the ground well behind the limb.

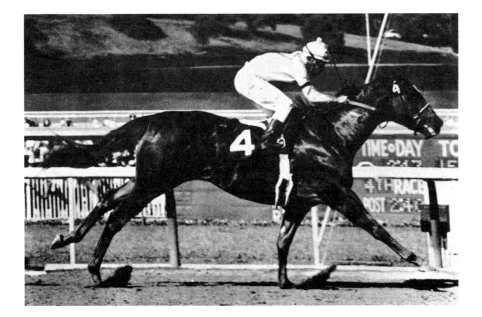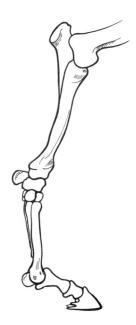

Fig. 2–20. Photograph of a Thoroughbred near the finish of a race. Note the backward deviation of the carpus, predisposing to chip fracture of the carpal bones. If a horse has a backward deviation of the carpus before limb fatigue forces it into this position, there is even greater possibility of carpal fracture. (Courtesy of Dr. W. Berkley.)

Excessive Angulation of the Hock Joints (Sickle Hocks) (Fig. 2–31)

When viewed from the side, the angle of the hock joint is decreased so that the horse is standing under from the hock down. The plantar aspect of the hock is under a greater stress, especially the plantar ligament. A horse so affected is predisposed to sprain and strain of soft tissue support structures on the plantar hock region. This is called "curby conformation."

Excessively Straight Limbs or "Straight Behind" (Fig. 2–32)

When viewed from the side, there is very little angle between the tibia and femur and the hock joint is correspondingly straight. This predisposes the horse particularly to bog spavin and upward fixation of the patella. The straight hock places increased tension on the dorsal aspect of the joint capsule, causing irritation and chronic distention of the joint capsule with synovia. This type of limb is easily injured by heavy work. It is not uncommon to find intermittent upward fixation of the patella accompanying this conformation. The pasterns will also be too straight.

Camped Behind (Fig. 2–33)

"Camped behind" means that the entire limb is placed too far caudally when viewed from the side. A perpendicular line dropped from the hip joint would hit at the toe, or in front of it, instead of halfway between the toe and heel. This condition is often associated with upright pasterns behind.

Base-Wide (Fig. 2–36)

Base-wide means that when viewed from behind, the distance between the center lines of the feet at their placement on the ground is greater than the distance between the center lines of the limbs in the thigh region. Base-wide conformation is not as frequent in the hindlimbs as in the forelimbs. The most common form of base-wide conformation is associated with cow hocks.

Medial Deviation of the Hock Joints (Cow Hocks or Tarsus Valgus) (Fig. 2–36)

"Cow-hocked" means that the limbs are base-narrow to the hock and base-wide from the hock to the feet. Cow-hocked conformation is a common defect. The hocks are too close, point toward one another, and the feet are widely separated. Viewed laterally, the horse may be sickle-hocked. Cow-hocked is one of the worst hindlimb conformations because there is excessive stress on the medial side of the hock joint, which may cause bone spavin.

Base-Narrow (Fig. 2–37)

Base-narrow conformation of the hindlimbs means that when the animal is viewed from behind, the dis-

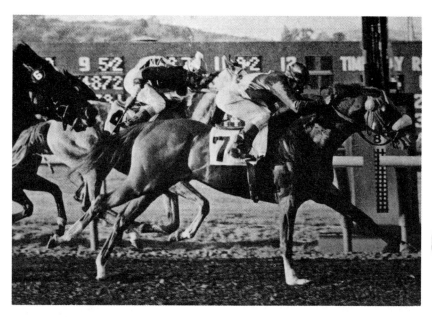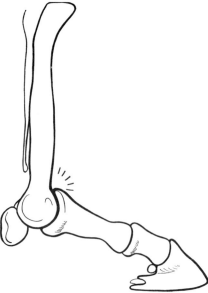

FIG. 2–21. Photograph of a Thoroughbred near the finish of a race. Note the backward deviation of the carpus and the extreme dropping of the fetlock. When the fetlock is in this position, there is a possibility of chip fracture of the proximal end of the long pastern bone. (Courtesy of Dr. W. Berkley.)

tance between the center lines of the feet is less than the distance between the center lines of the limbs in the thigh region. This is most commonly evident in heavily muscled horses in which there is excessive strain on the lateral aspect of the limb in the bones, ligaments, and joints. The feet may toe-in or have straight toes. Base-narrow conformation is often accompanied by bowlegs or a condition in which the hocks are too far apart. The limbs may appear fairly straight to the hock and then deviate inward. Most of the horse's weight is borne on the outside edges of the hooves. The hocks bow outward during movement. When a horse has good conformation in front and is base-narrow behind, many types of interference can occur between the fore- and hindlimbs.

Base-Narrow from Fetlocks Down

This conformation places stress on the lateral collateral ligaments of the fetlock, pastern, and coffin joints and similar strain on the bones and tendons in this area.

Conformation of the Foot

Principles of hoof conformation are discussed in detail in Chapters 1 and 6.

The Forefoot (Fig. 2–38)

Ideally, the forefoot should be round and wide in the heels, and the size and shape of the heels should correspond to the size and shape of the toe. The bars should be well developed. The wall should be thickest at the toe and should thin gradually toward the heels; the inside wall should be slightly straighter than the outside wall.

The sole should be slightly concave medial to lateral and front to back, but an excessive concavity is evidence of a chronic foot disease. There should be no primary contact between the ground and the sole, as it is not a weight-bearing structure.

The foot and pastern axes in the forefoot should be between 53 and 58°. The angle of the heel should correspond to the angle of the toe, and there should be no defects in the wall. The foot should show that the animal is breaking squarely over the center of the toe and not over the medial or lateral portion of the toe. The wall should show that it is wearing evenly.

The frog should be large and well developed with a good cleft, should have normal consistency and elasticity, and should show no moisture. It should divide the sole into two nearly equal halves, and the apex should point to the center of the toe. Unequal size of the two halves may indicate a base-wide or base-narrow conformation.

The Hind Foot (Fig. 2–39)

The hind foot should present a more pointed appearance at the toe than does the forefoot. It should

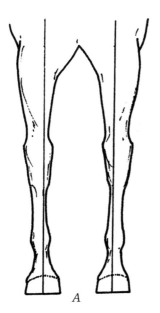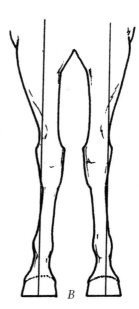

FIG. 2–22. Examples of poor conformation. Compare with Figure 2–6*A*. *A*, Bowlegs. *B*, Knock-knees.

show evidence of breaking straight over the toe, and the frog should divide the sole into equal halves. The foot axis should be 55 to 60°, and there should be no defects in the wall. The walls should show normal wear on the medial and lateral sides, and the sole should be slightly concave medial to lateral and front to back. The sole of the hind foot is normally more concave than that of the forefoot.

Abnormal Conformation of the Foot

Flat Feet

A flat foot lacks the natural concavity in the sole; it is not a normal condition in light horses but is present in some draft breeds. Flat feet may be heritable and are much more common in the forefeet than in the hind. The horse will often land on the heels in order to avoid sole pressure with this condition. Sole bruising and the lameness that results are common sequelae of flat feet. No remedy will cure a flat foot, but corrective shoeing can help prevent aggravation of the condition.

Contracted Foot or Contracted Heels (Fig. 2–40)

Contracted foot is a condition in which the foot is narrower than normal. This is especially true of the back half of the foot. This condition is much more common in the front feet than in the hind feet, and it may be unilateral or bilateral. Local or coronary contraction of the foot is a contraction at the heels confined to the horn immediately below that occupied by the coronary cushion. This term merely reflects an arbitrary subdivision of contracted foot.

One should bear in mind that certain breeds of horses normally have a foot that more closely approaches an oval than a circle in form. A narrow foot is not necessarily a contracted foot, and donkeys and mules normally have a foot shape that would be called contracted on a horse. Foot contraction is often present in the Tennessee Walking Horse and American Saddlebred when these horses are used for show because the hoof wall is allowed to grow excessively long.

Unilateral Contracted Foot

In some horses, a unilateral contraction of one forefoot is present. This may be congenital, and it is not known whether there is an inheritable tendency for this abnormality. The contracted foot may or may not eventually show lameness, but it should be regarded as an undesirable feature. A small foot on one side may also indicate a chronic lameness.

Bull-Nosed Foot (Fig. 2–41)

A foot that has a dubbed toe is called a "bull-nosed foot."

Buttress Foot (Fig. 2–42)

"Buttress foot" is a swelling on the dorsal surface of the hoof wall at the coronary band. This swelling may be from a low ringbone or the result of a fracture of the extensor process of the coffin bone. A conical deformity of the toe from the coronary band to the

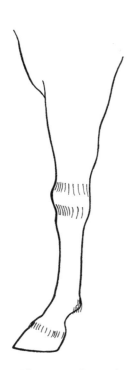

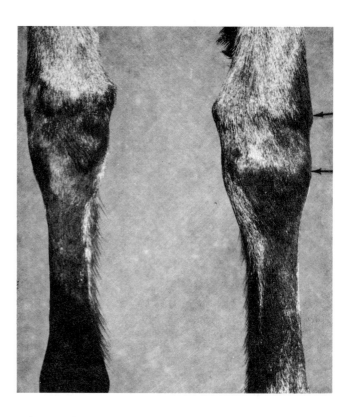

FIG. 2–23. Open knees. This term refers to the irregular profile of the carpal joints when viewed from the side, which is due to the enlarged distal physis of the radius and enlargement in the area of the carpometacarpal joint.

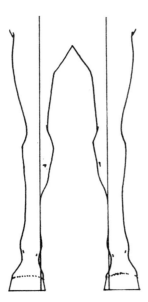
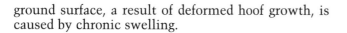

FIG. 2–24. Offset knees (bench knees). Note that the cannon bones are set too far laterally.

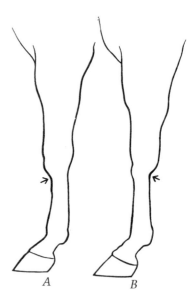

FIG. 2–25. Examples of poor conformation. *A,* Cut out under the knees, as indicated by arrow. *B,* Tied-in knees, as indicated by arrow.

ground surface, a result of deformed hoof growth, is caused by chronic swelling.

Thin Wall and Sole

Thin walls and sole accompany one another and are heritable. The conformation of the foot may appear to be normal, but the hoof wall either wears away too rapidly or does not grow fast enough to avoid sole pressure. This condition is especially noticeable at the heels, where the foot axis may be broken by the tendency of the heel to be too low.

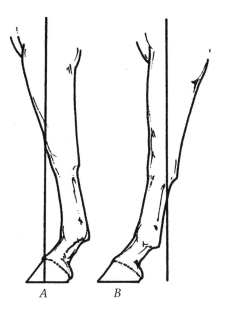

FIG. 2-26. Examples of poor conformation. *A*, Standing under in front. *B*, Camped in front.

Club Foot

A "club foot" is one that has a foot axis of 60° or more. When a club foot is unilateral, it is often due to some injury that has prevented proper use of the foot or from a flexural deformity involving the deep digital flexor tendon. It may be heritable or developmental. See Chapter 6.

Coon-Footed (Fig. 2-43)

The pastern of the coon-footed horse slopes more than the dorsal surface of the hoof wall. In other words, the foot and pastern axis is broken forward at the coronary band. It may occur in either the fore- or hind feet, and it causes strain on the flexor tendons, sesamoid bones, and distal sesamoid ligaments. There may also be strain on the common digital extensor tendon.

Movement

Movement is composed of a horse's travel and action. Although the lower limbs are the focal point of evaluation, movement is a combined effort of the horse's entire body. "Travel" refers to the flight of the hoof in relation to the other limbs and is often viewed from the front or rear. "Action" takes into account joint flexion, stride length, suspension, and other qualities and is usually assessed from a side view.

The Natural Gaits

The "walk" is a four-beat gait (Fig. 2-44) that should have a very even rhythm as the feet land and take off in the following sequence: left hind, left front, right hind, right front. A horse that is rushing at the walk might either jig or prance (impure gaits composed of half walking, half trotting) or might develop a pacey walk. The "pace" (Fig. 2-45) is a two-beat lateral gait in which the two right limbs rise and land alternately with the two left limbs. Although the pace is a viable gait for a Standardbred race horse, a pacey walk is considered an impure gait for most riding horses because the even four-beat pattern of the walk is broken.

The "trot" is a two-beat diagonal gait (Fig. 2-46). Traditionally, the trot refers to an English gait with a moderate to great degree of impulsion. The right front and left hind rise and fall together alternately with the diagonal pair left front and right hind. Often, the trot is a horse's steadiest and most rhythmic gait. The (western) jog is a shorter-strided trot with less impulsion. If a horse is jogged too slow, the gait becomes impure as the diagonal pairs break and the horse essentially walks behind and trots in front.

The "canter" or "lope" (Fig. 2-47) is a three-beat gait with the following sequence: one hind limb, then the other hind limb simultaneously with its diagonal forelimb, and finally the remaining forelimb. If a horse is on the right lead, the initiating hind will be the left hind, the diagonal pair will be the right hind (sometimes referred to as the supporting hind) and the left front, and the final beat will occur when the leading forelimb (the right front) lands. Then there is a moment of suspension as the horse gathers his limbs up underneath himself to get organized for the next cycle. When observing a horse on the right lead from the side, it is evident that the right limbs will reach farther forward than the left limbs. A change of lead (Fig. 2-48) should occur during the moment of suspension so that the horse can change both front and hind simultaneously.

The "gallop" or run is a four-beat variation of the canter (Fig. 2-49). With increased impulsion and length of stride, the diagonal pair breaks, resulting in four beats. The footfall sequence of a right lead gallop is left hind, right hind, left front, and right front. As in the canter, the right limbs will reach farther forward than the left limbs when the horse is in the right lead. There is a more marked suspension at the gallop than at the canter.

The "back," performed in its correct form, is a two-beat diagonal gait in reverse. The left hind and right front are lifted and placed down together, alternating with the right hind and left front.

The Phases of a Stride

The five phases of a horse's stride are landing, loading, stance, breakover, and swing (Figs. 2-50, 2-51, and 2-52).

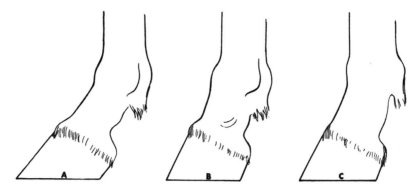

FIG. 2–27. Examples of pastern conformation. *A*, A normal angulation of hoof and pastern. *B*, A short upright pastern predisposing to injuries of the fetlock joint, ringbone of the pastern joint, and navicular disease. *C*, Long upright pastern predisposes to injuries of the fetlock joint and navicular bone. This type of conformation does not seem to predispose to ringbone as often as does *B*.

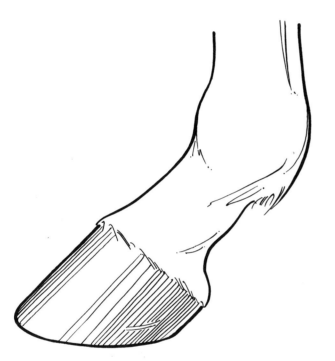

FIG. 2–28. Example of a long sloping pastern. The foot and pastern axes are less than normal (less than 45° in front or less than 50° behind).

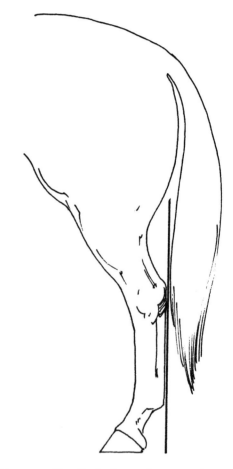

FIG. 2–29. Normal hindlimbs from side view. A line dropped from the point of buttock (tuber ischii) follows the cannon.

Landing (Fig. 2–50). The hoof touches the ground, and the limb begins to receive the impact of the body's weight.

Loading (Fig. 2–50). The body moves forward, and the horse's center of gravity passes over the hoof. Usually, this is when the fetlock descends (extends) to its lowest point, sometimes resulting in an almost horizontal pastern.

Stance (Fig. 2–51). The fetlock rises to a configuration comparable to the horse's stance at rest. The transition between the loading phase and the stance phase is very stressful to the internal structures of the hoof and lower limb. The horse's center of gravity moves ahead of the hoof. The flexor apparatus lifts the weight

of the horse and rider and the fetlock begins to move upward. The pastern straightens and the limb begins pushing up off the ground.

Breakover (Fig. 2–51). "Breakover" is the phase when the hoof leaves the ground. It starts when the heels lift and the hoof begins to pivot at the toe. The knee (or hock) relaxes and begins to flex. Breakover is

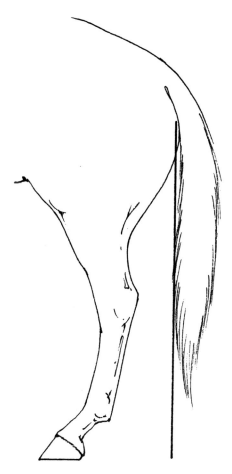

FIG. 2–30. Standing under behind. Compare with Figure 2–29.

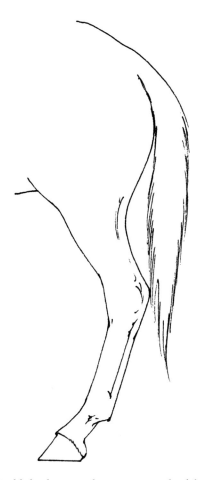

FIG. 2–31. Sickle hocks. Note the excessive angle of the hock joints. Compare with Figure 2–29.

measured from the time the heels leave the ground to the time the toe leaves the ground. The deep digital flexor tendon (assisted by the suspensory ligament) is still stretched just prior to the beginning of breakover to counteract the downward pressure of the weight of the horse's body.

Swing (Fig. 2–52). The limb moves through the air and straightens out in preparation for landing.

Stride Length

For years, it was believed that leaving the toe of a hoof long would increase a horse's stride length, thereby contributing to a smooth and efficient stride and less strides over a given distance. In the past, race horses, show ring hunters, and jumpers have mistakenly been shod with long toes and low heels to create a supposedly advantageous acute hoof angle. Research has shown that, contrary to popular opinion, horses with long toes and an acute hoof angle do not take longer strides. Long toes (often accompanied by low, run-under heels) put the pivot point of the hoof farther forward than normal. The long toe acts as a lever arm during breakover, making it more difficult for the heels to rotate around the · toe; consequently, tension

in the deep digital flexor tendon may be prolonged and/or exaggerated. Additionally, the navicular ligaments, which stabilize the navicular bone and which are already stretched to the maximum at the beginning of breakover in a normal hoof, are stressed excessively during the breakover of a hoof with an acute angle. The delayed breakover allows the mass of the horse's body to move farther forward over the horse's limbs before the limbs leave the ground.

Recent research (Fig. 2–53) has shown that the arc of hoof flight is not significantly changed by trimming. However, the approach to the loading phase and the landing phase were affected. With a normally trimmed hoof, the toe of the hoof elevated slightly prior to landing as the hoof prepared for a heel-first or flat-foot impact. The hoof with an acute angle approached the ground toe first, often landing with the toe impacting first. Such stabbing into the ground with the toes results in a broken, jarring motion rather than smooth action.

Research also showed that during the trot, when the fronts were trimmed normally and the hind toes were long, the hinds left the ground significantly later than their diagonal forefoot. However, the hindlimbs compensated for the delay in breakover by moving through

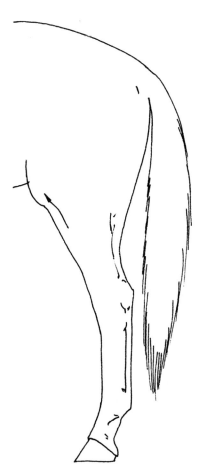

FIG. 2–32. Post legged too straight behind. There is too little angulation of the hock and stifle joints.

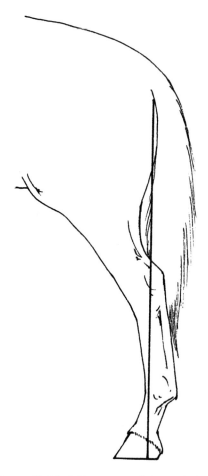

FIG. 2–33. Camped behind. Compare with Figure 2–29.

the air more rapidly so that they could catch up and land at the same time as their corresponding diagonal forefeet. This causes an unevenness in the gait; the horse is first delayed behind and then hurries the movement of the hindlimbs to catch up.

Research has also disproved the popular theory that long toes in the hind may make a horse reach farther forward. On the contrary, rather than the hind limbs reaching farther forward, the horse's mass moves further ahead of the weight-bearing limbs before they leave the ground. This tends to put the cycle of the forelimb movement further under the horse, thereby lessening the potential for (hindquarter) engagement.

Normal Movement

The straight foot flight pattern that is used as a basis when referring to deviations has often been termed "ideal." The fact is that such a foot flight is ideal only for a horse with ideal body and limb conformation. Horses with imperfections in their structural components, which includes virtually all horses, will have individual ideal foot flight patterns that compensate for imperfections; such an individual pattern may not be "textbook pretty," but it may well be functional. Instead of thinking of the straight foot flight as ideal, think of it as "standard," so that rather than representing a goal to strive for, the term indicates a baseline for comparison.

The standard for front limb movement starts with a straight bone column and a series of hinge joints all symmetrically conformed and working in a true forward-backward plane. Add to this a balanced hoof, and the result should be a straight foot flight.

Because hindlimbs nearly always turn out to some degree, the standard for hindlimb foot flight will be different than the front. Depending on the conformation of the hindquarters, this turning out of the limb facilitates a freer working of the stifle. The bone structure of a heavily muscled horse may, by genetic design, turn out in order to allow more drive and reach with the hindlimbs as well as to counteract the inward pull characteristic of a horse with heavy inside gaskin muscles.

Movement Abnormalities

"Gait defects" are movement abnormalities that consistently occur during regular work.

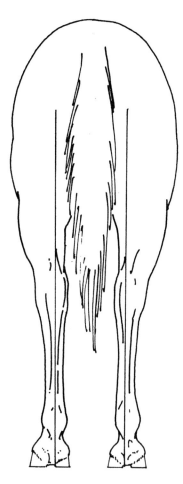

Fig. 2–34. Normal hindlimbs. A line dropped from the point of the buttock (tuber ischii) bisects the limb.

Forging

Forging is a gait defect that is commonly heard when a horse is trotting. Forging (Figs. 2–54 and 2–55) occurs when a hind foot contacts a front foot on the same side. Frequently, contact is made when the hind foot is gliding in for a landing and the front foot is beginning its swing phase. If the front foot is delayed in its breakover, the hind foot may arrive before the front foot has a chance to get out of the way. As the fetlock of the front foot begins hinging, the toe of the front shoe may swing back and slap the toe of the landing hind shoe. This creates a characteristic "clicking" as the shod horse trots and a dull "thwacking" if the horse is barefoot.

Forging is related to over-reaching. Forging customarily refers to the contact made between shoes or hoofs. A horse can receive sole bruises from a single blow or repeated tapping. Over-reaching (Fig. 2–56) usually indicates that a front shoe has been pulled off by a hind or that the hind has injured some part of the front limb such as the heel, bulb, coronary band, or even the fetlock or flexor tendons. A horse that forges or over-reaches may be more prone to stumble or fall, especially at the moment when the shoe is stepped on or pulled off. If the conditions that cause a horse to

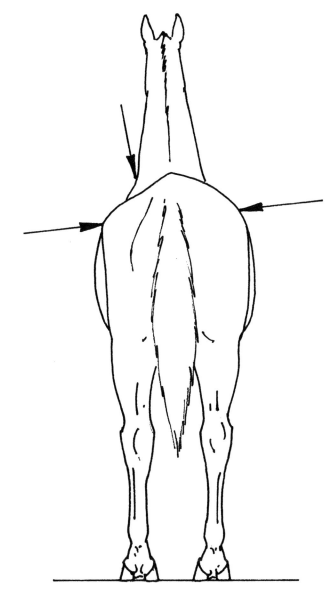

Fig. 2–35. Illustrates Asymmetry between peaks of the croup, points of the hip, and points of the buttock.

forge are ignored or inadvertently perpetuated, the stride imbalances may progress to over-reaching.

Forging and over-reaching are indications that the horse's movement is out of balance. Balance is customarily discussed in terms of dorsal–palmar (DP) balance, left–right (LR) balance, and medial–lateral (ML) balance.

DP balance can refer to the relationship between the front and rear of the horse's entire body as well as to the relationship between the toe and heel of the hoof. LR balance refers to the relationship between the left and right sides of the horse's body. There are inherent discrepancies in LR balance in most horses. ML balance is often used to describe the relationship between the two halves of a limb or hoof when viewed from the front or rear. Each limb and hoof is evaluated in-

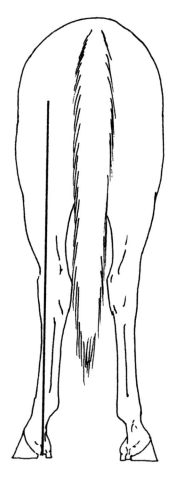

FIG. 2–36. Cow hocks accompanied by base-wide conformation. Such horses are usually base-narrow as far as the hocks, but base-wide from the hocks down. Compare with Figure 2–34.

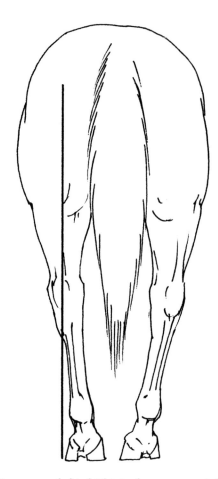

FIG. 2–37. Base-narrow behind. This is often accompanied by "bow-legs," as shown. Compare with Figure 2–34.

dividually for ML balance. The most graphic examples of ML imbalance are seen in the knees, hocks, fetlocks, and hoofs. These imbalances are implicated as causes of gait defects such as winging in and paddling. Although LR and ML imbalances can complicate a forging horse's problems, forging and over-reaching are mainly attributed to DP imbalances. Other movement abnormalities include cross firing (Fig. 2–57) and scalping (Fig. 2–58).

Causes of Forging. A horse's balance during movement is affected by many factors: conformation, condition, energy level, mental attitude, footing, level of training, gait or maneuver being performed, proficiency of rider, and shoeing. All of these factors affect breakover, but the theoretical discussion of breakover deals with the function of one limb at a time. To correct forging, the timing and direction of breakover of all of the hooves must be coordinated so that the limbs work in harmony and avoid collision.

Lateral Gait Defects

A lateral gait defect is one that involves a regularly occurring, abnormal sideways swing of a limb. Some

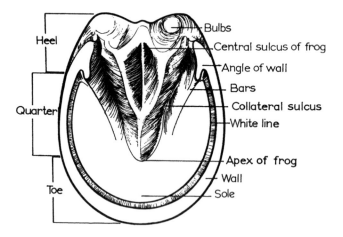

FIG. 2–38. Normal forefoot showing structures.

lateral gait defects result in actual physical contact with an opposite limb; others do not. Paddling or dishing, often seen with bow-legged, toed-in, or wide-chested and base-narrow horses, is a swinging out of the limb from the midline so that contact rarely results. In contrast, interfering is frequently associated

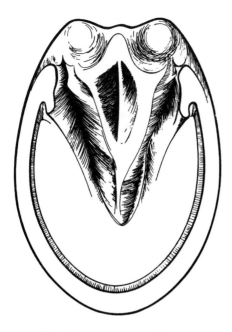

FIG. 2–39. Normal hindfoot. Compare with Figure 2–38. The toe of the hindfoot is more pointed than that of the forefoot.

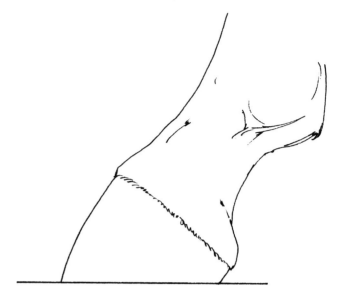

FIG. 2–41. Bull-nosed foot.

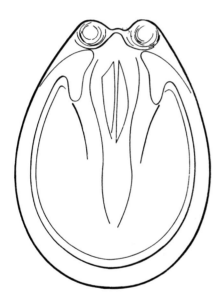

FIG. 2–40. Contracted foot. Note narrowing of the heels and quarters. Compare with Figure 2–38.

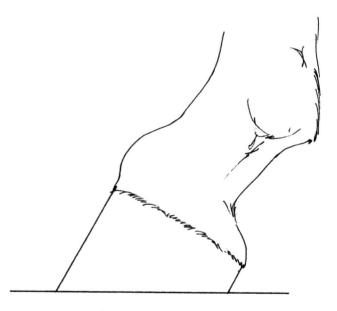

FIG. 2–42. Buttress foot.

with narrow and/or toed-out horses. Such chest conformation places the limbs closer together and the toed-out hoof predisposes the horse to winging, i.e., swinging the limb toward the midline during flight. As one limb swings inward, it passes the opposite limb, which usually is in a weight-bearing position. It is at this moment when contact might occur. The higher up the limb the turned-out deviation is located, the greater the torque is that is imparted to the limb and the worse the winging-in will likely be. Swinging in of the limb, often called "brushing," is commonly

referred to as "interfering" when contact between the two limbs is made.

Interfering occurs rarely at the walk. It appears most commonly at the trot and the other two-beat diagonal gait, backing up. The speed and energy level with which a horse moves its limbs has an affect on its tendency to interfere. One horse may interfere at the jog but not at the extended trot; another horse may move with adequate clearance at the jog but not at an energetic trot. Similarly, one horse performing a quiet rein back might place his limbs carefully, but if he were asked to speed up the back in a reining pattern, the limbs might swing from side to side and collide. Another horse may work his limbs with piston-like

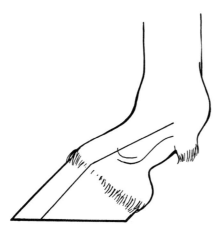

FIG. 2–43. Broken angle between hoof and pastern axis (coon-footed). The foot axis is steeper than the pastern axis.

precision while backing quickly and straight but might exhibit an altered foot flight if asked to slow down.

Interference can occur from the knee to the hoof of the front limbs and usually from the fetlock to the hoof of the hindlimbs. If a horse does not wear protective boots, the first signs of interference may be pain, heat, or swelling in the area of contact. The problem may escalate to include missing hair, bruises, cuts, lesions, chronic sores, and perhaps underlying bone damage.

Protective boots should be used, examined, and cleaned after each workout and points of contact noted. However, just because contact was made with a boot or leg wrap does not mean that contact would have been made without the protective gear because the thickness of the boot may be the safe tolerance in which the unbooted horse would work. Rather than take a chance of injury, however, it is best to use protective boots on all young horses and older horses with interference tendencies.

A horse sometimes will show reluctance to perform certain maneuvers that have caused him to hit himself in the past. The horse may try to avoid circular or lateral work by stiffening the back and working with short hopping strides with the hindlimbs. With a reining horse, interference problems in the front limbs may make him reluctant to add speed to his turn-around.

Factors that Affect Movement

There are many elements that affect a horse's movement. When lameness is a concern, the factors that are traditionally considered are lower limb conformation, pain, and shoeing. However, other factors should be considered because, in many cases, understanding the whole picture will result in a better treatment program and ultimately a more effective plan for lameness prevention.

Conformation

There are no absolutes when it comes to predicting whether a horse will paddle, wing-in, or travel straight. Generalizations related to stance, breed, or type are frequently proved wrong. Lateral gait defects can affect a pair of limbs or a single limb. Conformational components include (in the front limb, for example) shoulder to rib cage attachment, width of chest, width at knees, fetlock, and hoof, and straightness of forearm, cannon, and pastern.

The underdevelopment (hypoplasia) of one portion of a joint surface (particularly the knee and fetlock joints) can also cause a limb to exhibit a lateral gait defect. Normally, the fetlock and knee joints work in a hinge-like fashion, backward and forward in a straight line, parallel with the horse's midline. A hypoplastic joint tends to hinge in a swivel-like motion at an angle to the horse's midline. This arc causes the limb to deviate in flight.

Many factors influence how close a horse's front and hind feet come together when he is moving: the relationship between the height at the wither and the height at the hip; the amount of muscling and the width of the chest and hips; the length, proportion, and shape of the top-line components; the relationship between the length of the top line to the length of the underline; and, perhaps, most commonly, the length of underline to the length of the limbs. Horses with short backs and long limbs, and especially those with short front limbs and long hindlimbs, are the most likely to have contact between front and hindlimbs.

Pain

Even if a horse shows all of the conformational traits that theoretically add up to straight travel, if he experiences pain in a portion of his body, he may break all of the conformation rules as he attempts to use his limbs in a manner that creates the least stress and pain. An injury or soreness in a limb or an associated structure can cause a horse to protect one portion of the limb when landing, subsequently altering the arc of the foot's flight. For example, if the horse is sore in the navicular region of the front feet, instead of landing heel first and rolling forward, he may land toe first, which will shorten the stride.

When a horse is off in a part of the body other than the hooves or limbs, his balance during movement may be negatively altered as he compensates for the pain or soreness. Back soreness can mimic a lower limb lameness and alter foot flight. A variety of other factors can cause the horse to carry his body in a stiff or crooked fashion: muscle cramping, a respiratory illness, an ear infection, or poor fitting tack. Sometimes, the stiffness or pain is subtle but just enough to prevent the horse from tracking straight.

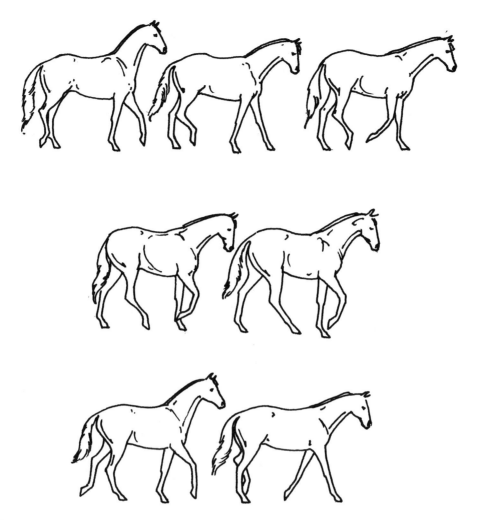

FIG. 2–44. The walk.

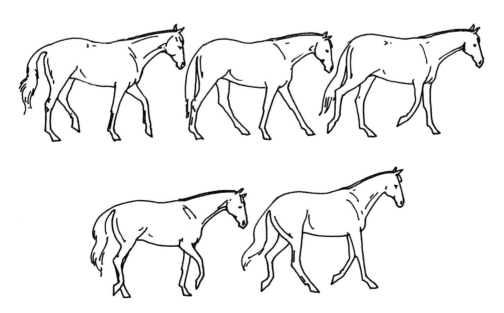

FIG. 2–45. The pace.

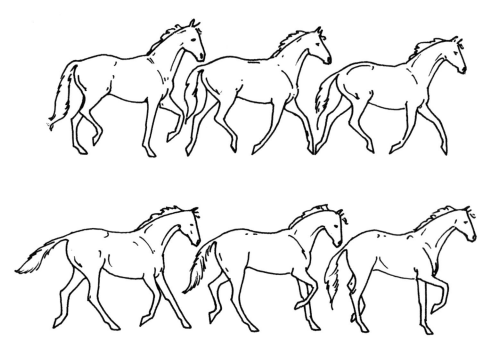

FIG. 2–46. The trot.

Imbalance

Gait defects often occur simply because the horse is trying to keep his balance. He is attempting to keep his limbs under his center of mass. Basically, there are three forces at work when a horse moves: the vertical force of the weight of the horse and rider, the horizontal force of the horse moving forward, and the swinging or side-to-side motion of the horse at various gaits. Exactly where under its body a horse places its limbs is determined in a large part by the interaction of these three forces and the direction of their composite. A barefoot horse moving free in a pasture rarely interferes. It is when a horse carries a rider and is asked to perform in collected and extended frames at both faster and slower speeds that interfering occurs.

A rider can make a horse move well or poorly. Rider proficiency will determine how the horse distributes its weight (from front to rear and from side to side), how the horse changes the speed of the stride or the length of a stride within a gait, and how the horse adapts the stride when turning, stopping, and performing such maneuvers as lead changes. Inadequate riding skills exaggerate the deficiencies in a horse's conformation and way of going. Because no horse is perfect or moves perfectly at all times, it takes a knowledgeable and competent rider to compensate for a horse's shortcomings. A rider's balance and condition, as well as talent, coordination, and skill at choosing and applying the aids, greatly affect a horse's coordination. A horse must be warmed up in a progressive manner before asking for more difficult work.

Inexperienced riders often ask a cold or poorly conditioned horse to do three things at once, such as come to a hard stop from a thundering gallop, make a sharp turn, and lope off in the opposite direction, without properly preparing the horse or helping him perform in a balanced fashion. When a horse is asked to do something he is not physically ready to do, such as a flying lead change, a deep stop, a fast burst out of the roping box, any kind of lateral work, a tight landing after a jump, or a sharp turn, he can easily over-reach or interfere.

An unskilled rider can easily throw off a horse's balance formula. Inexperienced riders often commit one or more of these imbalance errors: sit off to one side of the saddle, often with a collapsed rib cage; ride with one stirrup longer; ride with a twisted pelvis; lean one shoulder lower than the other; hold one shoulder farther back than the other; or sit with a tilted head. All of these postures can alter the horse's composite center of mass and can cause the horse to make adjustments in order to stay balanced. Riders that let their horses ramble on in long, unbalanced frames, heavy on the forehand, also seem to have more forging problems. Some horses are able to compensate for an imbalanced rider without forging or interfering and others are not.

Some horses simply have an imbalanced way of going. Certain horses are uncoordinated, inattentive, and sloppy, whereas others move precisely, gracefully, and balanced. Training, conditioning, and conscientious shoeing can improve a poor mover's tendencies, but some horses, no matter how talented the rider and farrier, will consistently move in an imbalanced fashion.

Shoeing

Recent but improper shoeing can be responsible for gait defects. If a farrier's shoeing style is the "long-toe,

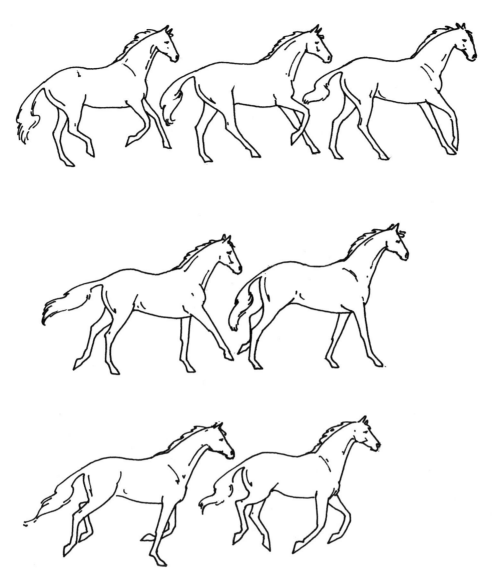

Fig. 2–47. The canter, right lead.

low-heel," a horse is set up to forge and possibly interfere. When a horse is overdue for a reset, even if it was shod by a world class farrier 8 weeks previously, its hoofs have probably grown so out of balance that it could easily exhibit gait abnormalities. Sometimes, just going a week past the horse's needs can adversely alter the gait synchronization. See Chapter 6.

Footing

The surface the horse is worked on will directly affect its movement. Traction on dirt occurs when the horse's weight descends through the bone columns of the limbs, causing the hoofs to drop 0.5 inch or more into the ground at the same time the soil is cupped upward toward the sole. This happens whether a horse is barefoot or shod. Shoes basically extend the hoof wall, creating a potentially deeper cup to the bottom of the hoof, therefore increasing traction potential in dirt or soft footing.

Ideal arena footing is light and does not stay compressed, so some dirt falls out of the hoof readily with every stride. During the work of a very active horse, dirt literally flies out of the shoes, but a placid horse may not move its limbs energetically enough to release some dirt with each stride. In dry arenas, the moderate amount of dirt in the shoe comes in contact with the dirt of the arena and results in good traction. However, if conditions are damp to wet and the footing is heavy, the hooves may pack and mound, thereby decreasing stability and traction. Packed dirt left in for prolonged periods of time creates constant pressure on the sole and can cause sole and frog bruises. Therefore,

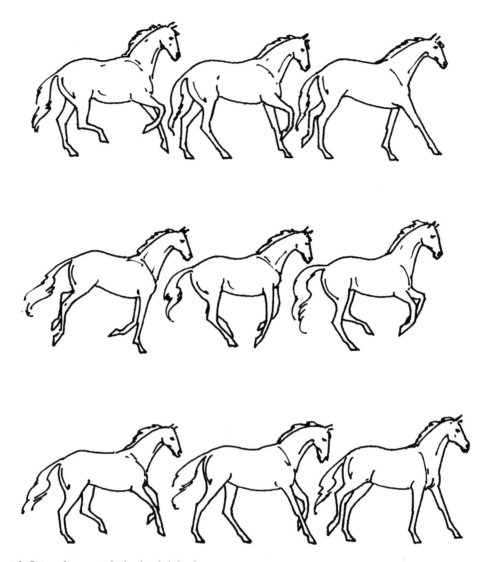

FIG. 2–48. Canter with flying change, right lead to left lead.

for work in soft, wet, and/or deep footing, it is important for shoes to be self-cleaning; they should allow mud, manure, or snow to move out at the base of the frog. This will ensure that the horse has an open sole and maximum traction potential for each stride.

Heavy footing (sand, mud, snow, long grass) generally delays front foot breakover. If a horse must be worked on footing he is unaccustomed to, protective boots may be helpful. Bell boots and scalping boots may prevent injury to the heels and coronary bands. Over-reach boots provide protection to the tendons.

Traction

In some instances, a horse requires greater traction than would be provided by a standard shoe. Generally, the wider the web of the shoe, the less traction the shoe provides. The extreme is the sliding plate, which

can be over 1 inch wide and allows the horse to "float" over the ground surface. Optimum traction can increase horse and rider safety, increase a horse's feeling of security so it will stride normally, and help a horse to maintain its balance in unstable footing such as mud, ice, snow, or rock.

Permanent calks, those driven into the shoe, forged into the shoe, or brazed or welded onto the shoe, provide good traction. However, such calks cannot be changed between shoeings and may lose their effectiveness as they wear down.

Removable screw-in calks (studs) may be the best answer when performance requirements or footing are constantly changing. Event riders can use large studs for the cross country phase of competition and take them out or replace them with smaller studs for dressage and stadium jumping.

Jar calks (either rectangular or triangular pieces of steel) can be brazed on the shoes to prevent sideways

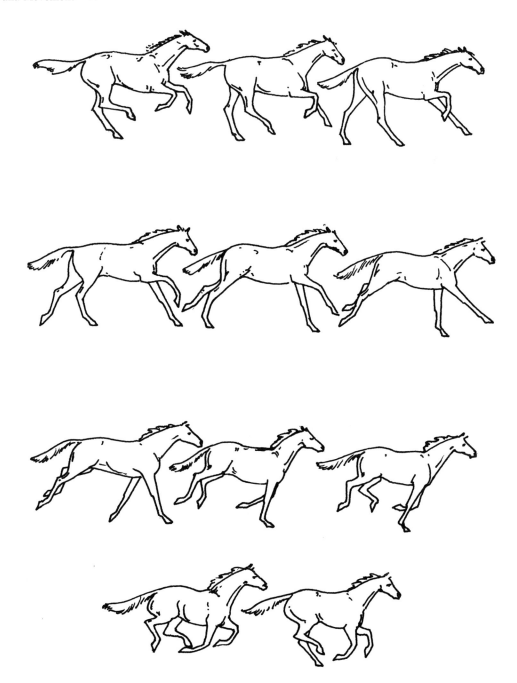

Fig. 2–49. The gallop, right lead.

slipping while allowing the hoof to slide forward on landing. They are usually applied at the heels and set in the direction of travel, not parallel to the sides of the shoe. However, if the goal is to decrease both sideways and forward/backward slipping, the jar calks can be placed parallel to the sides of the shoe.

Before additional traction devices are considered, the horse must be fit and in working condition. A conditioning program should be designed to strengthen the ligaments (via progressive, regulated stretching and exercise), muscles, and tendons. Adding traction to an unconditioned horse can result in injured ligaments and tendons.

Condition, Level of Fitness

A horse's level of fitness as well as energy level affects its movement. In general, a horse has 15 minutes of peak performance whether in a daily work session or at a competition. The horse either approaching that peak period or coming away from it. A rider must know how to properly warm up a horse to establish the most natural and efficient way of going for that horse; then the rider must assist (and not hinder) the horse in working in a balanced frame during the peak period. Finally, a rider must know how to gradually let the horse come down from his peak. A horse pre-

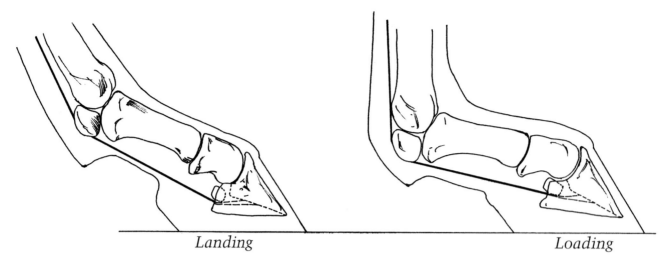

Landing   *Loading*

FIG. 2–50. Phases of the stride: landing, loading. From: Hill, C., Klimesh, R.: Maximum Hoof Power. New York, Macmillan Publishing, 1994.

disposed to forging or over-reaching may likely do so if he is allowed to dawdle around on the forehand during the warm-up, if the bridle reins are pulled up suddenly and the horse is put to work when he is "cold," if contact is "thrown away" all at once or engagement is allowed to slip away during work, or if the horse is allowed to fall on his forehand immediately following the completion of his peak performance.

If a rider asks too much in relation to a horse's current physical capabilities or fitness level, many horses will attempt to adapt while complying. If overworked, many horses will continue moving forward but will modify stride to minimize fatigue and discomfort to flexor muscles and tendons. When a tired horse adjusts the timing of the various phases of its stride, it can result in gait defects. If the hindquarters have not been properly conditioned and strengthened, a horse will rely heavily on the forehand for both propulsion and support. This makes it even harder for the already heavily weighted forehand to get out of the way of the incoming hindfeet.

Poor condition or fatigue will often cause a horse to fling its limbs aimlessly; the horse does not have the muscle strength or energy necessary to project its limbs in a controlled fashion. In some cases, when a lazy horse moves slowly at a trot, it may move sloppily and carelessly, causing him to occasionally interfere. Requiring such a horse to move out with more energy may smooth out gait defects. This situation can be interpreted as an exception to the general rule that an increase in speed usually brings an increase in the potential to interfere. The amount of weight that a horse is carrying can also exaggerate its lateral limb movements. An overweight horse or heavy rider may cause more side-to-side sway, which will alter the net force of forward movement.

Age and Stage of Development

Young horses that do not have fully developed muscles may lack the width of chest, stifle, or hip that will prevent them from interfering once they are adults. The relationship between the inside and outside muscles also can affect how the limb swings. A horse with heavy outside gaskin muscling and, in comparison, light inside gaskin muscling, especially if his hindlimbs toe-out, will tend to have trouble keeping its limbs under its body during a stop, which can be a major problem for a stock horse. There simply is not enough inside gaskin muscle power to counteract the outward rotation of the limb during the stop. To complicate things, this type of limb tends to wing inward during forward movement so interference might occur.

Training

One of the main causes of intermittent gait defects is asking a horse to perform something beyond his level of training. One of the first goals of training is to teach a horse to track straight. Until a horse learns to strongly and decisively step up underneath itself, its travel is often wobbly and inconsistent. Working on circles and lateral maneuvers before a horse is balanced and supple can cause it to make missteps and interfere. Asking a horse to perform advanced movements like the passage, canter pirouette, or turnaround before the horse is physically developed and trained can increase the possibility of interference. These movements are characterized by either higher action, greater speed, or a greater degree of joint flexion, all of which tend to increase rotational forces of the limb and the possibility of interference. Gait de-

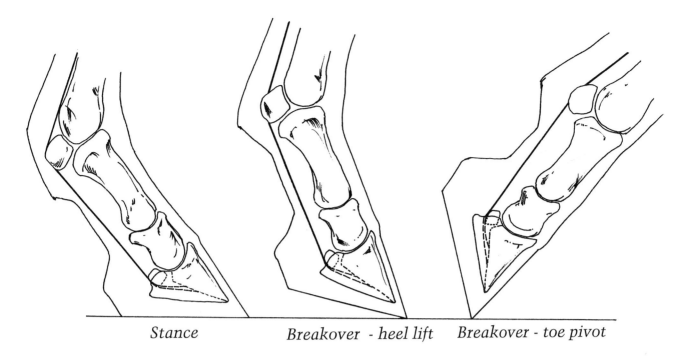

Stance   *Breakover - heel lift*   *Breakover - toe pivot*

FIG. 2–51. Phases of the stride: stance, breakover–heel lift, breakover–toe pivot. From: Hill, C., Klimesh, R.: Maximum Hoof Power. New York, Macmillan Publishing, 1994.

FIG. 2–52. Phases of the stride: swing. From: Hill, C., Klimesh, R.: Maximum Hoof Power. New York, Macmillan Publishing, 1994.

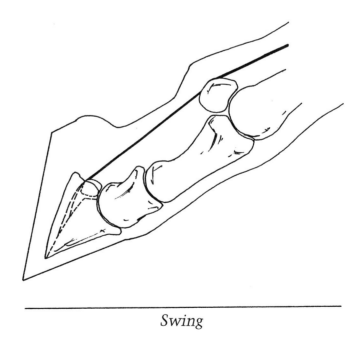

Swing

fects tend to surface with an increase in speed within a gait as well as the extension of a stride within a gait.

Tack

Poor-fitting saddles are a main cause of back pain and subsequently poor movement. If the tree is too narrow, it can cause pinching of the nerves and muscular pain. If the tree is too wide, it can cause the weight of the saddle and rider to be borne directly by the vertebrae.

Other

A host of other factors can cause a horse to move in an irregular fashion. Some mares move with extreme stiffness and tension during a portion of their estrous cycle. A horse with dental problems often carries its

Top

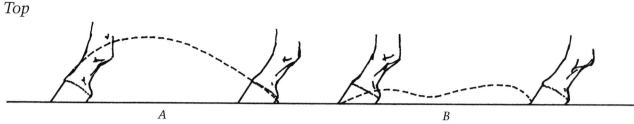

A

Normal hoof and pastern angle.
A. Proposed arc of foot flight.

B. Actual arc of foot flight shown
by recent research.

B

Bottom

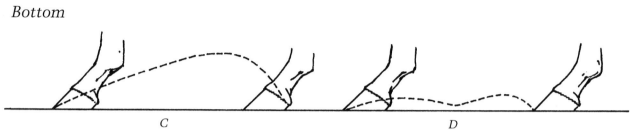

C

Long toe, low heel; acute hoof angle
C. Proposed arc of foot flight.

D. Actual arc of foot flight shown
by recent research.

D

Fɪɢ. 2–53. Arc of hoof flight.

head and neck in an unnatural position, which affects its movement. A sour, balky, or otherwise ill-tempered animal moves with characteristic resistance.

The horse owner should be involved in analyzing his/her horse's problem. Begin with an objective assessment of the horse's conformation, and then watch and listen to the horse as it is led and ridden on a smooth, level surface in a straight line at a walk and trot. View the horse from the front and the rear. Using a camera with a high-speed shutter, videotape the horse's limbs and hoofs moving at various forward gaits and backing. Play the tape in slow motion or in single-frame advance, and you will be able to see precisely when and where contact occurs or is most likely to occur. You can also note how the hoof lands and breaks over, which is critical information in formulating treatment.

Terms Associated with Movement

Action—the style of the movement, including joint flexion, stride length, and suspension; usually viewed from the side.

Asymmetry—a difference between two body parts or an alteration in the synchronization of a gait; when a horse is performing asymmetrically, he is often said to be "off."

Balance—the harmonious, precise, coordinated form of a horse's movement as reflected by equal distribution of weight from left to right and an appropriate amount of weight carried by the hindquarters.

Breakover—the moment between the stance and swing phases as the heel lifts and the hoof pivots over the toe.

Cadence—see "Rhythm."

Collection—a shortening of stride within a gait, without a decrease in tempo; brought about by a shift of the center of gravity rearward; usually accompanied by an overall body elevation and an increase in joint flexion.

Directness—trueness of travel, the straightness of the line in which the hoof (limb) is carried forward.

Evenness—balance, symmetry, and synchronization of the steps within a gait in terms of weight bearing and timing.

Extension—a lengthening of stride within a gait, without an increase in tempo; brought about by a driving force from behind and a reaching in front; usually accompanied by a horizontal floating called "suspension."

Gait—an orderly footfall pattern such as the walk, trot, or canter.

Height—the degree of elevation of arc of the stride, viewed from the side.

Impulsion—thrust, the manner in which the horse's weight is settled and released from the supporting structures of the limb in the act of carrying the horse forward.

Overtrack—"tracking up," the horse's hind feet step on or ahead of the front prints.

Pace—the variations within the gaits such as working trot, extended trot, collected trot; a goal (in dressage) is that the tempos should remain the same for the various paces within a gait. Pace also refers to a specific two-beat lateral gait exhibited by some Standardbreds and other horses.

Power—propelling, balancing, and sometimes pulling forces.

Rapidity—promptness, quickness; the time consumed in taking a single stride.

Regularity—the cadence, the rhythmical precision with which each stride is taken in turn.

Relaxation—absence of excess muscular tension.

Rhythm—the cadence of the footfall within a gait, taking into account timing (number of beats) and accent.

Sprain—injury to a ligament when a joint is carried through an abnormal range of motion.

Step—a single beat of a gait; a step may involve one or more limbs. In the walk, there are four individual steps. In the trot, there are two steps, each involves two limbs.

Stiffness—inability (pain or lack of condition) or unwillingness (bad attitude) to flex and extend the muscles or joints.

Strain—injury (usually to muscle and/or tendon) from overuse or improper use of strength.

Stride, length of—the distance from the point of breaking over to the point of next contact with the ground of the same hoof; a full sequence of steps in a particular gait.

Suppleness—flexibility.

Suspension—the horizontal floating that occurs when a limb is extended and the body continues moving forward; also refers to the moment at the canter and gallop when all limbs are flexed or curled up, reorganizing for the next stride.

Tempo—the rate of movement, the rate of stride repetition; a faster tempo results in more strides per minute.

Travel—the path of the hoof (limb) flight in relation to the midline of the horse and the other limbs; usually viewed from the front or rear.

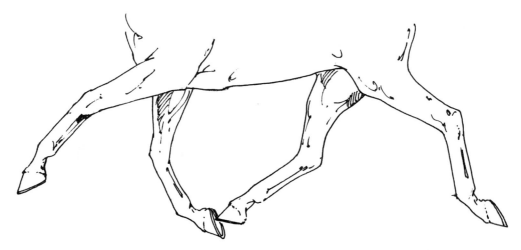

Fig. 2–54. Forging at the trot, hind foot and front foot on same side make contact.

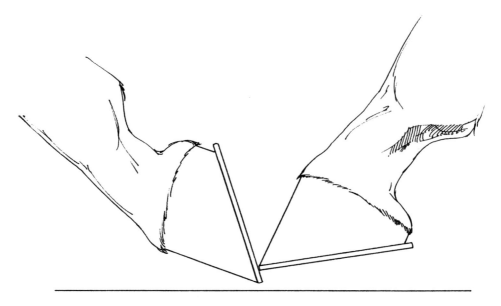

Fig. 2–55. Forging close-up. From: Hill, C., Klimesh, R.: Maximum Hoof Power. New York, Macmillan Publishing, 1994.

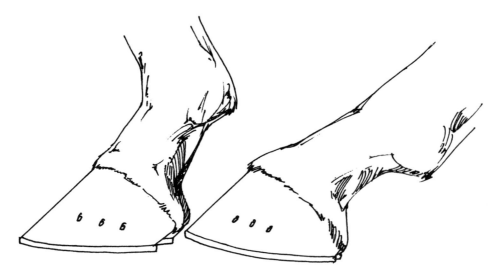

Fig. 2–56. Over-reaching close-up. Over-reaching or "grabbing" can occur when the front feet are delayed in breakover. From: Hill, C., Klimesh, R.: Maximum Hoof Power. New York, Macmillan Publishing, 1994.

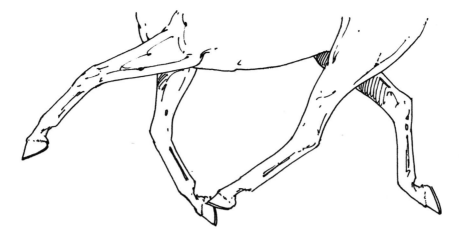

FIG. 2–57. Cross firing at the pace, hindlimb strikes opposite forelimb.

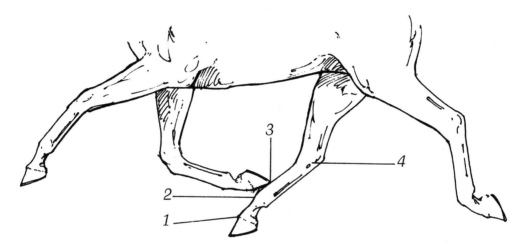

FIG. 2–58. Various forms of hindlimb contact at the trot. *1*, scalping; *2*, speedy cutting; *3*, shin hitting; *4*, hock hitting.

Defects in Travel

Paddling—the foot is thrown *outward* in flight, but the foot often lands *inside* the normal track; often associated with wide and/or toed-in conformation.

Winging—the foot swings *inward* in flight but often lands *outside* the normal track; often associated with narrow and/or toed-out conformation; dangerous because it can result in interfering.

Plaiting—also called rope-walking, the horse places one foot directly in front of the other; dangerous due to stumbling and tripping; associated with narrow, toed-out conformation.

Interfering—striking a limb with the opposite limb; associated with toed-out, base-narrow conformation; results in tripping, wounds.

Forging—hitting the sole or the shoe of the forefoot with the toe of the hindfoot on the same side; associated with sickle-hocked or short-backed/long-limbed conformation, a tired, young, or unconditioned horse, one that needs his shoes reset, or one with long toes.

Over-reaching—hitting the heel of the forefoot with the hindfoot on the same side before the forefoot has left the ground; also called "grabbing"; often results in lost shoes.

CHAPTER THREE

Examination for Lameness

TED S. STASHAK

Lameness is an indication of a structural or functional disorder in one or more limbs or back that is evident during movement or in the standing position. Lameness can be caused by trauma, congenital or acquired anomalies, (marked deviations from normal), infection, metabolic disturbances, circulatory and nervous disorders, or any combination of these. The diagnosis of lameness requires a detailed knowledge of anatomy, the physiology of the limb's movements, and an appreciation for geometric design and resultant forces. It is important to differentiate between lameness resulting from pain and nonpainful alterations in gait, often referred to as "mechanical lameness" and lameness resulting from neurologic (nervous system) dysfunction.

Classification of Lameness

Lameness can be classified as follows:

1. *Supporting Limb Lameness*: This type of lameness is apparent when the horse lands on the foot or is supporting weight on it. Injury to bones, joints, collateral ligaments or motor nerves, and the foot itself are considered causes of this type of lameness.
2. *Swinging Limb Lameness*: This lameness is evident when the limb is in motion. Pathologic changes involving joint capsules, muscles, tendons, tendon sheaths, or bursas are considered to be the cause.
3. *Mixed Lameness*: This is evident both when the limb is moving and when it is supporting weight. Mixed lameness can involve any combination of the structures affected in swinging- or in supporting-limb lameness.

    By observing the gait from a distance, one can determine whether it is supporting-limb, swinging-limb, or mixed lameness. Some conditions that cause supporting-limb lameness may cause the horse to alter the movement of the limb to protect the foot when it lands. This could lead to a mistaken diagnosis of swinging-limb lameness.
4. *Complementary Lameness*: Pain in a limb can cause uneven distribution of weight on another limb or limbs, which can produce lameness in a previously sound limb. A relatively minor condition in one foot, for example, can produce a more severe disorder in either the same limb or in an opposite limb. It is most common to have a complementary lameness produced in a forelimb as a result of a lameness in the opposite forelimb. For example, a lameness in the left forelimb can cause enough stress on the right forelimb to produce lameness.

    Even minor changes in weight-bearing can produce complementary lameness at high speeds, especially over long distances. The suspensory ligament, sesamoid bones, and flexor tendons seem to be the structures that suffer most. However, horses that are slightly calf-kneed often fracture both carpi in identical places, possibly shifting weight unevenly after one carpal bone is fractured. When lameness is in a forelimb, the horse often assumes a lead in the opposite forelimb to protect the unsound limb. The resulting stress on the lead forelimb may cause injury because normal change of leads does not occur.

    Moreover, one must always be alert to the possibility of an additional lameness occurring in a limb that already has a minor ailment. The cause of complementary lameness is increased stress on a sound limb resulting from an attempt to protect an unsound limb or, in the case of new injury in an unsound limb, stress to otherwise healthy structures trying to protect a painful region in that limb. This situation can lead to confusion.

    For example, a horse with navicular syndrome usually lands toe first. This constant landing on the toe can cause a bruised sole in the area of the toe and can result in localized x-ray changes indicative of pedal osteitis (inflammation of the coffin bone). In extreme cases, this soreness of the toe will be so painful that the horse will land excessively on the heel, because the toe bruise hurts more than the navicular region.

Character of the Stride

The character of the stride of a limb is also important to the diagnosis of lameness. When observing the stride, the following characteristics are noted:

1. *The Phases of the Stride* (Fig. 3–1): The stride consists of a cranial phase and a caudal phase. The cranial phase of the stride is in front of the footprint of the opposite limb, and the caudal phase is behind it. In lameness, the cranial or caudal phases may be shortened, although the length of the stride

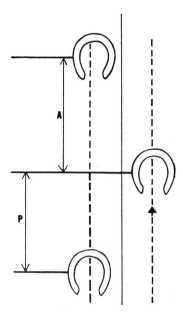

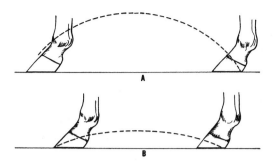

FIG. 3–2. Normal and abnormal arc of foot flight. *A*, Normal arc of foot flight. *B*, Low foot flight caused by lack of flexion in either the forelimbs or hindlimbs.

FIG. 3–1. Phases of a stride. *A*, Cranial phase of stride, which is that half of the stride in front of the print of the opposite foot. *B*, Caudal phase of the stride, which is that half of the stride in back of the print of the opposite foot.

must be the same as that of the opposite limb if the horse is to travel in a straight line. If the cranial phase is shortened, there must be a compensatory lengthening of the caudal phase, and vice versa.

Alterations in phase of the stride are best viewed from the side. Some causes for a shortened cranial phase of the stride include navicular syndrome (forelimb), chip fractures in joints, degenerative joint disease, trauma to the extensor tendons, shoulder problems, and gonitis (inflammation of the stifle) and bone spavin of the hindlimbs. Causes of shortened caudal phase of the stride include constriction by the palmar or plantar anular ligaments, tendinitis (inflammation of a tendon), and tendosynovitis (inflammation of a tendon and its sheath) of the flexor tendons.

2. *The Arc of Foot Flight* (Fig. 3–2): The arc of foot flight is changed when there is pain anywhere in the limb. The arc of one foot is compared to that of the opposite member when viewed from the side. In some cases, the arc is changed in both forefeet (bilateral navicular syndrome, laminitis) or in both hind feet (bilateral bone spavin). In the hindlimb, the arc may be changed enough to cause the toe to drag when the limb is advanced (bone spavin or gonitis) because of reduced flexion of the hock or stifle joints. Navicular syndrome, laminitis, nail punctures, degenerative joint disease of the phalangeal (coffin and pastern) joints, and other such conditions cause a lowering of the arc because of an effort to reduce pain when the foot lands. Painful conditions of the knee cause a lowering of the arc because of reduced flexion of the knee.

Most horses exhibiting a decrease in height of the foot flight arc also show alteration in their phase of stride. For subtle alterations in the hoof flight arc of the hindlimb, it is sometimes helpful to observe the horse from the rear and estimate and compare the duration that the horse presents the surface of the sole to the observer.

3. *The Path of the Foot in Flight*: If the foot travels inward, there may be an interference problem causing medial fracture of a splint bone or painful lesions of the knee. When the foot travels in an outward path (paddling), no special problem usually results. However, if paddling does develop, it is often a sign of pain in both knees. This is often seen in the young racehorse in training that develops carpitis (inflammation of the soft tissues in the knee).

4. *How the Foot Lands*: When a painful condition is present in the foot, the horse will usually indicate the pain by placing its weight opposite to the pain. For example, in navicular syndrome, the greatest pain is near the heel, so the foot is placed down toe-first. In a nail puncture of the toe, the weight is placed on the heel. If the lesion is on the lateral portion of the sole, the weight is carried on the medial side of the foot, and vice versa.

5. *Joint Flexion Angles*: Joint flexion angles are best viewed from the side and may or may not be associated with alterations in the hoof flight arc and phase of stride. In some cases, horses compensate with an increased flexion of the unaffected limb. One limb is compared to the other and the degree of flexion is assessed. In others, such as in bone spavin, a decreased height of foot flight arc and shortened cranial phase to the stride might be subtle, but an obvious decrease in hock joint flexion angle is noted.

6. *Symmetry and Duration of Gluteal Use*: To identify hindlimb lameness, it is helpful to observe the horse from the rear to compare the symmetry and duration of gluteal use and to correlate these findings with alterations in the character of the stride viewed from the side (see page 91; The Hindlimbs, for details).

Close observation of the above characteristics will aid in diagnosis of the lameness.

Other Lameness Factors

Most lamenesses are found in the forelimb and, of those in this region, 95% are in the knee or below. Approximately three lamenesses will be seen in the forelimb to every lameness in the hindlimb. However, in the Standardbred, hindlimb lameness is involved in approximately 40% of the lameness diagnoses, which is a result of the balanced gait characteristic of these horses. The greatest number of lamenesses occur in the forelimbs because they carry 60 to 65% of the weight of the horse and are thus subject to much greater concussion than the hindlimbs. The hindlimbs act as propelling limbs, while the forelimbs receive the shock of landing. Performance events such as dressage, cutting, and reining, which place greater stress on the hindquarters, result in a higher incidence of hindlimb lameness. In the hindlimb, most lamenesses occur in the hock and stifle. One must remember that the horse may be lame in more than one limb or may have more than one pathologic condition in the limb showing lameness. Lameness in one region of the limb may cause the horse to injure a second region in the same limb or to injure the opposite limb in an effort to protect the original injury.

Lamenesses in horses also varies according to the type of work performed (Table 3–1). Although there is considerable overlapping, the common lamenesses associated with the type of work should be suspected first. The diagnosis of lameness should eliminate the common sites of lameness and the common lamenesses first. In all cases, the foot should be suspected and eliminated as a cause of lameness.

At least 95% of lamenesses in the forelimb will occur from the knee down. Therefore, if the lameness is in the forelimb, all the common lamenesses from the knee down should be eliminated before considering other lamenesses, unless some other condition is obvious. In the hindlimb, approximately 80% of the lamenesses will be in the hock or stifle, so that after preliminary examination of the foot and lower limb, the hock and stifle are given primary consideration until conditions of those two joints can be eliminated. In difficult cases, nerve blocks are very helpful.

There are other factors to consider as the cause of lameness. Horses that are improperly or irregularly shod may become lame. Shoeing should be considered as a complementary aid to the way the horse goes; if not properly done, shoeing can produce lameness, especially at high speeds. The surface on which the horse works is frequently a contributing factor in lameness. Surfaces that are too soft, too hard, slippery, or rocky may aggravate conformational imperfections or may be the outright cause of lameness. Muscle fatigue is one of the most important predisposing causes of lameness. Even in horses that have good confor-

mation, muscle fatigue will allow relaxation of tendons and ligaments and perhaps will predispose to bone fracture, joint injury, tendon strain (e.g., bowed tendon), or sprain. Improper conditioning of horses is a common cause of performance problems, and many trainers do not fully understand the important concepts involved in proper conditioning of a horse. The age of a horse is often a factor in predisposition to lameness. With the emphasis on racing and showing 2-year-olds, many lamenesses are produced that would not occur in older, more mature horses. An immature skeletal system is not ready to accept the burdens of repetitive circling or continual high speed.

History

One should attempt to keep a detailed medical history of every horse. Records should be accurate and objective. It is very helpful to the veterinarian if specific information is provided regarding the duration and intensity of the lameness, the symptoms, the activity immediately preceding the lameness, and any previous treatments or therapies employed. The veterinarian may ask the following questions:

1. *How Long Has the Horse Been Lame?* If lameness has been present for a month or more, it can be considered a chronic condition, because permanent structural changes may have taken place that render complete recovery unlikely. The prognosis is usually guarded in this case. A young horse has a better chance for recovery from a chronic condition than a mature one.
2. *Has the Horse Been Rested or Exercised During This Lameness Period?*
3. *Has the Lameness Worsened, Stayed the Same, or Improved?* Those cases in which a marked improvement in the lameness has occurred will usually have a better prognosis than cases that have remained static or have worsened.
4. *What Caused the Lameness?* The owner may have removed a nail from the foot or may actually have seen the injury occur. This description should include the character of the lameness at the time first noticed. If the lameness was acute initially, this might indicate a condition such as a fractured coffin bone; if it developed insidiously, an arthritic type of disease might be present.
5. *Does the Horse Warm Out of the Lameness?* If so, muscular structures or arthritic joints (such as bone spavin) may be involved.
6. *Does He Stumble?* Stumbling may be the result of some interference with the synergistic action of the flexor and extensor muscles. It also may indicate that the animal has pain on heel pressure, as in navicular syndrome or heel puncture wounds, and thereby attempts to land on the toe, which causes stumbling. Painful conditions of the carpus and rupture of the extensor carpi radialis may in-

Table 3–1 Lamenesses Generally Associated with Specific Activities

Event	Movement	Lameness
Dressage	Sitting trot Weight carried rearward Increased joint flexion Great impulsion Collection Extension	Back Hip Early hock arthritis → bone spavin Gonitis Fetlock arthritis (synovitis/capsulitis)
Reining	Deep, sliding stops Fast spins Rollbacks	Hamstring tear → fibrotic myopathy Early hock arthritis → bone spavin PII fracture hind
Cutting	Balancing and turning on hindquarters with power and torque Lateral driving with forelimbs	Front bruised soles PI and PII fractures Early hock arthritis → bone spavin Gonitis
Roping	Explosive bursts Hard stops and abrupt change in direction	PII and PIII fractures Bone spavin Navicular syndrome
Racing (TB and QH)	Young horses Top speed Footing stresses Fatigue	Bucked shins Fatigue fractures Bowed tendons Carpitis Carpal chip and slab fractures Suspensory ligament injuries Fetlock arthritis and chip fractures Sesamoid fractures
Racing (SB)	Extended and fast pacing and trotting	Above racing lamenesses plus hock and stifle problems Cunean tendinitis
Barrel Racing Pole Bending	Speed with turning Torque and twist	Fetlock arthritis (synovitis/capsulitis) PIII fracture Navicular syndrome Ringbone Ligament sprain
Show Ring	Repetitive circular and arena work often on hard footing	Navicular syndrome Sprain trauma to fetlock and phalanges
Jumping Eventing	Fetlock hyperextension landing after jump Cross country footing	Navicular syndrome Bowed tendon Ligament sprain
Endurance	Long miles Often hard or rocky footing Fatigue	Bowed tendons Pedal osteitis Hoof injuries Sole bruises Fatigue fractures
Inactivity	Lack of movement Poor blood flow Overweight	Laminitis
Confinement	Over-exuberance Sudden outbursts	Trauma injuries

TB = Thoroughbred, QH = Quarter Horse, SB = Standardbred.

terfere with flexion and extension, enough to cause stumbling. Spinal ataxia (incoordination) should also be considered.

7. *What Treatment Has Been Done, and Was It Helpful?* This type of history may influence the prognosis of the case. If the horse has received certain types of recommended therapy with no results, the prognosis is guarded, because results from further treatment may be unsatisfactory. It is very important to record the names and dosages of drugs used in previous therapies and report this information to the veterinarian. Some drugs mask symptoms of lameness and give a false impression of recovery. If a horse has received corticoid injections in a joint, the veterinarian should be notified.

8. *When Was the Horse Shod?* Sometimes a nail is driven into or near sensitive tissue and then pulled out. In such case, signs of infection may not be evident for several days. In a case in which the nail remains in the sensitive tissue (a "hot nail"), the shoe must be removed to discover the potential cause of lameness. If a nail does not enter sensitive tissue, but is near it, it may cause lameness from pressure on the sensitive tissue. This is commonly called a "close nail" and the pressure will not be relieved until the nail is pulled (See Chapter 6).

Procedures for Examination

The following veterinary examination procedure for lameness is described in detail to provide horseowners and students with a thorough understanding of the process. Although some of the tests and observations can be performed by the horseowner, other tests require professional experience for proper administration and interpretation.

Visual Examination

At Rest

A careful visual examination of the horse is made at rest. This should be done at a distance and then up close, viewing the horse from all directions. From a distance, the body type is characterized (stocky vs. slender), conformation is noted, and body condition and alterations in posture, weight shifting, and pointing are also noted. For example, if the horse stands with the knee forward and the heel raised, the knee, palmer aspect of the fetlock, and heel regions should be examined closely. If the horse points with the affected foot, navicular syndrome or fracture of the extensor process of the coffin bone may be present. If a forelimb is held caudally and the knee is flexed with the toe resting on the ground, the shoulder on that side should be considered in the diagnosis. Elbow joint lameness will often result in the forearm being extended, the knee being flexed, and the foot being even

with or caudal to its opposite member. In addition, the elbow may have a "dropped" appearance. When the limb is nonweight-bearing, fractures, nail punctures, severe sprains, and septic (containing pus) arthritis or phlegmon (acute inflammation containing pus) are considered.

Compare the above findings with the normal attitude of the limbs. In the normal attitude, the forelimbs bear an equal amount of weight and are exactly opposite each other. In bilateral involvement of the forelimbs, the weight may be shifted frequently from one foot to the other, or both limbs may be placed too far out in front, called "camped in front." In the hindlimbs, it is normal for the horse to frequently shift the weight from one limb to the other. If the horse consistently rests one hindlimb and refuses to bear weight on it for a length of time or cannot be forced to bear weight on it at all, the possibility of lameness in that hindlimb should be considered.

At close observation, each limb is observed critically and compared to its opposite member. Feet are observed for abnormal wear, hoof cracks, imbalance, size, and heel bulb contraction. All joints and tendons are visually inspected for swelling and the muscles of the limbs, back, and rump are observed for swelling and atrophy (muscle shrinkage). Comparing one side to the other is most important.

At Exercise

Next, the characteristics of the gait of all limbs should be observed from a distance. In most cases, it is advantageous to observe the forelimbs first and follow this with observation of the hindlimbs. Once a person is able to accommodate his eye to observing all limbs at once, then each limb individually, the diagnosis of lameness is simplified. After a horse has been observed at exercise with shoes on, in some cases it is helpful to view the horse in motion without shoes. Removing the shoes is usually necessary when examining a horse wearing pads.

The main objective in exercising the horse is to identify the limb or limbs involved and the degree of lameness and incoordination in movement. To do this, the horse is observed at a walk, trot, and then, in some cases, at a canter under tack or at high speed on a treadmill. Proper examination includes watching the horse from the front, side, and rear. In general, forelimb lamenesses are best viewed from the front and side, and hindlimb lamenesses are best observed from the side and rear. The examiner is looking for head nodding, gait deficit, alterations in height of the foot flight arc, alterations in foot flight, phase of stride, joint flexion angle, foot placement, and symmetry in gluteal rise and use. To visualize these gait changes, it is best to look at the horse from a distance. The action of all four limbs is observed first, the limb in question is then isolated and observed closely, and then attention is shifted to the opposite limb for a comparison. For subtle gait changes, it may require visual shifting from one limb to the other for comparison, and in some cases it may be helpful to jog alongside, behind, or in front of the horse to get a better comparative appreciation.

How to Handle the Horse. The handler plays a very important role in assisting the veterinarian in diagnosis. In general, horses should be held loosely with their heads centered on line with their bodies and exercised as slowly as practical. If the head and neck are allowed to sway from one side to the other, an asymmetric gait will be created. If the handler holds the horse too tightly, subtle head nodding is difficult to observe. Fast trotting or cantering makes it more difficult to focus in on limb movement, but in some cases, it is helpful in identifying a neurologic deficit because it requires more coordination for movement at speed to occur.

Selection of Surfaces. In most cases, the evaluation of lameness is best carried out on a hard surface. It provides more concussion than a softer surface, and it affords the examiner the opportunity to listen to as well as visualize foot placement. There is usually an obvious difference in the horse's landing between the unsound and sound foot. The unsound foot makes less noise because less weight is taken on that foot. On the other hand, there is a louder noise elicited when the sound foot hits the ground because it is bearing more weight. This is true for both forelimbs and hindlimbs. Because hard surfaces typically do not apply good sole and frog pressure, horses with suspected foot problems can be exercised on dirt, turf, or gravel (short distance) surfaces to accentuate the lameness. This is particularly true of horses with chronic symmetric conditions involving the feet. When exercised on asphalt, they may travel with a stilted, shuffling-like gait but appear comfortable. When placed on gravel, bilateral lameness becomes quite evident. Foot placement is also best observed on hard surfaces because softer surfaces tend to envelope the foot, making placement more difficult to see.

The Forelimbs. As a result of lameness in a forelimb, the head will drop when the sound foot lands and rise when weight is placed on the unsound foot or limb. If acute lameness is not present, the trot should be used for diagnostic purposes, because most lamenesses evident in the walk will be increased in the trot because there is only one other supporting foot on the ground (Table 3–2).

At the trot one must be cautious not to confuse a left hind lameness with a left fore lameness, or a right hind lameness with a right fore lameness. This could happen when a hindlimb is lame at the trot, because the horse will often land more solidly on the sound opposite forelimb. For example, if a left hindlimb is lame at the trot, the horse will often lower its head when the left hind and right fore land and take more weight on the right fore (see Hindlimbs, page 91). On a hard surface, this gives the impression that the horse is yielding on the left fore, indicating lameness in that limb.

Occasionally, a situation arises in which a left hindlimb lameness is confused with a right forelimb lameness. This usually occurs in cases in which there is little or no head nodding at the trot. The sound diagonals (right hind and left fore) contact the ground with such force that it appears that the horse is protecting the right forelimb. Most confusion occurs in watching the horse from the side view. Watching it from behind would reveal the hip asymmetry typical of hindlimb lameness. Head movement may also be absent in bilateral involvement of the limbs or in mild lameness.

In the normal gait, the heel is lifted first when the limb is advanced. When the foot lands, the hoof should land flat or the heel should hit just before the toe. If there is pain on concussion to the heel, the horse will attempt to land on the toe, as in the navicular syndrome or a nail puncture in the heel region. If there is diffuse pain in the foot, such as with laminitis, the horse will make an exaggerated effort to land on the heel and thereby avoid concussion to the bottom of the foot. This is also the case when pain is present in the region of the toe. If pain is present in the lateral portion of the foot, the weight will be taken medially. In general, involvement in the toe of the foot or flexor surfaces will cause a shortened caudal phase of the stride, whereas involvement of the heel region of the foot or extensor surfaces will cause a short cranial phase of the stride.

The arc that the foot makes in flight should be observed (see Fig. 3–2). If it is too low in the forelimb, there is interference with flexion of the shoulder, knee, or fetlock due to pain or mechanical injury. Fixation of these joints will reduce the arc of the foot flight, limit the cranial phase of the stride, and lengthen the caudal phase. In shoulder involvement, the scapulohumeral joint usually remains semifixed during progression, and the head shows marked lifting and may be pulled toward the unaffected side. When involvement of both forefeet is present, the limbs show a stilted action that causes a false impression of shoulder involvement.

If interference of the limbs is suspected but cannot be seen, the hoof walls can be coated with chalk; the contact will leave a mark of chalk on the limb. This can be done for both the fore- and hindlimbs. Although "chalking" the hooves will work, a better approach is to use a video camera, which will identify interference as well as foot flight.

Various forms of limb contact are defined as follows: (see also Chapter 2)

1. *Brushing*: This is a general term for light striking, especially as in interfering.
2. *Cross-firing*: This is generally confined to pacers and consists of contact on the inside of the diagonal fore- and hind feet. It usually consists of the inside of the hind foot hitting the inside quarter of the diagonal forefoot (Fig. 3–3B).
3. *Elbow hitting*: This is when the horse hits the elbow with the shoe of the same limb. It rarely occurs except in those horses with weighted shoes.

Table 3–2 Supporting Limb Lameness

Head Movement at the Trot

Lame Limb	Head Down when these Limbs Land	Head Up when these Limbs Land
Right front	Left front/right hind	Right front/left hind
Left front	Right front/left hind	Left front/right hind
Right hind	Left front/right hind	Right front/left hind
Left hind	Right front/left hind	Left front/right hind

Note: Although not absolute, the above is true in many cases. Note the potential confusion between right front and right hind supporting lamenesses and left front and left hind supporting lamenesses when using head movement at the trot as the indicator.

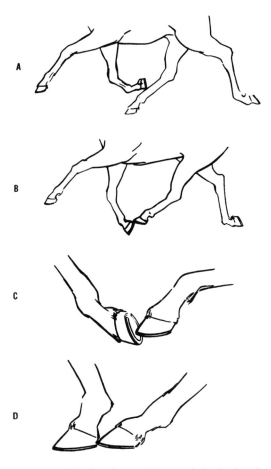

FIG. 3–3. *A*, Example of scalping. The toe of the forefoot hits the dorsal surface of the pastern or cannon of the hindlimb on the same side. *B*, Example of cross-firing. The inside of the toe of the hind foot and the inside of the forefoot on the opposite side make contact. This occurs in pacers. *C*, Example of forging. The toe of the hindfoot hits the bottom of the forefoot on the same side. *D*, Example of how over-reaching can cause pulling of the front shoe.

4. *Forging*: The toe of the hind foot hits the sole or shoe of the forefoot on the same side (Fig. 3–3*C*). Depending on the moment forging occurs; it can also be described as the front sole or shoe slapping the toe of the hind foot as it comes gliding in for a landing.
5. *Knee hitting*: This is a case of high interference, generally seen in Standardbreds.
6. *Interfering*: This occurs both in the forefeet and hind feet. It is a striking, anywhere between the coronary band and the cannon, by the opposite foot that is in motion.
7. *Over-reaching*: The toe of the hind foot catches the forefoot on the same side, usually on the heel. The hind foot advances more quickly than in forging, stepping on the heel of the forefoot. The toe of the hind foot may step on the heel of the shoe of the forefoot on the same side and cause shoe pulling (Fig. 3–3*D*).
8. *Scalping*: Here the toe of the front foot hits the hairline at the coronary band or above on the hind foot of the same side. It may hit the dorsal (front) face of the pastern or cannon bone. This is generally a fault of the trotting horse (Fig. 3–3*A*).
9. *Speedy cutting*: Speedy cutting is difficult to determine because it apparently has no positive definition. It may be the same as cross-firing or it may mean that the outside wall of the hind foot comes up and strikes the medial aspect of the front limb on the same side. Because there is no positive definition, it can literally be defined as any type of limb interference at the fast gaits.

Contact problems can occur in well-shod horses with good conformation as a result of the type of work they are performing. For instance, in barrel racing, cutting, pole bending, and reining, the horse's weight is suddenly shifted and the horse may be off balance.

The Hindlimbs. In observing the movement of the hindlimbs, the arc of the foot flight is best viewed from the side (see Fig. 3–2). Involvements of the hock and stifle joints reduce the arc of the foot flight and thereby shorten the cranial phase of the stride with a compensating lengthening of the caudal phase. Because of the reciprocal apparatus of the hock and stifle, incomplete flexion is characteristic of involvement of both joints. The toe may be worn excessively (dubbed off) with involvement of the hock or stifle, and the horse may kick up dirt or small stones when advancing the limb due to a reduced arc of foot flight.

Although head and neck movements can be observed from the rear, they are best viewed from the side at the trot. With mild hindlimb lameness, abnormal movements of the head and neck may not be evident. In moderate to severe lameness, the head and neck will rise as the unaffected hindlimb contacts the ground and lowers when the affected hindlimb contacts the ground (Table 3–2). In severe cases, horses will not only lower their head and neck but will also extend their heads. The lowering of the head and neck while the affected hindlimb is in the weight-bearing phase serves to reduce the weight on the affected hindlimb when it contacts the ground.

From the rear, the symmetry of gluteal rise and duration of gluteal use (movement of the croup) are evaluated. The rise is evident during the swinging phase of the stride; the use is evident during the support phase of the stride. This observation is best made on a level surface so that the examiner can visualize the uppermost excursion of the gluteal muscles. A symmetric gluteal rise as the hindlimbs are brought forward indicates that both limbs are swinging symmetrically and subsequently are elevated to the same height. On the other hand, the duration of gluteal use is a function of weight-bearing with subsequent contraction of the gluteal muscles as the limb moves from cranial to caudal during weight-bearing (supporting phase of the stride). In the painful situation, most horses attempt to get off the hindlimb more quickly and the gluteal muscle contraction is shortened, which leads to a shortened duration of gluteal use and a subsequent "hip roll" or hip "drop off." There are three different situations to recognize with regard to gluteal rise and use:

1. A depressed gluteal rise and a decreased use. This is usually seen in horses that are in pain during the swinging phase of the stride. Often, structures above the stifle are involved. Along with muscle atrophy, this type of gait is commonly seen with hip problems.
2. A symmetric gluteal rise but a decreased gluteal use of one limb. This is usually seen in cases with subtle hindlimb lameness. Head nodding is usually not a feature and only subtle changes in the height of the foot flight arc, phase of stride, and flexion angles may be observed.
3. An increased gluteal rise ("hip hike") in which the affected limb is brought higher than the normal limb but the duration of gluteal use is shortened. This situation is usually seen in horses that are in pain during the support phase of the stride. Varying degrees of head nodding will be seen, and the height of the foot flight arc, phase of stride, and flexion angles are usually altered.

Grading the Lameness

The degree of lameness should be recorded. Simply using mild, moderate, and severe may suffice. However, a more objective approach using a grading system may be more helpful. A grading system is not only beneficial because it standardizes the degree of lameness, but it makes record keeping easier and allows the examiner to come back at a later time to assess the degree of improvement. It is not important what grading system you use, but that each grade within the system helps differentiate it from another. The lameness grade is recorded and is used as an objective reference at reevaluation. The current AAEP Grading System is outlined below.

AAEP Grading System

0—Lameness is not perceptible under any circumstances.
1—Lameness is difficult to observe; not consistently apparent regardless of circumstances (i.e., weight-carrying, circling, inclines, hard surface, etc.).
2—Lameness is difficult to observe at a walk or in trotting a straight line; consistently apparent under certain circumstances (i.e., weight-carrying, circling, inclines, hard surface, etc.).
3—Lameness is consistently observable at a trot under all circumstances.
4—Obvious lameness: marked nodding, hitching or shortened stride.
5—Minimal weight-bearing in motion and/or at rest; inability to move.

Examination by Palpation and Manipulation

Following observation of the animal from a distance, a close visual examination of the limbs and palpation is in order. A systematic method of palpation is used so nothing will be overlooked. In palpating, start at the bottom of the foot and make a complete examination of the entire limb.

Examination of the Forelimb

Foot. The size and shape of the foot on the lame limb should be compared to its opposite member. The examiner is looking for asymmetry in hoof size, abnormal hoof wear, ring formation and heel bulb contraction, shearing of the heels and quarters, hoof wall cracks and swellings that are primarily associated with the coronet. Asymmetry in foot size may be a result of trauma, lack of weight-bearing leading to contraction, and congenital or developmental defects. In general, the limb with the smallest foot is usually the limb involved with lameness. Ring formation can be unilateral (trauma) or bilateral (from selenium toxicosis, laminitis, or a result from generalized systemic disease). Ring formation is not always associated with lameness. Heel bulb contraction is often misunderstood and in most cases results from decreased weight-bearing of the affected limb and is a symptom rather than the cause of the lameness. Visual examination of heel bulb contraction is best performed by the examiner standing or squatting near the flank and looking at both right and left heel bulbs at once. A more objective assessment can be made by checking the heel bulb spacing with finger measurements. Asymmetry in the heel bulb height (sheared heels) is recorded. This is most frequently associated with improper trimming and shoeing. Hoof wall cracks may or may not be associated with lameness but must be ruled out with a hoof tester examination and nerve blocks. Swellings around the coronet can result from superficial scar formation from wire cuts or constant bruising during exercise, keratoma, and dermatitis or from involvement of deeper structures (e.g., gravel and quittor).

After superficial cleaning of the sole, abnormal wear, heel bulb contraction, and frog atrophy are noted. If the heel bulbs are closer than normal, this is consistent with any condition that has resulted in decreased weight-bearing by that limb or improper trimming and shoeing. There is usually some frog atrophy associated with heel bulb contraction. However, heel bulb contraction associated with severe frog atrophy is more consistent with a long-standing navicular syndrome because the toe strikes the ground before the heel in an attempt to reduce heel pressure during weight-bearing. The shape of the sole is observed. A slightly concave shape is normal. Some horses are flat-footed and, therefore, predisposed to sole bruising. Convexity dorsal to the apex of the frog ("dropped soles" in front of the frog) is considered abnormal and may be associated with rotation of the coffin bone. If the foot has not recently been trimmed, it should be done at this time by a farrier or veterinarian. Some cases require only superficial paring with the hoof knife, whereas others require more extensive trimming. During this procedure, discoloration of the sole and/or a white line is noted. In some cases, the offending cause of lameness may be identified (e.g., a stick (Fig. 3–4) or nail wedged in the frog or pus exuding from a small hole in the sole). The clefts of the frog may have to be opened if the frog is overgrown and any indications of thrush are noted.

Hoof testers are applied by a veterinarian in a systematic manner to the entire sole and frog region. The examiner tries to identify and localize hoof sensitivity. This sounds simple but requires technique and experience. If sensitivity is encountered, it is absolutely necessary to confirm that it is a true sensitivity resulting from pain and not just a whimsical reaction by the horse. True sensitivity is identified by repeated intermittent hoof tester pressure that results in persistent (nonfatigable) reflexive withdrawal in association with hoof tester pressure. Obviously varying amounts of hoof tester pressure are applied to elicit a response, and this is dependent on sole thickness and the painfulness of the condition. Hoof tester responses are compared to those obtained from the opposite foot. In general, in those situations in which diffuse sole sensitivity is obtained, a sagittal fracture of the coffin bone, diffuse pododermatitis (inflammation of the corium) diffuse pedal osteitis and, in some cases, laminitis should be suspected. More localized hoof tester sensitivity is obtained with corns, sole bruising, non-articular fractures of the coffin bone, puncture wounds, localized subsolar abscesses and gravel. Hoof tester sensitivity over the central third of the frog usually indicates navicular syndrome and/or sheared heels. Sensitivity from other locations in the frog usually results from puncture. Any other region of sensitivity associated with cracks or abnormal discolorations of the sole should be thoroughly explored by a farrier or veterinarian with a hoof knife until normal tissue is observed. Additional tests might be used if navicular syndrome is suspected. One test is performed by placing a wedge underneath the frog of the affected foot while the opposite limb is held up. It is performed for 1 minute, after which the horse is trotted off. An increase in lameness indicates a positive test for pain in the frog region. In the other test, the toe is forced into an elevated position in relation to the heel by placing a wedge or some other object under the toe. This serves to increase the tension on the deep digital flexor tendon, causing an increase in pressure on the navicular bone. The opposite limb is elevated for 1 minute, and the horse is trotted off. Increase in lameness should make one suspicious of navicular syndrome or heel soreness.

After placing the foot on the ground, the hoof wall is struck with the hoof tester. If this is painful, laminitis or gravel may be the problem. If a hollow sound is heard over the dorsal hoof wall, there is probably a separation between the sensitive and insensitive laminae. The hoof wall is checked for cracks that may extend into the sensitive laminae (they are most common in the toe and quarter), uneven wear, and excessive dryness. Dishing (concavity) of the dorsal part (front) of the hoof wall is indicative of a prior rotation of the coffin bone or a chronic flexural deformity of the coffin joint.

The coronary band is palpated for heat, swelling, and pain on pressure. A generalized increase in the temperature of the coronary band of both limbs is consistent with laminitis, whereas selective swelling and pain on deep palpation over the extensor process region are consistent with an extensor process fracture

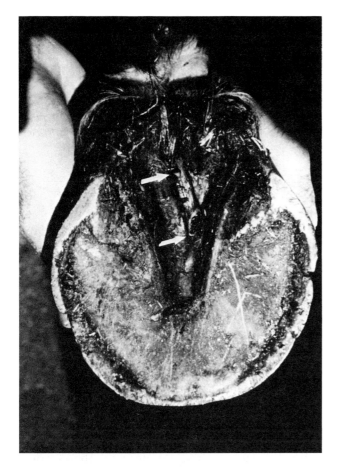 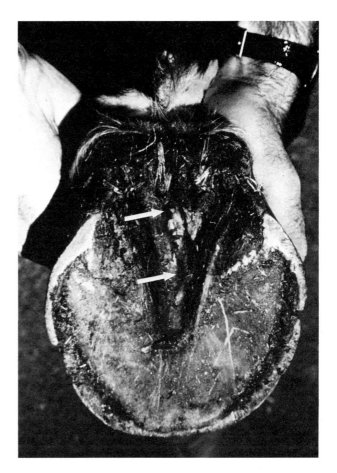

FIG. 3–4. This horse was presented with a history of hindlimb lameness of 3 weeks' duration. *A*, Examination of the ground surface of the hoof revealed a piece of wood buried in the frog (arrows). *B*, Frog after removal of the piece of wood. Notice that the sensitive corium is exposed (arrows).

of the coffin bone. Soft fluctuant swelling just proximal to the coronary bond involving one limb often indicates a coffin joint arthritis (Fig. 3–5). If firm, nonpainful swelling with hair roughening is present over the extensor process, it might indicate a developing low ringbone. Point swelling and pain with or without drainage at the midquarter region may indicate gravel (Fig. 3–6). If the heat and swelling are more diffuse, including the coronary band and the tissues above, quittor, and calcification of the collateral cartilages must be considered. Firm swelling of the dorsal hoof wall may be caused by a keratoma. Heat, pain, and swelling with or without drainage of one of the heel bulbs are consistent with a subsolar abscess (Fig. 3–7). Most subsolar abscesses not involving the white line eventually break out in the heel bulb region. Exclusive from this are nail punctures of the navicular bursa. In situations in which a small puncture hole in the sole has been identified, hoof tester applied pressure adjacent to the hole will not only cause pain but will often

be sufficient enough to force the pus out of the hole, which is diagnostic for subsolar abscesses.

Pastern. The dorsal (front) medial and lateral surfaces of the pastern joint are palpated for enlargement and a slight increase in temperature, possibly indicating ringbone (Fig. 3–8). If there is any question as to whether there is an enlargement, the opposite pastern is palpated. However, it is not too uncommon to have the lateral to medial dimensions of one pastern joint be larger than its opposite. Often, this slight enlargement is a result of disparity in phalangeal development, or soft tissue swelling, between the two. With the limb off the ground, the distal sesamoidean ligaments and flexor tendons (superficial and deep digital flexor tendons) are palpated deeply with thumb pressure for pain (Fig. 3–9). Low bows (tendinitis or tendosynovitis) of the deep digital flexor tendon are evidenced by thickening of the tendon and its sheath distal to the anular ligament. Deep palpation of the lateral and medial eminencies (wings) of the short pas-

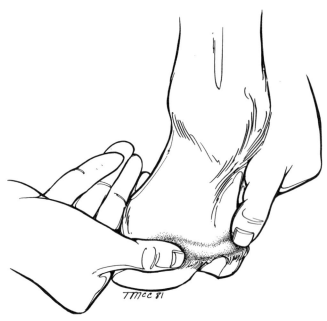

FIG. 3–7. Palpation of the heel bulbs to identify heat, pain, and swelling that may be associated with subsolar abscesses.

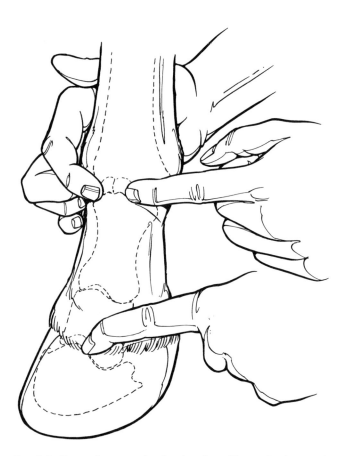

FIG. 3–5. Lower finger marks the site of swelling and pain associated with coffin joint (arthritis) and/or fracture of the extensor process. Upper fingers are applied over the dorsal surface of the fetlock to identify synovial distension and thickening of the joint capsule.

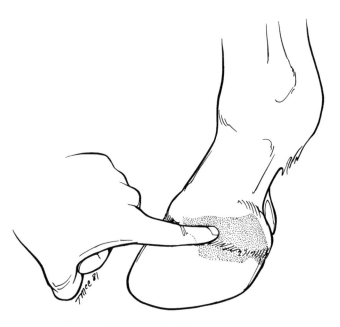

FIG. 3–6. Location where gravel and/or quittor occurs. Heat, pain, and swelling are palpated, and drainage of pus is common in the affected animal.

tern bone will elicit pain if fractures are present. With the fetlock held between the examiner's knees and the hands placed on the hoof wall, the pastern joint is rotated. Pain can be elicited if degenerative joint disease (articular ringbone) or if long pastern bone and short pastern bone fractures are present. Varying amounts of crackling can be felt with fractures, but it is dependent on the degree of fragmentation. The collateral ligament supports are checked both laterally and medially by placing one hand lateral or medial over the pastern joint while the other hand is used to pull the foot toward that side (Fig. 3–10). This bending force creates increased tension over the collateral ligament. If pain is present, it could indicate a sprain or fracture or nonarticular ringbone.

Fetlock. The dorsal aspect of the fetlock joint is palpated for joint capsule thickening and swelling, which may indicate a chronic proliferative synovitis/capsulitis (osselets or synovitis), chip fracture of the proximal articular margin of the long pastern bone or any long-standing articular fracture (see Fig. 3–5). The palmar recess of the fetlock joint capsule is palpated for distension (Fig. 3–11). If present, it may be associated with windpuffs or may indicate arthritis or an articular fracture if it is unilateral. Pressure is applied to the lateral and medial branches of the suspensory ligament just above their attachments on the sesamoid bones. If painful, it may indicate desmitis, sesamoiditis, or apex chip fractures of the sesamoid. The deep digital flexor tendon and sheath plus the superficial digital flexor tendon are palpated for heat,

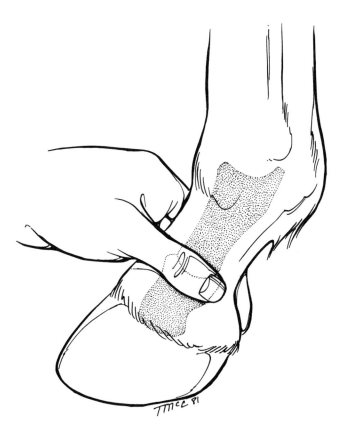

FIG. 3–8. Palpation of the pastern. Thickening in this region often indicates ringbone.

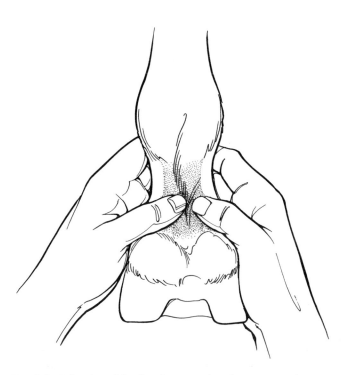

FIG. 3–9. Palpation of the distal sesamoidean ligaments and superficial digital and deep digital flexor tendons on the palmar aspect of the pastern.

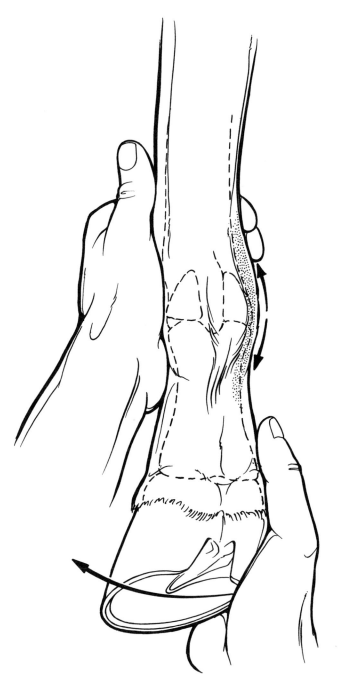

FIG. 3–10. Tension is being applied to the collateral ligament supporting the fetlock, pastern, and coffin joints in an attempt to identify sprain trauma.

pain, and swelling (Fig. 3–12). If present, they may indicate tendinitis and synovitis or tendosynovitis. Some distension of the deep digital flexor tendon sheaths of all four limbs is not uncommon in performance horses. This often is referred to as "windpuffs." The anular ligament is palpated for constriction. With the limb off the ground, finger pressure is applied to

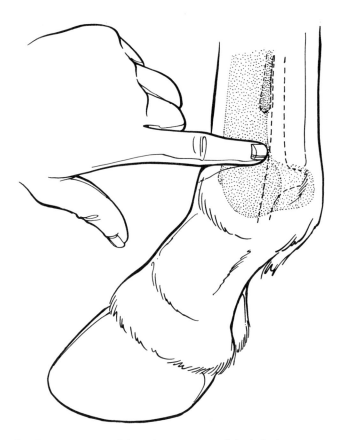

FIG. 3–11. Location of the palmar recesses of the fetlock joint capsule. Distension at this site results from synovial effusion, which is frequently referred to as "windpuffs."

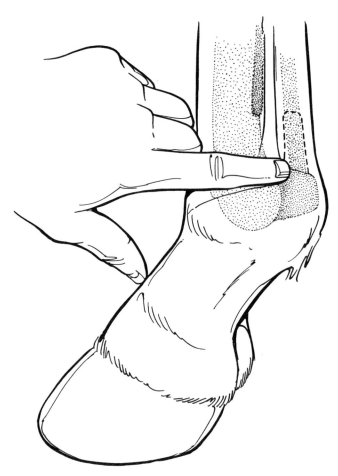

FIG. 3–12. Palpation of the digital synovial sheath around the superficial and deep digital flexor tendons. Synovial distension of this sheath is also referred to as "windpuffs."

the sesamoid bones (Fig. 3–13). Sensitivity and pain may indicate fracture. The fetlock is rotated and the collateral ligaments are checked in a similar manner to that of the pastern joint (see Fig. 3–10). Pain associated with this type of manipulation could indicate the same entities that are associated with the pastern. Additionally, the fetlock joint is intermittently flexed to identify pain and assess the degree of flexion. This is done by flexing the knee as little as possible and flexing the fetlock. Notice that one hand is placed on the pastern rather than on the hoof (Fig. 3–14). This technique flexes the fetlock joint separate from the pastern and coffin joints. If intermittent flexion is painful, a flexion test is performed by holding the fetlock in this position for 30 seconds to 1 minute, after which the horse is trotted off and lameness is observed. A marked increase in lameness with a decreased fetlock flexion angle may indicate a synovitis/capsulitis, sprain, intra-articular fractures, degenerative joint disease, osteochondrosis (in young animals) of the fetlock joint. If there is no lameness observed, the coffin, pastern, and fetlock joints are flexed by extending the knee and applying hand pressure to the toe region (Fig. 3–15). If painful, the examiner should be suspicious of involvement in either the coffin or pastern joint regions. Also, it is common for horses with the navicular syndrome to react painfully to this test. It is believed that excessive flexion of the coffin joint, as done with this test, many apply pressure to the navicular bone and at the same time stretch the soft tissue support structures (impar and suspensory ligament) of the navicular bone, which causes pain. Some horses with the navicular syndrome also have a coffin joint arthritis. Any painful signs should be checked with the opposite limb.

Cannon. The extensor tendons on the dorsal surface of the cannon bone are palpated for swelling and pain and manipulated with the thumb and forefinger to identify adhesions. This is particularly important if a history of trauma to the dorsal surface of the cannon bone is obtained and a reduced flexion angle to the fetlock is noted during exercise and the fetlock flexion

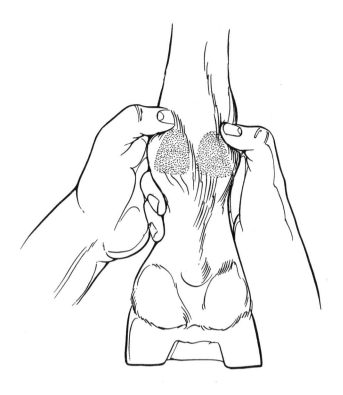

FIG. 3–13. Digital pressure is being applied to the apex of the proximal sesamoid bones located on the palmar aspect of the fetlock. Pain over this site may indicate fracture of the apex of the sesamoids. The midbody and basilar regions are palpated as well.

test is positive. Laceration involving the dorsal surface of the cannon bone will often involve the extensor tendons and periosteum and result in an adhesive scar formation to the adjacent soft tissue as well as to the bone. Selective heat, pain, and swelling over the dorsal middle third of the cannon bone may indicate dorsal metacarpal disease (buck shins) (Fig. 3–16).

The entire length of each splint bone is palpated. This is first done with the limb weight-bearing after which the limb is elevated with the fetlock flexed; the palmar and medial surfaces of the splint bone can be palpated by pushing the suspensory ligament to the opposite side (Fig. 3–17). Heat, pain, and swelling may indicate a splint fracture or a condition referred to as "splints." Splint fractures most commonly involve the medial splint bone in the forelimb and the lateral splint bone of the hindlimb. A chronic splint bone fracture associated with excessive swelling and pain presented with a history of recurrent drainage usually indicates a bone sequestrum (a piece of dead bone separated from healthy bone). The condition referred to as splints usually affects young horses and involves the proximal one-third of the medial splint bone in the forelimb. It is not uncommon to palpate nonpainful enlargements of the splint bones. These presumably represent sites of previous trauma.

Suspensory Ligament. The ligament (interosseus medius muscle) lies just palmar to the cannon (metacarpal) bone and between the splint bones in the metacarpal groove. It should be palpated both with the limb weight-bearing and with the limb flexed. Deep palpation with the thumb and forefinger is used to identify swelling and pain. Damage to this structure most often occurs in the distal third of the cannon associated with the suspensory ligament branches. However, desmitis (ligament inflammation) may be associated with a splint fracture that is healing by callus formation anywhere along its length. With the limb held in a flexed position and using the thumbs of both hands placed laterally and medially, the proximal attachment of the suspensory ligament to the cannon bone is palpated (Fig. 3–18). Painful withdrawal may indicate a tearing of the origin of the suspensory ligament with or without avulsion (separation) fracture.

Carpal (Inferior) Check Ligament. The carpal check ligament (accessory ligament of the deep digital flexor) originates from the palmar carpal ligaments and attaches in a cuplike manner to the deep digital flexor tendon at about the middle of the cannon. A painful, inflammatory process of the carpal check ligament picked up by digital exam is referred to as "check ligament desmitis."

Flexor Tendons. The deep digital and superficial digital flexor tendons are located palmar to the suspensory ligament and are intimately associated with each other. The proximal one-third of the flexors (associated with the knee) and distal one-third (associated with the fetlock) are encased in tendon sheaths, whereas the central one-third is covered by a paratendon only. Each region is palpated carefully for pain, swelling, and heat, and the degrees of tension are assessed if a flexure deformity is present. Palpation is first performed during weight-bearing. This allows the examiner to identify which structure is involved with inflammation or which structure is under the most tension. It is often helpful to push on the dorsal aspect of the cannon bone with one hand and palpate the tendons with the other. After this, the dorsal aspect of the limb is held in one hand with the fetlock flexed and an attempt is made to roll or separate the superficial flexor tendons off of the deep digital flexor tendons with the thumb and forefinger (Fig. 3–19). In their normal state, they can be easily separated and differentiated. In the pathologic situation, varying degrees of adhesions between the two, as well as thickening, will result in an inability of the examiner to separate them. Damage to these structures results in a tendinitis, synovitis, or a combination of both, referred to as "tendosynovitis (bowed tendon)." A painful swelling associated with minimal deformity of the tendon and synovial sheath structure is consistent with an acute or subacute tendinitis synovitis and/or tendosynovitis. A firm, sometimes painful swelling with or without heat associated with tendon deformity and thickening of the tendon sheath is consistent with chronic tendinitis, synovitis, and tendosynovitis.

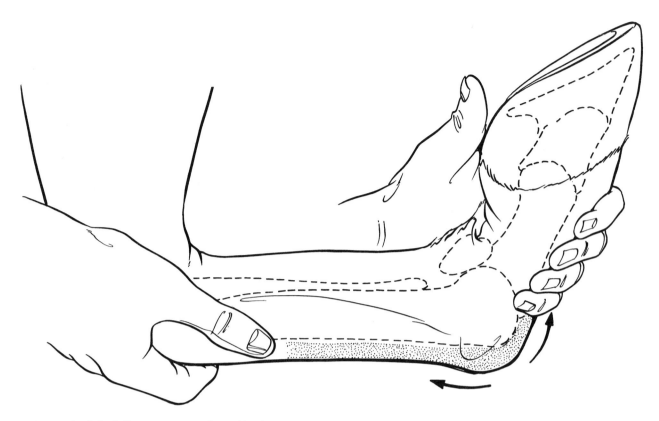

FIG. 3–14. The fetlock flexion test is performed by flexing the knee as little as possible and flexing the fetlock joint. Notice one hand is placed on the dorsal pastern to create fetlock flexion. The fetlock is flexed for 30 seconds–1 minute and lameness is evaluated. A positive test could indicate problems within the fetlock joint.

Knee. The knee is visualized for swelling on the dorsal and palmar surfaces. Point swelling associated with these joint spaces (the middle carpal and antebrachiocarpal joints) usually occurs medial to the extensor carpi radialis tendon and indicates chip fractures. More diffuse swelling of the carpal joints may indicate synovitis/capsulitis, articular slab fracture, degenerative joint disease, and proliferative exostosis (carpitis). The synovial sheaths of the extensor tendons overlying the carpus may also be distended, possibly indicating synovitis or tendosynovitis and/or rupture, particularly of the common digital extensor tendon in foals (Fig. 3–20). A diffuse moveable swelling over the dorsal surface of the carpus is consistent with acute hematoma/seroma or chronic hygroma (Fig. 3–21). Swelling on the palmar aspect, proximal and medial to the accessory carpal bone, may indicate accessory carpal bone fracture, tendosynovitis (carpal tunnel syndrome) or osteochondroma formation of the caudal distal aspect of the radius (Fig. 3–22). These regions are palpated individually. The carpal joints and bones as well as the integrity of the accessory carpal bone are best evaluated with the knee flexed. First, the degree of carpal flexion is evaluated. In most cases, the flexor surface of the cannon bone can approach that of the forearm when the knee is flexed in the normal horse (Fig. 3–23). In cases in which increased lameness associated with diffuse joint distension ex-

ists, flexion is performed very slowly. With rapid flexion, severely painful conditions such as slab fractures of the third carpal bone may result in the horse rearing and injuring itself or the examiner. Reduced degrees of flexion with pain are consistent with acute synovitis/capsulitis, chips or slab fractures, and tendinitis or tendosynovitis. Reduction in carpal flexion without pain is consistent with chronic degenerative joint disease and proliferative exostosis. After flexion assessment, the knee is rotated by swinging the cannon laterally and medially (Figs. 3–24 and 3–25). Associated pain may be seen with all acute entities plus damage to the collateral ligaments. With the knee held in flexion, the individual carpal bones are evaluated by deep digital thumb pressure along the dorsal articular surfaces (Fig. 3–26). The location of chip and/or slab fractures can often be discerned by using this technique. It is important to obtain consistent reflexive pain associated with the intermittent pressure. While the carpus is still flexed, the accessory carpal bone is manipulated and, with the tension of the ulnaris lateralis and flexor carpi ulnaris reduced, a fracture of the accessory carpal bone can be palpated (Fig. 3–27). In some cases, osteochondroma formation on the caudodistal aspect of the radius can also be palpated. However, this is dependent on the degree of synovitis present.

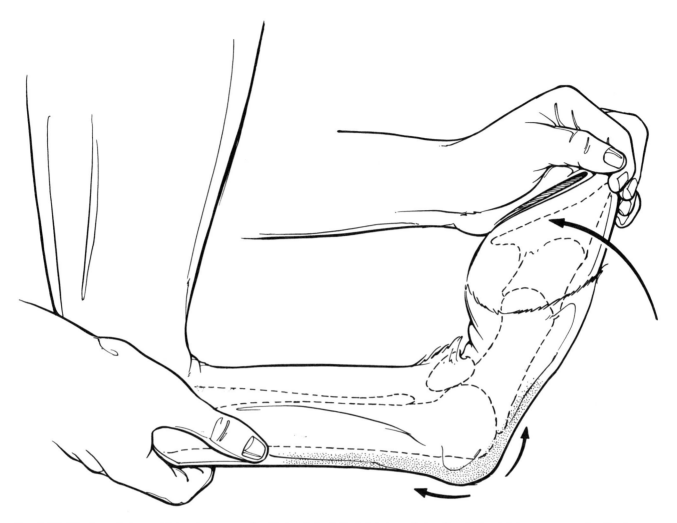

FIG. 3–15. The interphalangeal joints (pastern and coffin) and the fetlock joints are being flexed. A painful response can implicate any one of the joint spaces.

Forearm. The soft tissues between the knee and elbow are evaluated for inflammation. In some cases in which severe inflammation is present and a puncture wound is suspected, it is helpful to clip the hair over the region. A firm swelling associated with the flexor muscles may be consistent with a fibrotic or ossifying myopathy of these structures. The distal aspect of the radius is palpated for oblique articular fractures extending into the knee and avulsion fractures associated with collateral ligaments.

Elbow. The soft tissues surrounding the elbow joint are palpated. A firm, usually nonpainful but moveable swelling at the point of the elbow is consistent with elbow hygroma (olecranon bursitis). If increased swelling and a dropped elbow are present, a fracture of the ulna or olecranon process is likely. In some cases in which the olecranon fracture has not separated, elevating the limb into extension will cause pain (Fig. 3–28). Also it is helpful to palpate the olecranon process for swelling indicating the possibility of a fracture. The collateral ligament support structures as well as the fractured humerus can be evaluated by abducting and adducting the elbow (see Figs. 3–24 and 3–25). This is not a selective test because the shoulder joint is manipulated as well. However, with humeral fractures, crackling with increased pain response may be identified. The axilla (armpit) is also palpated for inflammation that may indicate a rupture of the serratus ventralis muscles.

Shoulder. The soft tissues around the shoulder joint (scapulohumeral joint) are observed and palpated for swelling and atrophy. Particular attention is paid to the bicipital bursa region (point of shoulder), and deep digital finger palpation is applied in an attempt to elicit pain (Fig. 3–29). If painful, bursitis or calcification of the bicipital bursa and biceps tendon may be present. Another test to evaluate this region is to flex the shoulder joint by placing one hand on the olecranon process and pulling the limb caudally (Fig. 3–30). Pain elicited by this manipulation is also consistent with the condition. This technique can also be used as a flexion test. The position is maintained for 60 to 90 seconds, after which the horse is trotted and the degree of lameness is evaluated. Young horses exhibiting an obvious shoulder lameness at exercise and evidencing variable degrees of pain on manipulation may be suffering from osteochondrosis of the shoulder joint. Degenerative change within the shoulder joint as well as fractures of the scapula and proximal humerus will also be painful on manipulation. Elevation of the limb as described for the elbow joint will also result in a painful response, particularly if a fracture or a lesion within the joint is present.

Scapula. The infraspinatus and supraspinatus muscles are observed for atrophy, which is consistent with suprascapular nerve paralysis (Sweeney), and swelling, which is consistent with external trauma resulting in fractures. Deep palpation and manipulation in conjunction with a stethoscopic examination are usually required to define these fractures. Extension or flexion and abduction or adduction of the shoulder joint will elicit pain.

Examination of the Hindlimb

Below the hock joint the hindlimbs are examined in the same manner as the forelimbs.

Hock (Tarsus). The hock is visualized and palpated for 1) tarsocrural (tibiotarsal) joint distension (synovitis, bog spavin), 2) thickening of the fibrous joint capsule (capsulitis), 3) bone proliferation of the distal tarsal joints (bone spavin), 4) distension of the tarsal sheath (thorough pin), 5) inflammation of the long plantar ligament (curb), 6) luxation of the superficial digital flexor tendon, and 7) capped hock. Cunean bursitis and inflammation of the distal hock joints are not identified until flexion tests and joint blocks are performed.

Generally, there are three types of swelling associated with the soft tissues of the hock. The first is palpated as a fluid distension of the tarsocrural joint. It results from synovitis and is referred to as "bog spavin." Synovitis can occur alone or in conjunction with osteochondritis dissecans of the distal intermediate ridge of the tibia, the trochlear ridges of the talus (tibial tarsal bone), and/or interarticular chip fractures. Most frequently, the synovial swelling can be forced from the dorsal medial pouch to distend the plantar-lateral reflection of this joint capsule and vice versa (Fig. 3–31). The second type of swelling (capsulitis) is a palpable firm distension of the tarsocrural joint capsule, and it is usually not possible to compress the synovial fluid from one pouch to another. The firmness results from an extension of the synovial inflammation or direct inflammation of the fibrous layer of the joint capsule (capsulitis). Chronic synovitis resulting from degenerative joint disease, chronic interarticular fractures, and sprain trauma to the fibrous joint capsule may be the cause. If the lameness is severe, chronic septic arthritis should be considered. The third type of swelling is a firm, diffuse swelling of the entire hock joint region. It is usually a result of severe sprain trauma to the fibrous joint capsule as well as the surrounding ligamentous support struc-

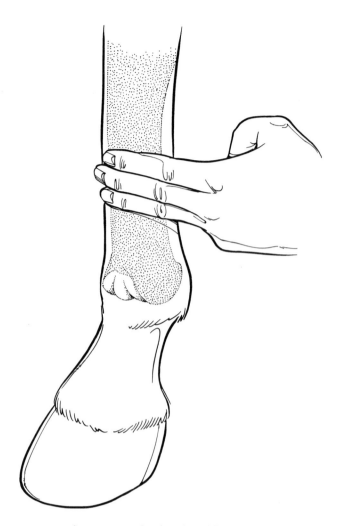

FIG. 3–16. Palpation over the dorsal middle third of the cannon bone to identify heat, pain, and swelling associated with the bucked-shin complex (dorsal metacarpal disease).

tures. In general, the greater the inflammation, the greater the reduction in hock flexion angle.

The distal tarsal joint region (distal intertarsal and tarsometatarsal joints) is palpated on the medial side (Fig. 3–32). In the normal horse, there is a smooth contour that tapers to the distal tarsal joints as they join the proximal cannon. This is easily seen from the rear and palpated from the side. If this region appears boxy and/or firmer with nonpainful, thickened projections, the examiner should be suspicious of degenerative joint disease of the distal intertarsal and/or the tarsometatarsal joints (bone spavin).

The tendon sheath of the deep digital flexor tendon is visualized and palpated for swelling. If swelling is present, it is a result of synovitis or tendosynovitis of the tarsal sheath and tendon (thorough pin) (Fig. 3–33). It should be noted at this time that this condition rarely causes lameness. The plantar aspect of the calcaneal tuber (point of hock) is palpated for inflammation of the plantar ligament (curb), displacement of and/or tendinitis of the superficial digital flexor tendon, and a fluid

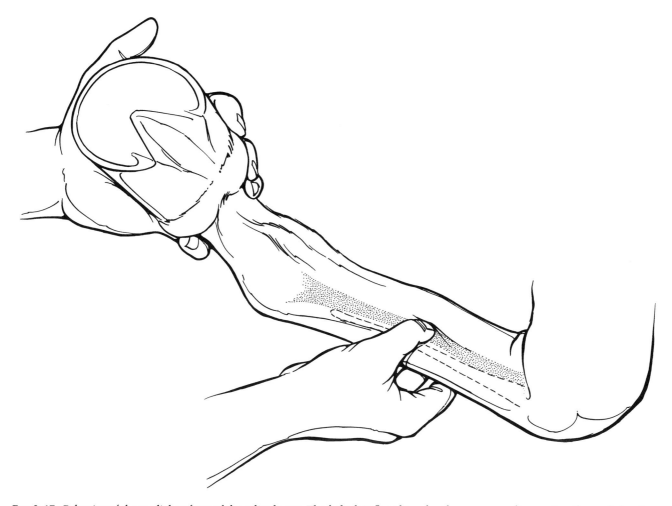

FIG. 3–17. Palpation of the medial surfaces of the splint bones. The fetlock is flexed to relax the suspensory ligament so the medial surfaces of the splint bones can be palpated.

swelling at its proximal limits of the calcaneal tuber referred to as "capped hock" (Fig. 3–34).

In most cases, palpation of the rest of the hindlimb is continued, but for the sake of continuity, the hock flexion test (spavin test) will be discussed now. With the hands placed on the plantar surface of the distal third of the cannon, specifically avoiding the sesamoid bones, the limb is elevated to flex the hock (Fig. 3–35). The hand placement as well as the grip pressure is important. This test should not be run by holding the foot, with the pastern and fetlock in a flexed position, or by holding the pastern or sesamoid bone region. The examiner should hold the limb with a loose grip. A firm grip may cause sufficient pressure to the flexor tendon and suspensory ligaments, causing withdrawal or result in a positive test. Alternatively, the tip of the toe can be held so the pastern and fetlock joints are extended and the hock is flexed. It is often beneficial to gradually flex the hock to its fullest extent over 15 to 30 seconds. This allows the sensitive or painful horse to accommodate to the flexion. In some cases in which the horse tends to lean away from the examiner, it is helpful to have the horse placed adjacent

to a solid support (i.e., wall or fence) or have an assistant provide counterbalance pressure to the tuber coxae of the opposite hip. Once the hock is in full flexion, it is held in this position for 60 to 90 seconds. If the horse forces the limb into extension, it is best to start the test over again.

As the end of the flexion test period nears, the handler should obtain a loose grasp on the lead shank. This is important because the person performing the flexion test should initiate the horse's movement. Far too often when the handler attempts to do this, the horse balks either standing still or backing up, which reduces the effectiveness of the test. Ideally, the examiner and the holder have selected an area to perform the flexion test in which the horse can be jogged away in a straight line. The examiner might need to initiate the movement by a gentle swat on the rump, which most horses accept very well. Of course, there are situations in which this would be undesirable. Experience is needed for this because, if the horse is swatted too hard, it may break into a gallop, negating the test.

The first few steps the horse takes after this test, in many cases, are the most important. A positive flex-

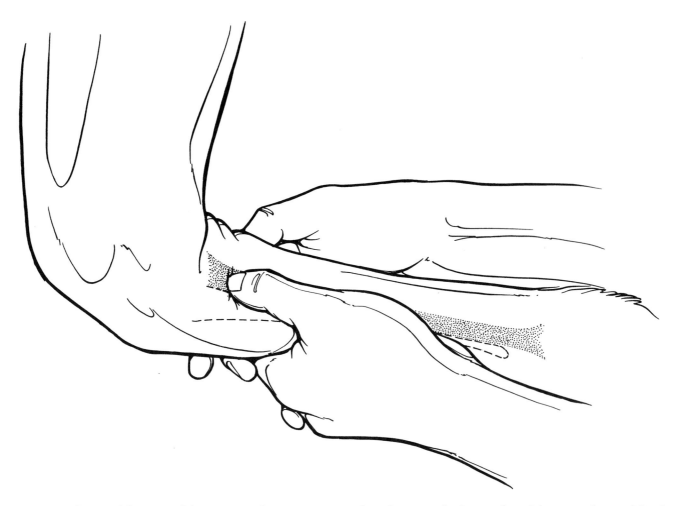

Fig. 3–18. Palpation of the origin of the suspensory ligament as it arises from the proximal palmar surface of the cannon bone and distal row of carpal (knee) bones. A painful response may indicate sprain trauma and/or avulsion fracture.

ion test is indicated by an increase in the asymmetry in the gluteal use, a more pronounced decrease in the height of foot flight arc, and a shortened cranial phase of the stride. Usually, a horse that tests positive will take very short strides and land primarily on the toe of the affected limb. For nonpalpable inflammatory diseases of the distal tarsal joints (tarsitis and bursitis), the increase in lameness may only be evidenced for the first 3 to 10 steps, after which the horse assumes its original gait. More prolonged lameness results from degenerative joint disease (bone spavin), incomplete tibial fractures, intra-articular fractures, and synovitis/capsulitis. Not all cases of osteochrondritis dissecans exhibit increased lameness after hock flexion tests.

If there is any question regarding the validity of the flexion test, it should be rerun. Two of the most common errors in performing this test are not obtaining full hock flexion and spooking the patient sufficiently enough that it balks at the onset of the test rather than jogging off at a smooth pace. Because the hip joint, stifle joint, fetlock joint, pastern joint, and coffin joint are flexed to a minor degree, this test cannot be con-

sidered definitive for the tarsal joints alone. For this reason, it is recommended that these other joints be examined before the hock flexion test is performed. An attempt can be made to extend the hock joint if clinical signs consistent with rupture of the peroneus tertius muscle are present during exercise. With the stifle flexed, the hock can be extended and a characteristic dimpling of the gastrocnemius tendon occurs (Fig. 3–36).

Tibia. The tibia should be observed from all angles for swelling, followed by deep palpation. Inflammation associated with the distal medial epicondyle region could be associated with a fracture or bruising of the bone and/or sprain to the medial collateral ligament. Swelling and pain with deep digital palpation of the distal third of the tibia associated with proximal tibial pain and severe lameness and a positive spavin test should alert the examiner to the possibility of an incomplete tibial fracture. A complete fracture of the tibia is associated with a nonweight-bearing lameness, severe swelling, and crackling on palpation and manipulation. The limb also appears somewhat shortened due to bone fragment overriding. Swelling and

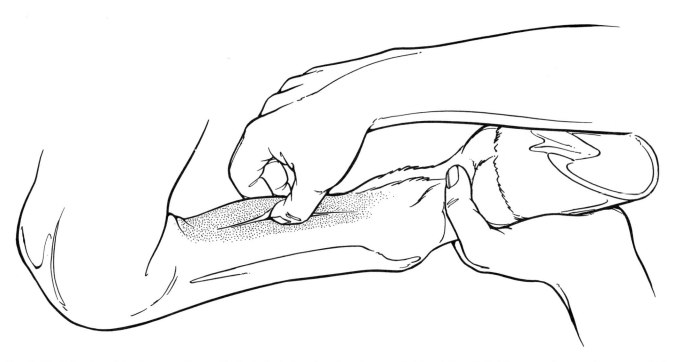

FIG. 3–19. Palpation of the flexor tendons with the fetlock flexed so that the superficial and deep digital flexor tendons can be separated. If they cannot be separated easily, it is most likely that adhesions have formed between the two tendons and a bowed tendon is present.

angular deformity of the limb associated with the tibia are common findings with physeal fractures.

Stifle. The stifle is observed for swelling and/or atrophy of the associated muscle groups. From a lateral view, an appreciation can be gained for distension of the femoropatellar joint capsule (Fig. 3–37). Next, the three distal patellar ligaments are palpated deeply for desmitis, and the medial patellar ligament is checked for scarring indicative of a previous desmotomy. The femoropatellar joint pouch is palpated for fluid distension and capsulitis (gonitis). If synovitis/capsulitis is present in the femoropatellar pouch, it indicates pathology within the femoropatellar joint or in the medial femorotibial joint. Results of this are compared to the opposite limb. In general, the more severe the fluid distension and the thicker the joint capsule, the more severe the pathology associated with it. Mild distension and capsulitis are normal for horses that are in active training or may be associated with partial upward fixation of the patella. Excessive fluid distension of the femoropatellar pouch associated with marked capsulitis is more indicative of cruciate ligament rupture, meniscal damage, medial collateral ligament sprain and/or rupture, intra-articular fracture, degenerative joint disease, and osteochondritis dissecans of the lateral trochlea. The patella should be palpated for peripatellar inflammation and crackling, which may indicate a fracture. The patella is also palpated for any displacement.

Manipulation tests of the stifle include the patellar displacement test, the flexion test, the cruciate test, and the evaluation of the medial collateral ligament. The patellar displacement test is performed with the base of the patella held between thumb and forefinger. The patella is then displaced proximally (upward) and laterally (outward) in an attempt to engage the medial patellar ligament over the medial trochlea. Many horses are sensitive to this manipulation and will attempt to flex the stifle to prevent the forced upward displacement of the patella. In some cases, the horse will attempt to kick. Because of this, it is helpful to grasp the tail in one hand in order to force the horse into weight-bearing on the limb that is being examined. In some cases, it is helpful to place the opposite side of the horse against a solid object so it cannot withdraw to that side. If the patella is easily displaced upward with apparent locking, the horse is walked off and its reaction is observed. With complete upward fixation, the horse will be unable to flex its stifle and will drag its limb behind in extension (Fig. 3–38). If the patella is easily placed proximally and does not lock, if crackling and femoropatellar capsule distension are present, and if there is increased toe wear, partial upward fixation of the patella should be considered. In some cases, repeated dorsal displacement of the patella 8 to 10 times will result in an increased lameness in the affected limb.

The stifle flexion test is performed by grasping the distal third of the tibial region while standing behind the horse. The limb is elevated to flex the stifle (Fig. 3–39). Although this test does somewhat selectively flex the stifle, the hock and fetlock are also flexed but more passively due to the reciprocal apparatus.

The cruciate test can be run in one of two ways. First, the examiner can stand behind the horse with his arms brought around the limb and the hands

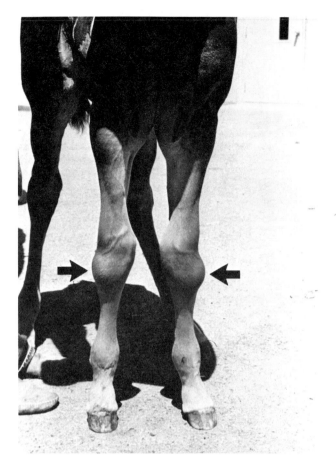

FIG. 3–20. Swelling over the dorsal surface of the knee typically seen with rupture of the common digital extensor tendon in foals (arrows).

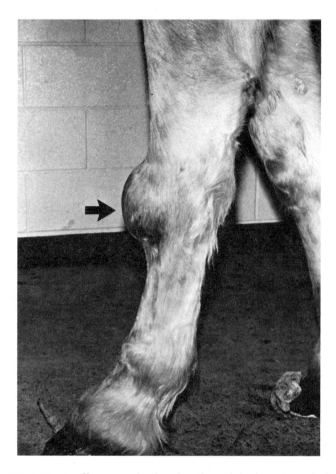

FIG. 3–21. Swelling over the dorsal surface of the knee typical of hygroma (arrow).

clasped together at the proximal end of the tibia. The examiner's knees or knee should be in close contact with the plantar aspect of the calcaneus, and the examiner's toe is placed between the bulbs of the heels. This position tends to stabilize the limb and protect the examiner from being kicked. In this position, the examiner pulls the tibia sharply caudally and releases it to go cranially, feeling for looseness and crackling that would indicate a cruciate ligament damage. If the caudal cruciate ligament is ruptured, the looseness and crackling are felt when the tibia is pulled caudally, whereas with a cranial cruciate ligament rupture, the looseness is felt as a sliding movement in a cranial direction (cranial drawer sign). In many cases, the only thing that is felt with this test is a generalized looseness, and it is difficult to identify which phase (caudal or cranial) it is felt in. In the normal horse, of course, no joint laxity is appreciated. This test is not routinely conducted on all horses but only those that are lame enough to indicate the possibility of a cranial cruciate ligament rupture. Still, it is important to select the case on which this test is performed.

For the second cruciate test, the examiner stands cranial to the affected limb and one hand is placed on the proximal tibial tuberosity to push caudally as quickly and forcibly as possible and let go. The other hand is used to pull the tail to that side to force the horse into weight-bearing. If an assistant is present, it is helpful for him to hold up the forelimb on the same side as the affected hindlimb. The caudal and rebound forces cause stress to the cranial and caudal cruciate ligaments (Fig. 3–40). This is done 20 to 25 times, after which the horse is trotted off and the degree of lameness observed. An increase in lameness may indicate a sprained cruciate ligament; however, other entities such as degenerative joint disease, interarticular fracture, and medial meniscal damage cannot be ruled out.

The medial collateral ligament test is performed by placing the shoulder over the lateral aspect of the femorotibial joint and abducting the distal limb (Fig. 3–41). This also can be performed in two ways. In cases of medial collateral ligament rupture, this manipulative test usually elicits enough pain to cause the horse to fall to the opposite side. In situations in which the ligament is sprained, the limb is abducted 5 to 10 times, after which the horse is trotted and the degree of lameness is noted. Medial meniscus damage is frequently associated with rupture of the cranial

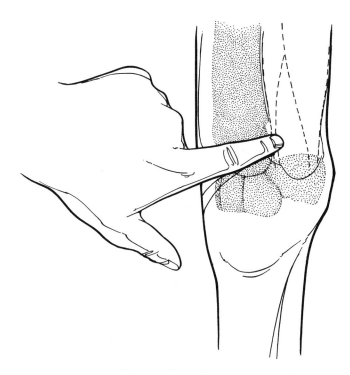

FIG. 3–22. Location of the carpal canal. Distension can be associated with tendosynovitis, a fractured accessory carpal bone or osteochondroma of the distal radius. The carpal tunnel syndrome may also be present.

cruciate ligament and rupture of the medial collateral ligament (terrible triad). As would be expected, these horses are usually severely lame. The lateral collateral ligament is tested by forcing the limb medially.

Finally, the semimembranosus and semitendinosus muscles are palpated for any evidence of a painful swelling (hamstring injury) or for firm scarring that would indicate either fibrotic or ossifying myopathy.

Femur. The muscles surrounding the femur are examined for inflammation and atrophy. The femoral artery is palpated for the quality of pulsations on the medial side of the thigh in the groove between the sartorius muscle cranially and the pectineus muscle caudally. If the pulse is weak or nonexistent, thrombosis of the iliac artery may be the cause. Pressure can be applied to the greater trochanter, and, if painful, trochanteric bursitis (whorlbone disease) should be suspected. Standardbred horses evidencing pain in this region may also have hock or stifle problems. Complete fractures of the femur result in nonweight-bearing lameness associated with swelling. Sometimes, it is difficult to discern crackling, and often it is helpful to place a stethoscope over the region of suspected fracture to pick up any audible crackling. Femoral neck fractures can be particularly difficult to diagnose. However, if they are examined shortly after the fracture has occurred, associated swelling will be localized to the hip region, and the hip joint can be rotated more easily than in the normal state. An x-ray examination is obviously very important in this region.

Hip. The hip is examined for asymmetry and muscle atrophy associated with muscle groups. The examiner can estimate the location of the greater trochanter of the femur in relationship to the other structures by using finger-hand measurements, checking the distance from the tuber ischiadicum to the greater trochanter and the tuber sacrale to the greater trochanter. With luxation of the hip, there will be a disparity in these measurements. Because the head of the femur usually luxates cranial and dorsal to the acetabulum, the distance between the tuber ischiadicum and greater trochanter will be greater, whereas the distance between the tuber sacrale and the greater trochanter will be decreased as compared to the opposite side. At a walk, a stifle-out, hock-in, toe-out gait is frequently observed, with an apparent shortening of the limb length evidenced by the horse stepping down to the affected limb. While standing from the side, the affected limb will be straighter than the contralateral limb. On manipulation, the limb cannot be rotated medially. In cases in which the round ligament is ruptured without coxofemoral (hip) luxation, the horse will still walk with the stifle out, hock-in, and toe-out appearance. With the cannon held in hand, the coxofemoral (hip) joint is manipulated into extension, flexion, and abduction. Additionally, the hip can be intermittently flexed and auscultated (listened to) with a stethoscope at the same time to identify any crackling. If crackling is present, the examiner should be suspicious of a femoral neck fracture with nonweight-bearing lameness, acetabular fractures, and/or degenerative joint disease. It is important to compare the sounds heard on one side to those heard on the other. At times, it is also helpful to auscultate over the coxofemoral joint while the horse is being walked. However, it is important that the examiner only interpret those sounds that emanate from this region as being abnormal when the foot is off the ground in flight. A myriad of sounds are heard as the horse places the foot on the ground and progresses through weight-bearing to lift off. These are difficult to interpret. Perceived abnormal sounds should be compared to the opposite side. If a fracture of the acetabulum is suspected, this may be diagnosed by examination of the region per rectum.

Pelvis. The pelvis is examined externally. First, the symmetry of the tuber coxae and tuber ischiadicum on each side is checked. Asymmetry in the tuber coxae or tuber ischiadicum should make the examiner suspect fracture of these prominences. If swelling is present in the perivaginal tissues in the mare, along with edema of the vaginal mucosa, one should be suspicious of a symphyseal fracture of the pubis. In the mare, this can be confirmed by a vaginal examination in conjunction with manipulation of the hindlimb by an assistant. If present, crackling and separation of the pubis can be palpated. Fractures of the ileum and acetabulum can also be picked up by rectal examination, which is covered in greater detail later in this text.

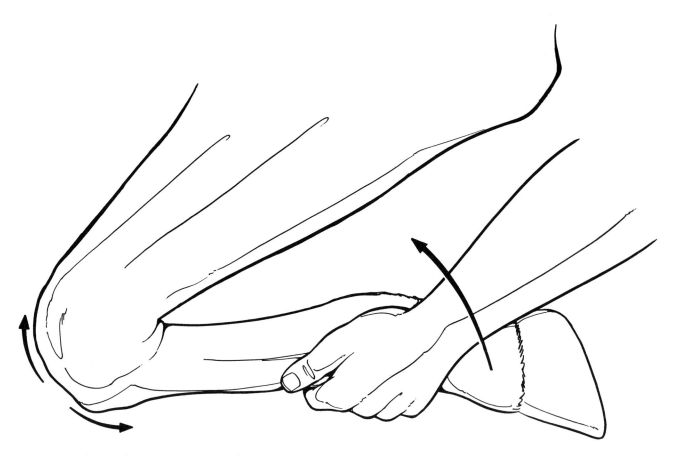

Fig. 3–23. The knee is flexed to identify a painful response. This should be done slowly in horses suspected of having slab fracture of the carpal bones and acute painful synovitis-capsulitis. In the normal horse, the flexor surface of the cannon approaches that of the forearm.

Examination of the Back

First, the horse's reaction to gentle running of the fingertips of both hands down the back from the withers to the base of the tail is assessed. Thin-skinned, hypersensitive horses will tend to cringe when this is done, but, without a dramatic response such as rearing or kicking or withdrawal, it should not be considered clinically significant. Any muscle swelling, atrophy, or asymmetry is noted. Following this, with the fingers flattened and held together, firmer pressure is applied to the dorsal muscles in the same manner as mentioned (Fig. 3–42). Most horses respond to this pressure in the lumbar region by ventroflexing (hollowing) their backs. However, after a few repeated applications of hand pressure, this response fatigues and withdrawal is not prominent. Special attention is paid to the insertion of the longissimus dorsal muscles on sacral vertebrae 2 and 3. This is particularly important when dealing with the harness horse. For horses that appear to be sensitive, a gradual increase in finger-applied pressure is in order. If back sensitivity continues and minimal reduction in response is observed, this should be considered clinically significant. As with any of these tests, each animal responds somewhat differently and, therefore, the assessment requires clinical experience for the subtle case. In some cases,

tightening (muscle spasms) of the longissimus dorsi muscle is felt rather than withdrawal. This usually signifies that the horse is attempting to fix the vertebral column because ventroflexion (hollowing) and withdrawal from pressure is painful. Next, the tips of the dorsal spinous processes are palpated for axial alignment, protrusion or depression, and interspinous distance (Fig. 3–43). Malalignment of these processes may indicate fracture and luxation or subluxation or overlapping of the dorsal spinous processes.

Flexion and Manipulative Tests. With these tests, the examiner is attempting to gain an appreciation of the horse's willingness to ventroflex (hollow), dorsiflex (raise), and lateralflex (bend sideways) its thoracic and lumbar vertebrae. Assessment of the horse's ability to ventroflex the back is obtained by alternately pinching the horse in the thoracolumbar area. For dorsiflexion of the back, the horse is either pinched over the croup or a blunt instrument is run over this area (Fig. 3–44). This creates a dorsal arching of the thoracolumbar region and a coupling under of the croup. Lateral flexion is assessed by firm stroking of the lateral lumbar musculature and/or lateral thoracic area. This procedure is performed on both sides with a blunt instrument (Fig. 3–45). Skin sensation assessed by using a sharp object causes withdrawal rather than flexion and is undesirable. Horses normally resent a test

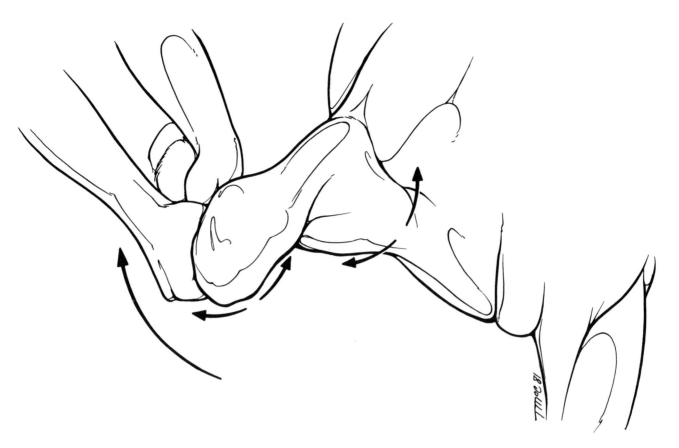

FIG. 3–24. Abduction (movement away from the median line) of the elbow joint and knee to place stress on the medial support structures. Pain may indicate strain or sprain trauma.

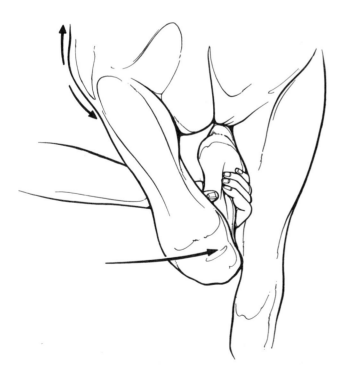

FIG. 3–25. Adduction (movement toward or beyond the median line) of the elbow joint and knee to place stress on the lateral support structures. Pain may indicate strain or sprain trauma.

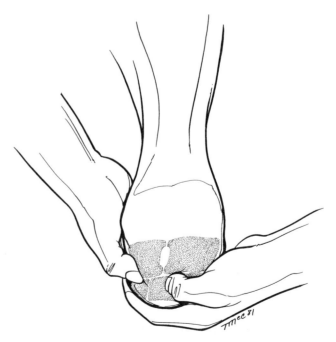

FIG. 3–26. The dorsal articular margins of the carpal bones can be palpated after the carpus is flexed. If pain is elicited, it could mean that a carpal chip is present and/or acute synovitis-capsulitis is present.

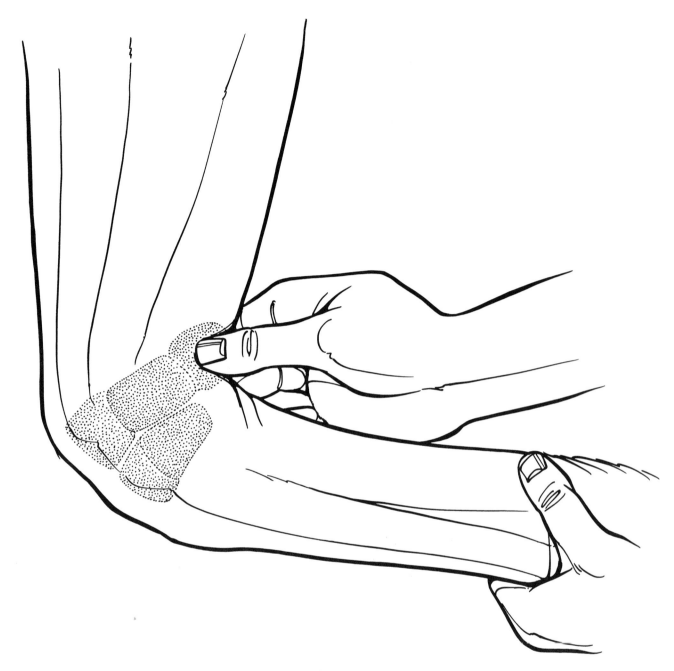

Fig. 3–27. Palpation of the accessory carpal bones to identify a fracture. This is best done with the knee flexed to decrease the tensional influence created by the tendinous insertions of the ulnaris lateralis and flexor carpi ulnaris muscles.

with a sharp object and the desired flexure is not observed. Reluctance to flex associated with muscle tightening and back rigidity often indicates a soft tissue or bony lesion in the thoracolumbar spine. In some instances, the location of pain can be localized by selective finger pressure, but frequently x-rays or nuclear scintigraphy of this region are needed. Tail elevation usually causes the horse to couple under behind. With damage of the sacrococcygeal region, however, the dorsal lifting of the tail often results in a camping out behind.

A rectal examination should be performed on all cases of suspected upper hindlimb involvement and back problems to rule out luxations or fractures of the sacral vertebrae and fractures of the pelvis. Often, a painful response can be elicited by palpation of the sublumbar muscles in those horses suffering from myositis.

Rectal Examination. The rectal examination can be an important part of the lameness evaluation, particularly if myositis, fractured vertebrae, thrombosis of the iliac arteries, or pelvic fracture is suspected. The

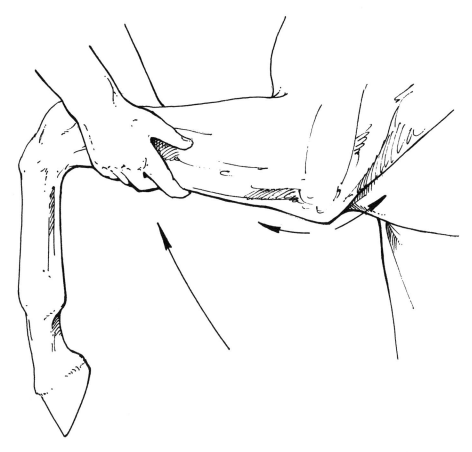

FIG. 3–28. Elevating the limb into extension to flex the elbow joint serves to increase the tension of the triceps brachii tendon, as it inserts on the olecranon process, and to extend the shoulder joint. Pain associated with this manipulation may indicate a nondistracted fracture of the olecranon process or problems within the shoulder joint (i.e., osteochondrosis and fractured scapula).

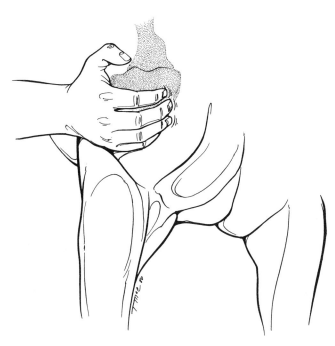

FIG. 3–29. Palpation over the point of the shoulder may cause pain from bicipital bursitis or ossification of the biceps tendon and bursa.

horse is first examined while standing still and the examination begins in a cranial-to-caudal direction. Pressure is applied to the iliopsoas muscle located cranial to the pelvic brim (Fig. 3–46). If painful, with the horse assuming a splinting (muscular fixing) position, local myopathy, or fracture of the lumbar vertebrae should be suspected. In some cases of fracture, there will be ventral swelling associated with the lesion. The aorta is checked for pulsation. If a strong pulse is not present in one of the iliac arteries, thrombosis should be suspected. In the older horse, the sublumbar lymph nodes are checked for any asymmetry that may indicate metastasis of a tumor, particularly in the lightly pigmented horse. The symmetry of the entire pelvis is checked by comparing one side to the other (Fig. 3–47). With displaced ileal fractures, an obvious asymmetry is present. If a hairline pelvic fracture is present, manipulation of the limbs may cause crackling or result in enough separation in the fragments so that this can be felt digitally. The ventral aspect of the sacral vertebral bodies are checked for alignment and any depression or protrusion into the pelvic canal, which may indicate fracture or dislocation. If any question still exists, the examination continues first

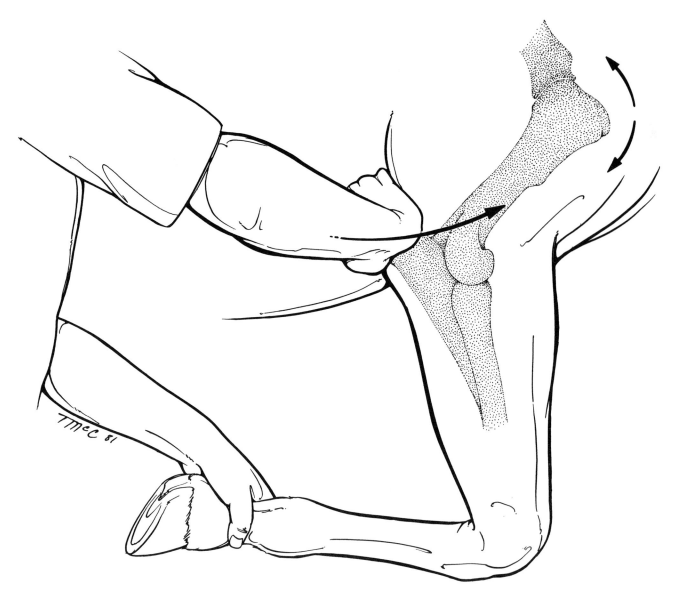

Fig. 3–30. Another test that flexes the shoulder and increases the tension on the biceps tendon to produce pressure on the bicipital bursa. Horses with bicipital bursitis are very reluctant to have their shoulder joint flexed as would horses with fracture of the supraglenoid tuberosity. This can be run as a flexion test as well if held in this position for 60 to 90 seconds.

with the horse being rocked from side to side by alternate pressure applied to each tuber coxae. In some cases, it is beneficial to walk the horse while the hand is still in the rectum to identify the disease.

Sway Response. The horse is checked for weakness in the hindlimbs that may indicate ataxia (wobbler syndrome). It can either be pushed from one side to the other or pulled by its tail (Fig. 3–48). Normal horses resist this pressure or pull effectively. Ataxic horses on the other hand appear relatively weak and do very little to resist swaying from one side to the other.

Additional Palpation Considerations

Hyperthermia (increase in body heat) is best checked by testing the area with the back of the hand and comparing this with the opposite limb. One should bear in mind that an area that has been clipped will feel warmer than an unclipped area, and the sun's rays on one limb will make it feel warmer.

Crackling may be produced in normal joints, and there is more movement in the pastern and coffin joints of some horses than in others. One should always compare the lame limb with the opposite limb to determine whether abnormalities are present.

Areas of both limbs may appear to show pain on pressure, so the examiner must determine whether the animal is actually exhibiting pain or, through nervousness, is pulling away. Young animals are more difficult to examine than horses that are well disciplined. Some mature horses, though, have nervous temperaments that hamper examination procedures,

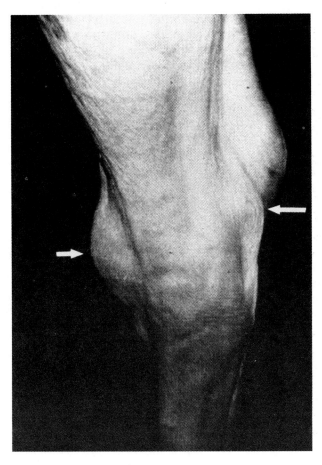

FIG. 3–31. Synovial swelling of the medial and lateral pouches of the tarsocrural joint capsule in a horse with bog spavin (arrows).

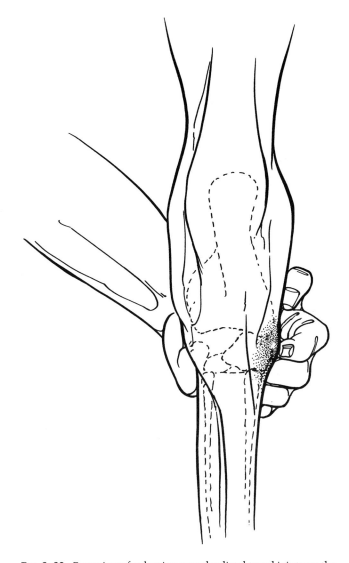

FIG. 3–32. Rear view of palpation over the distal tarsal joints on the medial side of the hock. This is the site where firm swelling is located that gives the hock a boxy appearance in cases of bone spavin.

so some allowances should be made for nervousness or fear. Tranquilization may be necessary, or at least helpful, in conducting a thorough examination.

One cannot judge the seriousness of enlargements in the limbs by palpation alone but must be able to evaluate carefully the importance of these swellings and the proximity to articular or other structures.

Other Examination Procedures

Local Anesthesia

Local anesthesia is commonly used in lameness diagnosis because it helps identify the site or sites of pain in horses that do not show an obvious problem. The site for local anesthesia may be prepared by clipping; in all cases, scrubbing with an antiseptic agent is performed. In addition, for joint blocks, the area is generally clipped and the scrubbing procedure is more thorough. For the veterinarian to perform local anesthesia, the horse should be restrained by a capable handler. A twitch may be necessary to prevent movement of the limb as the needle is inserted and the an-

esthetic is injected. If a horse moves quickly during this time, it could cause injury to the veterinarian or handler or could cause the needle to be broken off. When working on the hindlimbs, it is often helpful to wrap the tail and tie it out of the way.

The veterinarian should manipulate the region and observe the horse at motion before anesthesia and after each stage of anesthesia.

There are various means of local anesthesia.

Nerve Block (Perineural Infiltration). Nerve blocks are used to localize the source of pain causing lameness to a certain *region* and must therefore be performed in a systematic manner, starting with the lower (distal) limb and progressing upward (proximally). When several regions of one limb contribute to the lameness, systematic nerve blocking allows the veterinarian to determine what percentage of the lameness is contributed by each region. After each re-

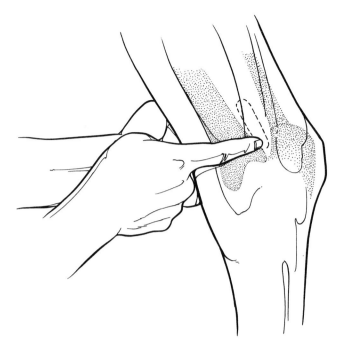

Fig. 3–33. This represents the site where tendosynovitis of the tarsal sheath and deep digital flexor tendon occurs. When distended, it is referred to as "thoroughpin."

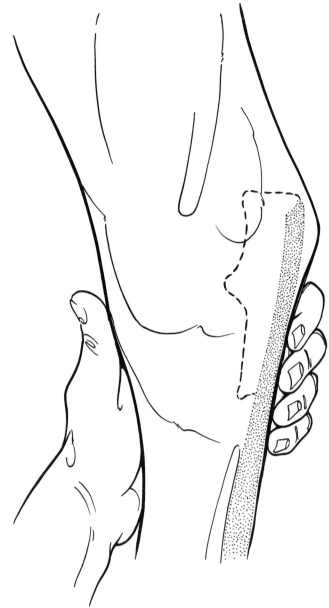

Fig. 3–34. Palpation of the long plantar ligament over the plantar surface of the calcaneous. Swelling here is referred to as "curb." Foals that have a curby appearance may have collapse of the central and third tarsal bones.

gion is blocked, it is necessary to wait approximately 10 minutes before working the horse in-hand or on the longe for the veterinarian's observation. Therefore, a complete forelimb evaluation may require several hours.

Ring Block (Field Block). Like a nerve block, a ring block is used to identify a specific region. A common field block, the low pastern ring block, deposits anesthetic subcutaneously around the pastern and localizes the problem to the foot region. A ring block takes more time to perform but is often more region-specific than a series of systematic nerve blocks.

Direct Infiltration. To identify sensitive areas such as tendons, ligaments, or bony prominences, anesthetic is directly infused into the region.

Joint Block (Intrasynovial Anesthesia). To identify problems in joint capsules, tendon sheaths, or bursae; after 10 to 30 minutes, the block is evaluated.

X-Ray Examination (Radiography)

Conventional X-Rays

X-rays are frequently required in lameness diagnosis and prognosis. Without x-rays, it is sometimes impossible to differentiate between fibrous tissue swellings and bony growths. X-rays are also helpful in determining the location of new bone growth in relation to joint surfaces. Although x-rays are an important part of a lameness diagnosis by themselves, they do not provide a definitive diagnosis. Changes that appear on x-rays do not necessarily indicate lameness, and all

lamenesses do not show x-ray changes. X-rays are used in conjunction with an accurate history, clinical examination, and other tests.

X-ray machines can be portable, mobile, or fixed. A veterinarian making a farm call uses a portable machine that can produce x-rays of varying quality due, in part, to the proximity of the examination area to a power source (therefore, the length of extension cord is important) and fluctuations in line voltage on the farm. Large equine hospitals use mobile or fixed machines that usually produce uniform, high-quality x-rays.

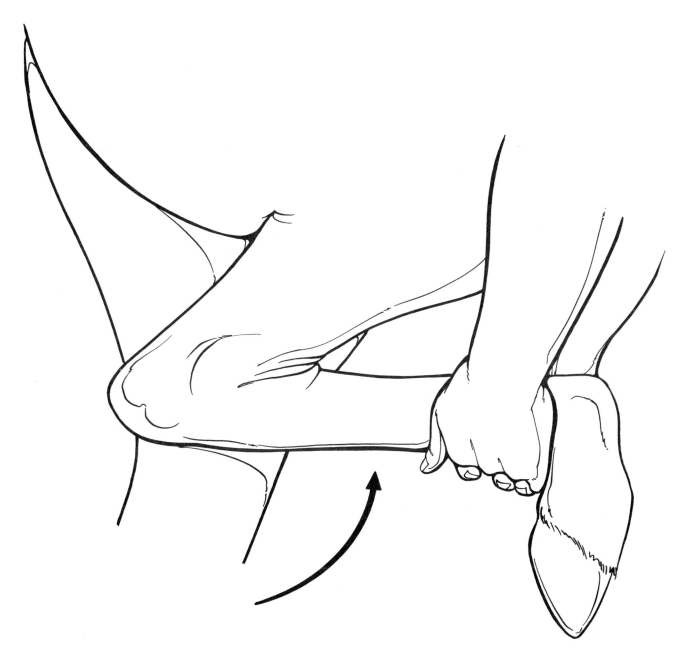

FIG. 3–35. Hock flexion test (spavin test). The hindlimb is flexed so that the metatarsus is approximately parallel to the ground surface. It is held in this position for 60 to 90 seconds, and the horse is observed for increased lameness. Increased lameness is considered a positive test but is not pathognomonic for spavin because the stifle and fetlock joints are also flexed.

X-ray film is put in strong, durable metal cassettes. The cassettes are placed behind the limb being x-rayed, and the x-ray machine is positioned a specific (critical) distance from the limb (Fig. 3–49). It is important that the horse does not move during the x-ray procedure. If it is necessary for the owner to hold the horse while it is being x-rayed, radiation safety procedures should be followed by standing away from the primary x-ray beam and wearing a lead apron and gloves.

To provide a complete diagnostic picture, it is often necessary to take two to eight x-rays. After the x-ray films are developed, the x-rays can be evaluated on a viewing screen. Bone changes usually stand out dramatically to the trained eye. Some soft tissue changes are evident when the film is viewed with a very bright light. The veterinarian may point out areas of significance to the horse owner.

Special X-Ray Examinations. A *sinus tract injection* involves injecting a contrast material in a draining tract to help identify a foreign body, bone sequestrum, chronic infection, or tissue necrosis. *Arthrography* involves injecting contrast material into a joint to provide more information related to articular carti-

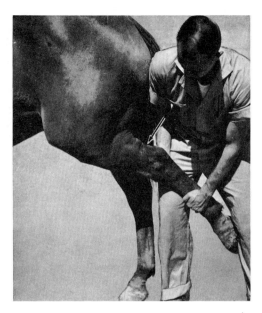

FIG. 3–36. Rupture of the peroneus tertius. The arrow indicates a dimpling in the tendon of Achilles when the limb is extended. Note that the hock is extended but the stifle is flexed; this cannot be done in a normal limb.

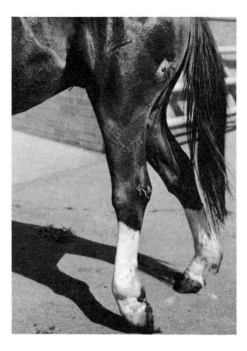

FIG. 3–38. Typical attitude of upward fixation of the patella. Extension of the stifle and hock joints and flexion of the fetlock joint are evident.

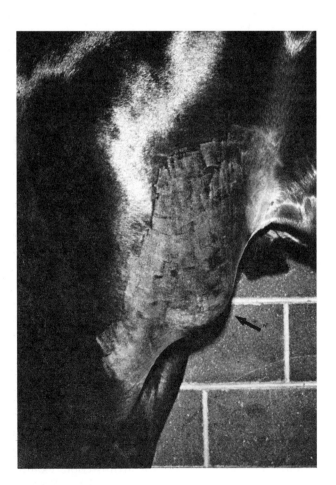

FIG. 3–37. Lateral view. Notice the distension of the femeropatellar joint pouch, indicating gonitis (arrow).

lage, subchondral bone, and lesions of the synovial membrane. *Myelography* involves injecting contrast material into the space surrounding the spinal cord to substantiate suspicion of neurologic damage.

SCINTIGRAPHY (NUCLEAR SCINTIGRAPHIC EXAMINATION)

When standard x-ray procedures cannot identify injuries, scintigraphy may be helpful. A radioactive isotope is administered intravenously. It infiltrates soft tissues first and an image is taken with the gamma camera of the suspected area 2 to 3 minutes after injection. The isotope becomes attached to bone within 30 minutes and is cleared from soft tissue within 2 hours. Therefore, 3 to 4 hours after injection of the agent, another image of the suspect area is taken. By doing this, soft tissue injury can be separated from bone injury. Equipment costs for scintigraphy are high, materials must be carefully handled, and procedures must be followed carefully by licensed personnel. However, scintigraphy provides an early sensitive means of detecting soft tissue inflammation, increased bone turnover, and new bone formation, as soon as 12 hours after injury. It is also provides a means of monitoring fracture healing.

XERORADIOGRAPHY

A specialized plate is exposed by x-ray and is processed in a unique manner. The result is a bluish im-

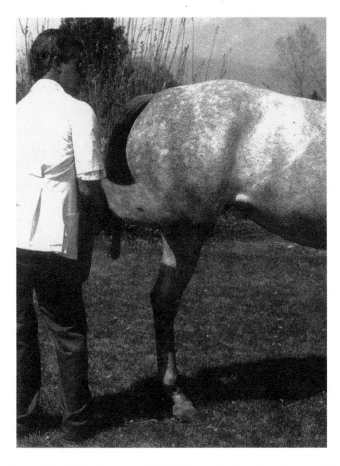

FIG. 3–39. Stifle flexion test. With the hands placed on the cranial surface of the distal tibia, the limb is elevated to flex the stifle. The stifle is held in this position for one minute, after which the horse is trotted.

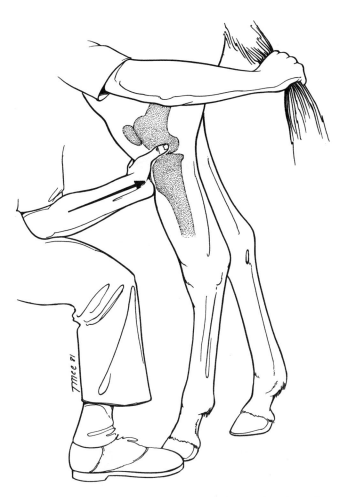

FIG. 3–40. Cruciate test. The examiner stands cranial to the stifle. With one hand placed on the proximal tibia, it is forced caudally and released cranially 20 to 25 times. During this manipulation, the horse's tail is pulled to the side of the examiner to force the horse into weight bearing. With cruciate rupture, joint laxity is associated with severe pain. With sprain trauma of the cranial cruciate ligament, increased lameness will be observed at exercise.

age on paper that provides good visualization of soft tissue structures and bony lesions (Fig. 3–50). Although xeroradiography is costly, the image obtained is superior to conventional x-rays.

Other Methods of Visual Imaging

VIDEOGRAPHY

Filming a horse's movement at various gaits can be an important part of a lameness evaluation. A videotape is a permanent record that can be viewed repeatedly and used as reference when reevaluating a lameness. Videos can be played in slow motion and the frames can be frozen to allow photography or measuring if desired. With the rapid advances in video technology, portable equipment is affordable and easy to operate. To get the best quality image, a portable video camera with a high-speed shutter (1/500 minimum) and a tripod should be used. The tripod will help the operator produce a smooth, sharp image that will be clear when used at slow motion, freeze-frame, and single frame advance. The quality of the video cassette player that the tape is played on will determine the range of special functions available. For gait analysis, a video cassette player with at least four heads is necessary to provide the above-mentioned functions.

ARTHROSCOPY

Arthroscopy allows examination of a joint by arthroscope to evaluate the condition of the synovial membrane and articular cartilage. The arthroscope is passed through a small incision (Fig. 3–51) that can be closed with a single suture after examination. Fiberoptic lighting allows the examiner to view the interior structures (Fig. 3–52). The veterinarian may record the findings via a verbal description, drawings, or photographs. Some joints, such as the knee, stifle, and shoulder, are more suitable for arthroscopic examination. The hock and fetlock have some spots that are blind to examination. A sample (biopsy) of the synovial membrane may be taken to characterize the

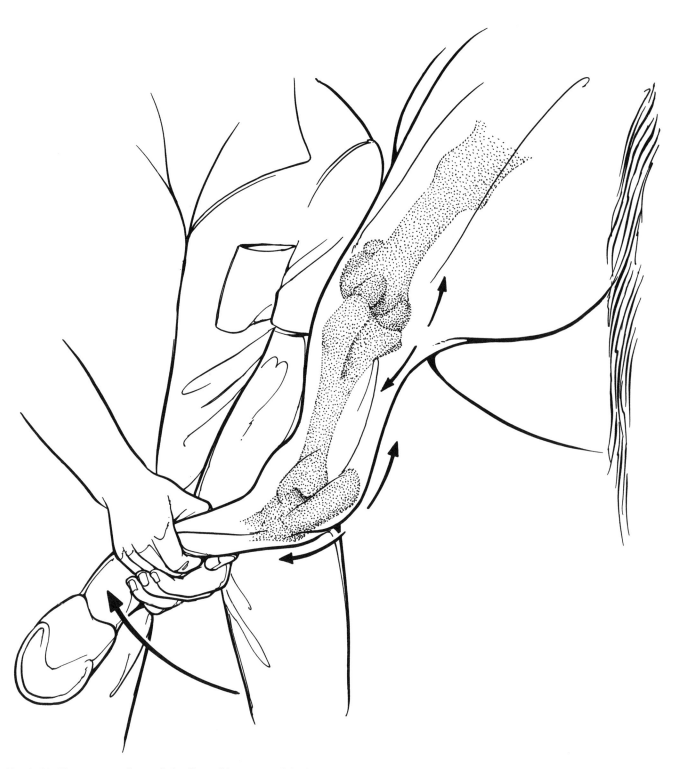

FIG. 3–41. Test to stress the medial collateral ligaments of the hock and stifle. Alternatively, one hand can be placed on the medial aspect of the distal end of the tibia to stress more selectively the medial collateral ligament of the femorotibial joint. Also, the examiner's shoulder can be placed over the middle of the tibia and both hands on the distal cannon to create selective tension on the medial collateral ligament of the hock. A painful response could indicate sprain trauma.

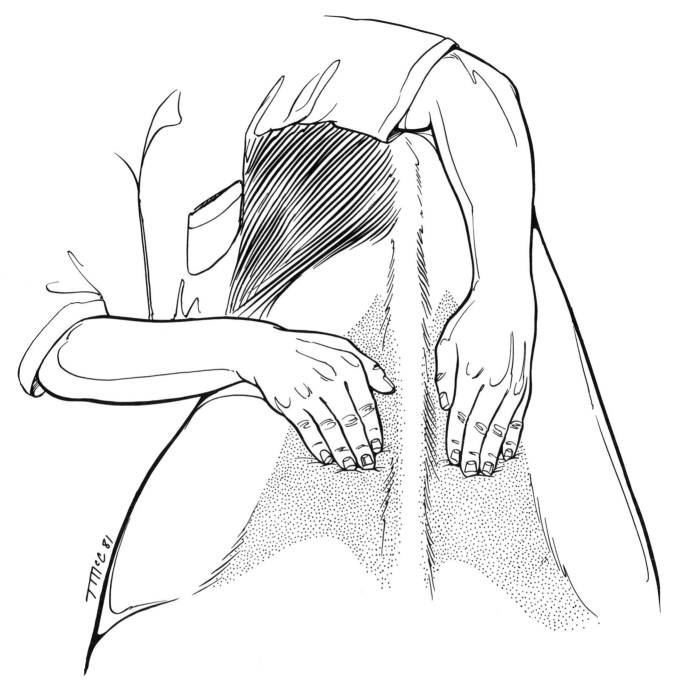

FIG. 3–42. Firm pressure is applied to the back muscles, along their entire length from the withers to the tuber sacrale, to identify a painful response. Notice that the fingers are held flat.

changes and to identify cellular changes that may provide insight into the problem. If joint infection is a concern, the synovial biopsy may be submitted for culture and results of antibiotic sensitivity.

THERMOGRAPHY

A thermograph measures skin surface temperature. An infrared scanning device converts radiation emitted from the skin into electrical impulses that are transferred to a color visual image (thermogram) on a video screen (Fig. 3–53). The greatest clinical value of the thermograph is the early identification of inflammation of soft tissue and bone and the monitoring of the healing process. Inflammation in stressed tendons can be picked up 1 to 2 weeks earlier than by routine clinical evaluation. Thermography is not harmful to the examiner or the horse.

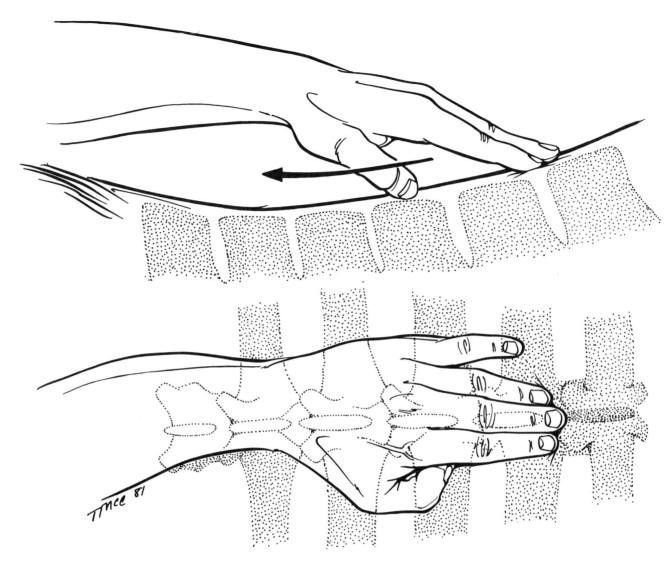

FIG. 3–43. *Top*, Palpation of the summits of the dorsal spinous processes for depressions or protrusions that may indicate subluxation or fracture. *Bottom*, Palpation of the axial alignment of the dorsal spinous processes.

ULTRASOUND

An ultrasonic image is formed by ultrasound waves reflecting from tissue interfaces that are converted and displayed on a television monitor (Fig. 3–54). Ligaments and tendons that cannot be differentiated by conventional x-rays can be imaged with ultrasound. Importantly, the degree of damage to the structures can be documented objectively. Ultrasound is also an important tool for the assessment of healing and often determines when a horse is capable of returning to work.

Other Methods of Diagnosis

PORTABLE INFRARED THERMOMETER

A hand-held portable infrared thermometer measures body surface temperature by converting the in-frared radiation to electrical signals that are displayed on a temperature dial (Fig. 3–55). The examination is conducted indoors in a cool area. The horse should have blankets and bandages removed 30 minutes before measurement and the area to be measured should be very clean. Infrared thermometry is a simple means of detecting early inflammation of the limb so that a treatment or an adjustment in the training program can be employed.

ANGIOGRAPHY

Angiography involves injecting dye into any artery or vein to evaluate blood flow. Usually, the horse is under general anesthesia and the flow of the dye is monitored by x-ray. This technique may be helpful in assessing blood supply to various portions of the

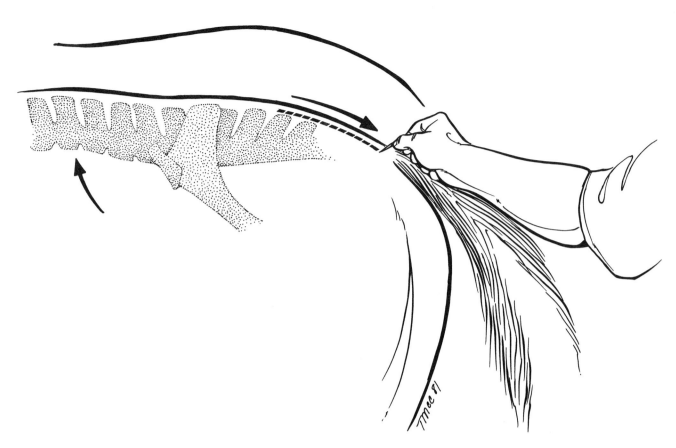

FIG. 3–44. A blunt instrument such as a ballpoint pen is run over the croup to create dorsiflexion in the back region. Reluctance to dorsiflex may indicate a problem of either the soft tissues or vertebral column associated with the back region.

horse's limb after trauma from wire cuts, laminitis, or carpal tunnel syndrome.

SYNOVIAL FLUID ANALYSIS

Synovial fluid is secreted by the synovial membrane and is contained in joint cavities, bursae, and tendon sheaths for lubrication. Hyaluronic acid, a constituent of synovial fluid, provides its viscous, lubricating properties. Synovial fluid analysis is routine in arthritis evaluations to provide an indication of the degree of synovitis and metabolic changes within the joint.

The site for sampling is prepared aseptically. The sample is collected using a sterile needle and syringe (Fig. 3–56). Normal synovial fluid is pale yellow, clear, and free of clouds, shreds, or particles of debris. Although streaks of blood may occur from needle puncture, uniformly distributed blood in the sample indicates trauma. Laboratory tests check for clot formation, protein content, viscosity, white blood cell count, increased enzyme activity, particle analysis, and other factors.

Diagnosis of Muscle Disease

Diagnosis of muscle disease includes visual observation, palpation, clinical pathologic examination, muscle biopsy, and electromyography. For more information, see page 140.

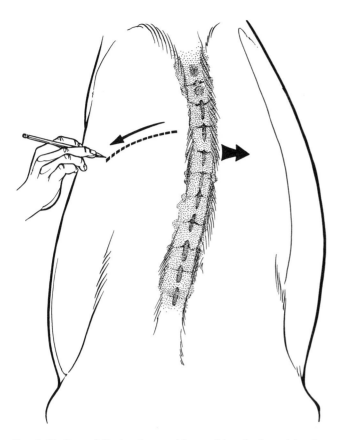

FIG. 3–45. Lateral flexion is tested by stroking the lateral lumbar and thoracic area with a blunt object such as a ballpoint pen. Normal horses are usually quite expressive and flex readily.

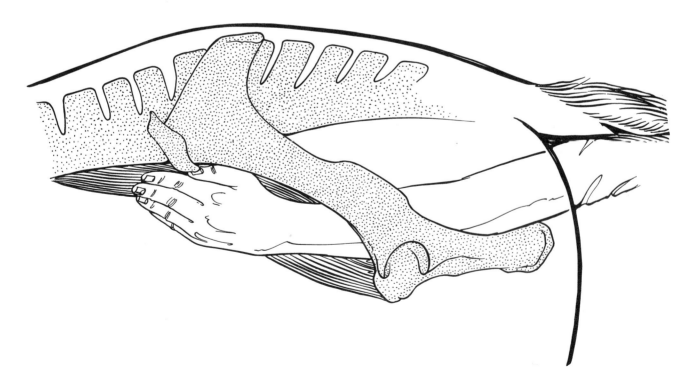

FIG. 3–46. Rectal examination, lateral view. The iliopsoas muscles just cranial to the pelvic brim are being palpated.

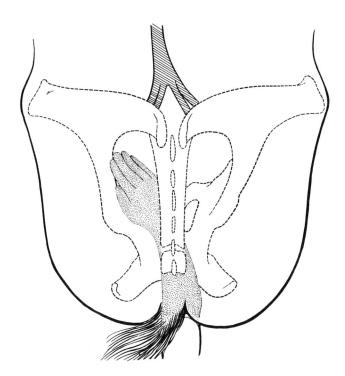

Fig. 3–47. Rectal examination, dorsal view. The symmetry of the pelvis is being evaluated. One side is compared to the other. The pelvis is also palpated for crackling while the horse is being swayed from side to side while standing or during movement.

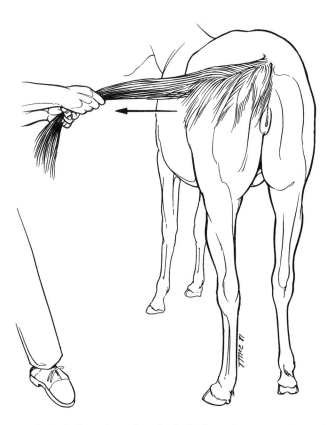

Fig. 3–48. Pulling the tail to check the horse's response. Normal horses resist this, whereas ataxic ("wobblers") horses can be pulled toward the examiner with varying degrees of ease.

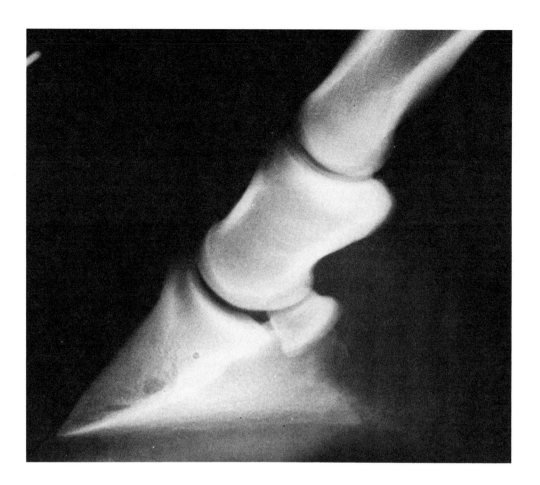

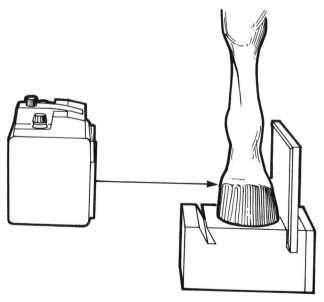

(Legend Appears on Facing Page)

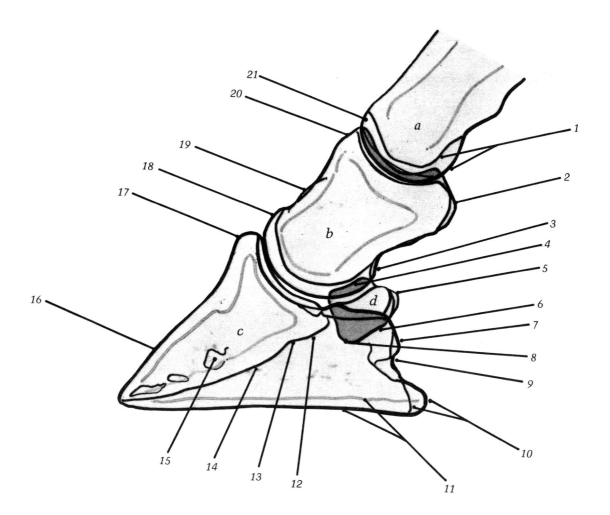

FIG. 3–49. Distal Phalanges And Navicular Bone (Foot). Lateromedial View.

1. Palmar aspect of the medial and lateral condyles on the distal extremity of the long pastern bone.
2. Transverse bony prominence on the proximopalmar aspect of the short pastern bone.
3. Superimposed medial and lateral condyles on the distopalmar aspect of the short pastern bone.
4. The articular surface of the navicular bone.
5. Proximal border of the navicular bone.
6. Flexor surface of the navicular bone.
7. Superimposed medial and lateral proximal parts of the palmar process on the coffin bone.
8. The distal border of the navicular bone.
9. Palmar process incisure.
10. Superimposed distal parts of the medial and lateral palmar processes on the coffin bone.
11. Medial and lateral distal borders of the coffin bone.
12. Flexor surface of the coffin bone. The deep digital flexor attaches on this area.

13. Semilunar line on the solar surface of the coffin bone.
14. Opaque line representing the concave solar surface of the coffin bone.
15. Solar canal of the coffin bone on end. This canal makes a semi-circular loop in the coffin bone.
16. Dorsal surface of the coffin bone.
17. Extensor process of the coffin bone.
18. Dorsal extent of the distal articular surface on the short pastern bone.
19. Eminence for collateral ligament attachment from the pastern joint.
20. Extensor process of the short pastern bone.
21. Distal dorsal articular surface of the long pastern bone.
a = Long pastern bone.
b = Short pastern bone.
c = Coffin bone.
d = Navicular bone.

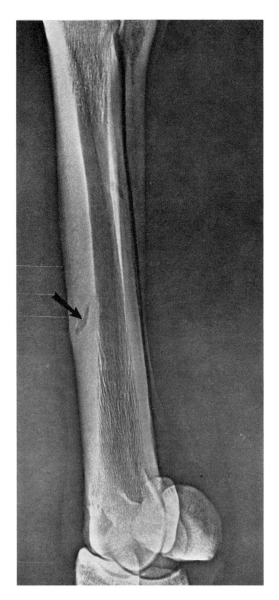

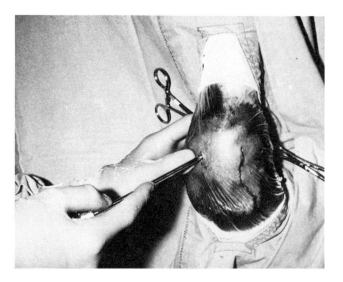

FIG. 3–51. Insertion of arthroscopic cannula through joint capsule.

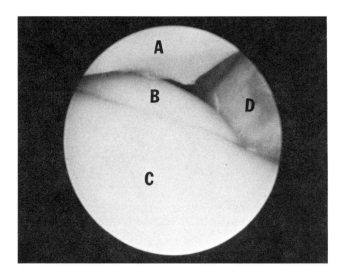

FIG. 3–50. A dorsomedial-palmarolateral oblique (D45M-PaLO) metacarpal xeroradiograph. A fracture through the dorsal lateral metacarpal cortex can be seen (arrow) on this xeroradiograph. (Courtesy of Dr. C. F. Reid, University of Pennsylvania, Philadelphia, PA.)

FIG. 3–52. Arthroscopic anatomy of medial aspect of midcarpal joints. Radial carpal bone (A), second carpal bone (B), third carpal bone (C), and synovial membrane (D).

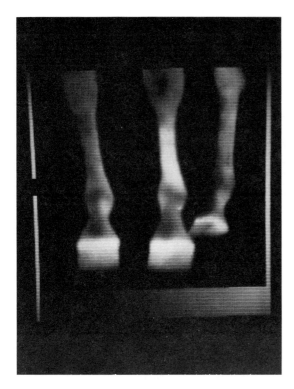

FIG. 3–53. A normal thermogram of bilateral forelimbs in a horse. The warmer vascular areas are lighter areas on the thermogram. (Courtesy of Dr. Ram C. Purohit, Auburn University, Auburn, AL.)

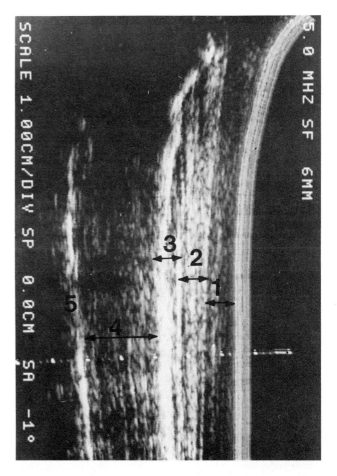

FIG. 3–54. A sagittal ultrasound scan of the palmar aspect of the metacarpus, proximal to the suspensory ligament bifurcation (1), the superficial digital flexor tendon (2), deep digital flexor tendon (3), accessory ligament of the deep digital flexor tendon (4), the suspensory ligament. All are characterized by small intense internal linear echos. There is an intermittent line depicting the acoustic impedance interface between the tendons. A bold white line is present between the margin of the third metacarpal bone and soft tissues of the metacarpus (5).

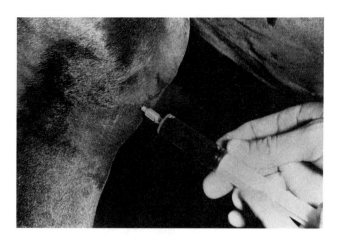

FIG. 3–56. Synovial fluid sampling.

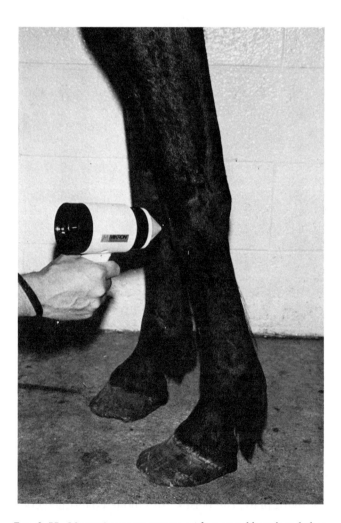

FIG. 3–55. Measuring temperature with a portable infrared thermometer.

CHAPTER FOUR

Selected Diseases of Bones, Joints, and Related Structures*

*Some of this material has been extracted from: Turner, S.: Diseases of Bones and Related Structures; and McIlwraith, C.W.: Diseases of Joints, Tendons, Ligaments, and Related Structures; *In* Adam's Lameness In Horses, Stashak, T.S., ed., 4th Ed. Philadelphia, Lea & Febiger, 1987.

Bone Growth

The longitudinal growth of a bone results from a series of events occurring at highly specialized regions at one or both ends of the bone. These regions are referred to as the "physis," the "growth plate," or more correctly, the "metaphyseal growth plate." The process occurring at the growth plate (endochondral ossification) is characterized by rapidly differentiating and maturing cartilage cells and the replacement of cartilage by bone (Fig. 4–1).

Injury to growth plates, either by excessive pressure, direct trauma, traction, circulatory loss, or shearing forces, can cause arrest in longitudinal growth and potentially can cause an angular limb deformity or a bony malformation.

One of the hallmarks of bone growth is that it is highly dependent on resorption (disappearance of bone) as well as bone formation. If, for example, bone resorption did not occur and bone only grew in length, then the bone would be disproportionately long and thin. Similarly, in the diaphysis, if bone did not become resorbed from the inner surface, then continued apposition of bone from the periosteum would produce a bone that was too thick with inadequate marrow cavity.

The blood supply to the growth plate comes from epiphyseal circulation, metaphyseal circulation, and perichondral circulation (vessels surrounding the growth plate). Transphyseal vessels (vessels crossing the growth plate) are found in the large epiphyses and present a route for spread of infection from the metaphysis to the epiphysis. The metaphyseal circulation provides a sluggish pattern of blood flow that predisposes this region to bacterial numbers and osteomyelitis inflamation of the bone marrow.

Although the exact mechanism is incompletely understood, tension and compression (with a certain physiologic range) on the growth plates are essential for continued orderly development. Each growth plate has a biologic range of both tension and compression within which it will respond. Within this range, increasing tension or compression will accelerate growth while decreasing tension or compression will decrease growth. Beyond the physiologic limits of tension or compression, growth may be significantly decreased or even stopped. This principle has an important practical application in the management of foals with angular limb deformities. Assume that a foal with an angular limb deformity of the carpus (e.g., carpus valgus) is exerting an asymmetric load on the growth plate of the distal extremity of the radius. Clearly, unrestrained exercise, such as would occur running on pasture with a mare, would increase the likelihood of producing excessive asymetric pressure due to concussion that is greater than the physiologic range. This would retard any autocorrection of the angular limb deformity that the foal may have been able to elicit, increasing the likelihood that surgical correction will be required. That is why confinement is often the recommendation for treatment of angular limb deformities.

Apart from the effects of pressure and tension on the growth plate, the periosteum (bone covering) acts as a mechanical restraint to bone growth. This ex-

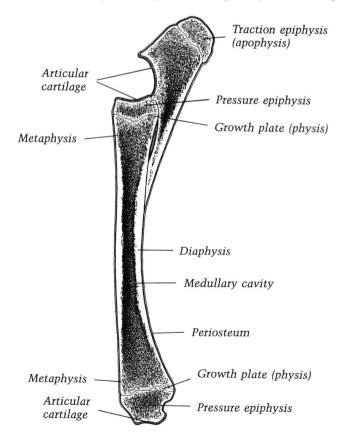

Traction epiphysis (apophysis)

Articular cartilage

Pressure epiphysis

Growth plate (physis)

Metaphysis

Diaphysis

Medullary cavity

Periosteum

Growth plate (physis)

Metaphysis

Articular cartilage

Pressure epiphysis

Fig. 4–1. Sagittal section of the radius and ulna of a foal.

plains why the technique of hemicircumferential transection ("stripping") of the periosteum and periosteal elevation produces dramatic results when used to correct angular limb deformities in foals. Following periosteal stripping, the tension on that side of the bone is relieved, allowing bone growth to continue at an increased rate. When the limb is straight, the periosteum reattaches or regrows and presumably begins to reexert tension. This is a possible explanation as to why limbs with angular limb deformities have been observed not to overcorrect following this surgery.

Cessation of Growth

As growth of the bone ceases, the growth plate becomes progressively thinner, and finally the epiphysis and metaphysis fuse. The cartilaginous growth plate is thus replaced by bone, making it incapable of correcting any angular limb deformity, either by autocorrection or surgical correction. The timing of the closure of the growth plate will depend on the bone (and even the limb). Some close early in life, while others may be present for several years (see Table 1–1). Most data on epiphyseal closure are based on x-ray interpretation. However, it is well known that functional physeal closure occurs well before closure is evident on x-rays, and it will have an important bearing on the timing of surgery used to correct angular limb deformities.

Injuries of Bones

The Effect of Physical Force on the Epiphysis: Epiphyseal Injuries

When a severe force is applied to a joint and its nearby epiphyses, an epiphyseal injury is likely to occur. This is because the cartilaginous epiphyseal (growth) plate is weaker than bone, surrounding ligamentous structures, and the joint capsule. Injuries that would produce a torn ligament or dislocation in an adult may produce a traumatic separation of the growth plate in a growing bone.

CLASSIFICATION OF GROWTH PLATE (PHYSEAL) INJURIES

A diagrammatic representation of growth plate injuries is shown in Figure 4–2.

Type 1. In this injury, there is complete separation of the growth plate without any fracture through bone. The prognosis varies drastically in foals.

Type 2. This is the most common type of physeal injury. The line of fracture separation extends along the physeal plate to a variable distance and then out through a portion of the metaphysis, producing a triangular metaphyseal fragment. In foals, the distal cannon bone physis commonly incurs this injury when the mare steps on the foal.

In foals, there is no real evidence to indicate to what degree this injury interferes with growth. Obviously, if the injury involves a physis that has virtually no residual growth left (such as distal physis of the cannon bones, or the proximal physis of the long pastern bone), then the potential for interference with growth will be minimal.

Type 3. The fracture is intra-articular and extends from the joint surface to the deep zone of the physeal plate and then along the plate to its edge. In foals, this injury is extremely rare. If it does occur, fixation would best be achieved with bone screws.

Type 4. This fracture is intra-articular, extending from the joint surface through the epiphysis, across the entire thickness of the physeal plate, and through a portion of the metaphysis. Fixation with bone screws is necessary. The prognosis for growth may be poor unless perfect alignment is achieved and maintained.

Type 5. This injury results from a severe crushing force applied through the epiphysis to one region of the physeal plate. The prognosis in a child is poor because it causes premature closure of the growth plate and subsequent cessation of growth. It is difficult to assess the retardation effect on growth in a foal.

Type 6. This injury occurs when a periosteal bridge forms between the metaphysis and epiphysis (Fig. 4–3). This acts as a restraint to growth of that side of the growth plate.

Bone Healing, Fracture Repair and Complications

When a fracture occurs, there is usually a loss of structural continuity of the bone and its function is impaired to some degree. The degree of impairment and the particular bone that is fractured determines the type of lameness. For example, a displaced fracture of the olecranon process or a fracture of one of the load-bearing bones such as the radius or tibia usually produces a severe lameness. Conversely, a chip fracture of a carpal bone produces a mild lameness that may resolve with rest, although it may initiate a synovitis and set the stage for degenerative joint disease and produce a lameness in a secondary manner.

In the past, fracture healing in horses often resulted in altered function and/or a certain amount of arthritis. Because of the nature of the horse and what man uses it for (e.g., athletic performance), a greater demand for improved techniques for fracture repair has evolved. For example, there have been improved techniques in internal fixation of particularly long bone fractures with emphasis on improving the implants to withstand massive functional forces and not to fail due to mechanical overload. Such implants must also be strong enough to maintain their integrity until the bone has united, without breaking under fatigue. Herein lies one of the main obstacles of fracture repair in horses, and that is an inability to maintain fixation, especially during recovery from anesthesia.

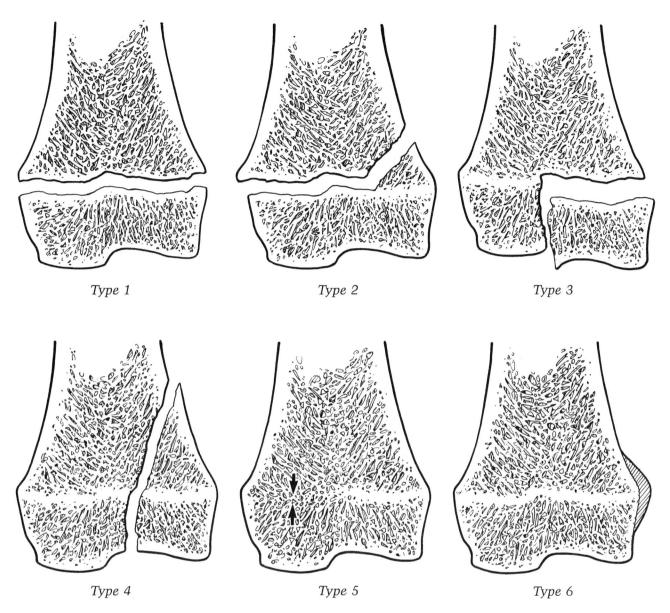

FIG. 4–2. The Salter-Harris classification of physeal injuries. (From Salter, R. B., and Harris W. R.: Injuries involving the epiphyseal plate. J. Bone Joint Surg., 45A:587, 1963).

COMPRESSION FIXATION

The use of various methods of compression in the treatment of fractures in man and animals has become widely accepted. The function of an implant (plate and/or screws) is to hold the bone fragments under compression, enabling the bone and neighboring joints to function more normally until fracture union has occurred.

One method used to compress a fracture is to use a lag screw, a basic technique used routinely by carpenters and engineers. It is particularly suited for the horse that has an intra-articular fracture, in which accurate anatomic alignment at the level of the joint surface is essential to avoid secondary degenerative joint disease

(Fig. 4–5). The lag screw is virtually never used to repair major long bone fractures in horses or even small foals, because it is simply not strong enough. It is ideally suited, however, for fractures such as slab fractures of the third carpal bone, lateral condylar fractures of the distal third cannon bone, sagittal fractures of the long pastern bone, and certain coffin bone fractures. The lag screw can be used in conjunction with plates for the repair of comminuted fractures where the fracture reconstruction is repaired with screws and a so-called "neutralization plate" is applied.

Joint laxity, especially in young animals, with fractures treated with casts seems to be much more common than joint stiffness.

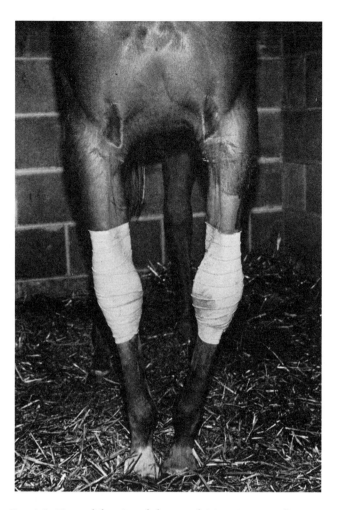

FIG. 4–3. Varus deformity of the carpal joints in a weanling as a result of a type 6 injury to the medial side of the distal radial metaphysis-epiphysis region.

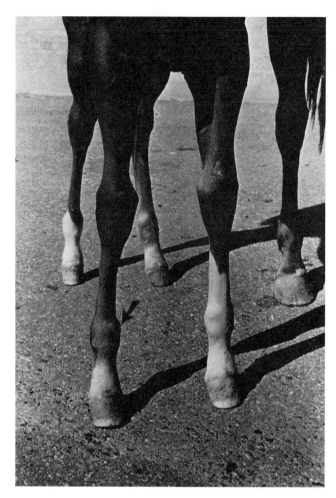

FIG. 4–4. Varus deformity of the right fetlock joint in a foal due to excessive weight-bearing. Some metaphyseal flaring is also present (arrow).

Tendon and associated muscle flaccidity is also seen in horses with fractures treated with external immobilization such as casts. Other aspects of so-called "fracture disease" in young horses are angular limb deformities in the weight bearing limb due to excessive axial loading on active growth plates. A common deformity is a fetlock varus (Fig. 4–4). Carpus valgus and carpus varus are also seen. Complications in the weight-bearing limb during the healing of a fracture (i.e., the opposite limb) can lead to permanent lameness. Stretching of flexor tendons and associated muscles as well as atrophy of unassociated muscles can also cause potentially irreversible complications. Laminitis with coffin bone rotation can occur in the limb opposite to a fracture. This is often referred to as support limb laminitis.

Following a fracture, there is a certain amount of inflammatory response that is eventually replaced by scar tissue. Subsequently, adhesions can impair tendon function or produce stiffening of neighboring joints.

Infection is a serious complication of fractures that can eventually lead to permanent lameness or a non-union of the fracture necessitating euthanasia. Open (compound) fractures that eventually heal are accompanied by considerably more fibrosis with a greater chance of loss of function of surrounding structures. The limb may be permanently thickened because of scar tissue, which would be a handicap for show animals.

Diseases of Bones

Osteitis and Osteomyelitis

Osteitis and osteomyelitis are terms used to describe inflammation of bone. If the process begins in the periosteum, the term "osteitis" or "osteoperiosteitis" is used. If it begins in the medullary (marrow) cavity, the term "osteomyelitis" is used.

INFECTIOUS OSTEITIS

Osteitis commonly occurs in the extremities of the horse, especially in the cannon bone because of a mea-

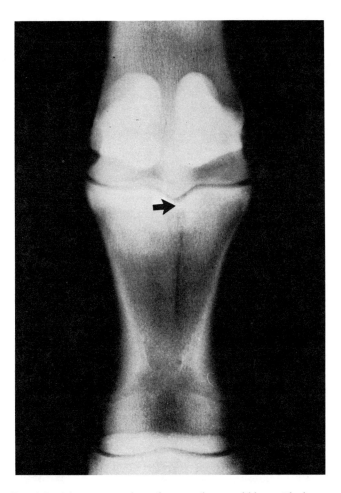

FIG. 4–5. A long pastern bone fracture that would be an ideal candidate for lag screw fixation. This would minimize the chances of secondary degenerative joint disease (arthritis) of the fetlock joint by accurately reconstructing the intra-articular component of the fracture (arrow).

ger soft tissue covering and lack of natural protection. Lameness due to pain in cases of osteitis is usually a result of infection from a nearby septic process or from a break in the skin. Osteitis is seen frequently when a horse is kicked with or without breaking the overlying skin.

Occasionally, an osteitis may resolve spontaneously, especially if there is no infectious component. If bacteria are present, the wound may discharge indefinitely until a sequestrum (layer of dead bone) is removed. Wound debridement involving dissection of unhealthy scar tissue and dead bone is usually required. Although small bone sequestra may resorb spontaneously due to the inflammatory process, larger ones usually require surgical removal. Removal of bone sequestra is often performed with the animal recumbent under general anesthesia.

The prognosis for osteitis is usually excellent unless the nearby vital structures are involved or are injured at the time of surgery.

OSTEOMYELITIS

Osteomyelitis is a more extensive inflammation of the bone that begins within the medullary (marrow) cavity. Osteomyelitis in newborns is usually blood borne (hematogenous), whereas in adults this form is very rare. Osteomyelitis may also result from penetrating wounds, from open fractures, and from internal fixation of a closed fracture where there has been a break is aseptic surgical technique.

Hematogenous Osteomyelitis. Hematogenous osteomyelitis is frequently part of a generalized disease with an infected focus elsewhere in the foal's body, such as the umbilicus, gastrointestinal tract, or lungs. Foals with a compromised immune system (i.e., failure of passive transfer) are predisposed to neonatal osteomyelitis. The animal may have multiple sites of the same bone involved as well as involvement of multiple bones. Bone infection due to *Salmonella spp.*, for example, typically has multiple involvement. In severe cases of osteomyelitis, the infection can spread to the synovial membrane, resulting in infectious arthritis.

Hematogenous osteomyelitis may be missed in its early stages. It may seem that the lameness is due to a sprain or that the mare stood on the foal. There is usually a very severe lameness with swelling in the nearby soft tissues. The animal may be so lame that it resembles a fractured bone. Fever will be present with pain on manipulation of the joint. X-ray changes in the bone are not visible until 30 to 50% of the bone mineral has been absorbed. This is usually evident 10 to 14 days after the onset of infection.

Because the lameness is frequently attributed to a sprain by the owner and veterinarian alike, by the time the osteomyelitis shows obvious signs on x-rays, it is usually too late to treat medically. If acute hematogenous osteomyelitis is suspected and there are still no x-ray signs, then broad-spectrum bacteriocidal antibiotics are administered.

Surgical curettage (a scraping to remove abnormal tissues) is indicated if the osteomyelitis is not close to an adjacent joint and when mechanical stability of bone is not jeopardized. The infected bone is removed when possible. Bone grafting is used often to accelerate the consolidation of the hollow space left by the curettage.

The prognosis for hematogenous osteomyelitis is extremely poor, especially if multiple sites are involved.

Osteomyelitis Following an Open Fracture or Penetrating Wound. Osteomyelitis may also occur following an open (compound) fracture or following a penetrating wound. Here, the pathogenic organisms penetrate the medullary cavity. There is usually some degree of trauma to the skin and surrounding soft tissues as well. Occasionally, hematogenous arthritis is seen in fractures without any external evidence of breaks in the skin. In such situations, the dead tissue provides a medium for bacterial proliferation and infection develops from a hematogenous source.

Treatment of an open fracture without providing absolute stability is usually futile unless the fragments can be removed or reincorporated into the healing fracture, where they can be revascularized. Infection spreads through the bone in a similar manner described for hematogenous osteomyelitis.

Osteomyelitis Following Internal Fixation. The cause of osteomyelitis following internal fixation is usually contamination following an open fracture or at the time of surgery, despite meticulous aseptic technique.

The clinical signs of osteomyelitis following internal fixation include lameness, retarded wound healing over the implants, and drainage. Signs can be present as early as 7 to 10 days or be delayed for 3 to 4 weeks.

The first priority for treatment must be to achieve stability. This usually means compression plating or the use of external fixation devices. Bone will heal in the face of infection if the fracture site is stable. If it is impossible to stabilize the fracture either with internal fixation, external fixation, or both, euthanasia is the only practical and humane alternative. Bone grafts are often placed in healthy tissue away from the infection. Other factors that aid in successful treatment include good nursing, nutrition, and husbandry. Additionally, the patient's temperament is important, and the animal should be receptive to daily treatment and confinement. The prognosis of osteomyelitis following internal fixation of a fracture in a horse is poor.

OSTEOPOROSIS

In osteoporosis, the mineral density of the bone is usually not altered but the amount of bone tissue is reduced. The bone becomes porous, light, and fragile and is prone to fracture.

Generalized Osteoporosis. The generalized osteoporosis seen in postmenopausal women has no counterpart in the aged horse. Osteoporosis is seen occasionally with undernutrition rather than actual deficiencies of calcium, phosphorus, or vitamin D. A condition first recognized in Thoroughbred foals may be a manifestation of generalized osteoporosis. The condition is characterized by fractures of the proximal sesamoid bones and typically occurs when foals gallop to exhaustion trying to keep up with the dam. Foals seem more prone to the condition if they are confined after birth. During this time of relative inactivity, the bones are not subjected to stresses required to strengthen them and are a potential weak link in the skeletal system.

Localized Osteoporosis. *Disuse Osteoporosis.* This condition is fairly common, especially in horses with rigid external immobilization devices on their limbs, such as casts. With the lack of stress on that portion of the limb that is in the cast, there is increased resorption of bone and decreased bone formation. It is more severe in young animals because of the inherent rapid turnover of bone compared with the adult horse.

Bones become thinner and more porous. Localized osteoporosis is essentially identified by x-ray diagnosis. Fortunately it is easily reversed when the external immobilization device is removed and the animal commences normal weight-bearing.

OSTEOPETROSIS

Osteopetrosis is a rare skeletal disease of horses characterized by an imbalance of bone apposition and resorption. It is an inherited disease of people, rabbits, mice, and cattle and may be an inherited disease in horses. The underlying problem is a failure of bone resorption resulting in a complete closure of the marrow cavity. Since there is no evidence of bone marrow in affected bones, an anemia commonly accompanies this condition. Osteopetrosis has been reported in a Peruvian Paso foal. Although evidence is circumstantial, it may be an inherited condition in this breed.

FLUOROSIS

Fluorosis is occasionally seen in horses that ingest small but toxic amounts of fluorine in diet or drinking water. It produces an osteoporosis. The source of the fluorine is usually contamination from nearby industries. Plants can become contaminated from industrial fumes and wells may become contaminated from an industrial effluent. The exostosis (excess bone) formation is usually first observed in the cannon bones. (Fig. 4–6, *A* and *B*).

The horse may be intermittently lame and show signs of generalized unthriftiness. The gait may be stiff. The lameness is not one the horse will warm out of. Horses may stand with their feet abnormally placed and shift their weight on the feet to relieve pain. Bones are easily fractured, and there is usually a classic mottling of the teeth. The dental lesions occur if the animal is exposed to fluorine during development of the teeth. Teeth are generally regarded as sensitive indicators of fluorosis. Tooth loss is increased.

The diagnosis usually rests on the clinical and x-ray findings and is confirmed by analysis of fluorine in bone and urine. Also, a diagnosis should be confirmed by examining animals exposed to a similar environment. The treatment is directed toward prevention as well as general symptomatic treatment of the affected horse.

HEREDITARY MULTIPLE EXOSTOSIS

Hereditary multiple exostosis (HME) is a skeletal disorder characterized by numerous abnormal projections from growing bones that result in an abnormal bone contour. The condition affects most of the long-bones as well as the ribs and pelvis. It is an hereditary condition and transmitted by a single dominant autosomal (not sex-linked) gene. Affected individuals

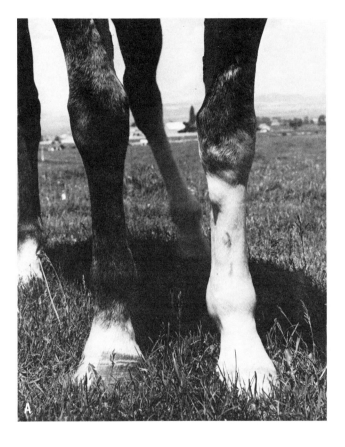
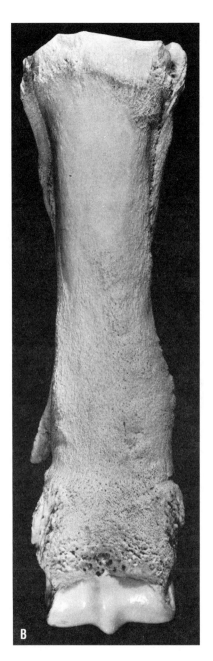

FIG. 4–6. *A,* Enlargement of the cannon due to fluorosis. *B,* Fluorosis of the cannon bone. (Courtesy of Dr. J. L. Shupe, Utah State University.)

transmit the trait to approximately 50% of their progeny. It is used as a model for the condition in man.

Signs. The characteristic swellings of HME are usually present at birth, and the lesions are probably initiated during fetal bone development. They are usually bilaterally symmetric and consist of multiple bony enlargements of various shapes and sizes that are firmly attached to the bone. They are easily palpable in regions of thin skin. Swellings on the limbs do not appear to enlarge as the animal matures, but others such as those located on the ribs and scapulae usually enlarge until maturity is reached (about 4 years of age) (Fig. 4–7 *A, B,* and *C*). Such animals may be lame, but

it is usually very mild. The lameness is caused by infringement on various tendons and muscle groups. Some horses have various joint swellings and tendon sheath swellings. The tumors adopt a variety of shapes, ranging from conical to spurlike. They occur in regions of most active bone growth and regions of stress or strain. Lesions on the ribs may be quite extensive, especially on the medial surfaces.

Diagnosis. X-ray examination of the affected region, as well as the opposite limb, is recommended. The condition is rare.

Treatment. There is no known treatment for hereditary multiple exostosis. The genetic background of

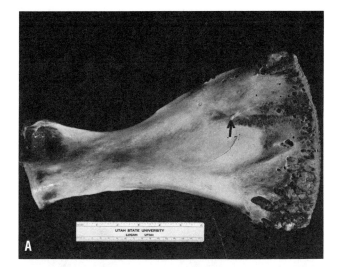

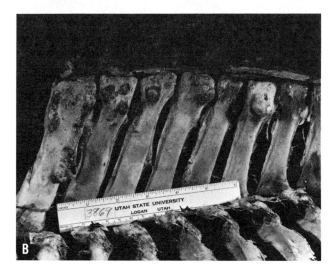

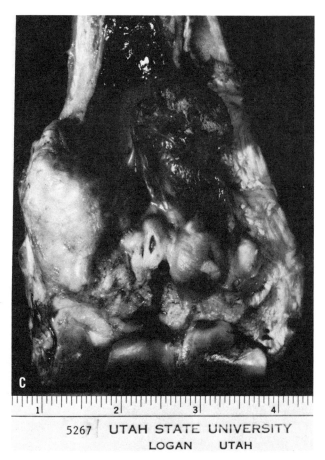

FIG. 4–7. Hereditary multiple exostosis involving the *A)* scapula, *B)* spinous processes of the thoracic vertebrae, and *C)* caudal aspect of the distal extremity of the radius. (Courtesy of Dr. J. L. Shupe, Utah State University.)

the disease should be seriously considered. Cases of solitary osteochondromas causing a lameness may require surgical excision.

TUMORAL CALCINOSIS (CALCINOSIS CIRCUMSCRIPTA)

Tumoral calcinosis is the formation of calcified, granular deposits in the subcutaneous tissues that induces fibrous tissue formation. The deposits usually occur near joints and tendon sheaths. It occurs infrequently in the horse, although it may be more common than is actually recognized. The cause of the condition is unknown.

The horse is presented most frequently because of an unsightly swelling that is becoming progressively larger. There is a low incidence of associated lameness with this condition. The swellings are firm and pain-less, and the skin is usually intact and movable over the swellings. A history of trauma is rarely reported. The most common location for tumoral calcinosis lesions is the lateral aspect of the stifle.

The treatment for calcinosis circumscripta is surgical excision. This should be performed only in cases in which lameness can be directly attributed to the lesion.

BRAN DISEASE AND BIGHEAD (OSTEODYSTROPHIA FIBROSA)

Bran disease is a generalized bone disease caused primarily by a dietary calcium deficiency in the face of a phosphorus excess. Presently, the classic form of this disease is rare due to improved knowledge in feeding practices in the horse. It occurs in horses that have been fed cereal and cereal by-products (which contain high levels of phosphorus) such as bran, hence the name "bran disease." "Bran disease" can be reproduced with a dietary calcium to phosphorus ratio of 1:3 or greater irrespective of the amount of calcium intake. It is seen in horses with diets high in phosphorus and low in calcium, such as would occur with grain or bran feeding or indiscriminate force feeding high phosphorus mineral. Addition of a legume hay high in calcium can prevent the disease. It is also seen in horses grazing plants high in oxalates, which chelate the calcium and interfere with the absorption of calcium.

Cause. The underlying cause is defective mineralization of bone. The diet high in phosphorus leads to increased absorption of phosphorus and elevation of serum phosphate levels. This tends to lower serum calcium and stimulate the parathyroid glands to increase secretion of parathyroid hormone. Parathyroid hormone increases activation of remodeling, leading to resorption of bone. With bone resorption there is a compensatory replacement with fibrous tissue. This results in poorly mineralized bone that is eventually replaced with a cellular connective tissue. Horses of both sexes and all ages are susceptible. Lactating mares and foals are more at risk.

Signs. The classic form of osteodystrophia fibrosa is called "bighead" because of the predilection of the jaws and flat bones of the skull to respond to parathyroid hormone. The classic clinical signs of the disease include a symmetric enlargement of the mandible and facial bones (Fig. 4–8 *A*). There is loss of bone around the teeth, which is one of the first signs of the disease. The teeth may eventually loosen. Swelling initially begins just above the facial crest and in the mandible producing a reduction in intermandibular space (Fig. 4–8 *B*).

If oxalate-containing plants are suspected, then such plants should be analyzed for levels of oxalate. Oxalate levels in certain plants have been shown to vary, being the highest during active growth after rain.

HYPERTROPHIC OSTEOPATHY

Hypertrophic osteopathy is a progressive bilaterally symmetric proliferation of subperiosteal bone and fibrous connective tissue on the appendicular and axial skeleton and facial bones. It is a relatively rare disease in the horse. It occurs in man and dogs more commonly and is usually associated with pulmonary tumors.

The cause of hypertrophic osteopathy is still unclear at present. Classically, the disease is associated with a space-occupying lung lesion such as a neoplasm or chronic pus-producing process such as a large abscess, tuberculosis, or a fractured rib with pleural adhesions. Hypertrophic osteopathy has been reported in a mare with a dysgerminoma (a neoplasm of ovarian primordial germ cells) that had abdominal metastases but was free of thoracic lesions.

The clinical signs include obvious symmetric enlargement of the longbones of the limb. All bones in the limb are affected. There is pain and edema of soft tissues.

On x-rays, there is a generalized increase in soft tissue swelling as well as a periostitis. Irregular new bone growth occurs, especially at the proximal and distal ends of the longbones. The differential diagnosis should include fluorosis, but the gross appearance of bones, absence of dental lesions, as well as blood and urine fluorine levels can rule fluorosis out. With the new high-powered x-ray machines, it may be possible to localize a lesion on lateral radiographs of the chest.

EPIPHYSITIS (PHYSEAL DYSPLASIA)

Epiphysitis is a very important generalized bone disease of young growing horses characterized by enlargement of the physeal regions (growth plates) of certain longbones and the cervical vertebrae. Two syndromes have been recognized. The first occurs in young rapidly growing horses such as foals and weanlings, with a peak incidence of 4 to 8 months. The second is seen in young horses that are beginning training (yearlings and horses up to 2 years of age). The term "epiphysitis" is a misnomer as there is no active inflammation of the epiphysis, physis, or metaphysis. Because the lesion is more directly related to changes in the growth plate rather than the epiphysis, a preferable term would be dysplasia (abnormal tissue development) of the growth plate. The condition is a self-limiting one, disappearing as the growth plates close.

Epiphysitis has also been called rickets, which is also somewhat of a misnomer. Rickets classically results from a vitamin D deficiency, which in turn causes reduced calcium and phosphorus levels. Some of the manifestations of epiphysitis are similar to rickets, but because an overt vitamin D deficiency is uncommon or rare in horses, the term rickets should not be used. Most equine clinicians agree that the syndrome of epiphysitis has increased in incidence. Many of the aspects of epiphysitis are related to excessive or imbalanced feeding, especially high grain rations, without regard to mineral balance and, therefore, certain aspects of the condition are man-made. The condition is also seen in horses on high protein intakes.

The exact cause of epiphysitis is unknown, but popular theories include nutrition, rapid growth rate, genetic predisposition, and trauma. In essence, diets low in calcium and high in phosphorus are responsible. This is similar to "bran disease", although a high grain, low roughage component also seems to be involved. However, simply feeding a high quality ration does not reproduce the disease. Several other factors, such as the trauma component and perhaps certain trace minerals, may also be involved. Epiphysitis does have a certain mechanical as well as nutritional component. Individuals are frequently heavily muscled. The condition is often seen in overweight, active foals

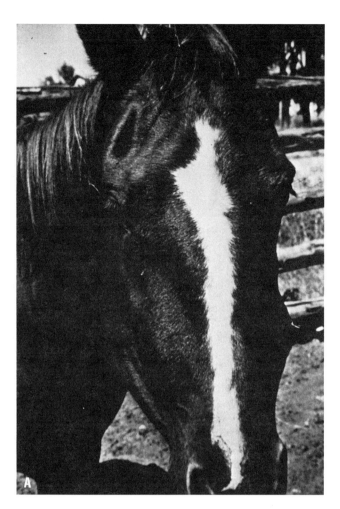 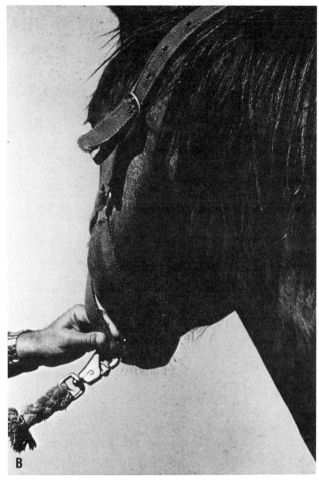

FIG. 4–8. *A*, Symmetric enlargement of the facial bones in a horse with nutritional secondary hyperparathyroidism. (Courtesy of Dr. R. A. McKenzie, Animal Research Institute, Yeerongpilly, Queensland, Australia.) *B*, Mandibular swelling in a horse with nutritional secondary hyperparathyroidism.

and yearlings. Similarly, a foal with severe lameness in one limb may develop an epiphysitislike condition of the contralateral weight-bearing limb as well as an angular limb deformity. The term epiphysitis is often referred to as epiphyseal "compression," which emphasizes the mechanical component of epiphysitis. Epiphysitis may be compounded since breeders are selecting sires and dams that produce rapidly growing offspring that hopefully will do better in the show ring. The Quarter Horse seems more prone to epiphysitis, although there is no statistical evidence to back up such an observation. It is a disease of the well cared for animal in most cases.

The clinical appearance of a horse with epiphysitis is metaphyseal flaring, which is enlargement of the ends of the longbones, especially the distal extremities of the radius, tibia, and cannon bones (Fig. 4–9). This results in an hourglass shape to such bones. Frequently, all limbs are affected to some degree. There is a variable degree of lameness. The lameness may be mild and intermittent. Severe cases may have increased warmth and pain to deep palpation over the affected regions. These are usually the lamest of the epiphysitis cases. The lameness may be no more than a generalized stiffness. Affected individuals may not play as actively as other members of the herd. Epiphysitis may be sporadic in nature, affecting one or two horses in an entire herd, or may involve the entire herd. It is often seen in conjunction with other developmental orthopedic conditions as well. Epiphysitis and osteochondrosis (p. 149) may also be related to various malformations of the vertebral column that can lead to various abnormalities of the gait and make up part of the general "wobbler syndrome" in horses. The affected individual, especially the younger group involved, may have concurrent angular limb deformities (Fig. 4–10). Some horses may have certain manifestations of osteochondritis dissecans as well as subchondral cystlike lesions. Frequently, the affected individual has an upright conformation in the fetlock joints and may periodically knuckle forward. Severe cases may have degenerative joint disease in one or more joints, such as bone spavin and ringbone. Epiphysitis has also been associated with a toe-in confor-

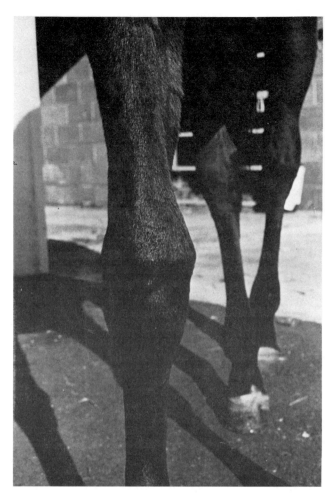

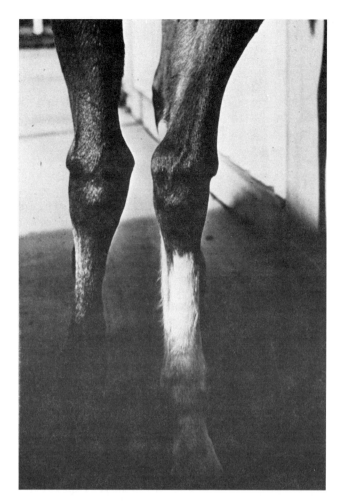

FIG. 4–9. Epiphysitis in a 2-year-old Thoroughbred colt with metaphyseal flaring of the distal radius.

FIG. 4–10. A 5-month-old foal with an angular limb deformity (carpus valgus) and concurrent epiphysitis. There is noticeable metaphyseal flaring of the distal extremities of the radii.

mation that increases the compressive load on the medial side of the forelimb. This produces a more prominent metaphyseal enlargement on the medial side of the affected physis. The so-called contracted tendons or flexure deformities have also been associated with epiphysitis.

X-rays are useful for evaluating the degree of epiphysitis and for identifying other irregularities associated with it.

The first step in treating epiphysitis is to evaluate the ration. Many times, a geographic nutritional deficiency may exist, and this needs to be corrected. Usually an entire herd is involved if there is a geographic nutritional deficiency.

The horse should be prevented from becoming overweight and a general reduction in body weight is advisable if the animal is obese. This decreases the trauma component of the epiphysitis. Associated mineral imbalances should be corrected, which usually requires dietary analysis.

Nonsteroidal anti-inflammatory drugs are used in certain cases in which the animal is stiff. This will help diminish pain and prevent the further development of flexure deformities. Nonsteroidal anti-inflammatory drugs may be required on a low-level, long-term regime. Generally, cases of epiphysitis resolve spontaneously and the horse "grows out of it," but often the horse is left with a residual problem that can be severe enough to limit future athletic soundness.

ANGULAR LIMB DEFORMITIES (SEE CHAPTER 5)

Diseases and Injury of Muscle

Three major muscle types in equine skeletal muscle have been identified. These three muscle types have been designated Type 1, Type 2a and Type 2b. In man, the capacity for muscle performance (i.e., athletic performance) can be related to the individual's type of fiber profile. Studies have shown that long-distance runners usually have a higher proportion of slow twitch (Type 1) fibers than the general population, while athletes who have a predominance of fast twitch (Type 2) fibers are more likely to excel in sprinting.

Type 1 Fibers

These are slow twitch (ST), high oxidative red fibers and have lower glycogen storage capacity. They have a slow speed of contraction, exhibit little or no fatigue, are good for slow speeds, and are equipped for aerobic metabolism. These fibers retain their slow twitch aerobic capacity throughout the animal's life. Horses with the highest proportion of these fibers usually have the best performance record in endurance events.

Type 2 Fibers

These are fast twitch white fibers (FT) and have a well-developed glycolytic pathway but few mitochondria. They fatigue rapidly but are called upon for short-term powerful activity. There are also fast twitch high oxidative red fibers (FTH) or Type 2b that have large glycogen storage capabilities, a well-developed glycolytic pathway, and many mitochondria. These resist fatigue better than FT fibers and are suited more to sustained activity.

In horses, the proportion of fibers in the middle gluteal muscle may be related to the breed and the type of work that the breed has been selected for. Quarter Horses or Thoroughbreds involved in sprinting events have fewer ST fibers and a high proportion of FTH and FT fibers compared to a breed such as the Arabian, which is used for endurance events.

To some degree, the proportion of fibers can be altered by training, whereby FT and FTH fibers can undergo interconversion. However, a training stimulus does not seem to affect the ratio of ST to FT and FTH fibers. Training has been shown to increase the cross-sectional area of all three fiber types, similar to what has been observed in human athletes.

Glycogen depletion within muscle can also provide information about performance and muscle fiber composition. The pattern of glycogen depletion during exercise is as follows: ST fibers are the first to be depleted at lower intensity exercise levels because these are the fibers involved in endurance training. As these become depleted, the FTH fibers follow. This is the same pattern of glycogen depletion as occurs in long distance running. Success at endurance rides probably requires a high proportion of ST fibers and adequate muscle glycogen. Repletion of glycogen occurs in the reverse pattern to depletion, with a preferential repletion of FTH (Type 2b) fibers relative to Type 1 fibers. The practical implication of this is that exercise should be restricted in this postride period to allow sufficient repletion of muscle glycogen.

Muscle Response to Injury

Degeneration

Cloudy Swelling. This is a mild form of injury that is only visible microscopically. Cloudy swelling may be caused by mild deviations in cellular metabolism such as would be seen in cases of tying-up syndrome in the horse (discussed later).

Hyaline (Zenker's) Degeneration. This is a response of the muscle cell in a variety of different conditions, such as white muscle disease and azoturia. Hyaline degeneration affects the cytoplasm.

Granular Degeneration. This is a more severe grade of degeneration. Many nuclei die making regeneration difficult. In cells that have viable nuclei, regeneration is possible.

Fatty Degeneration. This is an irreversible change seen following granular degeneration.

Regeneration

Skeletal muscle has the capacity for regeneration if certain structures are intact. The regenerative process can be classified into three basic types: 1) regeneration by budding; 2) regeneration by proliferation of cellular bands; and 3) regeneration by recombination of muscle fibers along adjacent surviving sarcoplasm (muscle cytoplasm). Regeneration by budding occurs when segments of fiber are destroyed as would occur in a clean incision. The crucial factor is the size of the gap between the free ends of the tube with large buds forming at the ends of the muscle cells that advance across the gap, making contact with similar growths from the other side of the incision. These buds grow just over 1 mm per day, and a certain amount of cross over and interlacing of fibers inevitably occurs. If the gap is greater than 5 mm or infection or fibroblastic (scar) tissue is present, then bridging may be retarded. A certain amount of fibroblastic tissue will be seen in such gaps.

If the injury to the muscle cell is milder, regeneration occurs by proliferation of cellular bands. Macrophages (scavenger cells) clear away the degenerating substances, nuclei proliferate, and new sarcoplasm appears. Longitudinal and cross striations are restored. Regeneration by fusion of muscle fibers with the same sarcoplasm is seen in fibers undergoing granular degeneration. In certain conditions, the ability of muscle to regenerate is lost. This is seen with the very chronic (over 1 year) denervation muscle atrophy such as in sweeney in horses.

Atrophy

Muscle atrophy is a decrease in the volume of muscle due to a decrease in size of individual muscle cells. It occurs when a muscle is not subjected to sustained periods of tension. It is a potentially reversible phenomenon because artificial stimulation can reverse the atrophy. Muscle atrophy is seen predominantly in the muscles of the locomotor system.

Generalized Muscle Atrophy. Generalized muscle atrophy is associated with poor nutrition, malnutrition, or senility. Muscle atrophy due to senility in the horse is rare because horses do not reach the same equivalent age as human beings. Generalized muscle atrophy is also seen in horses with severe systemic illnesses and is occasionally seen in hospitalized patients that have suffered surgical complications (e.g., peritonitis). In addition to generalized muscle atrophy, there will be a loss of fat from the depots as well as a decrease in body weight. Usually, the loss of muscle is symmetric in distribution but not all muscles are affected to the same degree.

Localized Muscle Atrophy. Localized muscle atrophy is seen associated with paralysis (e.g., sweeney) or from immobilization of a limb in a cast or following an injury such as an episode of rhabdomyolysis (potentially fatal skeletal muscle disease). Localized muscle atrophy is commonly seen in horses with casts or other forms of external fixation. Such immobilization will produce a hyperextension of the limbs due to a lack of tone of the flexor muscles and associated tendons. Muscle atrophy following a full limb cast application is very rapid and, for this reason, if casting is to be prolonged, the cast will be changed frequently so the cast does not become too loose. Return of muscle volume is slow with this type of atrophy. Localized muscle atrophy is also seen following a tendon rupture or fracture of a bone that is required for muscle function such as triceps atrophy that occurs with fractures of the olecranon or atrophy of the extensor carpi radialis following transection of its tendon due to, say, a wire cut. If atrophy persists, the muscle will eventually be replaced with fibrous and adipose (fat) tissue.

Atrophy of Denervation (Neurogenic Muscle Atrophy). This is usually a localized phenomenon as well and is characteristic of a few well-recognized syndromes in the horse, the best known of which is denervation atrophy due to paralysis of the suprascapular nerve (sweeny). The involvement of the suprascapular nerve is usually due to pressure from a poor-fitting collar in working horses, kicks, falls, and scapular fractures. Following denervation, paralysis of the respective muscles will result. Paralysis of the radial nerve following fractures of the humerus may also result in severe muscle atrophy in the forearm.

Lesions within the central nervous system (CNS) (brain and spinal cord) can produce denervation atrophy. The muscles that are atrophied here are those that receive innervation from the particular region of the CNS that is damaged. Brain tumors, although rare in horses, have the same effect. Protozoal myeloencephalitis also results in localized muscle atrophy.

In contrast to generalized atrophy, atrophy of denervation occurs in groups of fibers supplied by the nerve. Ultimately, the muscle is replaced with adipose and fibrous tissue.

Denervated muscle fibers can be reinnervated if the neural sheaths are not injured. If injury is mild, then most nerves can regenerate (at about 4 mm per day) and the original continuity to the muscle can be reestablished. If severe nerve injury occurs (e.g., transection) following a wire cut or other type of trauma, regrowth of the nerve ending to the muscle is delayed and concurrent muscle atrophy may be so severe that even when a functional connection is made, there may be only a limited number of fibers available for reinnervation. A more significant cause of debility seen in horses with muscle atrophy, particularly of the limbs, is contracture or shortening of the musculotendinous unit. In addition, joint capsule contracture may occur in the involved limb.

Calcification and Ossification of Muscle

Calcification. This occurs when calcium salts are deposited in degenerating muscle tissue. The muscle fibers first undergo granular degeneration, at which stage they are apparently highly susceptible to calcification. The most common instance of muscle calcification is seen in degeneration due to nutritional causes, such as white muscle disease associated with vitamin E/selenium deficiency.

Ossification. This is the formation of bone in the connective tissue of muscle. It is seen in muscles that have been chronically traumatized or inflamed. It may occur as a result of metaplasia (abnormal tissue transformation), which is common, or may be seen in long bone fractures where there has been displacement of periosteum.

Ossification of muscle is seen primarily in two instances in horses: 1) ossifying myopathy of the semitendinosus muscle, and 2) ossification of the biceps brachii muscle.

In horses, trauma that occurs with repeated tearing or straining of the muscle fibers will result in ossification. Such trauma occurs in the semitendinosis of horses that use their hindlimbs excessively. For this reason, the condition of ossifying fibrotic myopathy is seen more frequently in the Quarter Horse involved in ranch work as well as in horses used for reining. The end result of repeated tearing or straining of muscle is gradual replacement by fibrous tissue and ultimately irregular jagged plaques of spongy bone are produced with loose fibrous tissue in the interstices. Muscle fibers in the region become atrophic. There may also be adhesions to adjacent muscles, including biceps femoris and semimembranosus. Because the muscle lacks elasticity, it results in a typical goose-stepping gait, characterized by a shortened cranial phase of stride with the limb being pulled back before the sole hits the ground. The gait is most evident at the walk. Palpation usually reveals a firm, hard scar tissue and x-rays may identify ossification in the affected muscle, although this is relatively uncommon. If the biceps brachii muscle is involved, the horse has a shortened cranial phase of stride tending to land on the toes similar to navicular disease.

The treatment of such a condition involves either surgical removal of the affected scar tissue and muscle or transection of the tibial insertion of the semitendinosus muscle. This has been performed when the ossification involves the semitendinosus but has not been performed in cases in which the biceps brachii has been involved. It is highly unlikely that surgery is indicated for ossification of the biceps brachii since the tendon and bicipital bursa are usually involved.

Inflammation of Muscle

The term "myositis" is often applied to degeneration of muscle. Strictly speaking, myositis is a reactive inflammation. A certain amount of inflammation, however, is seen with true degeneration of muscle. Inflammation of skeletal muscle is quite common in horses because of the frequent occurrence of trauma such as lacerations and wire cuts.

Causes of myositis associated with wire lacerations are usually bacterial. Muscles are highly susceptible to bacterial invasion by spore-forming organisms of the genus *Clostridia*. The bacterial exotoxin (poisen) causes further muscle swelling that produces ischemia (reduction in blood supply), resulting in an anaerobic environment conducive to further bacterial proliferation and toxin production. Death can occur from toxemia. The types of wounds often associated with clostridial myositis in horses are usually small and benign. If the wound edges seal over, an anaerobic environment results. This is conducive to growth of clostridial organisms. Bacterial spores then commence vegetative growth. The species of *Clostridia* involved are commonly found in spore form in soil and feces. Because of the environment of the horse, any penetrating wounds may potentially result in an anaerobic infection. Fortunately, most limb wounds in horses are large and open enough so that clostridial myositis is not a major problem.

Sites affected with myositis are painful on palpation and have variable swelling and firmness. Some horses may have systemic signs, fever, and lameness to a varying degree. Sometimes the lameness is extremely severe and resembles a fractured bone or an abscess in the foot. If clostridial organisms are involved, the horse will be severely lame and have severe systemic signs, and the outcome may be fatal if toxemia results. Chronic cases of bacterial myositis may result in muscle wasting.

Viral myositis is rare in the horse but is occasionally seen in certain viral respiratory infections. Myositis is occasionally caused in horses by injection of irritating substances. Such substances include oxytetracycline, phenylbutazone, chloral hydrate, iron injections, and others. If iron injections are given over the gluteal muscles, myositis may be so severe that grave consequences, such as abscessation and fibrotic myopathy, will result.

Circulatory Disturbances of Muscle

Circulatory disturbances of muscles in horses can occur in a number of ways. If there is swelling of a particular muscle, then this may result in collapse of capillaries. Such collapse is predisposed by the fact that capillaries run parallel to surrounding muscle fibers. Another circulatory disturbance of muscle occurs when there is obstruction of a major artery of the limbs but this is a relatively infrequent cause of lameness.

Direct injury to the artery supplying a muscle, such as would occur with a wire cut when the vessel is actually severed, may also result in muscle ischemia.

With venous occlusion (blockage of blood flow), the muscle becomes congested and there is a much greater inflammatory response than with arterial occlusion. Healing of muscle damage due to venous occlusion results in more scar tissue. Such an injury is seen in horses subjected to prolonged sternal recumbency such as occurs with problems of the central nervous system. The lesions are seen in the limb that is "down" and may involve the semitendinosus and part of the proximal gastrocnemius muscles. The cause is sustained pressure on muscle leading to venous occlusion and thrombosis.

Diagnosis of Muscle Diseases in the Horse

Examination of muscles should be included as part of the overall lameness examination.

Physical Examination

Examination with respect to muscles begins with visualization for symmetry. The symmetry of the muscle is best determined by comparing it with the opposite side of the animal. Are the abnormalities unilateral or bilateral? Symmetry is observed from a distance. The horse should be examined at various gaits and any lameness noted. The suspected regions are examined for soreness and palpated for degree of firmness, pain, and temperature. If atrophy is from sweeny or disuse, the various muscles affected must be identified. The muscles should be palpated to see if they are flaccid or tense. Muscle enlargement may be due to fat or scar tissue accumulation rather than an increase in diameter of individual muscle cells. Some muscles are more susceptible to denervation than others.

Muscle pain may be difficult to determine in horses unless it is severe. It occurs in response to overexertion similar to the situation in man. Viral respiratory diseases as well as other systemic diseases can cause muscular pain.

Clinical Pathology

When any tissue is damaged, certain enzymes leak into the blood stream and the degree of tissue damage is reflected in the measured levels.

Interpretation of muscle enzyme values is made in light of the clinical situation, including the animal's daily training routine and stage of fitness. Acute muscle damage causes marked elevations in serum enzymes, whereas slow progressive damage may have levels within normal ranges. In some cases, horses are exercised vigorously on the treadmill, after which samples are taken to identify abnormal elevations in muscle enzymes.

Electromyography (EMG)

Electromyography refers to changes in electric potential associated with motor unit twitch. Needle electrodes inserted into the muscle are used to pick up action potentials that are displayed on a cathode ray oscilliscope. This technique is useful to indicate muscle damage and is used to identify muscle diseases originating in the nervous system from those of disuse.

Biopsy

Microscopic examination of muscle can be used for diagnosis of pathologic conditions as well as assessment of athletic potential in normal animals. It is useful to check for inflammation or edema. The middle gluteal muscle is the one usually biopsied for studies in exercise physiology, although in disease states, the muscles that are actively involved are selected.

Systemic Diseases of Muscle

Exercise-Related Myopathies (Exertional Myopathies)

Exercise-related or exertional myopathies have been grouped under one general heading and include such terms as "paralytic myoglobinuria," "exertional rhabdomyolysis," "Monday morning disease," "myositis," "tying-up," and "azoturia." Although these terms encompass a wide range of diseases that are associated with exercise, in all probability they are related and represent varying degrees of the same condition. Azoturia is the most severe form of the conditions; tying-up denotes the mildest form.

Exercise-related myopathies are usually seen in fit working and performance horses. Classically, the disease was described as occurring following exercise after a period of inactivity in which the horse has been on a full ration. A high carbohydrate ration is usually implicated. Causes of inactivity may be bad weather, lameness, or injury. Monday morning disease was seen when the horse was rested over the weekend, maintained on full ration, and resumed work on Monday.

A similar exertional myopathy is also seen in unfit horses in which there has been inadequate conditioning for the degree of exercise attempted. This form of the disease is seen occasionally in horses competing in endurance events (trail rides, etc). However, this type of myopathy is consistent with energy (glycogen) depletion within the muscles rather than an energy abundance. The condition is also commonly seen in nervous or excitable animals and heavily muscled horses. It occurs more frequently in cold, damp weather. Mares and fillies seem to be affected more than colts or geldings, which has led to the speculation that a hormonal abnormality may be involved. It has been noted that a correlation exists between previous corticosteroid administration and tying-up.

Causes and Progression. Although the basic underlying mechanisms of exercise related myopathies is poorly understood, they are possibly related to ischemia (a localized reduction in blood flow). Classically, the horse that succumbs to the condition known as azoturia is one that has been maintained on a high grain diet during a period of rest. This apparently leads to glycogen accumulation within the muscle and the horse appears to have a greater ability to store glycogen than other species. When the animal is exercised, and subjects certain muscle groups to anaerobic metabolism, excessive lactic acid is produced, which results in swelling of the affected muscle fibers. Affected individuals accumulate excessive glycogen. The fibers most commonly affected are the fast twitch fibers (FTH and FT fibers). These have higher glycogen stores than the slow twitch fibers. The reduction in cellular oxygen causes increased local levels of metabolic by-products, including lactic acid, to be released.

Tying-up seen in the horse that is involved in endurance related activities occurs in the later stages of competition and is a result of an energy (glycogen) depletion. Such a depletion causes a similar clinical picture (pain, stiffness) but with a different cause and progression. Other causes include dietary deficiency in vitamin E and/or selenium, artery damage due to blood worms, deviations in intracellular calcium metabolism and toxic levels of certain antibiotics (ionophores such as monensin).

Hypothyroidism (depressed thyroid function) may also be involved in exertional myopathies. Causes may include stress due to training, infectious disease, transport, adverse weather conditions, as well as the demands of growth. All of these may occur simultaneously in a young racehorse that is beginning a training program.

Clinical Signs. For the sake of simplicity, the clinical signs of exertional-related myopathies will be divided into three syndromes: Azoturia, tying-up, and endurance-related myopathy.

Azoturia. Azoturia is the more severe form of exercise-related myopathy. It is seen in heavier breeds and occurs shortly after the horse begins to work. Muscle stiffness and muscle spasms of the loin and hindlimbs, profuse sweating, tachycardia (rapid heart beat), hyperventilation, a slight fever, and an anxious facial expression are common. Because this resembles or mimics abdominal pain, it may lead to a diagnosis of colic. The horse is often reluctant to move, and the symptoms may be confused with laminitis, tetanus, hypocalcemia (lactation tetany), or pleuritis. In some cases, the horse may become recumbent. If exercise is continued, it will further exacerbate the problems associated with ischemia and pressure on affected muscles.

Urine will vary from a red brown to black depending on the amount of myoglobin content (myoglobinuria). Varying degrees of myoglobinuria occur due to the escape of myoglobin from damaged muscle cells. Because the renal threshold for myoglobin has been exceeded, it is excreted in the urine. Myoglobinuria is a useful sign to help rule out other conditions that may mimic azoturia.

Tying-up. Tying-up is considered a mild form of azoturia with some signs similar but not to the same degree as azoturia. Affected horses may or may not have myoglobinuria, although some feel that if myoglobinuria is present, the disease should be called azoturia. Tying-up is commonly seen when the horse is cooled out after vigorous exercise. Clinical signs include local or diffuse sweating, anxiety, stiffness, myalgia, and muscle tremors. The muscles may be hard and the horse is usually reluctant to move and has a short, stilted gait.

Endurance Related Myopathy. The clinical signs of this exertional myopathy are similar to tying-up but typically occur in a poorly or inadequately conditioned horse that has been ridden long distances. This may occur in trail rides and endurance events and is an important reason why veterinary supervision at such competitions is mandatory. As well as having stiffness, muscle tremors, and muscle pain, the horse may show signs of severe electrolyte disturbances (thumps or synchronous diaphragmatic flutter). The patient may be severely dehydrated (reduced skin turgor, dry coat). The condition may become so severe that the horse will refuse to move at all. This resembles the energy depleted state of the marathoner known as "hitting the wall."

Myositis of the Longissimus Muscles. This is also an exercise myopathy. It is most frequently seen in Standardbreds as well as hunters and jumpers but can be seen in other breeds. The condition is essentially a localized exertional myopathy of this muscle group. The resultant muscle spasms lead to a gait alteration in the hindlimbs resembling bilateral hindlimb lameness and begins with a shortening of the stride. The

condition unfortunately serves as a catchall for undiagnosed hindlimb lamenesses in many horses with afflictions elsewhere. It is an integral part of the sore back syndrome in horses and may be seen secondary to conditions of the stifle or hock. Poor jumping technique as well as the horse twisting itself over the jumps is a common complaint. The signs are usually vague and are frequently mistaken for problems in the limbs. Because of the vagueness of the condition, many remedies such as chiropractic, physiotherapy, ultrasound, and faradism have benefited in reputation with treatment of this condition.

Diagnosis. Laboratory tests are useful to confirm the diagnosis of exertional myopathies. Muscle enzymes usually rise rapidly when there is acute muscle damage. Some horses may have low serum potassium and low serum chloride.

Treatment. Treatment of azoturia and tying-up is directed toward several fronts and is primarily supportive in nature. The main aim should be to minimize further movement if at all possible, particularly in the severely affected horse. This is often difficult if the horse suffers an attack some distance from the stable or accessible transportation. Horse owners have a natural tendency to want to "walk the horse out of it" in an attempt to "free up" affected muscles or when the condition has been mistaken for colic. This should be condemned especially in severe cases.

Tranquilizers are useful to relieve anxiety in some cases. They also produce a small vessel dialation (vasodilation) that not only increases circulation to the affected muscles but also may aid in the removal of deleterious by-products of anaerobic metabolism. Because of this peripheral vasodilating effect, they should only be administered to hydrated horses.

Aggressive intravenous fluid therapy is often undertaken in severe cases. Such therapy will treat dehydration as well as encourage urination and minimize myoglobin precipitation in the renal tubules. (Myoglobin is toxic to the tubules.)

Analgesic and anti-inflammatory drugs are most useful and, in mild cases, may be the only therapy required. Corticosteroids have been implicated in precipitating tying-up and laminitis.

Muscle relaxants may be used in severe cases. Analgesia with narcotic agents are used in the severely distressed horse that is struggling and exacerbating the condition.

Other forms of supportive therapy play an important role especially in the severe case. The horse should be kept away from cold drafts and blanketed. Massage of affected muscles with hot towels may also be of some benefit. The horse should be left in recumbency until it has the strength and confidence to stand. Horses with malignant hyperthermia (extreme heat sensitivity) usually require alcohol or ice baths and ice water enemas to reduce their temperature.

Following the initial episode of azoturia or tying-up, several measures are usually recommended. Some may be of benefit. Oral electrolyte therapy is advocated, especially supplementation with potassium chloride (KCl) (1 oz daily). There are no controlled studies to justify this procedure, although it does appear to be safe. Vitamin E/selenium supplementation is frequently advocated. Although controlled studies proving its efficacy are lacking, anecdotal evidence has indicated that certain horses will be spared exertional myopathies while on this medication indefinitely. Monthly injections of vitamin E/selenium preparations or continuous low-level feeding of the drug is recommended. If a definitive diagnosis of hypothyroidism is made (based on T_4 levels in a blood test) then supplementation of these horses with thyroid hormone may be of benefit. However, it is important to remember that horses being treated with phenylbutazone typically have lowered T_4 levels, which may cause an erroneous diagnosis of hypothyroidism. Dietary sodium bicarbonate supplementation (1% to 4% of dry matter) has been shown in one study to be beneficial in the treatment of recurrent exertional myopathies.

Other Myopathies

Nutritional Myopathy

In foals nutritional myopathy is classically recognized from birth to 7 months of age and is believed to result from a vitamin E/selenium deficiency. Factors associated with a vitamin E/selenium deficiency include rancid feed, addition of fish or plant oil to the feed, poor quality hay, and lush pastures. The condition is also seen in adult horses but with a different clinical manifestation. Nutritional myopathy is seen in various parts of the world when soil and pastures are low in selenium. Horses residing in these areas may be more prone to azoturia, although this observation has not been substantiated with statistical analysis and only anecdotal evidence is available. Nutritional myopathy is also seen if pastures have high sulfur levels.

The exact role of vitamin E/selenium is unclear.

Generalized Myopathy Associated with Prolonged Recumbency or General Anesthesia

Myopathy associated with extended periods of prolonged recumbency or general anesthesia is seen occasionally in horses. The condition was originally thought to be a primary neurologic problem due to nerve compression and dysfunction. Most evidence now supports the hypothesis that the condition is primarily a myopathy caused by local hypoxia of various muscle groups. Although it is referred to as myositis, this is probably a misnomer and the word myopathy should be used. The condition commonly occurs in a localized form, although a generalized myopathy involving all muscle groups is occasionally seen. Localized myopathies related to general anesthesia or recumbency are believed to be due to compression of the muscle groups that compromise circulation. Therefore, those muscles that are lowermost are affected and include the triceps brachii, quadriceps femoris, hindlimb extensors, masseter, and flank muscles. For horses positioned in dorsal recumbency, the muscles of the back—longissimus, iliocostalis, gluteal medius, as well as the vastus lateralis—are affected. In most cases, the down limb is affected. Occasionally, the upper limb is involved, in which case the cause is felt to be compromised circulation. This occurs when the limb overhangs the edge of the table or is allowed to assume a crisscrossed position.

Cause. The condition is seen following general anesthesia of greater than $2\frac{1}{2}$ hours duration and in horses positioned in recumbency on hard surfaces. It is also seen following very deep anesthesia for procedures requiring muscle relaxation, such as ovarectomy and surgery of the eye. Deep anesthesia reduces blood pressure, cardiac output, and oxygen supply to tissues. Postanesthetic myopathy is also seen following other disorders that may cause recumbency such as CNS diseases. It is seen in heavily muscled breeds, draft breeds, Quarter Horses, and especially in horses taken out of training and placed under general anesthesia for one reason or another (e.g., fracture repair). Patient position and type of padding under the horse is also involved. The condition does limit recovery from certain conditions such as long bone fractures and certain CNS diseases.

Signs. In the localized form of the condition, the horse will usually stand from the anesthetic and is initially unaffected. Either in the recovery stall or back in its stall, a syndrome of muscular weakness develops and the horse adopts a dropped-elbow appearance. This appears superficially like radial nerve paralysis, but horses are usually able to use extensors. If the hindlimb is involved then the horse will show knuckling of the fetlock. If the quadriceps femoris is involved, the stifle will drop and the horse will be unable to stand. Most horses that develop these problems have a long recovery time. The discomfort usually persists for 2 to 3 days postoperatively in uncomplicated cases. The affected muscle masses may become hard and swollen. If the condition is very painful, it may invoke fear and pain and produce struggling, which only compounds the problem.

In horses with a generalized myopathy, there is usually involvement of the limbs that were not dependent. It has been seen regardless of the time involved in general anesthesia and does not affect muscles under pressure. Muscles become rigid even before the horse stands from the anesthetic. There may be anxiety, sweating, and even signs of colic. The animal may not be able to stand, making management of the condition very difficult. Myoglobinuria, renal failure, shock, and death are frequent sequelae. This syndrome may be caused by the actual anesthetic agent itself resembling malignant hyperthermia rather than purely pressure on affected muscles.

Diagnosis. Serum enzymes are usually elevated due to leakage from muscle cells. A rise in muscle enzymes is frequently seen without clinical signs of muscle damage and, therefore, rises in serum enzymes must be correlated with clinical signs. Enzymes are useful to evaluate the severity of the muscle damage as well as to establish a prognosis on horses that develop the condition. Decreased serum calcium levels have also been reported.

Treatment. Treatment is similar to what has been described for exertional myopathies and therefore is essentially symptomatic. The initial aim of treatment should be directed at preventing further muscle damage. Mild cases require nothing more than observation, whereas others require nonsteroidal antiinflammatory drugs. For muscle pain, more potent analgesics may be indicated if the horse appears anxious and looks as if it may panic and compound the situation. Tranquilizers to produce vasodilation to the affected muscles is also advocated by some. In addition the horse should have "support" bandages on the opposite limb and be placed in a stall with good footing. Slinging is indicated in severe cases, but not all horses tolerate this method of restraint and it may, in fact, exacerbate the problem if the horse fights the sling. Glucocorticoids are avoided due to the ability of these agents to potentiate laminitis. Fluid therapy is instituted. In some cases muscle relaxants are used. The key to a quick recovery is good nursing care. The horse should be turned frequently and kept clean and dry to minimize the development of sores. Adequate food and water should be available. Much will depend on the personality of the horse. Despite aggressive and heroic measures, some horses tend to give up and succumb to the condition.

Diseases of Joints

General Anatomy of a Synovial Joint

A synovial joint consists of the articulating surfaces of bone covered by articular cartilage, a joint capsule, a cavity within these structures containing synovial fluid, and associated ligaments (Fig. 4–11). The joint capsule is composed of two parts: the outer fibrous layer, which is continuous with the periosteum (membrane covering bone), and the inner synovial membrane, which lines the synovial cavity where articular cartilage is not present. The fibrous portion of the joint capsule is composed of dense fibrous connective tissue that provides some mechanical stability to the joint. It also has numerous nerves that are sensitive to painful stimuli.

The principal functions of the synovial membrane include phagocytosis (engulfing foreign substances by the white blood cells), regulation of protein and hyaluronate content of the synovial fluid, and regeneration. Unwanted materials are engulfed and become contained within phagocytic vacuoles and are digested. Excessive phagocytic activity releases enzymes to the synovial fluid (characteristic of synovitis). The synovial membrane acts as an important

permeability barrier that, in turn, controls synovial fluid composition. In traumatic swelling, the changes in protein content and composition of synovial fluid have been associated with both increased vascular permeability and increased protein synthesis. Hyaluronate arises from the synovial membrane. The synovial membrane has the ability to reform following synovectomy (surgical removal of the synovial membrane).

Another property of synovial membrane important in joint function is its ability to stretch and contract. Using the example of a fetlock joint as illustrated in Figure 4–12, it can be seen that synovial membrane gathers at the dorsal aspect of the joint in extension and at the palmar aspect in flexion. This property of gathering has been termed "redundancy." Inflammation and fibrosis (abnormal formation of fibrous tissue) will impede this property and result in joint stiffness. Adequate lubrication of synovial membrane is

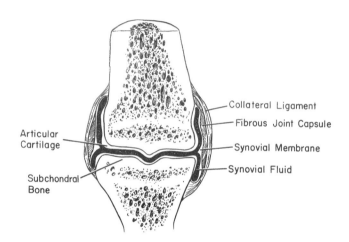

FIG. 4–11. Diagram of a typical synovial joint.

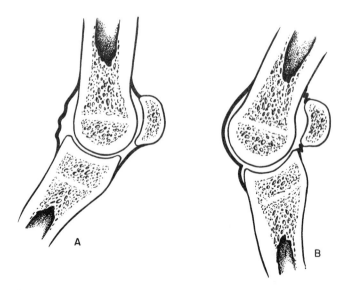

FIG. 4–12. Diagram of a fetlock joint demonstrating how redundant synovial membrane gathers at the dorsal aspect on extension (*A*) and at the palmar aspect on flexion (*B*).

also important for normal joint function, and this is discussed below.

The synovial joint contains two systems that require lubrication: a soft tissue system, involving the sliding of synovial membrane on itself or other tissues, and a cartilage-on-cartilage system. Lubrication of the synovial membrane is by boundary lubrication, and hyaluronate is the important component in the synovial fluid that performs this function. The hyaluronate molecules stick to the surface of the synovial membrane and allow sliding of synovial membrane over the opposing surface. This function is important because a major part of the frictional resistance in joint movement is in the synovial membrane and fibrous joint capsule.

Cartilage-on-cartilage lubrication is independent of hyaluronate and uses two systems: boundary lubrication and hydrostatic lubrication. Boundary lubrication operates at low loads, the necessary component being a glycoprotein lubricating fraction. At higher loads, boundary lubrication fails because the lubricant is sheared off the articular cartilage, and the joint is lubricated by hydrostatic or squeeze-film lubrication. In hydrostatic lubrication, the cartilage surfaces are kept apart by a fluid film made of joint fluid and interstitial fluid that weeps from the articular cartilage itself.

In the past, it was considered that articular cartilage was the main shock absorber of the joint. However, force attenuation studies have shown that the bone and periarticular soft tissues are the primary shock absorbers of the joint.

The Reaction of Joints to Injury

Joint Capsule Inflammation

The synovial membrane is a modified connective tissue and, as such, manifests a typical inflammatory response. Some degree of synovitis is present in most types of equine joint disease. Synovitis results in excess production of synovial fluid with distension of the joint capsule. In mild synovitis, the synovial fluid differs little from normal except that there is more of it; in more severe cases, there is among other changes, a decrease in viscosity.

Inflammation of the synovial membrane is important for the following reasons.

1. It is a source of enzymes potentially destructive to articular cartilage. These enzymes can cause degradation of the proteoglycans and glycosaminoglycans in the cartilage matrix and can digest collagen.
2. Prostaglandins released by inflamed synovium may also cause a decrease in proteoglycan and glycosaminoglycan content of the cartilage matrix in inflamed joints.
3. In an inflamed joint, large amounts of superoxide anions are released into the joint, which has a po-

tent capability to degrade hyaluronic acid, cartilage proteoglycans, and collagen.

4. It is a source of joint pain. Most sensitivity is in the fibrous joint capsule and the associated ligaments. However, stimuli from the synovial membrane can be transmitted to the capsule, and it is recognized that inflammation of the synovial membrane also involves the fibrous joint capsule and causes direct stimulation to the pain sensitive receptors of that structure. If the synovitis is low grade (as occurs in bog spavin), it is feasible that some inflammation may be present without causing pain.
5. The swelling from inflamed synovial membrane may be worsened by the joint capsule distension. The increased intra-articular pressure may also shunt blood, thereby decreasing the effective blood flow to the joint.

Reaction of Articular Cartilage to Injury

The reaction of the articular cartilage to injury is fairly consistent. Trauma can cause an immediate physical defect or initiate a degenerative process. Degeneration of articular cartilage includes softening, fraying, and erosion (see Degenerative Joint Disease (Osteoarthritis) section in this chapter). Loss of glycosaminoglycans and proteglycans constitute "lesions" of the articular cartilage.

In discussing the repair of articular cartilage, it is appropriate to consider two situations: 1) superficial defects that do not penetrate the full thickness of the cartilage; and 2) full-thickness defects. It has been shown that superficial defects in equine articular cartilage do not heal, whereas full-thickness defects can potentially heal through granulation tissue that arises at the articular margin or in the subchondral marrow spaces.

Diagnosis of Joint Disease

Disease changes in a joint can be detected and evaluated in a number of ways. These include clinical examination to detect pain and swelling, synovial fluid analysis, thermography, x-ray examination, arthroscopy, and nuclear medicine. Prior to evaluating specific joints, a general lameness examination is indicated to localize the problem. Refer to Chapter 3 for a discussion of these various diagnostic techniques.

Specific Joint Diseases

Effective management of joint diseases in the horse necessitates the classification and definition of the various disorders. In some instances, however, a joint condition may progress from one classification to another and the treatment and prognosis must change accordingly. For example, a case of traumatic arthritis or septic arthritis may progress to degenerative joint disease.

Idiopathic Synovitis (Bog Spavin and Articular Windpuffs)

Idiopathic synovitis refers to a chronic synovial effusion of a joint of uncertain pathogenesis and unassociated with lameness, tenderness, heat, or radiographic changes. This is commonly seen with bog spavin of the tarsocrural (tibiotarsal) joint (Fig. 4–13). and with windpuffs of the fetlock (Fig. 4–14). See Chapter 5 for more information on bog spavin.

Arthritis

Arthritis is a general term for joint inflammation that describes a range of conditions affecting any joint in the body. It is usually chronic but often has acute signs. "Osteoarthritis," also called Degenerative Joint Disease (DJD) and usually considered synonymous with arthritis, refers to a group of disorders with the common end stage of a progressive deterioration of the articular cartilage accompanied by changes in the bone and soft tissues of the joint. Synovitis is often associated with arthritis. There are various names for arthritis in specific joints, for example: hock arthritis (jack spavin or bone spavin), dorsal fetlock arthritis (osselets), pastern and/or coffin arthritis (ringbone), knee arthritis (carpitis) (Fig. 4–15).

Causes. The chain of events leading to arthritis can be complex and interrelated. The initial causes include hard, heavy, or fast use, a slip or fall, a direct blow to the joint, poor conformation, inadequate conditioning, poor footing, inadequate farrier care, nutritional inadequacies or imbalances, and faulty joint injections. Continued, repeated trauma through hard use, especially if it is coupled with inadequate condi-

tioning, leads to fatigue and overextension of joints. Conformational defects can result in asymmetric stresses to the joints, causing abnormal distribution of weight on joint surfaces and weight being borne by bone edges (Fig. 4–16). Improper or irregular shoeing that results in hoof imbalance causes abnormal joint loading as well. In addition, excessive hoof traction devices (such as toe grabs, stickers, and calks), which prevent normal hoof slippage on landing, can result in joint trauma.

The previously mentioned primary insults result in a variety of intermediate conditions that are often precursors to arthritis. These include joint strain, joint sprain, chip fracture, osteochondrosis, and joint infection. Joint strain occurs from wear and tear, often occurring in the fetlock and hock. It is usually slow and insidious but can be sudden in its onset. Joint strain includes synovitis, the inflammation of the synovial membrane, and capsulitis, inflammation of the fibrous joint capsule. Joint sprain is a stretching or tearing of a supporting ligament associated with a joint

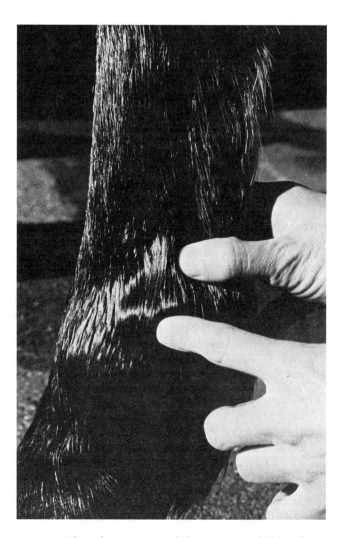

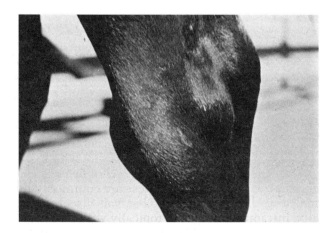

FIG. 4–13. Idiopathic synovitis of the tarsocrural (tibiotarsal) joint (bog spavin).

FIG. 4–14. Idiopathic synovitis of the metacarpophalangeal joint (windpuffs).

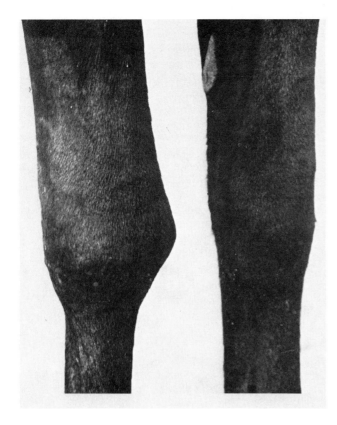

FIG. 4–15. Acute carpitis. The limb is held in a partially flexed position.

when the joint has experienced movement beyond its normal range. This is especially common with young race and futurity horses. Chip fractures can be caused from biomechanical forces within the joint or by direct trauma to the joint. See later sections in this chapter for a discussion of osteochondrosis and infectious arthritis.

Following joint trauma, the synovial membrane exhibits an inflammatory response and releases chemicals that contribute to cartilage breakdown. Subsequently, the toxic by-products of cartilage degradation are released into the synovial fluid and contribute to a self-perpetuating cycle that can eventually destroy the joint. Healthy cartilage that is firm, thick, white, smooth, and glistening changes to that which is soft, yellow, dull, and contains blisters, pits, fragments, overall thinning, or full-thickness sites of erosion (Figs. 4–17 and 4–18). These changes are due in large part to the decrease in one or more of the glycosaminoglycans, important cartilage constituents that give it its firm, tough, yet resilient, quality. In addition to cartilage destruction, bone proliferation changes also occur with arthritis. Osteophyte (bone spur) formation and periosteal proliferation are steps leading to ankylosis.

Signs. The lameness associated with arthritis is a decreased range of motion. For example, with bilateral osselets, the gait would be short and choppy. With carpitis, there would be a shortening of the cranial phase of the stride due to decreased knee flexion. In addition to various degrees of lameness, there is often heat and joint swelling, pain on palpation and flexion of the joint, and a palpable thickening of the dorsal aspect of the joint in such cases as carpitis and osselets. By the time signs appear, arthritis may already be well established.

Diagnosis. Diagnosis includes a thorough clinical examination, x-rays, synovial fluid analysis, joint blocks, thermography, and arthroscopy. The synovial fluid from an arthritic joint is thin and watery because of its decreased viscosity. X-rays of arthritic joints can show a narrowing of the joint space, bony proliferation (osteophytes and periosteal thickening), increased density of subchondral bone, and chip fractures (Fig. 4–19). For more details on these diagnostic techniques, refer to Chapter 3, Examination for Lameness.

Treatment. The goals of arthritis therapy are to relieve pain, prevent further joint degradation, preserve what function remains, and possibly repair damage. Arthritis is a result of a number of different conditions and the choice of treatment and its effectiveness will depend on the stage of the disease and the degree of active inflammation present. For a more thorough discussion of the therapies presented below, refer to Chapters 6 & 7.

Farriery. In some cases, farrier adjustments are necessary to remove the primary cause of arthritic pain. Balancing the hoof and removing traction devices are the most common adjustments made in cases of arthritis.

Rest with Controlled Exercise. Taking a horse out of work and giving it time off is helpful. Exercise should be moderate and controlled, such as short periods of daily hand walking. Passive manipulation (repeated flexion of the limb) and massage are also helpful.

Physiotherapy. Hydrotherapy can be used in the early stages of joint trauma: cold up to 48 hours after injury to retard the inflammatory process, and hot after 48 hours to relieve pain and reduce tension in tissues.

Joint Lavage. Lavage involves washing degradation debris out of the joint capsule with large volumes of fluid with the horse under general anesthesia.

DMSO. A topical application of DMSO with or without corticosteroids can reduce acute joint inflammation. Diluted DMSO solution can also be used for joint lavage.

Corticosteroids. Corticosteroids are potent anti-inflammatory agents that help the synovial membrane return to normal and reduce the level of harmful enzymes in the synovial fluid. These are commonly injected directly into the joint but can also be used orally, intramuscularly, and topically with DMSO.

NSAIDs. Non-steroidal anti-inflammatory drugs (NSAIDs) act as a pain reliever and control the inflammatory response in soft tissues but cannot reverse or

FIG. 4–16. *A*, Fetlock joint, used as an example in the accompanying arthritis progression. *B*, Healthy joint with shock-absorbing cartilage, synovial fluid. *C*, Infection or injury causes inflammation, which results in a thinning of the synovial fluid and eventually a thickening of the capsule and erosion of the cartilage. Excess bone is also produced. *D*, End-stage arthritis with complete loss of cartilage, bone spur formation, and, subsequently, an asymmetric joint and/or crooked limb.

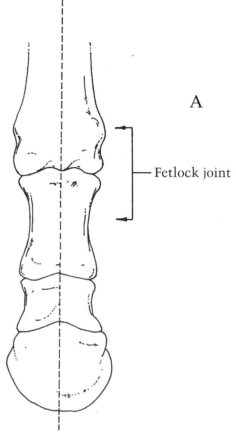

A

Fetlock joint

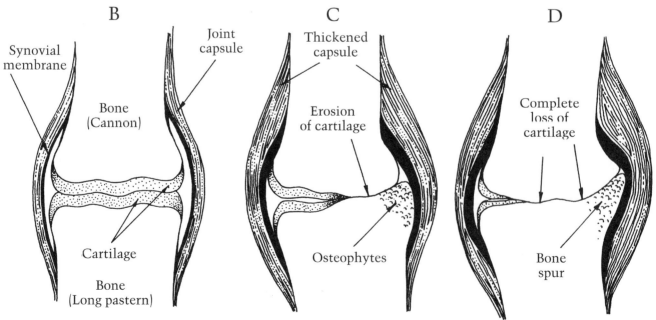

B

Synovial membrane

Joint capsule

Bone (Cannon)

Cartilage

Bone (Long pastern)

C

Thickened capsule

Erosion of cartilage

Osteophytes

D

Complete loss of cartilage

Bone spur

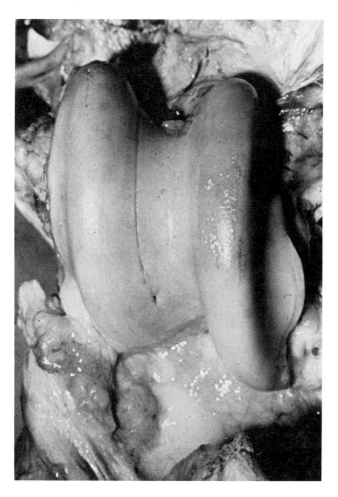

FIG. 4–17. Early degenerative joint disease with discoloration and blister formation in the articular cartilage.

heal cartilage damage. NSAIDs can be given orally or intravenously.

Palosein. Palosein (Orgotein) is a copper-zinc protein with powerful anti-inflammatory properties. Generally, it is injected into the joint and results in a marked reduction in synovial inflammation. However, in some cases it has caused a prominent chemical synovitis or "joint flare."

Hyaluronic Acid. Hyaluronic acid (HA) is a natural constituent of synovial fluid that is useful for treating synovitis but does not help repair cartilage degeneration. Sodium hyaluronate (the acid salt of hyaluronic acid), which is a very thick fluid, is injected directly into the joint. In the appropriate cases, 80 to 90% of the horses treated experience a beneficial effect (often immediately) for up to several months. There are no side effects. This fluid is available in several viscosities; the higher the molecular weight, the more effective and the more expensive.

Polysulfated Glycosaminoglycan. Polysulfated glycosaminoglycan (PSGAG) is also naturally occurring in synovial fluid and is partially responsible for the resiliency of cartilage. Treatment of an arthritic joint with PSGAG not only improves the viscosity of the synovial fluid, but it also arrests or delays further cartilage damage in chronic or recurrent arthritis. More frequent injections may be necessary with PSGAG than HA and the beneficial effects from PSGAG treatment may not show up for several weeks. However, it has been used orally and intramuscularly as well as intra-articularly. The former two methods have the added benefit of treating more than one joint at the same time.

Synovectomy. The surgical removal of the synovial membrane in a chronically arthritic joint results in a decreased production of destructive enzymes.

Counterirritation. Application of rubefacients, blisters, firing, diathermy, and ultrasound are means of counterirritation.

Surgery. The removal of chips, cartilage fragments, and osteophytes via arthroscopy or arthrotomy is sometimes necessary and beneficial (Figs. 4–20 and 4–21).

Joint Fusion. For end-stage arthritis, particularly in the pastern and distal hock joints, surgical arthrodesis is an option. Work is under way to develop a means of initiating arthrodesis in the distal hock joints via an injection of an irritating chemical.

Radiation Therapy. This controversial treatment is rarely used. When it is employed, special facilities are required.

Cartilage Repair. Drugs such as PSGAG and others under study can be used to simulate or aid cartilage in healing and repair. Work is also under way to resurface a joint with cartilage that has been lost.

Prognosis. Generally, the earlier the diagnosis is made and treatment begins, the better the chances for preserving joint function and a horse's useful life. If a young horse shows early signs of arthritis and it is given rest and good treatment, it should have a good chance of recovery. In chronic cases, the prognosis is guarded and continued treatment is often necessary to maintain performance. For end-stage arthritis, the prognosis is poor for return to function with the exception of the joints (pastern and small tarsal joints) that can be surgically fused so the horse can return to performance.

Osteochondrosis

Osteochondrosis refers to a disturbance in the cellular differentiation of cartilage in growing horses resulting in a failure of normal ossification (bone formation) and a persistence of cartilage. It occurs at the growth centers. The first sign is a thickening of the cartilage at the growth center, the growth plate (physis), or the deep layers of the articular cartilage. As a result, endochondral ossification (the normal process of cartilage changing to bone) does not proceed normally. The subsequent cartilage defects can include (Fig. 4–22) a separation of the cartilage from the underlying bone, the death of cartilage before it turns into bone, a progressive breakdown of the cartilage resulting in wrinkling, cracking, and weak spots as well

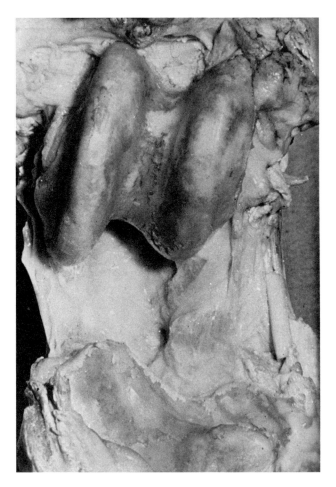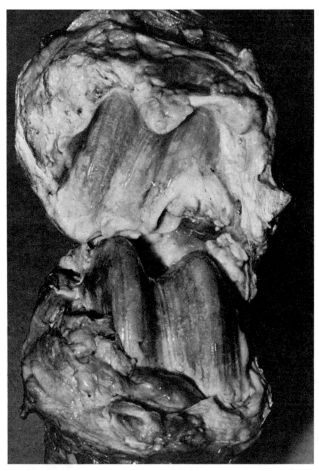

FIG. 4–18. Degenerative joint disease with partial-thickness and full-thickness erosion of articular cartilage.

as flaps, and loose bodies, which are referred to as "osteochondritis dessicans" (OCD). (Fig. 4–23), or bony (osseous) cysts (Figs. 4–24, 4–25, and 4–26). These joint defects result in various levels of pain and lameness and can eventually lead to arthritis.

The most commonly affected joints are the stifle (Fig. 4–27), hock (Fig. 4–28), shoulder, and fetlock. Racing Thoroughbreds and Standardbreds and futurity Quarter Horses most frequently affected because they are put to work at a young age and have no time off to spontaneously heal as do horses on a less rigorous training schedule.

Causes. Factors that may lead to osteochondrosis include nutritional imbalances involving calcium, phosphorus, copper, and zinc. For example, young horses that lick or chew lead-based paints then have a too-high zinc intake. A low copper intake is also suspect.

Selective breeding and unwise management can contribute to osteochondrosis. Individuals bred for fast growth and large size that are pushed nutritionally to attain an abnormal size for the age and maturity of their bones and joints are most likely to have osteochondrosis. Also, an obese horse has an abnormally high weight for its size and therefore experiences increased stress on joint cartilage.

Trauma and stress from early and aggressive training can result in separation of already-defective cartilage tissue. Stress is caused by such factors as the excess weight borne by the joint surfaces, being forced to work when fatigued, and hyperextension of joints.

Signs. Indications may be apparent as early as 3 months, but most lamenesses appear between 6 months and 2 years, coinciding with the onset of training. Signs may include generalized "bad" behaviors such as a reluctance to work, bucking, and rearing. The lameness may be gradual and insidious or acute. The gait may be asymmetric and awkward with specific characteristics pointing to the location, such as a rolling outward of the stifles if a bilateral stifle problem or a stumbling and shortened cranial phase of the forelimb stride if a shoulder problem. Joint swelling may be apparent if the conditions affect the stifle or hock.

Diagnosis. Lameness often worsens from flexion tests and is eliminated by either nerve or joint blocks. X-rays are not absolute proof that a horse does or does not have osteochondrosis. Often, arthroscopy will uncover lesions that were not discernible with x-rays.

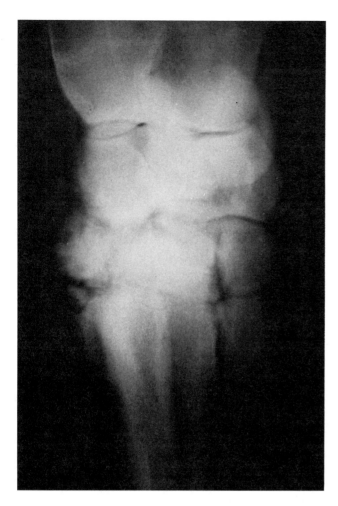

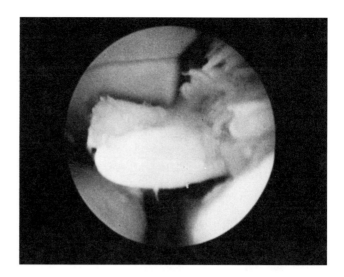

FIG. 4–21. Removal of carpal chip fracture under arthroscopic visualization.

FIG. 4–19. Severe degenerative joint disease of the midcarpal (intercarpal) and carpometacarpal joint. There is loss of joint space and considerable periosteal bone proliferation.

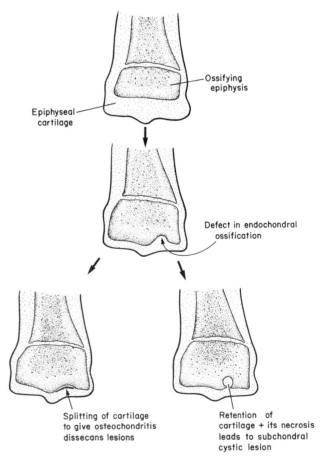

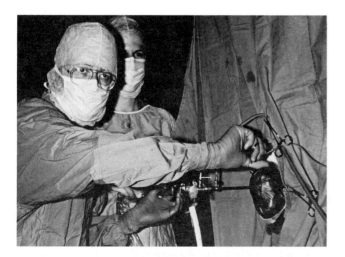

FIG. 4–20. Performing arthroscopic surgery for carpal chip fracture removal.

FIG. 4–22. Diagram of pathogenesis of osteochondritis dissecans and subchondral cystic lesions in relation to the generalized condition of osteochondrosis.

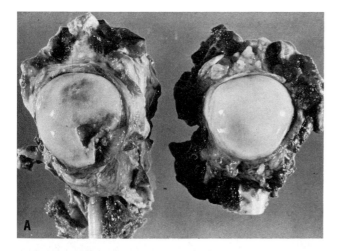

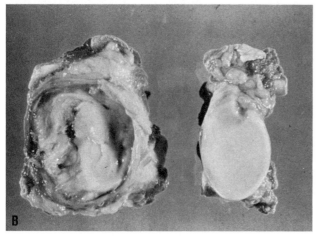

FIG. 4–23. Postmortem specimen of osteochondritis dissecans of the shoulder with normal joint for comparison on the right. *A*, Humeral head, *B*, Glenoid.

Treatment. The two primary treatment approaches are conservative management and surgical intervention. Certain cases diagnosed early may respond to a conservative treatment of turn-out and attention to diet and exercise. It may require a 6- to 12-month postponement of training to see any beneficial effect. Meanwhile, there should be a restricted feed intake with concentrates eliminated or greatly decreased in the diet. The entire ration should be evaluated for mineral imbalances. Osteochondrosis of the stifle does not respond favorably to conservative therapy; osteochondrosis in the hock may if the horse is not destined for demanding work. Although conservative therapy cannot reverse osteochondrosis, it may prevent the condition from getting worse. Some benefit has been seen with injections of HA and steroids in the affected joints in certain cases.

Surgical intervention includes arthrotomy (surgical incision of a joint) and arthroscopy. Arthrotomy is a more traumatic surgery than arthroscopy, requires a longer recovery period, and results in a smaller percentage of horses returning to work. Bone cysts may

be surgically removed and the defect may be packed with a bone graft.

Prognosis. Overall, the prognosis is guarded. With conservative therapy for a stifle lameness, the problem can persist for years and most horses will not return to work. The prognosis for conservative therapy with a shoulder problem is not good because of the high incidence of arthritis. Conservative therapy for hock problems may result in the horse returning to a moderate work level. Bone cysts in any location treated with conservative therapy may not show improvement for 2 years or more. With moderate exercise, the cysts may resolve more quickly. However, moderate exercise could also cause worse problems, such as bone collapse. Fairly good results have been obtained by arthroscopic removal of bone flaps and loose bodies. Surgical removal of cysts followed by implanting the defect with bone cells has also proved to be an effective treatment.

Incomplete or Defective Ossification of Carpal or Tarsal Bones

This condition is characterized by an angular deformity of the carpus (knee) or a flexure deformity of the tarsus (hock) (Fig. 4–29). X-rays will reveal incomplete ossification of one or more carpal or tarsal bones, resulting in a deformed shape. Normally, these bones begin ossifying during the last 2 months of gestation and ossification is complete shortly after birth. Therefore, premature births are associated with increased incidence of this condition. Treatment includes manual straightening (under general anesthesia) followed by casting (Figs. 4–30 and 4–31).

Synovial Osteochondromatosis

This describes bone or cartilage nodule formation within the synovial membrane. These nodule pieces may detach and exist as loose bodies in the joint cavity. The masses may or may not show up on x-rays. Treatment involves surgical removal of the bodies and the portions of the affected synovial membrane.

Infectious Arthritis

Infectious (septic) arthritis is caused by bacterial infection in a joint. The synovial membrane responds with an inflammatory reaction that can range from mild to severe and can be characterized by extensive swelling, heat, and pus production. Joint function can be markedly disturbed due to granulation (formation of rounded, fleshy connective tissue projections on the surface of inflamed tissue) and rapid cartilage destruction (Fig 4–32). Collagen loss leaves the cartilage vulnerable to physical trauma because it has lost its stiffness.

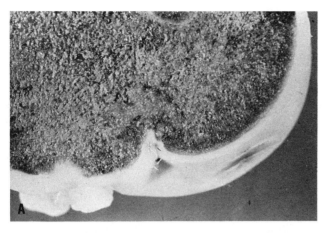
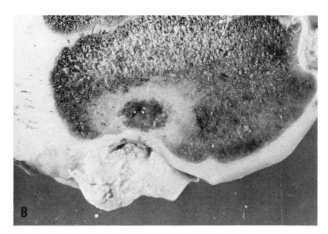
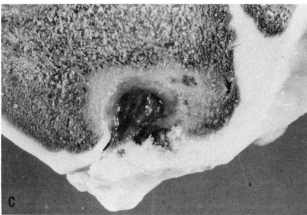

FIG. 4–24. *A, B,* and *C,* Cross-sectional views of subchondral cystic lesions at different stages of development.

Causes. Bacteria that cause joint infections can be carried to the joint by the blood (hematogenous) or can be introduced to the joint via traumatic injury or via nonsterile joint therapy injections. Hematogenous joint infection is most commonly observed in foals ("joint ill" or "navel ill") but the umbilical cord is not the only avenue of infection. The disease can arise from systemic infection, such as pneumonia, and it has also been linked to an incomplete passive transfer of immunity through colostrum. Certain structures in the synovial membrane tend to trap circulating microorganisms, thereby promoting joint infection. Direct penetration of a joint, as well as trauma to structures surrounding a joint, can lead to joint infection. Intra-articular injections of corticosteroids and other solutions is a cause of therapy-related joint infection.

Diagnosis. Joints such as the hock, stifle, knee, and fetlock may be enlarged and hot. Lameness may be mild initially but can rapidly progress to nonweight-bearing (Fig. 4–33). The horse may have an elevated body temperature. Pus may or may not exude from the joint (Fig. 4–34).

Synovial fluid analysis (Fig. 4–35) is one of the best means to confirm the presence of infectious arthritis. The synovial fluid is often filled with pus and blood. A sample of fluid is taken to document the white blood cell count and total protein. Bacterial stains of the fluid are examined and cultures are grown to identify the offending organism and to determine the appropriate antibiotic therapy. Infectious arthritis is an emergency condition, so it requires treatment before the results of the culture and antibiotic sensitivity are available.

X-rays are necessary to identify bony lesions of osteomyelitis and to monitor changes in the joint and bone, which can develop quickly with this condition and even proceed to ankylosis.

Treatment. The goal of treatment is to eliminate the bacteria and remove harmful enzymes that cause cartilage damage. Initially, a combination of broad-spectrum antibiotics are used systemically until culture results are available. Antibiotic therapy is usually continued for 4 to 6 weeks. Systemic antibiotic administration is preferred to intra-articular administration.

It is sometimes necessary to surgically open a foal's umbilicus to search for an abscess. In cases that do not respond to antibiotic therapy, drainage and joint lavage with sterile salt solutions and diluted DMSO solution (Fig. 4–36) may be required. In chronic cases, open arthrotomy and joint debridement may be necessary to remove large fibrin clots and diseased syno-

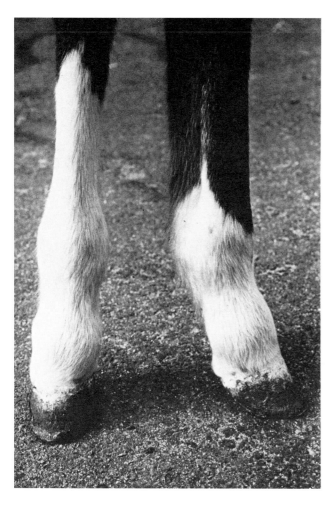

FIG. 4–25. Clinical presentation of subchondral cystic lesions of the distal aspect of the long pastern joint.

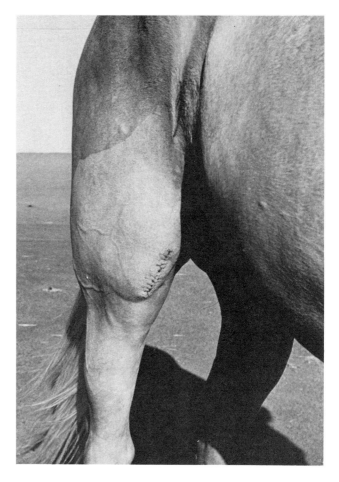

FIG. 4–26. Typical postoperative appearance after removal of cystic lesion or stifle.

vial membrane. The accompanying use of HA and NSAIDs is appropriate in some instances.

It is important that, following treatment, the horse be allowed a prolonged period of rest before exercise begins in order to allow soft tissues and articular cartilage to become completely restored.

Prognosis. The presence of marked changes on x-rays generally indicates irreversible joint damage and a poor prognosis. In any case of infectious arthritis, even with early and correct treatment, problems can develop, so in general the prognosis is not good. Young horses have a greater chance of joint healing than adults. However, even after successful treatment, some horses have a sudden relapse.

Synovial Hernia, Ganglion, and Synovial Fistula

A synovial hernia protrudes through a defect in a joint capsule or tendon sheath (Fig. 4–37). A ganglion is a cystic swelling containing mucus located near a joint or tendon sheath. A synovial fistula is an abnormal passage usually between a joint and a tendon sheath. Treatment is surgical removal.

Congenital Joint Anomalies

Although not common, congenital joint deformities include flexure deformities, underdeveloped and malformed joints, lateral dislocation of the patella (Fig. 4–38), hip dysplasia (rare), and "two-part" sesamoid bones and "three-part" navicular bones.

Tumors

Tumors associated with joints of the horse are very uncommon. Treatment involves surgical removal.

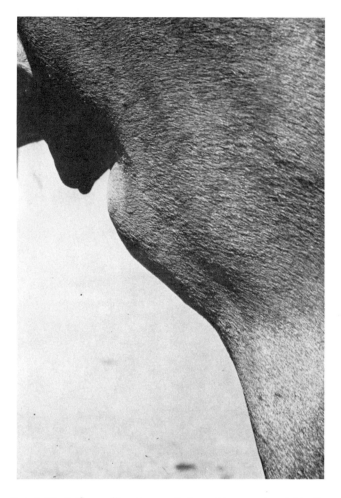

FIG. 4–27. Stifle swelling in association with osteochondritis dissecans.

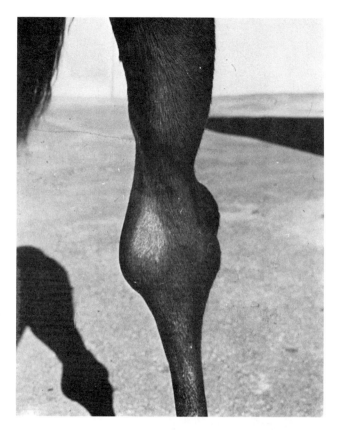

FIG. 4–28. Swelling of the hock with osteochondritis dissecans.

Diseases of Tendons, Ligaments, and Tendon Sheaths

Tendon Anatomy and Function

A tendon is a dense band of fibrous connective tissue that acts as an intermediary in the attachment of muscle to bone. Tendons are composed of dense, regular connective tissue and have a specific arrangement that reflects the mechanical requirements of this tissue. The chief constituents of tendons are thick, closely packed parallel bundles of longitudinally oriented collagen. Fibroblasts (specialized cells that produce collagen) are arranged in long parallel rows in the spaces between the collagenous bundles. The basic unit of tendon structure, the primary tendon bundle, is grouped together to form secondary bundles and these, in turn, are aggregated into larger tertiary tendon bundles. The complex structure of the collagenous bundles results in considerable lateral cohesion within the tendon, which makes slippage between fibers and fibrils difficult. Tendon fibroblasts do not actually contribute to tendon strength, but they are necessary for the formation of new collagen

fibrils. Tendon, being a dynamic structure, renews all its collagen every 6 months. As fibrils are broken down, the fibroblasts replace them.

Knowing tendon structures is important to gain an understanding of both normal tendon function and tendon damage (Fig. 4–39). Endotendon lies between tendon bundles and carries vessels, nerves, and lymphatics. The endotendon is an extension of the paratendon, a specialized loose tissue that fills the space between a tendon and the compartment through which the tendon moves. Elastic and pliable with long fibers, the paratendon allows the tendon to move back and forth. However, because the paratendon is attached to the tendon, it does not allow a true gliding mechanism like a sheath but rather it moves with the tendon.

A tendon sheath is composed of two layers: an inner synovial lining that covers the tendon fibers and an outer fibrous sheath that lines the tunnel through which the tendon glides. In some locations, the two layers converge to form mesotendon.

Anular ligaments, which are tough, fibrous, thickened portions of the sheath, encircle the tendon at the top and the bottom to maintain the tendon in its correct position.

A tendon may receive blood from four sources: the muscle or bone to which the tendon is attached, a mesotendon within a synovial sheath, and the paratendon if no sheath exists. It has been shown that the

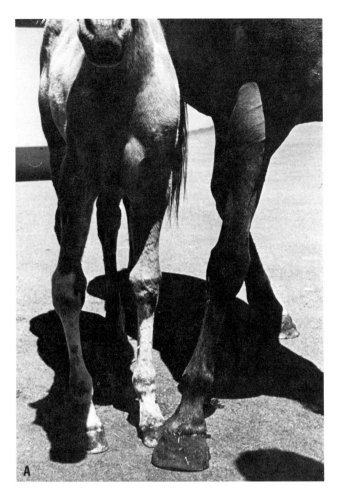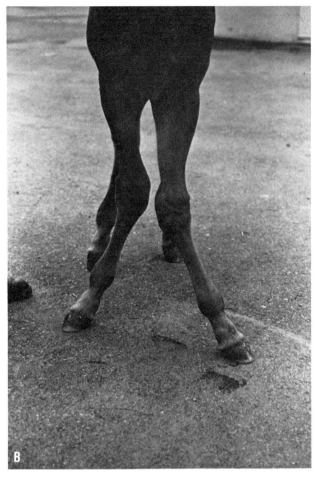

Fig. 4–29. *A,* A carpal varus deformity of the right front limb associated with collapse of radial carpal bone. *B,* Bilateral carpal valgus deformity associated with collapse of the fourth carpal bone and the lateral aspect of the third carpal bone.

muscle and bone only supply the proximal and distal 25% of the tendon with blood, and it can be assumed that the paratendon plays an important role.

Tendons possess great tensile strength (resistance to lengthwise stress) and limited lengthening ability. In mechanical terms, the tendon is a force transmitter. Other mechanical functions include that of a dynamic amplifier during rapid muscle contraction, an elastic energy store, and a force attenuator (dilutor) during rapid and unexpected movement.

Initially, a tendon appears highly compliant, but on further extension there is a stiffer region of response (Fig. 4–40). This transition occurs at approximately 3% extension. Beyond this initial elastic phase, the mechanical characteristics of the tendon change and irreversible structural changes take place. Under constant load, the tendon extends progressively with time (creep) (see Fig. 4–40).

Response to Injury and Tendon Healing

Both extrinsic (from outside the tendon) and intrinsic (from within the tendon) components can be in-

volved in tendon healing. Maximization of the intrinsic healing and minimization of extrinsic healing will potentially lead to fewer problems with adhesions.

As with wound healing elsewhere in the body, tendon healing begins with an inflammatory reaction proportional to the size of the wound and the amount of trauma. A greater inflammatory reaction is a significant stimulus for the formation of excessive granulation tissue and collagen deposition.

The contribution of capillaries from the paratendon is important in tendon healing. They contribute oxygen for cellular survival, affect synthesis of collagen, deliver inflammatory cells for removal of debris, and supply the amino acids essential for protein synthesis. However, the tendon can and does contribute significantly to its own healing. Unfortunately, many tendon injuries in the horse involve contamination as well as loss of tendinous tissue so primary intrinsic repair is overshadowed by an extensive response from the peritendinous tissues. This response causes massive adhesions in addition to tendon healing and precludes restoration of normal gliding function.

While limited passive motion aids in longitudinal orientation of collagenous fibrils and bundle forma-

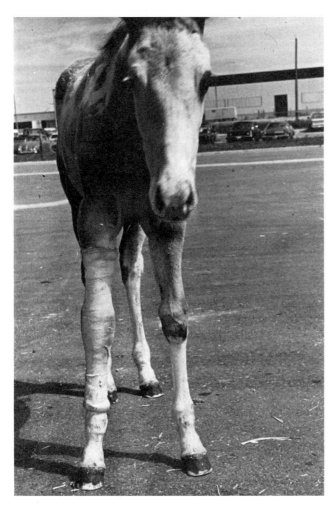

FIG. 4–30. Tube-casting of carpal collapse seen in Figure 4–29.

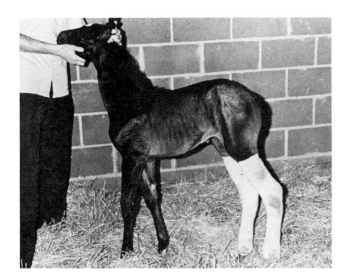

FIG. 4–31. Tube-casting for treatment of tarsal bone collapse.

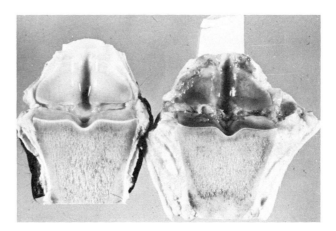

FIG. 4–32. Severe loss of articular cartilage in right fetlock joint in a case of infectious arthritis that did not respond to treatment.

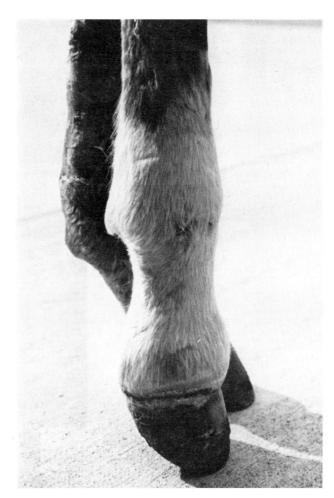

FIG. 4–33. Nonweight-bearing lameness and swelling over the coronary band in a case of infectious arthritis of the coffin joint.

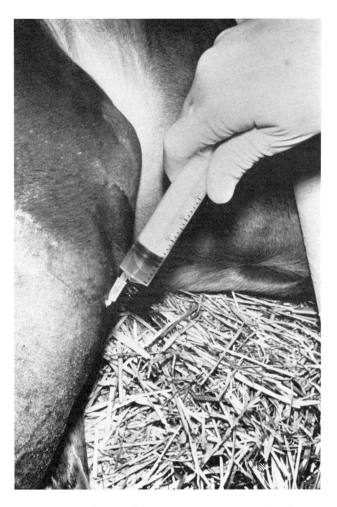

FIG. 4–34. Open drainage from a septic joint associated with external soft-tissue injury.

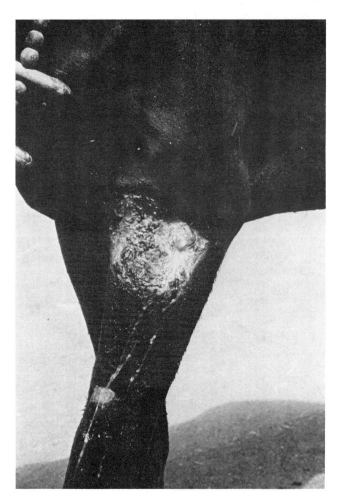

FIG. 4–35. Aspiration of turbid synovial fluid in a case of infectious arthritis.

tion in tendon repair, more severe active motion inhibits early repair of the tendon. This situation constitutes the major dilemma in the management of equine tendon injuries.

Developmental Problems

Flaccidity or Weakness of Flexor Tendons in Foals

This is a common condition in newborn foals generally affecting only the hindlimbs, but sometimes all four limbs. It usually corrects itself spontaneously and can almost be considered a physiologic variant rather than a disease. However, the problem has been associated with systemic illness or a lack of exercise. The affected foals walk on the palmar (plantar) part of the hoof and do not bear weight on the toe (Fig. 4–41). They essentially rock back on the bulbs of the heel.

In foals that do not correct themselves within a few days, the treatment involves corrective trimming and exercise. The heels are trimmed to eliminate the

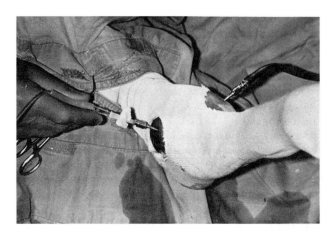

FIG. 4–36 . Through-and-through lavage of tarsocrural (tibiotarsal) joint of foal with septic arthritis.

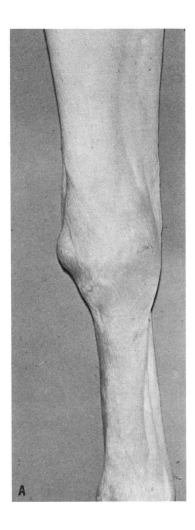

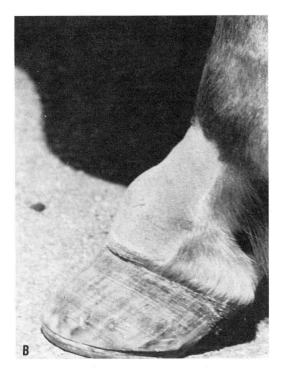

FIG. 4–37. External appearance of synovial hernia of (*A*) midcarpal (intercarpal) joint and (*B*) coffin joint.

"rocker" effect and to provide a flat weight-bearing surface (Fig. 4–42). The toes should not be trimmed. If the heels are not trimmed, the problem can persist, and with further rocking back on the heels, partial dislocation of the coffin joint may result. The use of protective bandages or casts will worsen the tendon weakness. Special shoes are not generally necessary but may be beneficial in severe cases.

Digital Hyperextension in Foals

This condition is apparent at birth or shortly after birth and is characterized by extreme extension of the fetlock and pastern joints. It is a rare condition. It appears as an extreme form of the flaccid tendon problem but must be considered as a separate entity. Severely affected animals bear weight on the palmar or plantar surface of the phalanges (long and short pastern bones) and sesamoid bones (Fig. 4–43). The cause is unknown.

Conservative methods of treatment such as the use of elongated shoe branches or support bandages are not successful. A surgical procedure for shortening of

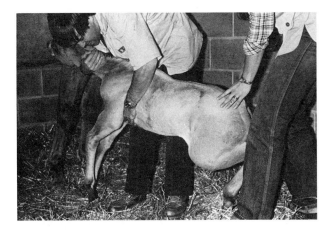

FIG. 4–38. Foal with bilateral congenital lateral luxation of the patella. The foal was unable to stand.

the superficial and deep digital flexor tendons has variable results.

Foal Limb Deviations

Foal limb deviations can be divided into three categories: angular deformities, rotational deviations,

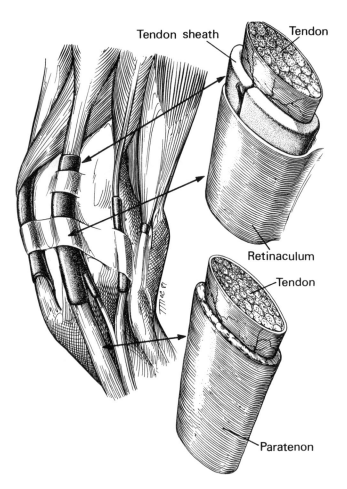

FIG. 4–39. Diagram of tendons and their relationship to paratenon (paratendon) and tendon sheaths.

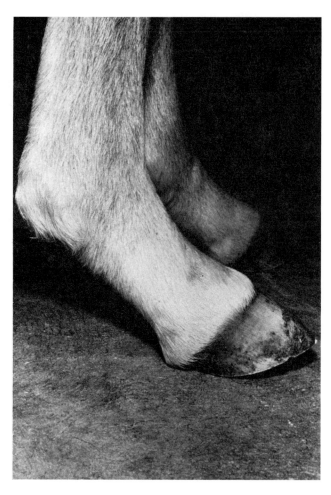

FIG. 4–41. Flaccid flexor tendons in a foal. The feet have been trimmed. The problem resolved in a short time.

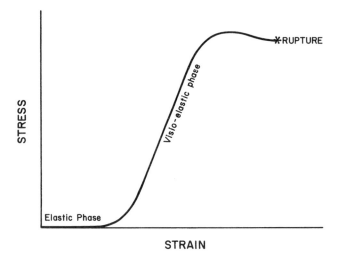

FIG. 4–40. Diagram of stress-strain characteristics of a tendon. An initially lax response (elastic phase) precedes a stiff, near linear region (visco-elastic phase). Rupture occurs at about 8% elongation. (From Evans, J. H., and Barbenel, J. C.: Structured and mechanical properties of tendon related to function. Eq. Vet. J., 7:5, 1975.)

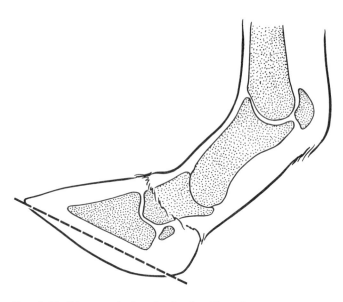

FIG. 4–42. Diagram of trimming for flaccid tendons.

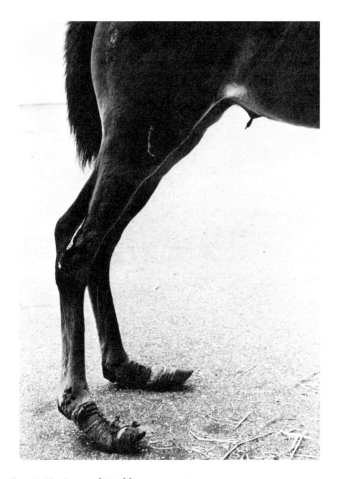

FIG. 4–43. Severe digital hyperextension.

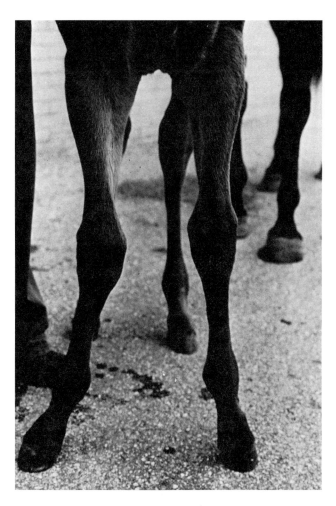

FIG. 4–44. Carpus valgus deformity (right front) in a 2-month-old foal.

and flexure deformities. These deviations can appear separately or in conjunction with each other. A deviation may affect a single limb, a pair of limbs, or all four limbs. Limb deformities can be congenital (present at birth) or acquired (developed after birth).

Angular limb deformities are medial or lateral deviations that are evident when a foal is viewed from the front or rear. Angular deviations are termed "valgus" or "varus." Valgus is a tilt toward the midline (of the limb or body) of the bone or joint distal to the site of the deformity (Fig. 4–44). Varus is a tilt away from the midline (of the limb or body) of the bone or joint distal to the site of the deformity (Fig. 4–45). Therefore, "carpus valgus" refers to a deformity of the knee (carpus) in which the bone (cannon) distal to the knee is tilted toward the midline of the limb. Angular limb deviations are covered in the sections on the carpus fetlock in Chapter 5 for more information.

Rotational deviations are evident when looking down the foal's limb from the point of the shoulder perpendicular toward the ground. The normal limb and hoof point forward; the rotated limb faces outward (most common) or inward. In many cases, a rotated limb is relatively straight with horizontal physes and joint surfaces but the limb itself faces outward.

Flexure deformities are cranial-to-caudal deviations in the limb that are evident when the foal is viewed from the side. Flexural deformities include, but are not limited to, upright hoof and pastern, club foot, the knuckled-over hoof (as in the foal that walks on front of the fetlocks) and flexion of the fetlock and/or carpus. Although these conditions have commonly been attributed to "contracted tendons," this is a misnomer. Tendons themselves do not actually contract; however, the muscles to which they are attached are capable of contraction. So, more accurately, there is a contraction of a muscle/tendon unit.

"Contracted Tendons" or Flexure Deformities

The term "contracted tendons" has been traditionally used to represent various flexure deformities in the limbs. However, the amount a tendon can actually contract is very limited. The primary defect is not necessarily in the tendon itself. In many instances, the effective functional length of the musculotendinous unit (the combination of the tendon and muscle(s) to which it is attached) is less than necessary for normal limb alignment to be maintained, but this should not imply a primary defect in the tendon itself. The term contracted tendons has become a common means of describing the condition. However, other possible pathogenetic mechanisms are probably involved.

Flexure deformities are considered congenital (apparent at or close to the time of birth) or acquired (developing during the growth period). Various causes have been incriminated in each group.

Congenital Flexure Deformities

Causes. Many cases of this condition have been attributed to uterine malpositioning. Although this concept is plausible and may occur in many instances, it is also considered that a number of cases are associated with more complex influences, including genetic factors and disturbed fetal growth during the embryonic stage of pregnancy.

There was one report of eight foals with severe fetlock flexion considered to result from a recent dominant gene mutation in the sire, and another report of three cases of congenital flexor contracture in foals from mares on a farm where an influenza outbreak occurred while the mares were pregnant. Congenital limb deformities have also been found in association with ingestion of locoweed by the pregnant mares. Although such evidence is often circumstantial, it does point out the need for continuing investigation into the role of toxic and infectious agents in congenital deformities. Another reported contracted foal syndrome was hypothesized to originate from joint instability associated with bony malformations that resulted in compensatory muscle contracture. Congenital flexure deformities have also been associated with equine goiter.

A condition appearing clinically similar to arthrogryposis (a congenital limited range of joint motion) occurring as a result of the mare ingesting hybrid Sudan grass pasture has been reported.

Signs. Congenital flexure deformities may affect one or more limbs. The most common are either fetlock or carpal flexure deformities. With fetlock flexure deformities, the foals may be able to stand but knuckle over at the fetlock (Fig. 4–46). In severe instances, the foals will walk on the dorsal surface of the fetlock. Generally, both the superficial and deep digital flexor tendons are shortened in these cases. It has been suggested by some authors that the suspensory ligament (interosseus medius muscle) is the primary structure involved. Involvement of the deep digital flexor tendon alone may result in a flexure deformity of the coffin joint. Congenital flexure deformities of the carpus are common (Fig. 4–47).

Rotational deformities may also accompany flexure deformities (Fig. 4–48).

Treatment. Some foals improve spontaneously and this category would include most of the foals in which

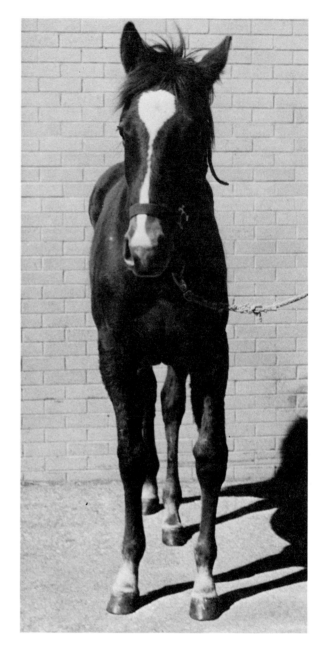

FIG. 4–45. Carpus varus deformity (left front) in a 5-month-old foal.

the deformity is associated with uterine malpositioning. The remainder of this group will generally respond to splinting if they have not been neglected. The basic principle of treatment is forced extension of the limb in order to induce the stretch reflex and consequent relaxation of the flexor muscles. Various splints and devices have been used, such as polyvinyl chloride (PVC) tubing (Figs. 4–49 and 4–50). All splinting devices require proper placement of padding, constant evaluation, and changing of the splints to prevent skin necrosis. Even more severe problems can result from faulty use of splints and bandages (Fig. 4–51).

Successful results have been experienced with the intravenous administration of oxytetracycline. Com-

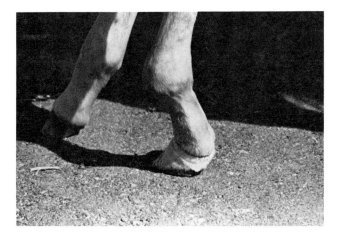

FIG. 4–46. Congenital flexion deformity of joint. A toe extension has been placed on the hoof but is not helping the condition.

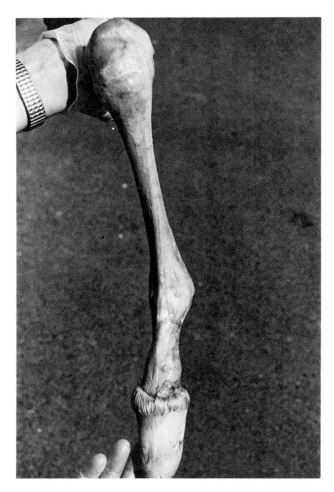

FIG. 4–48. Rotational deformities may accompany flexion deformities.

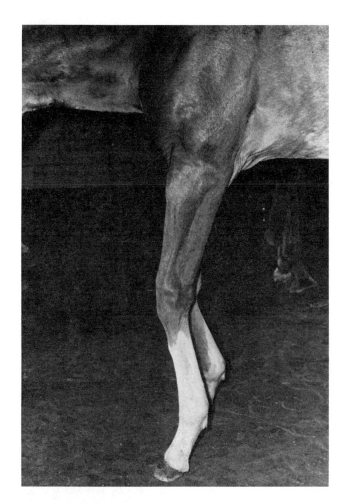

FIG. 4–47. Mild congenital carpal flexure deformity. This case recovered spontaneously.

plete resolution of early cases has been seen with a single dose; in other cases, a second dose was necessary. Although the mechanism whereby these patients are helped is unknown, it is logical that it may be related to calcium binding by oxytetracycline, presumably at the muscular rather than bone level because the responses have been seen quickly.

If the conservative methods are not successful, casts may be used to provide extension, but their indications are limited to severe contractures that cannot be extended completely. In this instance, casting may weaken the muscles enough to allow sufficient extension after the cast is removed. The prognosis is generally poor in cases that necessitate cast application. Cast management is particularly difficult in foals. Corrective shoes may be useful in some instances (see following section on treatment of acquired flexure deformities). The final alternative in treatment of congenital tendon contractures is surgery. Flexor tendon tenotomies (severing tendons) and carpal (inferior) check ligament desmotomies (severing ligaments) have been used successfully but are not common. The

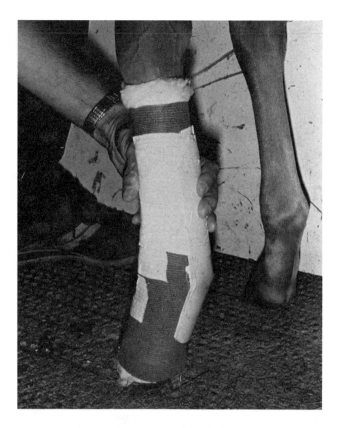

FIG. 4–49. Splinting of a congenital fetlock flexion deformity. Limb is bandaged and prebent PVC splint is in position.

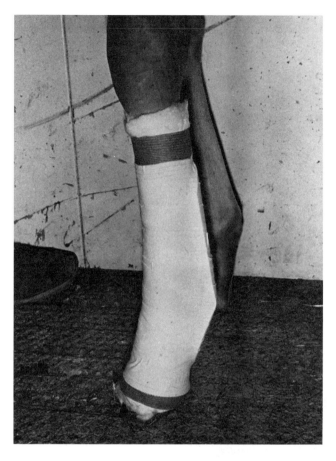

FIG. 4–50. Splint held in place with adhesive tape.

difference between congenital and acquired flexure deformities should always be recognized.

Acquired Flexure Deformities

Cause. Acquired flexure deformities can be unilateral or bilateral and usually occur as flexure deformities of the fetlock or coffin joint.

The underlying cause of acquired flexure deformities is frequently related to pain. Any pain in the limb will initiate a flexion withdrawal reflex, which results in flexor muscle contraction and an altered position of the joint. Pain can arise from physitis (inflammation of the growth plate), osteochondritis dissecans, septic arthritis, soft tissue wounds, or hoof infections with or without involvement of the coffin bone. Epiphysitis (physitis) is commonly observed in animals with flexure deformities. Flexure deformities have also been associated with osteochondritis dissecans in the shoulder and stifle joints.

Poor nutritional management has been incriminated as a common cause of flexor deformities in young growing foals.

The major nutritional imbalances that appear to be related to musculoskeletal disorders in the growing horse are a deficiency or excess of energy, protein, calcium, phosphorus, zinc, and/or vitamins D and A and

a deficiency of copper and possibly manganese. The major effect of these imbalances is an interference with endochondral ossification, which then can result in malformations, including angular limb deformities and acquired flexure deformities.

The factors that predispose the growing horse to alterations in endochondral ossification are rapid growth, trauma to the growth plates or cartilage, genetic predisposition, and nutritional imbalances. A combination of two or more of these factors may increase the incidence or severity of the condition.

Rapid growth appears to be the major factor in causing alternations in endochondral ossification and it is prompted by a horse's genetic predisposition, high-energy intake, and feeding for maximum growth after a period of stunting. Not providing adequate amounts of properly formulated creep feed to the suckling but then providing an excess of feed following weaning can result in a growth spurt that leads to flexure problems. The bones may grow too fast for the tendons to accommodate; thus, there is a relative shortening of the muscle tendon unit.

Trauma to endochondral ossification centers is greater in a foal of excess body weight. The weight is concentrated on the proportionally small growth plate and articular cartilage and can result in alterations in endochondral ossification. Horses with short upright pasterns and faster-growing, larger, finer-boned breeds are affected more frequently.

Genetic predisposition to alterations in endochondral ossification that is unrelated to growth rate, bone size, or conformation may be a factor in some cases. As previously mentioned, nutritional imbalances may lead to ossification problems as well.

Excess dietary energy from the intake of large amounts of grain resulting in rapid growth is one of the major factors responsible for alterations in endochondral ossification and can lead to poor bone quality. To prevent this, a good rule is to feed a maximum of 1 lb. of concentrate/day for each month of age up to a maximum of 8 to 9 lbs. daily.

Inadequate protein in the ration interferes with proper bone growth and development and decreases the growth rate. Feeding excess protein does not increase the growth rate above that achieved when requirements are just met. However, increasing protein without adequate minerals such as calcium and phosphorus to support faster growth rate can lead to bone development problems. The protein content of the ration should be met and not exceeded by more than 2%. In the total ration, the dry matter protein per-centage that is recommended is 18% for nursing foals, 16% for weanlings, 13% for yearlings, and 10% for 2-year-olds.

The growing horse must have adequate amounts of available (capable of being absorbed) calcium and phosphorus. The phosphorus present in grains, wheat bran, and other concentrates is less available to the horse than the phosphorus in roughages and minerals. Excessive phosphorus can decrease calcium absorption. Excess calcium can decrease absorption of trace minerals.

Providing the amount of calcium and phosphorus are adequate, the ratio of Ca:P can vary from 0.8:1 to 8:1 in the mature horse and from 0.8:1 to 3:1 in the growing horse without problems. If the amount of either calcium or phosphorus is inadequate or if the ratio is outside these limits, alterations in endochondral ossification may occur. Trace minerals that may alter bone development include zinc, copper, and possibly manganese.

Suggested pathogenetic pathways for acquired flexure deformities are illustrated in Figure 4–52.

The mechanism by which suggested causes produce flexure deformities is still uncertain. It has been suggested that rapid bone growth without exercise results in a failure of tendons and ligaments to develop at the same rate as bone lengthening. Flexor muscles are stronger than extensor muscles, and the foal consequently develops a flexion deformity. Another explanation relates the mechanism of flexure deformity development to discrepancy between bone growth and the capacity for lengthening of the check ligaments. These theories are not entirely compatible with bone growth of the distal limbs. Bone growth from the mid-cannon distally is very limited beyond 2 months of age and many cases of flexure deformities develop following this period.

True tendon contracture of a flexor tendon can occur following some cases of severe traumatic tendi-

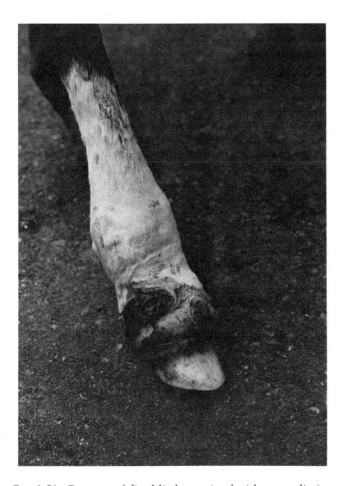

FIG. 4–51. Gangrene of distal limb associated with poor splinting technique and failure to remove splint when lameness developed.

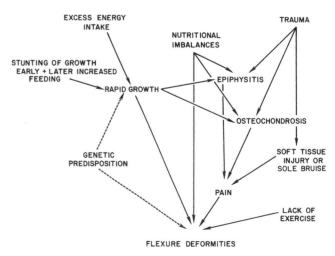

FIG. 4–52. Suggested pathogenetic pathways for acquired flexure deformities.

nitis. This is associated with contraction of fibrous tissue in the reparative process but is a relatively infrequent occurrence.

Clinical Signs. Clinically, there are two distinct entities. Flexure deformity of the coffin joint or so-called deep digital flexor (DDF) contracture results in a raised heel and a club foot (Fig. 4–53). For purposes of prognosis and therapy evaluation, this deformity has been subdivided into Stages I and II. Stage I contracture is used when the dorsal surface of the hoof does not pass beyond vertical (Fig. 4–54). When the dorsal surface of the hoof passes beyond vertical, the situation is classified as Stage II (Fig. 4–55). A grading system has also been used to classify the severity of this deformity. Refer to page 168.

The primary abnormality with DDF contracture would appear to be a relative shortening of the deep digital flexor musculotendinous unit. However, once the problem has progressed to that of a Stage II contracture, pathologic changes develop in the joint capsule and other tissues of the coffin joint, resulting in an irreversible state of fibrous ankylosis if these cases are not treated promptly.

The other clinical entity, flexure deformity of the fetlock joint, has been classically referred to as contracture of the superficial digital flexor (SDF) tendon. It is characterized by knuckling at the fetlock with the hoof itself remaining in normal alignment (Figs. 4–56 and 4–57). These cases should be called "fetlock flexure deformities" (the clinical problems are usually in the forelimbs) because the use of the term SDF contracture is a gross oversimplification. Deep digital flexor involvement is commonly present in these cases as well, and it would be more appropriate to describe the condition as combined superficial and deep digital flexor contracture. In long-standing cases, the suspensory ligament becomes involved secondarily, and degenerative changes in the fetlock joint occur.

Flexure deformities of the coffin joint have been typically described as occurring in foals and weanlings, and fetlock flexure deformities have been considered more typical of 1- to 2-year-old animals. Such a distribution was believed to be related to the suspensory ligament (interosseus medius muscle) losing muscle fiber content and, therefore, elasticity during the first year of life. In foals, the extensor branch of the suspensory ligament stretches and the coffin joint flexes under the influence of deep digital flexor contracture. After 1 year of age, the extensor branch of the suspensory ligament cannot stretch and the extensor tendon can only stretch proximal to its junction with the extensor branches of the suspensory ligament. In these cases, fetlock knuckling will occur. Some of these assumptions are controversial, and the sequence of events requires investigation. The relationship between age and the type of flexure deformity is not absolute. Fetlock knuckling does tend to occur in older animals, but flexure deformities of the coffin joint are also observed in animals over 12 months of age.

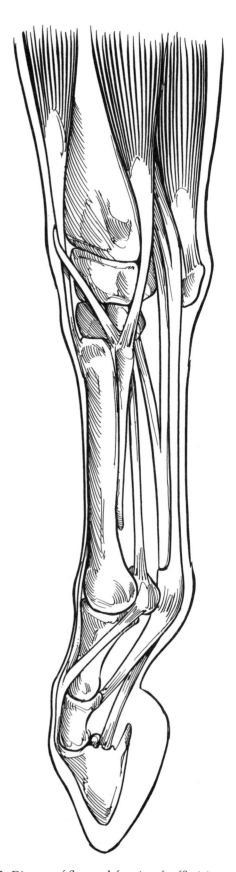

FIG. 4–53. Diagram of flexure deformity of coffin joint.

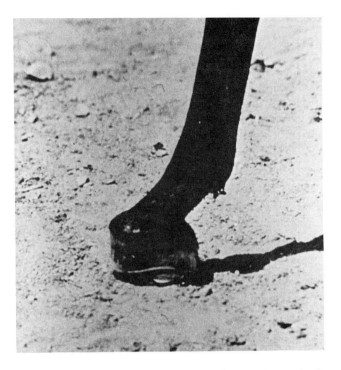

FIG. 4–54. Acquired flexure deformity of coffin joint (Stage 1). The elongated heel gives the typical "club-foot" appearance.

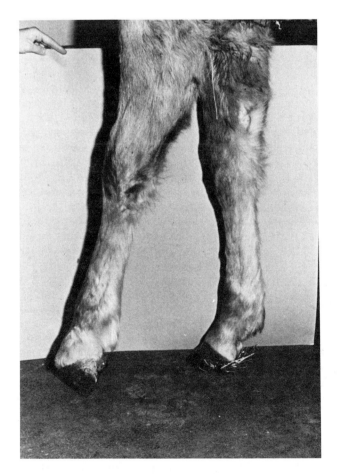

FIG. 4–55. Stage 2 acquired flexure deformity of coffin joint.

In all cases of flexure deformities, careful palpation of the limbs in both the standing and flexed positions to determine which structures are involved is necessary. With flexure deformities of the coffin joint, the structures involved are easily ascertained. However, with fetlock flexure deformities, it is important to ascertain which tendon seems to be primarily affected. This determination is very important regarding treatment.

Treatment. Conservative methods of treatment, including dietary changes, exercise, and hoof trimming are appropriate if affected animals are presented early.

The major feeding practices responsible for nutritional imbalances in the growing horse are feeding too much grain, feeding alfalfa hay without adding phosphorus to the ration, or feeding a grain mix that is inadequate in calcium, phosphorus, and protein when grass hay is fed. To treat problems resulting from alterations in endochondral ossification, alfalfa and grain are removed from the diet and as much good quality grass or cereal grain hay as the horse will eat is provided. The lower energy and protein content slows the growth rate and allows recovery to occur. However, these hays are deficient in both calcium and phosphorus, so 4 oz. of 12:12 Ca:P mineral mix must be fed daily. This can be mixed with a minimal amount of grain containing molasses.

Although exercise is often detrimental for cases of acute angular deformities, it is usually beneficial for treatment of flexure deformities.

A club foot results when a malfunction of the muscle-tendon unit (composed of the deep flexor muscle and the deep digital flexor tendon) of the limb causes an abnormal state of contracture. To varying degrees, this contraction takes weight off the heel of the hoof and loads the toe. The result is irregular horn growth and abnormal hoof shape. Characteristically, the hoof develops a high heel and a steeper-than-normal hoof angle. The hoof may develop a dish in the dorsal hoof wall and may exhibit other changes. More often, one hoof is involved rather than both hooves.

Foals with mild to moderate deviations that are diagnosed and treated early have a fair chance to perform unencumbered as adults. However, it is difficult to predict which foals will respond to treatment. Yearlings that have had extensive corrective trimming and shoeing may appear normal upon cursory visual examination. However, x-rays may reveal an undesirable relationship between the hoof wall and the coffin bone, demineralization of the coffin bone, or proliferation of bone at the tip of the coffin bone.

To devise an effective treatment plan, the age of the horse is considered as well as the severity of the deformity. During diagnosis, a horse with upright pastern-hoof conformation should not be mistaken for a bilaterally club-footed horse. Similarly, a horse with narrow heels should not be confused with a club-footed horse.

The goals for dealing with a club foot are to unload the toe, load the heel, allow adequate space between the sole and the ground surface, perhaps increase

CLASSIFICATION OF STAGE II DEFORMITIES

A **Grade I** club foot appears mismatched with the other hoof. The angle of the affected hoof is usually 3° to 5° greater than the opposite hoof. Because of the slight luxation (dislocation) of the short pastern bone and the coffin bone, there is a characteristic fullness at the coronary band.

The angle of the hoof of a **Grade II** club foot is approximately 5° to 8° greater than the opposite foot. The heel of the hoof will not touch the ground when it is trimmed to a normal length. The sole will touch the ground and the bulbs of the heels will appear thickened. Growth rings are wider at the heel than at the toe. When viewed from the bottom, it is evident that the bars tend to invaginate (curl inward).

The sole of a **Grade III** club foot shows signs of direct weight-bearing in the toe area just forward of the apex of the frog. An impression of the coffin bone can often be seen on the sole as well as bruising in many cases. The hoof wall is dished and the growth rings are twice as wide at the heel than at the toe. When viewed from the bottom, the hoof may exhibit a rectangular or pear shape (wider at the heels), and the bars curl inward. The dorsal face of the long pastern bone is directly in line with the face of the dorsal hoof wall, which causes the coronary band to bulge over the face of the dorsal hoof wall. Radiographic examination of the coffin bone often reveals lipping and demineralization along the apex.

The hoof angle of the **Grade IV** club foot is 80° or more and may be extremely dished. The coronary band at the heel is on the same plane as the toe or it may be higher at the heel than the toe. Because the sole in front of the apex of the frog actually supports weight, it is now below the ground surface of the hoof wall. On x-rays, the apex of the coffin bone will appear rounded because of extensive demineralization and may also show several degrees of rotation relative to the dorsal hoof wall.

One procedure to help separate the grades is to trim the heel of the affected hoof to a normal length and set it down in line with its limb but slightly behind the opposite hoof. If the heel of the affected hoof is not touching the ground, then the foot is Grade II or greater.

---

the ease of breakover, and encourage horn growth at the toe.

To decrease the incidence of toe abscesses and to help maintain a normal hoof-pastern axis, the toe of a club foot should be protected from excessive wear. All club feet should be evaluated and trimmed every 2 to 3 weeks because heel growth (and toe wear) would be excessive by 30 days. Frequent trims allow the farrier to monitor the results of treatment and implement appropriate changes if necessary.

Traditionally, treatment has consisted of lowering the heel and preventing wear at the toe. A tip shoe (half shoe) can prevent wear at the toe and is often used in conjunction with lowering the heel. The "heel" of the tip shoe is located approximately at the midpoint of the hoof. The "heel" of the shoe is either tapered or the hoof is notched to accept the shoe so that the result is a flush surface. Often the tip shoe is set slightly forward (0.25 to 0.5 inch) on the hoof to act as a toe extension, which further stretches the flexor tendon during a prolonged rather than eased breakover. This shoeing method, along with rasping of the bare heels, results in tension on the deep digital flexor tendon. In some mild cases, this treatment shows a favorable response. However, some cases progress rapidly to a severe club foot when the traditional heel-lowering treatment is used. The negative results may be due to the restriction on the vascular tissues, which results from the compression of the digital cushion that is caused by the increased pull of the deep digital flexor tendon.

The dorsal-palmar balance of more severely affected club feet (those in which the heel does not touch the ground) should be adjusted in order to prevent permanent damage to the toe area. The goal is to move the load off the toe and toward the heel. One technique to accomplish this is to apply a shoe with a raised heel to allow the heels to be weight-bearing. Mechanically raising the heel on more severely affected club feet is designed to reduce the continuous pull of the deep digital flexor tendon. If a horse stands with 0.25 inch of space between his heel and the ground, adding a 0.5-inch raised heel shoe to the hoof will essentially "pitch slack" to the deep digital flexor tendon while allowing the heel to load. Such an adjustment may break the cycle of continuous muscle contraction that perpetuates the condition. Nail-on raised-heel shoes work best on horses 1 year of age or older. Glue-on shoes are available for treating younger horses whose hooves would not tolerate the frequent nailing required for treatment.

For fetlock flexure deformities, it has been generally recommended in the past to raise the heels by corrective shoeing. It was believed that raising the heel creates a relative relaxation of tension in the deep flexor tendon, which in turn leads to selective overloading of the remaining support structures and dropping of the fetlock. Some research indicates that although mean tendon strain in the deep digital flexor tendon changes with hoof angle, there is no significant difference in strain in either the superficial digital flexor tendon or suspensory ligament with changing hoof an-

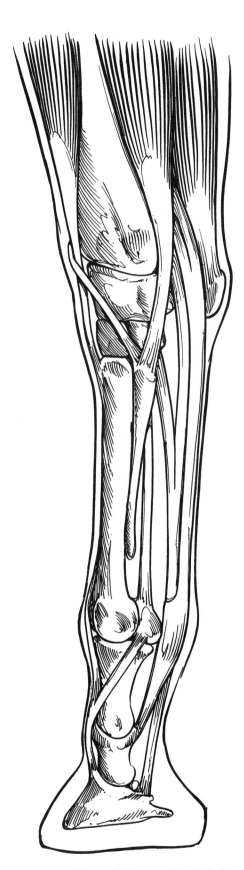

FIG. 4–56. Diagram of flexure deformity of the fetlock joint. It is to be noted that the deep digital flexor tendon has to span a decreased distance when the fetlock is in this position.

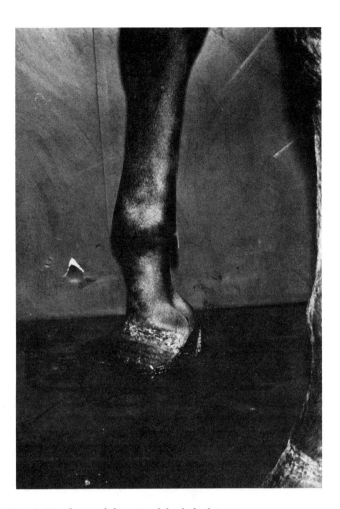

FIG. 4–57. Flexure deformity of the fetlock joint.

gle. This finding, coupled with the realization that the deep flexor tendon is involved in some instances of fetlock flexure deformities, makes rationalization of raising the heel and increasing the hoof angle difficult. However, it is a common observation that clinical cases respond to this regimen.

Surgical intervention can be considered in cases unresponsive to conservative methods of therapy. Immediate surgical intervention is also indicated on initial presentation of cases in which rapid correction of the flexure deformity is necessary to prevent the development of permanent degenerative joint changes.

Stage I DDF contracture (coffin joint flexure deformity) should be treated by carpal (inferior) check ligament desmotomy (Fig. 4–58). Normal limb alignment is usually obtained immediately following surgery, but in some cases, flexor relaxation progresses for 7 to 10 days postoperatively as the digital flexor muscles relax. Some cases in which the dorsal surface of the hoof is beyond vertical (mild Stage II) may respond to carpal check ligament desmotomy.

If surgery is part of the treatment, postoperative shoeing is usually required. Corrective shoeing should accompany and follow the surgery for 12 to 18 weeks. It is necessary to shoe the horse in a manner that will

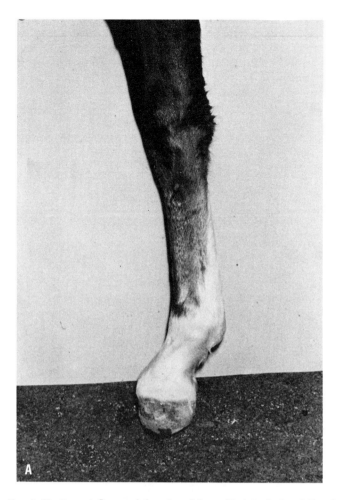 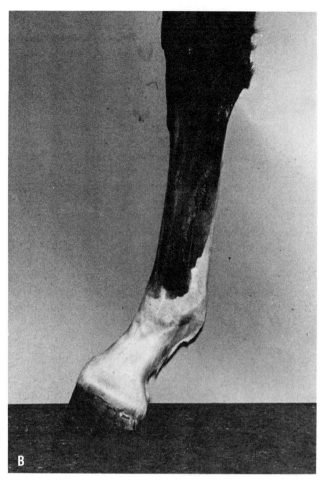

FIG. 4–58. Stage 1 flexure deformity of the coffin joint before (*A*) and after (*B*) carpal (inferior) check ligament desmotomy.

hold the ligament ends apart or scar tissue will form rapidly in the old configuration. Postoperative shoeing techniques include a tip shoe with regular rasping of heels or a toe extension shoe with or without a toe elevator.

Deep flexor tenotomy is indicated for severe long-standing cases of DDF contracture, including most Stage II cases (Fig. 4–59). This surgery corrects the flexure deformity in some animals but, in others, fibrosis and contraction of the joint capsule and associated ligaments does not permit proper realignment (Fig. 4–60). The cosmetic appearance following tenotomy is sometimes unsatisfactory, and the functional ability of the limb is often limited because of the drastic nature of the surgery. However, satisfactory cosmetic and functional results following deep flexor tenotomy have been obtained (Fig. 4–61). An alternative to a tenotomy is a tendon-lengthening procedure. The actual functional differences between these two techniques is uncertain, and the cosmetic appearance does not appear to be improved significantly by the tendon-lengthening procedure compared to tenotomy.

Although the prognosis for full functional soundness is poor, tendon contracture following severe ten-

dinitis can be treated by tenotomy to restore normal limb alignment.

The results of surgical treatment of flexure deformities of the fetlock joint or SDF-DDF contracture are less predictable than for flexure deformities of the coffin joint. A number of surgical treatments are available. If the SDF tendon is the most taut, either superficial flexor tenotomy or radial (superior) check ligament desmotomy may be performed. Superficial flexor tenotomy is simple and not as drastic in terms of cosmetic appearance and postoperative functional ability as deep flexor tenotomy. Radial (superior) check desmotomy is more difficult than carpal (inferior) check ligament desmotomy.

More recently, it has been found that carpal check ligament desmotomy has been most useful for the treatment of this condition particularly when the DDF tendon seems the most taut on clinical examination. Following the performance of the carpal check ligament desmotomy, a PVC splint is used to hold the fetlock in position as an additional measure (Fig. 4–62).

A final surgery that may be considered when the condition is resistant to the previous treatments is

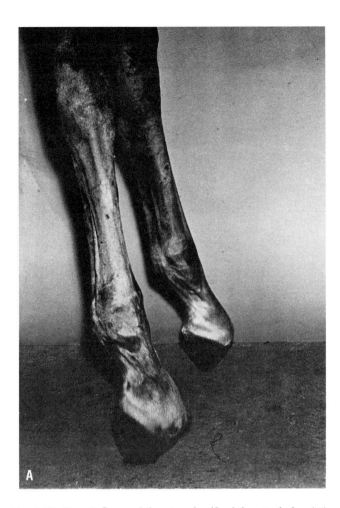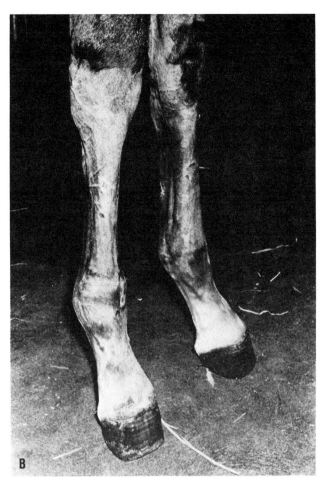

FIG. 4–59. Stage 2 flexure deformity of coffin deformity before (*A*) and after (*B*) deep digital flexor tendon tenotomy.

that of suspensory ligament desmotomy (Fig. 4–63). Suspensory ligament contracture may be a final secondary effect of a prolonged flexure deformity of the fetlock joint. Probably more often, the failure to respond to other surgical procedures is due to fibrosis and contraction of the fetlock joint capsule, sesamoidean ligaments, and other associated structures in the region. Suspensory ligament desmotomy is a drastic final measure and partial dislocation of the pastern joint is an anticipated sequel.

Traumatic Problems of Tendons and Ligaments

STRAIN

Strain has been defined as damage to a tendon or muscle caused by overuse or overstress. Strain of a tendon can range from minor inflammation to disruption of the tendon or avulsion (a tearing away) of the tendon from its bony attachment. There are various specific entities in the horse that could be classified as strains and they are described separately. Tendinitis or tenosynovitis may range from a simple to a severe strain. Rupture of a tendon is obviously a severe strain. Stress injuries of the suspensory ligament are also classified as strains because this particular structure is a vestige of the third interosseous muscle rather than being a true ligament.

TENDINITIS, TENDOSYNOVITIS, TENOSYNOVITIS, AND DESMITIS

Tendinitis is inflammation of tendon and tendon-muscle attachments. In the horse, it refers specifically to inflammation of the flexor tendons due to excessive strain. The term tendinitis, if used correctly, applies to strain-induced inflammation involving tendon that is surrounded by paratendon and not tendon sheath. If the region of involved tendon is associated with a tendon sheath the term "tendosynovitis" is used (the use of the term "adhesive tendosynovitis" could also be used). Tenosynovitis implies inflammation of the tendon sheath alone and is considered separately later. As previously noted, inflammation of a ligament is referred to as "desmitis" and, therefore, injury to the suspensory ligament is referred to as "suspensory ligament desmitis."

With tendinitis, the tendon becomes thickened at the site of injury as a result of fibrosis within the tendon itself and in the surrounding paratendon and/or

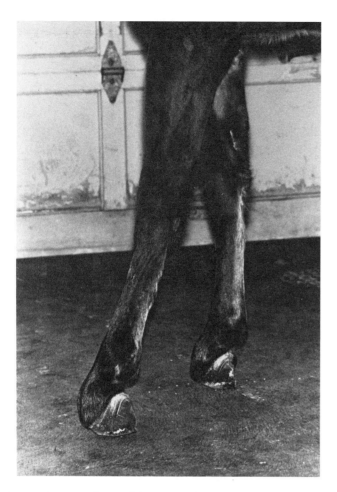

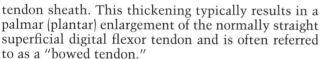

FIG. 4–60. Severe flexure deformity of the coffin joint not amenable to treatment.

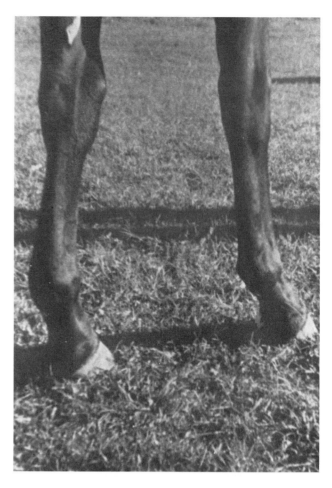

FIG. 4–61. Horse 1 year after bilateral deep flexor tenotomy with good cosmetic results (the horse was also sound as a riding animal).

tendon sheath. This thickening typically results in a palmar (plantar) enlargement of the normally straight superficial digital flexor tendon and is often referred to as a "bowed tendon."

Tendinitis and tenosynovitis are most common in the forelimb in racing Thoroughbreds and Quarter Horses hunters, jumpers, and event horses and typically involve the superficial digital flexor tendon (SDF). The suspensory ligament of the hindlimb is the most commonly affected structure in Standardbred race horses, followed by relatively equal incidences in the suspensory ligament and SDF in the forelimb. Tendinitis in the SDF of the hindlimb is uncommon in all breeds but does occur to some extent in the Standardbred. Desmitis of the carpal (inferior) check ligament can also occur independently or in association with these other conditions.

Tendinitis or tenosynovitis has also been classified according to position:

1. High—just distal to the knee or hock.
2. Middle—in the middle third of the cannon.
3. Low—distal third of the cannon and in the region of the palmar or plantar anular ligament. The deep digital flexor tendon may also be injured distal to

the fetlock joint. This has been referred to as a low-low bow.

Causes. Tendinitis or tenosynovitis usually results from a severe strain to the flexor tendons that is associated with excessive loading and overstretching of the tendon. (However, tendinitis can also occur in any horse as a result of striking the tendon.) The higher incidence of the disease in race horses and hunters compared with other horses confirms that the injuries are directly related to excess physical stress. Because the most common site of injury is in the central area of the cannon of the front limb where the SDF has its smallest cross-sectional area, it has been suggested that the primary cause is an excessive force per unit area on the tendon. Various predisposing causes have also been incriminated. These include inadequate training and muscle fatigue at the end of a long race. In common with other connective tissues, rapidly repeated loading (such as occurs with conditioning) tends to stabilize the mechanical response of tendon. In this tensed, stabilized position, the tendon is more nearly elastic and slightly stiffer, and this is desirable. On the other hand, muscle exhaustion results in poor muscle response and loss of tendon stabilization.

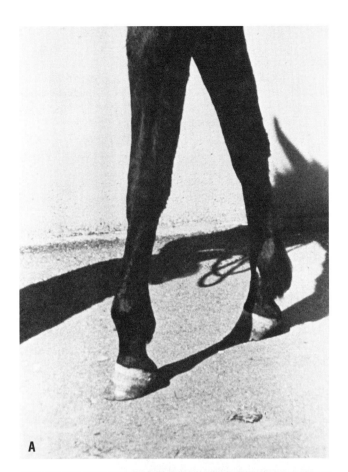

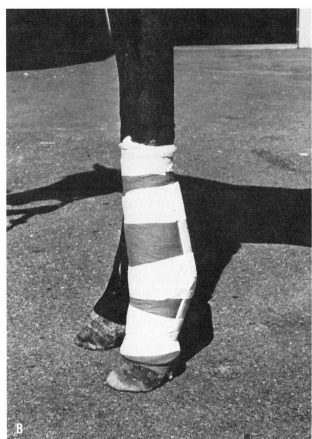

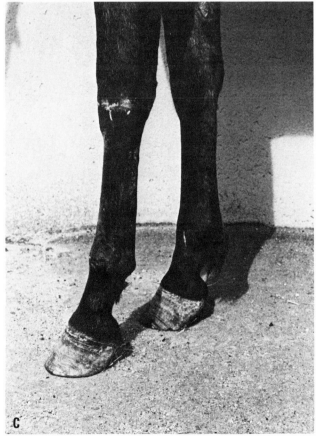

FIG. 4–62. Flexure deformity of fetlock joint before (*A*) and after (*B*) carpal (inferior) check ligament desmotomy and additional splinting. The splint was removed after 10 days with an excellent result (*C*).

Abnormal angulation of the fetlock associated with muscle weakness or conformation increases the stresses on the tendon. Excessive pastern slope, short shoeing, shoeing with long toe/low heel, a low hoof angle, or toe grabs may also place extra stresses on the tendon. Muddy tracks increase the workload on the tendon and tight-fitting bandages or boots have also been implicated. Incoordination and disproportion between body weight and tendon strength can also be incriminated.

Course of the Disease. Tendon injury and degeneration occur in all degrees of severity, ranging from slight subclinical injuries that may be detected only by ultrasound to those sustaining complete tendon rupture. Loads above the safe limit may produce minor fiber displacement and rupture. This separation results in capillary hemorrhage within the tendon. Typically, acute tendon injury is accompanied by hemorrhage, edema, and local swelling. Hemorrhage and leakage of fluids into the tendon separates and weakens remaining normal fibers. Enzymes are also released and can cause further damage. Disruption of

blood supply in the damaged region also occurs. The amount of necrosis occurring in the region can be related to the degree of vascular compromise.

Healing following severe tendon injury involves the formation of granulation tissue, which is followed by organization into fibrous tissue. In the course of repair, residual regions of hemorrhage may persist for a long time. The healing process results in the formation of collagenous scar tissue that also may contain cartilaginous or calcified regions. Peritendinous fibrous and adhesion formation also occurs, unless the lesion is small and restricted to the center of the tendon.

Diagnosis. In the acute phase, there is diffuse swelling over the region with heat and pain on palpation. Severe lameness is present. Major disruption of tendon fibers or stretching of the tendon will result in a "dropped fetlock."

The chronic stage is characterized by fibrosis and hard swelling on the palmar or plantar aspect (Fig. 4–64). Some acute inflammatory changes may still be present, depending on the stage of healing or if reinjury has occurred. The horse may be sound at the walk and trot but becomes lame with hard work. Anular

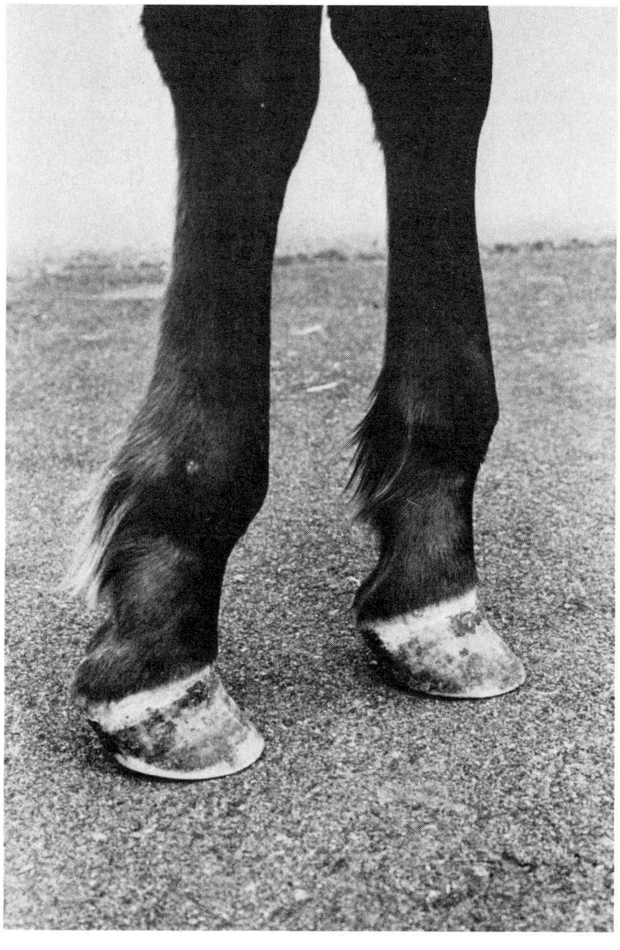

FIG. 4–63. Severe flexure deformity of fetlock joints that required sectioning of the carpal (inferior) check ligament, superficial digital flexor tendon and branches of the suspensory ligament to return fetlock to normal position.

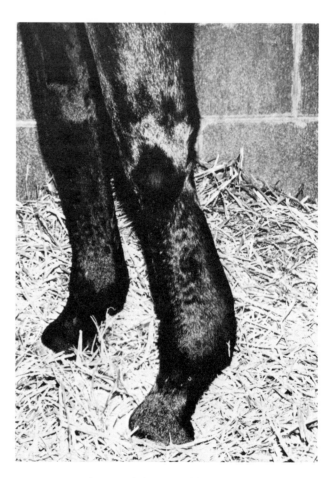

FIG. 4–64. Tendinitis of the superficial digital flexor tendon ("bowed tendon").

ligament constriction may be present in association with a chronic bow at the level of the fetlock.

Diagnostic ultrasound is used to define the degree of damage in a tendon and to monitor tendon healing.

ACUTE TENDINITIS (WITHIN 48 HOURS OF INJURY)

Treatment for an acute bowed tendon involves reducing the swelling and inflammation with pressure, ice, and anti-inflammatory drugs. Cold therapy should be administered for 24 hours, along with absolute confinement for at least 48 hours.

Ice is an effective inhibitor of inflammation. It constricts injured vessels, slows hemorrhage, reduces the effect of inflammation (inflammatory mediators), and provides some relief of pain. Application of cold for 30 minutes three to four times per day is preferable. Bandaging between treatments provides counterpressure against subcutaneous swelling. Complete rest for 48 hours is recommended to eliminate the possibility of worsening the damage. In most cases, it is best to remove the shoes, balance the feet, and possibly apply egg-bar shoes if the heels are low and underrun.

NSAIDs are often used to reduce the prostaglandin mediated inflammation resulting from tissue destruction. Banamine is often administered first because of its rapid onset and this is followed by the appropriate doses of phenylbutazone ("bute"), which are administered until inflammation subsides.

Corticosteroids should not be used for treatment of tendinitis because they can delay healing and can result in soft-tissue calcification if injected locally. Additionally, some steroids are implicated in the development of laminitis.

The use of DMSO is rational for the treatment of acute inflammation. It not only has fluid-dispersing properties but it also has the ability to scavenge harmful chemicals (superoxide radicals), which can further damage the affected tendon. Diluted DMSO is often given intravenously, but it can also be given through a nasogastric tube. Topical application is also used.

Hyaluronic acid (HA) injected peritendinously in man has been shown to reduce adhesion formation. Its use in horses has been questioned because research studies have not found a clear benefit. However, tendons injured within their sheath may benefit from injection of HA directly into the sheath.

SUBACUTE TENDINITIS (48 HOURS AFTER INJURY)

The treatment of subacute tendinitis is aimed at stopping the unnecessary spread of inflammation into normal tendon to reverse the effects of inflammation and to facilitate the repair process.

Alternating temperature therapy is begun 48 hours after injury and is continued for 4 to 6 days. The warm interval should be three times as long as the cold treatment and this can be done at least 3 to 4 times during the day. Warm therapy is continued after 6 days to improve circulation and healing. Topical medication is used for prolonged warm treatment. Pressure bandaging is continued in some cases for as long as 3 weeks.

Surgical treatment includes tendon splitting, radial check ligament desmotomy, and anular ligament desmotomy. Tendon splitting has recently regained value in treating certain bowed tendons. It has been discovered that tendons that have a "liquid center" (i.e., a pocket of accumulated serum and debris) can be drained, thereby accelerating healing and reducing the amount of scar tissue required to heal the injury. Tendon splitting is best done within the first week after injury although some benefit is seen at 3 weeks.

Radial (superficial) check ligament desmotomy is generally done within the first month after injury, although some benefit is seen in those cases done at a later time. Cutting the check ligament to the SDFT essentially lengthens the muscle-tendon unit, allows the tendon to heal with a more elastic function, and minimizes reinjury of the torn tendon. After the surgery, the horse is stalled for 2 weeks before a carefully monitored exercise program is started. This allows the check ligament to grow back longer than it was previously, giving the horse a more stretchable tendon unit. The amount of the elastic tissue in the tendon does not change, but the place at which the check ligament attaches does change.

Anular ligament desmotomy is recommended if the anular ligament becomes thickened or is restrictive to the free movement of the tendons within the fetlock canal.

Carefully monitored exercise can be beneficial during the healing period. After the initial 2 weeks of stall rest, the horse is hand-walked for 6 to 8 weeks. Then, a light jogging program (under tack, if possible) can be implemented for 1 month. Healing progress should be closely monitored with ultrasound examinations. Some horses can go back into regular training 90 days postinjury; others require more time. Depending on the severity of the injury, it takes from 6 to 10 months for a horse to return to its previous level of performance.

A relatively recent treatment proposed for acute tendinitis is the use of carbon fiber implants. The material is implanted in a longitudinal direction within the tendon. In experimental cases, collagen fibers align along the carbon fibers. The carbon fibers later disintegrate, leaving the aligned collagenous tissue. Experience in treating clinical cases of tendinitis using carbon fiber has not been very encouraging.

In transected and lacerated tendons, the results are even less encouraging.

No panacea is available for the treatment of tendinitis and tenosynovitis and it is a major cause of wastage in the racehorse and performance horse. To reduce the incidence of the problem, a gradual approach to training should be used and work should minimize excessive forces on an unconditioned musculotendinous unit.

Desmitis of the Suspensory Ligament

Desmitis of the suspensory ligament is considered in this section because of its similarity to tendinitis and because the suspensory ligament is really a vestigial tendon. Suspensory desmitis is a problem of racehorses and is most common in the Standardbred, in which it is often associated with periostitis and/or fracture of a splint bone or sesamoiditis (see Chapter 5). It is also seen in horses that are used for endurance and jumping.

Causes. There are three primary regions of involvement: 1) In one or both suspensory branches. This is the most common site of primary desmitis, and the causes are similar to those of tendinitis and tenosynovitis. The tendency for stress-induced injury to occur predominantly in the suspensory ligament in Standardbreds has been related to the relatively long cranial phase of their stride when the suspensory ligament has its primary support function. 2) In the main body of the ligament. This form of desmitis is often considered to be secondary to periostitis or fracture of the splint bones. 3) The proximal attachment of the ligament to the cannon bone. This is less common. The cause is presumed to be excessive stress.

Diagnosis. The problem can be generally recognized by visual inspection and palpation. As with tendinitis, there will be acute or chronic inflammatory signs, depending on the stage of the injury. The lameness may be exaggerated by deep palpation, flexion, or picking up the contralateral limb to cause increased tension on the affected ligament. Local infiltration of analgesic solution is often necessary to confirm high suspensory desmitis. X-rays will assess associated lesions in the splint bones or sesamoid bones and in the case of high suspensory desmitis, to eliminate avulsion fractures of the origin of the suspensory ligament. Ultrasound is used to document the degree of damage to the suspensory ligament.

Treatment. The treatment regimes are essentially the same as for tendinitis. It is important to cease all training with painful suspensory desmitis and accompanying sesamoiditis in the racing Thoroughbred because of the risk of suspensory rupture or sesamoid fracture and fetlock dislocation if work is continued on symptomatic therapy. The results of tendon-splitting surgery (as well as other treatments) are generally better with suspensory desmitis than they are with tendinitis and tenosynovitis. Of course, check ligament desmotomy is not recommended as it is for tendinitis. Ultrasound examination is used to document healing and is the deciding factor when horses are put back into full work. The overall prognosis for suspensory desmitis in Standardbreds is fair for racing; results are not quite as good in Thoroughbreds. Generally, the prognosis for horses used for purposes other than racing is good for return to their intended use as long as sesamoiditis and splint fracture are not a problem.

Traumatic Tendon Rupture

Tendon rupture can occur in association with excessive stress. As mentioned before, some degree of loss of integrity may occur in association with tendinitis or tenosynovitis, but complete rupture of the flexor tendons is not usually observed unless there is previous infection or degeneration. Some specific instances of complete traumatic rupture of tendons include rupture of the peroneus tertius and gastrocnemius, superficial digital flexor tendon in the hindlimb, and/or rupture of the extensor carpi radialis tendon in the forelimb.

Cause. The peroneus tertius is an important part of the reciprocal apparatus, mechanically flexing the hock when the stifle is flexed. Rupture is associated with overextension of the hock. This may occur in association with struggling to free a trapped limb or in traumatic injury to the region.

The gastrocnemius and superficial digital flexor tendons of the hindlimb are intimately associated. Proximal to the point of the hock, the combined tendons are known as the "common calcaneal tendon." Rupture of the gastrocnemius tendon may occur in one or both limbs in association with trauma due to strenuous effort. Incidents that may cause the problem include a fall with the hindlimbs flexed and underneath the body, being pulled up sharply and thrown back on the hocks, or making violent efforts to avoid slipping when going down a hill. The gastrocnemius muscle apparently ruptures before the superficial digital flexor tendon. Rarely, both structures will rupture (rupture of common calcaneal tendon) and this injury is particularly serious.

Rupture of the extensor carpi radialis tendon may also occur, but it is rare. The condition is too uncommon to make a valid observation regarding the cause. The occurrence of rupture of the common digital extensor tendon in foals has been discussed previously.

Diagnosis. The signs of rupture of the peroneus tertius muscle are classical. The hock joint does not flex as the limb moves forward, and the distal limb tends to hang limp. The horse will bear weight and pain is not a feature. On picking up the limb, the hock can be extended without extending the stifle (this cannot be done in a normal limb) and there is dimpling in the common calcaneal tendon (Fig. 4–65).

With gastrocnemius rupture, the hock is dropped so there is excessive angulation at the hock joint. If the entire common calcaneal tendon is ruptured, the horse cannot bear weight.

The signs of extensor carpi radialis rupture are more subtle, but careful observation of the gait will reveal that the carpus on the affected forelimb flexes more than the carpus of the normal limb. Consequently, the arc of the hoof in flight is significantly higher in the affected limb than in the sound limb. This is most noticeable at the trot. The problem is confirmed by palpation.

Treatment. Rupture of the peroneus tertius muscle is treated with rest. After stall rest for 1 month, the

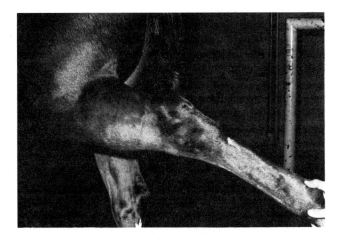

FIG. 4–65. Rupture of the peroneus tertius demonstrated by simultaneous extension of the hock and flexion of the stifle.

horse may be turned out to pasture. Most cases will heal well and surgical intervention is unnecessary.

Casting may be performed for a rupture of the gastrocnemius or the calcaneal (Achilles) tendon. The prognosis is guarded for gastrocnemius rupture and poor for calcaneal tendon rupture. Suturing the ends of the ruptured tendons may improve the success rate in these cases.

In the rare instances of rupture of the extensor carpi radialis muscle, treatment has not been attempted. The animal is still usable. If treatment is considered warranted in an athletic horse, implantation of carbon fiber could be considered.

Degenerative Rupture of Tendons

Prior damage to a tendon can weaken it to the extent that spontaneous rupture can occur with normal tensile forces. Typical examples of this situation are rupture of tendons secondary to septic tenosynovitis, advanced navicular disease following palmar digital neurectomy, or a sequel to repair of severed tendons. Septic tenosynovitis is associated with high levels of lysosomal enzymes as in septic arthritis. These enzymes can cause a chemical digestion of the tendon material and loss of its strength. Rather than a rupture, it is probably more accurate to describe the process as dissolution.

Rupture of the deep digital flexor tendon has been associated with the deep flexor tendon being weakened by degeneration in proximity to the navicular bone. Following palmar digital neurectomy, the horse starts using the limb in a normal fashion, adhesions between the deep flexor tendon and navicular bone are broken down, and a weakened deep digital flexor tendon may rupture. This may occur at a variable time following neurectomy. It is uncommon. In rare instances, rupture of the deep digital flexor tendon may occur in association with advanced navicular disease, even when neurectomy has not been performed. Rup-

ture of the deep digital flexor tendon may also follow severe, long-standing suppurative navicular bursitis.

Diagnosis. Loss of integrity of the tendon will be recognized by the particular limb conformation and gait. These signs usually occur after other disease has been recognized.

Treatment. In most instances, rupture due to degeneration is an indication for euthanasia.

Tenosynovitis

Tenosynovitis implies inflammation of the synovial membrane of the tendon sheath, but the fibrous layer of the tendon sheath is usually involved as well. The condition is characterized by distension of the tendon sheath due to synovial effusion (fluid leakage from blood vessels into synovial tissue). The condition has various causes and clinical signs manifestations. The various types of tenosynovitis in the horse will be classified as follows: 1) idiopathic tenosynovitis, 2) acute tenosynovitis, 3) chronic tenosynovitis, and 4) septic (infectious) tenosynovitis. There is some overlap in this classification system, but it is appropriate for an effective discussion of treatment.

IDIOPATHIC TENOSYNOVITIS

Idiopathic tenosynovitis may be defined as tenosynovitis with synovial effusion but without inflammation, pain, or lameness. The cause of the condition is vague. In the adult, tendon sheath effusion without other signs will typically develop insidiously and the most common sites affected are the tarsal sheath, the digital flexor sheath, and the extensor tendon sheaths over the carpus.

Tenosynovitis of the tarsal sheath is also called "thoroughpin." The tarsal sheath encloses the deep digital flexor tendon of the hindlimb. Thoroughpin is a structural description of the swelling, and while most cases would be an idiopathic synovitis, the presence of other clinical signs may cause it to be classified in one of the other categories. The term "wind puffs" or "wind galls" has been used as a general term to describe synovial swelling of various joints and tendon sheaths that do not cause lameness but is most commonly used to describe tenosynovitis of the digital flexor tendon sheath.

Cause. In idiopathic tenosynovitis that develops with time, the cause is presumed to be chronic low-grade trauma in many cases, but this is generally undefined. Conformation has been incriminated with tenosynovitis of the tarsal sheath. There is usually no previous history of injury or inflammation.

Diagnosis. Distension of the tendon sheath due to effusion is the typical clinical sign (Figs. 4–66 and 4–67). There is no inflammation, pain, or lameness. Distension of the tarsal sheath may be confused with bog spavin. Tenosynovitis of the digital sheath (wind puffs) distension that may be palpated between the

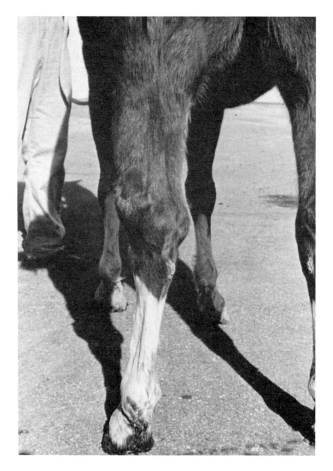

FIG. 4–66. Thoroughpin.

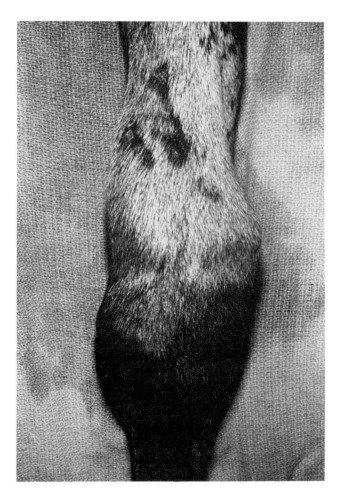

FIG. 4–67. Tenosynovitis of the common digital extensor tendon sheath overlying the carpal joint.

suspensory ligament and the flexor tendons. Tendon sheath distension may also be palpated on the palmar or plantar aspect of the pastern.

These lesions should be considered blemishes as they are not causing a clinical problem. Treatment by synovial fluid aspiration and injection of a corticosteroid has been used successfully. Alleviation following steroid injection is often temporary. However, the use of bandaging following injection may improve the success rate. Unless the presence of the blemish is of concern, no treatment is necessary. The application of a limb brace or sweat under cotton or bandage at the end of the day can be used if there is particular concern. These measures will control the distension but will not cause a permanent resolution. Distension will also become less evident with exercise. If lameness develops at any stage, the cause should be ascertained by appropriate examination.

ACUTE TENOSYNOVITIS

Acute tenosynovitis is characterized by a rapidly developing effusion within a tendon sheath accompanied by heat, pain, and possibly lameness.

Cause. There may be a history of trauma, but this is not always the case. The occurrence of tenosynovitis in the extensor sheath over the carpus has been associated with falling or hitting a jump with the carpus. Direct trauma could be a cause in other sites as well. Acute tenosynovitis often develops in association with acute tendinitis (tenosynovitis). Other proposed causes include friction between layers of the synovial sheath, peritendinous pressure, or acute direct trauma to the tendon and its sheath.

Diagnosis. Diagnosis is based on the presence of tendon sheath effusion accompanied by acute inflammatory signs. The presence of associated tendinitis should be differentiated. In tenosynovitis of an extensor tendon over the carpus the differential diagnosis may include acute carpitis, hygroma, cellulitis and synovial hernia. Ultrasound examination is used to document changes in the synovial membrane and to determine whether the tendon is involved.

Treatment. Treatment includes rest, the use of cold hydrotherapy or ice initially and the administration of NSAIDs. Astringent dressings and braces or sweats may be used at a later stage. Aspiration of fluid and injection of anti-inflammatory agents may be used but are generally reserved for cases that do not respond within a week.

The prognosis is favorable if the horse is rested, if damage to the tendon is not present, and appropriate treatment is commenced immediately. With inappropriate treatment, chronic tenosynovitis may develop.

CHRONIC TENOSYNOVITIS

Chronic tenosynovitis is characterized by a persistent synovial effusion and fibrous thickening of the tendon sheath. It is often accompanied by a constriction within the sheath or adhesions between the layers of the tendon sheath and the tendon.

Cause. The condition commonly follows acute tenosynovitis that has not resolved satisfactorily, but it can develop from trauma that is multiple and minor. Direct trauma and/or inflammation can lead to the formation of adhesions. Again, direct tendon damage may also be present.

Diagnosis. The clinical signs include a persistent synovial effusion in the affected tendon sheath generally accompanied by constriction or adhesions within the sheath. Inability to flex the carpus is the most common complaint with chronic tenosynovitis of the extensor tendon sheaths of the carpus, and pain is not a major factor. Tenosynovitis in the tarsal sheath could rarely be classified as chronic because lameness is uncommon. Chronic tenosynovitis of the digital sheath can be accompanied by anular ligament desmitis. In all cases, ultrasound examination should be performed to document changes.

Treatment. As an initial treatment method, drainage and injection of anti-inflammatory agents may be attempted. In clinical cases unresponsive to drainage and injection and in which lameness is present, surgical exploration of the tendon sheath may be performed. This procedure has been generally restricted to carpal extensor tendon sheaths. In cases of chronic tenosynovitis of the digital sheath in which the anular ligament is thickened and is restricting free movement of the flexor tendons through the fetlock canal, an anular ligament desmotomy is performed. A guarded prognosis is given if surgical exploration of a chronic tenosynovitis is necessary. A good prognosis is given if anular ligament thickening (desmitis) is the case and the anular ligament desmotomy is performed.

SEPTIC (INFECTIOUS) TENOSYNOVITIS

Septic tenosynovitis is characterized by marked synovial effusion, heat, pain, swelling, severe lameness, and suppurative synovial fluid.

Cause. As in septic arthritis, septic tenosynovitis can be the result of blood-borne infection, or trauma (punctures and lacerations). The severe inflammatory process can progress quickly to adhesion formation. In addition, enzymes released by the inflammatory process can cause digestion of the tendon structure.

Diagnosis. Septic tenosynovitis is recognized by a severe lameness with associated tendon sheath effusion accompanied by heat, pain, and swelling. The diagnosis is confirmed by synovial fluid analysis. Ultrasound examination is recommended to document changes. The temperature may be elevated.

If such a case does not receive treatment immediately, the disease may already have progressed to the stage of degenerative tendon rupture.

Treatment. The principles of treatment are the same as those described for infectious arthritis. Broad-spectrum antibiotics are used and synovial fluid aspiration with irrigation and drainage is usually appropriate. An aggressive approach includes opening the tendon sheath and implanting irrigation devices and drains. The prognosis is guarded to poor unless the case responds to treatment rapidly. Adhesions quickly form within the tendon sheath.

Diseases of Bursae and Other Periarticular Tissues

Anatomy and Physiology

A bursa is a closed sac lined with a cellular membrane resembling a synovial membrane that is interposed between moving parts or at points of unusual pressure such as between bony prominences and tendons. According to position, they have been classified. (Table 4–1 and Fig. 4–68).

The walls of the true bursae are lined with connective tissue membrane that is practically identical to the synovial membrane of joints.

Bursitis

Bursitis is defined as an inflammatory reaction within a bursa. This may range from a mild inflammatory reaction to a septic bursitis. Most instances of bursitis are of irritative or traumatic origin.

As with other entities of synovitis, bursitis may be manifested as an acute inflammation or in a chronic form. Examples of acute bursitis include bicipital bursitis and trochanteric bursitis in the early stages. A chronic bursitis may follow the acute form but is more frequently due to repeated injuries that subsequently become clinically unacceptable. Examples of this type of bursitis include capped elbow, capped hock, and carpal hygroma. The condition is characterized by the accumulation of excessive bursal fluid and a thickening of the wall of the bursa by fibrous tissue. Fibrous bands or septa may form within the bursal cavity, and generalized subcutaneous thickening usually develops. These bursal enlargements develop as cold, painless swellings, and unless they become greatly en-

TABLE 4–1. *Examples of Bursae*

Bursa	Position	Significance or Clinical Condition
Subcutaneous		
Olecranon bursa	Over olecranon tuberosity	Capped elbow
Subcutaneous calcaneal bursa	Above tuber calcis on plantar aspect of superficial digital flexor tendon	Capped hock
Subligamentous		
Atlantal bursa	Between ligamentum nuchae and rectus capitis dorsalis major muscle	Poll evil
Supraspinous bursa	Beneath ligamentum nuchae and over 3rd and 4th thoracic vertebrae	Fistulous withers
Subtendinous		
Bicipital bursa (Bursa intertubercularis)	Under tendon of biceps brachii muscle on the central ridge of the bicipital groove of the humerus. Bursa extends around tendon	Bicipital bursitis

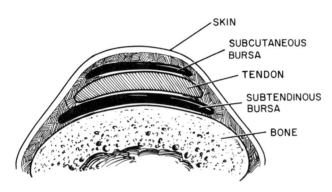

FIG. 4–68. Diagram of synovial bursa and the various positions in which it may occur.

larged, they do not severely interfere with function. If they become infected (particularly in the elbow or carpus), they may enlarge and rupture. The lesion is then characterized by exuberant granulation tissue, discharging sinuses and excessive fibrous tissue formation.

Bursitis can be classified as traumatic or septic.

Traumatic Bursitis

Most cases of bursitis fall under this classification. This group includes bicipital, trochanteric, and cunean bursitis as well as bursitis associated with the olecranon (capped elbow, shoe-boil), hock (capped hock), and carpus (carpal hygroma).

Causes. The trauma that causes the bursitis can either be direct or associated with racing stresses. Bicipital bursitis may be associated with a direct injury to the point of the shoulder. Trochanteric and cunean bursitis occur typically in Standardbred racehorses and are associated with racing stresses. Trochanteric bursitis is a poorly defined entity but is commonly considered to arise secondarily to hock lameness and presumably the change in gait due to the primary lameness causes abnormal stresses in the region of the trochanteric bursa. Cunean bursitis usually occurs in conjunction with inflammation of the distal tarsal and/or tarsometatarsal joints and is referred to as cunean tendon bursitis-tarsitis. Direct trauma is the cause of the other traumatic bursitis entities. Olecranon bursitis is an acquired bursitis caused by the shoe on the foot of the affected limb traumatizing the point of the olecranon during motion or when the horse is lying down. Bursitis of the hock (traumatic calcaneal bursitis) is usually associated with trauma from the horse kicking a wall or trailer gate. Direct trauma or stall door banging is also associated with carpal hygroma.

Clinical Signs. Bicipital, trochanteric, and cunean bursitis are characterized by lameness. Localizing pain to palpation is usually present with bicipital bursitis and sometimes present with trochanteric bursitis. Cunean bursitis requires local blocking to define, although there are certain characteristic clinical signs. The other bursitis entities are characterized by local fluctuant swelling in the region (Fig. 4–69). The relative amount of fluid and thickened soft tissue varies with the stage of the condition.

Treatment. The treatment methods vary considerably. Rest is the preferred method of treatment with bicipital bursitis. Cold applications in the acute stage and counterirritation during later stages have been used. Treatments for cunean tendon bursitis-tarsitis include cunean tenectomy, rest, local anti-inflammatory injections, or phenylbutazone.

With bursitis associated with the elbow, hock, or knee, the first principle of treatment is the prevention of further trauma to the region (not always easy or possible). Local injection of anti-inflammatories and pressure bandaging have been used with variable results. In resistant cases, the implantation of drains allows fluid drainage and acts to enhance fibrosis and obliteration of the cavity. Another method involves injection of the cavity with an iodine compound or incision into the cavity and packing it with gauze soaked in Lugol's iodine. No one treatment is a panacea. Surgical removal of the mass and primary closure is the final treatment of choice. Results of this treatment can be good if immobilization of the region is also performed.

Septic Bursitis

This term is restricted to bursitis that results from induction of infection into the bursa. The classic ex-

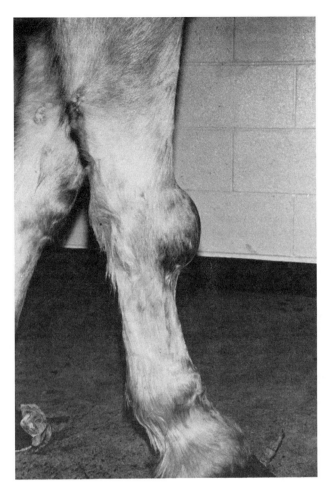

FIG. 4–69. Carpal hygroma.

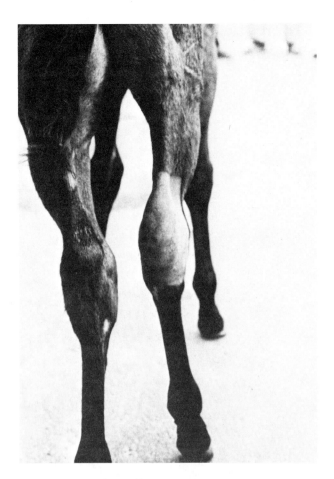

FIG. 4–70. Septic calcaneal bursitis.

ample is septic navicular bursitis following nail penetration. Supraspinous bursitis (fistulous withers) may be considered as a septic bursitis when it is associated with *Brucella abortus* infection for instance. This group does not include cases of traumatic bursitis that become secondarily infected.

Causes. Septic navicular bursitis is usually associated with penetration by a nail or similar foreign body through the frog. Establishment of infection in the region of the navicular bursa causes severe lameness, and the septic process can rapidly involve the neighboring navicular bone and deep digital flexor tendon. Acquisition of septic bursitis of the supraspinous bursa can be by a systemic (occasionally) or a direct penetration.

Clinical Signs. Septic navicular bursitis is characterized by severe lameness that is usually associated with recognition of foreign body penetration of the hoof. Drainage above the bulbs of the heel may develop. Septic bursitis can occur over the point of the

hock (Fig. 4–70). Fistulous withers is characterized by swelling over the withers with or without drainage (Figs. 4–71 and 4–72).

The principle of treatment for septic bursitis involves surgical drainage with removal of infected and necrotic tissue. In both examples given here, the surgical techniques are radical and the prognosis for complete recovery is guarded.

Bursal Fistula

As has been described in the section on joints, intersynovial fistulae may develop between a bursa and a joint or tendon sheath. The typical site of occurrence for this problem involves the bursae under the common digital extensor tendon at the level of the fetlock joint (over the dorsal capsule of the fetlock joint) or at the level of the pastern joint where the common digital extensor tendon unites with the branches of the suspensory ligament. These bursae may develop fistulae with the fetlock and coffin joints, respectively.

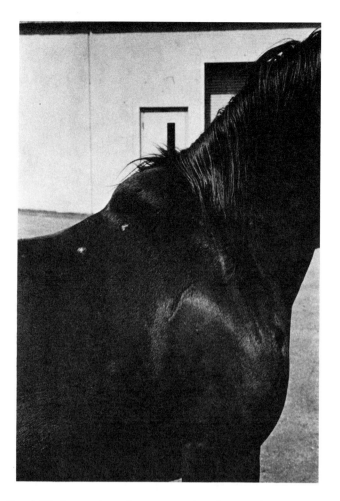

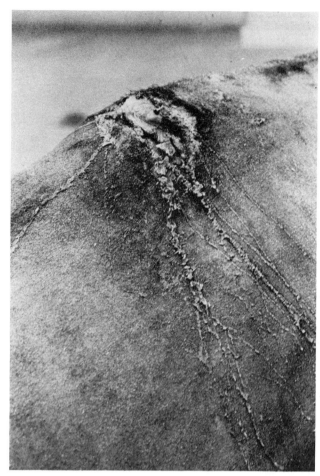

Fig. 4–71. Supraspinous bursitis manifested as swelling over the withers.

Fig. 4–72. Supraspinous bursitis with drainage from the withers.

CHAPTER FIVE

Lameness

The Foot

Laminitis

Although laminitis may be defined as an inflammation of the laminae of the foot, that definition is a gross oversimplification of a complicated, interrelated sequence of events that results in varying degrees of foot disease. Research suggests that laminitis is a disease characterized by a decrease of blood flow through the capillaries within the laminae, a passage of blood directly from arteries to veins (arteriovenous shunting) bypassing the capillary network and resulting in death of the laminae, and pain.

Research in the last decade also indicates that the foot disease is only a local expression of a much broader, systemic problem that can affect the circulatory and hormonal systems, the kidneys, the blood-clotting mechanism, and the horse's overall acid-base balance. Although many of the predisposing factors that cause laminitis have been identified, it appears that they all trigger a final common pathway that results in foot disease. In some cases, the damage is severe enough to result in rotation and possibly "sinking" of the coffin bone. With laminitis, the tone and the size of the blood vessels are altered and the blood-clotting mechanism is affected. These factors are believed to be responsible for the decreased capillary blood flow and tissue death occurring in the laminae of the foot.

The *developmental phase* is initiated when a horse comes in contact with factors that trigger the mechanisms that cause laminitis. This phase ends at the first sign of lameness. The *acute phase* begins at the onset of lameness and lasts for variable periods of time, depending on when or if rotation of the coffin bone occurs. All four feet can be involved, but more frequently, just the forefeet are involved. Signs of extreme pain, pounding digital pulse, and warm feet are most common. The *chronic phase* begins either when the signs of lameness are continual for longer than 48 hours or when there is evidence of rotation of the coffin bone. This phase may last for a period of weeks or may continue for the rest of the animal's life. It is characterized by intermittent or continual lameness and diverging growth patterns of the hoof wall.

Although one study indicated that all breeds of horses are affected equally (with the exception of the pony, which is at a higher risk), another study on 91 cases of laminitis found a higher incidence in Quarter horses (Quarter horses, 22; Arabs, 14; Thoroughbreds, 13; Standardbreds, 11; and Morgans, 7). Other studies suggest that both male and female horses are at equal risk; however, females are at a higher risk between 4 and 7 years of age, whereas males are at a higher risk between 7 and 10 years of age. A significantly greater number of stallions founder than mares or geldings.

Causes

The predisposing factors that trigger the development of laminitis are multiple and varied and include overeating (grain and lush green pasture), ingestion of cold water, trauma, systemic infections, and certain corticosteroid therapies.

Ingestion of a Toxic Amount of Grain (Grain Founder). Grain founder is caused by ingestion of greater quantities of grain than can be tolerated by the horse. The amount varies, because a certain degree of tolerance develops in those horses accustomed to eating large quantities of grain. Signs of laminitis may occur suddenly in a horse that has been eating considerable quantities of grain as a daily ration, or the laminitis may result from accidental exposure of the horse to excessive amounts of grain, as when the horse gains access to open grain bins. The grains most commonly involved are wheat, corn, and barley. Ingestion of oats usually is not as serious, and signs of laminitis from overeating oats will be mild or may not appear at all. Many other grains and grain-based feeds are capable of causing the disease, including rabbit feed, chicken feed, and pig feed.

The intake of high carbohydrates (grain) has been shown to alter the bacterial balance within the cecum, resulting in increased lactic acid producing bacteria, primarily *Lactobacillus* and *Streptococcus*. The increase in lactic acid and decrease in pH break down the cell wall of the bacteria, resulting in the release of endotoxins. A combination of decreased pH and increased endotoxin is believed to be responsible for the alteration in the inner lining of the intestines, allowing absorption of these substances into the systemic circulation. Endotoxins and lactic acid have a profound systemic effect, and it is believed that lactic acid may contribute to the onset of laminitis. Changes in cecal lactic acid and endotoxin levels occur within 3 hours after carbohydrate overload and lameness is usually observed 16 to 24 hours postingestion. The common association of colic or diarrhea with endotoxemia and laminitis is undeniable.

Ingestion of Large Amounts of Cold Water (Water Founder). Ingestion of large amounts of cold water by an overheated horse is considered a cause of laminitis. Although the phenomenon is not fully understood, it may be due to irritation of the stomach and intestines.

A horse that is overheated should be allowed only small amounts of water until he is cooled.

Concussion (Road Founder). This type of laminitis is the result of concussion to the feet from hard work or fast work on a hard surface. Unconditioned animals are especially subject to this type of laminitis, as are those horses having thin walls and soles. This is a traumatic laminitis, and sole bruising inflammation of the coffin bone (pedal osteitis) will also result if the cause persists.

Endometritis or Severe Systemic Infections. A mare may develop this type of laminitis shortly after foaling as a consequence of an infection resulting from retention of part of the fetal membranes or of a uterine infection without retention of fetal membranes. Always a serious form of laminitis, it also may occur as a sequel to severe pneumonia or other systemic infections.

Obesity and Ingestion of Lush Grass Pasture (Grass Founder). Grass founder is common among horses grazed on summer grass pastures. Pastures containing clover and alfalfa apparently are more likely to cause the condition than grass pastures. However, cases resulting from grass pastures, usually lush pastures, have been recorded. Horses that develop grass founder usually are overweight, and affected horses have a heavy crest on the neck caused by fatty tissue. Shetland ponies, Welsh ponies, and fat horses of other breeds are especially subject to the disease.

The cause of this type of laminitis is unexplained. It is not uncommon for horses that previously have been affected with grass founder to show recurrence of laminitis in winter when fed legume hay. However, laminitis can occur in obese horses fed legume hay during the winter with no previous history of grass founder. Hormonal factors may be the cause in some cases, if the grasses or legumes contain estrogens. Such estrogens, if present, cause obesity.

Inadequate production of the thyroid hormone (hypothyroidism) has also been considered a possible cause of this type of laminitis. However, recent studies indicate that laminitis may be the cause rather than the result of hypothyroidism. Thyroid function is monitored by blood analysis, specifically T3 and T4 uptake levels. Typically, T3 and T4 levels fall to hypothyroid levels during the acute phase of the disease and may return to normal or remain low in the chronic phase. Preliminary results indicate that the thyroid gland is structurally normal and exhibits a normal response to thyroid stimulating hormone (TSH) stimulation. Thus, the problem may be in an altered brain function or altered metabolism of the thyroid hormone. Of real interest is a report that identified significant decreases in T3 and T4 levels (hypothyroid levels) in normal horses treated with phenylbutazone for 5 days. Because most horses suffering from laminitis are placed on phenylbutazone therapy, it may be that treatment is influencing the thyroid results as well.

Miscellaneous Causes. Laminitis has been recorded in mares that had absolutely no exposure to any of the above causes. In some cases, these mares did not show estrus; once brought into heat, the laminitis ceased almost immediately. In other cases, mares that were in continuous estrus developed laminitis. It has been noted in a few cases that if this persistent heat was corrected, the laminitis ceased. It is possible that, in some cases, hormonal influences other than those in grass founder are the cause. In these types of laminitis, permanent changes in the feet do not seem to occur as rapidly as from other causes. There are other miscellaneous causes of laminitis, one of which is overeating of beet tops. It is common practice in some areas to turn horses into beet fields following harvest. It is not uncommon for these horses to develop "beet top founder." Additionally, other stress-related factors (e.g. severe lightning storms, separation from barnmate) have also been implicated.

Laminitis may be seen following viral respiratory disease or following administration of some drugs. In these cases, the wall changes are not as marked as they are in other types of laminitis. The sole shows extensive changes, and rotation of the coffin bone may occur within 72 hours. In some cases, portions of the sole slough out, exposing the coffin bone in as little as 10 days. Some horses lose the hoof wall completely before typical laminitis rings are present. This loss begins as a crack at the coronet, eventually extending completely around the hoof wall; the hoof wall loosens and comes off. Several weeks may elapse before slough of the hoof finally occurs.

Some horses showing this type of laminitis have a history of viral respiratory disease 2 to 6 weeks before onset of the laminitis. Others have a history of having been wormed or having received large doses of corticoids or phenylbutazone derivatives.

It has been demonstrated that high doses of steroids predisposed horses to more severe episodes of laminitis. Studies on the effect of steroids on the circulation of the foot have shown that administering steroids increases the response of the foot's vessels to normal circulating levels of hormones that can cause vessel constriction.

The Progress (Course) of the Disease

Before embarking on a complete discussion of the course of the disease, a brief review of the anatomic concepts of the foot is helpful. The coffin bone is suspended inside the hoof wall by interlocking laminae that surround it (see Figs. 1–4, 1–5, and 1–6). For practical purposes, the laminae has been classified as sensitive and insensitive, however, dermal and epidermal (respectively) are more correct designations. Dermal laminae originate on the wall surface of the coffin bone and project outward toward the epidermal laminae, which line the inside of the hoof wall and project inward. The secure "Velcro-like" interlocking attachments of the dermal and epidermal laminae are responsible for bearing most of the weight of the horse.

The growth of the hoof wall is from the coronary band downward. Coronary papillae that project downward from the coronary corium are responsible for the formation of tubular horn (insensitive papillary sockets), which provides structural strength to the hoof wall (Fig. 5–1, *A* and *B*). The growth of the wall progresses at a rate of 6 mm per month, taking 9 to 12 months to grow out. This region may be damaged with severe laminitis, which can result in altered function of the hoof wall due to damage of the coronary papillae and altered growth. The microcirculation of the dermal laminae is illustrated in Figures 5–2 and 5–3. Alteration in blood flows through the arteriovenous anastomosis (AVAs or AV shunts) is important in the development of laminitis.

In laminitis, the tissue changes are believed to result from two interrelated mechanisms involving a change in the tone and size of blood vessels and an alteration in clotting. The reduced capillary flow in the laminae is observed in all horses with acute laminitis and the degree of the reduction in blood flow is proportional to the lameness and is reversed when the horse recovers. Accompanying this is an overall increase in the blood flow to the foot. It is ironic that, although there is an increase in blood flow in the foot, the blood does not actually reach the capillaries in the laminae in laminitis. Instead, the blood flow is diverted away from the capillary beds in the dermal laminae through arteriovenous anastomoses (AVAs). This deprives the epidermal cells in the epidermal laminae of necessary nutrients and oxygen, which eventually results in separation of the epidermal and dermal laminae. This can result in rotation or sinking of the coffin bone (Fig. 5–4). The pain that develops stimulates the adrenal gland to release hormones, which cause constriction of the vessels and decrease blood flow in the digit.

An alteration in the clotting mechanism is also thought to be involved for the following reasons: 1) There is a correlation between causes of disseminated intravascular coagulopathy (DIC) in man and laminitis in horses; 2) alterations in the coagulation system have been identified in the developmental phase of laminitis; and 3) heparin therapy used as a preventative treatment markedly decreases the incidence of laminitis from 90 to 20% in horses fed laminitis diets, and none of the horses developed rotational laminitis.

It is difficult to separate the changes in the vessels from those in the clotting mechanism because each can secondarily affect the other.

Tissue studies of the foot in the early acute phase of laminitis indicate that the epidermal laminae are affected first. In severe progressive cases, congestion within the dermal laminae is noted; the dermal-epidermal junction becomes fluid filled and the epidermis begins to undergo (tissue) death. As laminitis progresses in the chronic phase, the tissue death extends to the dermal structures and causes a loss in suspensory support between the dermal and epidermal laminae. Additionally, an extensor tendon inserts on the extensor process of the coffin bone, functioning to extend the foot, and a larger stronger flexor tendon inserts on the palmar or plantar surface of the coffin bone, functioning to produce flexion of the digit (see Chapter 1). A combination of pulling forces of the deep digital flexor tendon and the rotating (pivotal) forces that focus on the toe serve to mechanically separate the coffin bone from the hoof wall (Fig. 5–5).

Microscopic evaluation of the chronically affected digit reveals an increase in tissue mass of the epidermal laminae to the point that it creates a wedge of tissue of sufficient magnitude that it forces the epidermal and dermal laminae apart (Fig. 5–6). It is hypothesized that this wedge of tissue, in part, is the reason the rotation persists.

Systemic Changes

The systemic manifestations of laminitis include alterations in the cardiovascular and endocrine systems, alterations in acid base imbalance, and coagulation. During the acute phase, variable degrees of hypertension, and elevation in lactic acid levels are observed. As the disease progresses into the chronic phase, approximately 80% of the horses remain hypertensive. Although the degree of hypertension is varied, some cases remain high as long as 6 months after the onset of lameness. Other horses return to normal blood pressure within a week or so after the onset of lameness.

Another frequent finding with chronic laminitis is kidney disease. A mild inflammation of kidney capillaries is usually present. Death of kidney tissue also occurs and is believed to be a side effect of the prolonged use of nonsteroidal anti-inflammatory analgesic drugs. Although the clinical significance of these changes is largely unknown, they may contribute to the long-term hypertensive state, fluid and electrolyte imbalance, and cresty neck appearance in some horses. These metabolic alterations may also predispose some horses to future episodes of laminitis, which substantiates the idea that once a horse experiences laminitis it has a higher risk for recurrence.

Signs

Signs of laminitis from all causes are similar; therefore, they will be described here as "acute" and "chronic." Signs for a specific cause will be described in detail.

Acute Laminitis. Acute laminitis may affect both front feet or all four feet. If all four feet are affected, the horse tends to lie down for extended periods. When standing, a horse so afflicted places its hind feet well up under itself and places the forefeet under its belly so that there is a very narrow base of support. Most commonly, only the two front feet are involved. In this case, the hind feet are carried well up under the body and the front feet are placed forward, with the

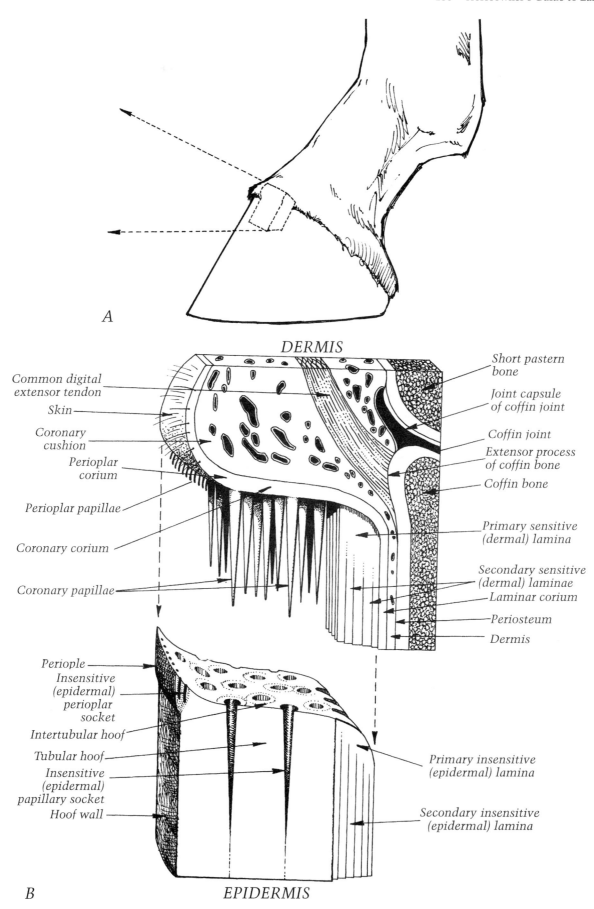

DERMIS

Common digital
extensor tendon

Skin

Coronary
cushion

Perioplar
corium

Perioplar papillae

Coronary corium

Coronary papillae

Short pastern
bone

Joint capsule
of coffin joint

Coffin joint

Extensor process
of coffin bone

Coffin bone

Primary sensitive
(dermal) lamina

Secondary sensitive
(dermal) laminae

Laminar corium

Periosteum

Dermis

Periople

Insensitive
(epidermal)
perioplar
socket

Intertubular hoof

Tubular hoof

Insensitive
(epidermal)
papillary socket

Hoof wall

Primary insensitive
(epidermal) lamina

Secondary insensitive
(epidermal) lamina

B *EPIDERMIS*

Fig. 5–1. *A*, A section of the coronary region of the hoof. *B*, Expanded diagrammatic view of the coronary region of the hoof.

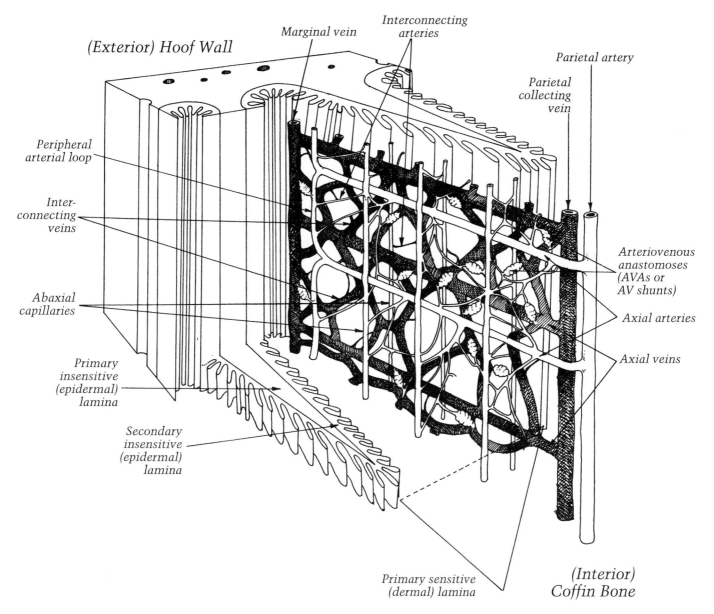

(Exterior) Hoof Wall

Marginal vein

Interconnecting
arteries

Parietal artery

Parietal
collecting
vein

Peripheral
arterial loop

Inter-
connecting
veins

Abaxial
capillaries

Arteriovenous
anastomoses
(AVAs or
AV shunts)

Axial arteries

Axial veins

Primary
insensitive
(epidermal)
lamina

Secondary
insensitive
(epidermal)
lamina

Primary sensitive
(dermal) lamina

*(Interior)
Coffin Bone*

Fig. 5–2. Microcirculation of the sensitive (dermal) laminae. From Pollitt CC: A scanning electron microscopical study of the dermal microcirculation of the equine foot. Equine Vet J. 22: 79–87, 1990.

weight on the heel of the foot (Fig. 5–7). The horse shows great reluctance to move.

The severity of lameness can be graded by the following criteria:

Grade 1: At rest, the horse will alternately and incessantly lift the feet. Lameness is not evident at a walk, but a short stilted gait is noted at a trot.

Grade 2: Horses move willingly at a walk, but the gait is stilted. A foot can be lifted off the ground without difficulty.

Grade 3: The horse moves very reluctantly and vigorously resists attempts to have a foot lifted.

Grade 4: The horse refuses to move and will not do so unless forced.

Heat is present over the wall and the coronary band. There is an increased digital pulse. Many horses show anxiety, muscle trembling from severe pain, increased respiration, and variable elevation of temperature. The vessels of the mucous membranes (such as gums) are visibly distended with blood. It is often difficult for the horse to lift one foot from the ground as it throws additional weight on the other affected foot or feet. If a person uses a hoof tester, a uniform tenderness will be noted over the entire area of the sole.

Signs of grain founder usually do not appear for 12 to 18 hours after ingestion of the grain, often leading the

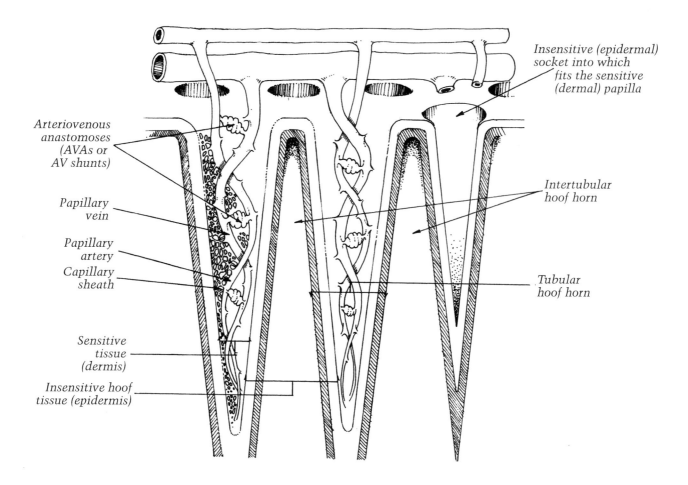

FIG. 5–3. Microcirculation of the sensitive (dermal) papillae. From Pollitt CC: A scanning electron microscopical study of the dermal microcirculation of the equine foot. Equine Vet J. 22: 79–87, 1990.

owner to believe that the horse will not be affected. After this interval, however, laminitis, diarrhea, muscular tremors, and increased pulse and respiration appear, and there is a variable rise in temperature.

In mares suffering from laminitis resulting from uterine infection, the temperature will often be high (104° to 106° F), the mucous membranes will be deep red, and considerable increase in pulse and respiration will be present. Uterine examination will reveal a dark watery fluid in variable quantities, and portions of the fetal membranes may be found.

Death may result from acute laminitis, but it is not common. In severe laminitis, the hoof may slough.

Chronic Laminitis. Laminitis becomes chronic after 48 hours of continual pain or when rotation of the coffin bone occurs. Severe lameness may not be present after the acute phase, but an acute recurrence may occur. Ponies and fat horses that have had laminitis will often experience recurrence with sudden changes in pasture, as the lush green grass returns in the spring. Show horses have a higher risk of laminitis in the late summer and early fall, which is the peak of the show season. During this time, horses are often under a lot of stress and are usually being fed high carbohydrate (grain) diets.

If and when rotation of the coffin bone occurs, it can vary from mild to severe. Severe rotation may be accompanied by separation of the coronary band over the extensor process region and serum will ooze out through this defect (Fig. 5–8). Upon examination of the ground surface of the foot, a semicircular separation of the sole just dorsal to the apex of the frog may be noted, indicating that the tip of the coffin bone is beginning to penetrate the sole (Fig. 5–9). This is a very serious situation, and horses rarely recover or can be salvaged from this. With mild to moderate chronic rotation of the coffin bone, diverging rings on the hoof wall will be evident. Typically, the space between the rings at the heel are wider than those at the toe (Fig. 5–10). This represents a differential growth pattern in which the heel grows more rapidly than the toe. Horses suffering from chronic laminitis with rotation of the distal phalanx have a tendency to land on the heel, followed by an exaggerated toe slap. This is to be expected, because the distal phalanx is not in normal alignment within the hoof wall or sole.

"Seedy toe," resulting from separation of the laminae, is usually present in chronic laminitis. Enough separation of the white line may occur to allow infection to penetrate the laminae (see the puncture

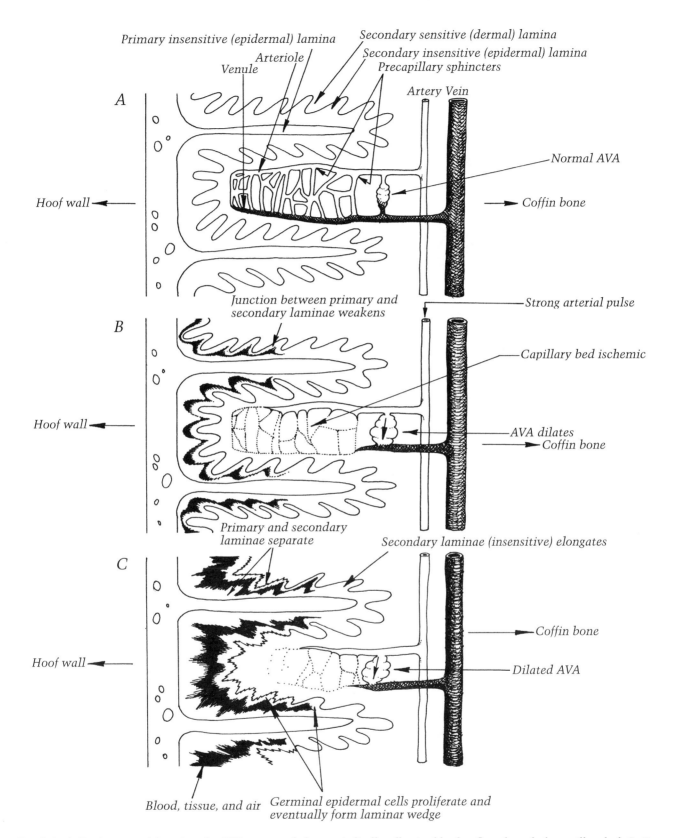

Primary insensitive (epidermal) lamina
Secondary sensitive (dermal) lamina
Arteriole
Secondary insensitive (epidermal) lamina
Venule
Precapillary sphincters
Artery Vein

A

Hoof wall

Normal AVA

Coffin bone

Junction between primary and secondary laminae weakens

B

Hoof wall

Strong arterial pulse

Capillary bed ischemic

AVA dilates
Coffin bone

Primary and secondary laminae separate

Secondary laminae (insensitive) elongates

C

Hoof wall

Coffin bone

Dilated AVA

Blood, tissue, and air
Germinal epidermal cells proliferate and eventually form laminar wedge

FIG. 5–4. *A,* During normal function, the AVAs open and close periodically, allowing blood to flow through the capillary bed. Optimum blood flow maintains the health of the dermal/epidermal cells and the strength of the bond between the coffin bone and the hoof wall. *B,* As laminitis develops, the AVAs can remain dilated for long periods, which shunts (diverts) the blood away from the capillary bed. Deprived of necessary nutrients, the epidermal cells deteriorate. *C,* As laminitis progresses, the primary and secondary laminae separate and the hoof wall tears away from the sensitive laminae overlying the coffin bone. Without its supportive attachment, the coffin bone can rotate or sink in the hoof capsule.

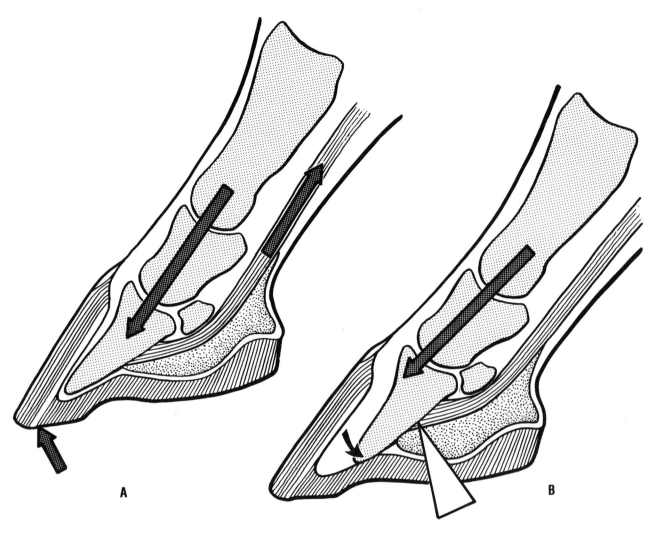

FIG. 5–5. *A*, Arrows indicate the various forces that contribute to rotation of the coffin bone. The pull of the flexor tendons overrides the pull of the extensor tendons, contributing to the rotation of the coffin bone. *B*, As the coffin bone begins to rotate, the horse's weight becomes focused on the extensor process (large stippled arrow), which theoretically increases the tendency to rotate. Large triangle points to the attachment of the deep flexor tendon on the coffin bone.

wounds of the white line (gravel) section in this chapter). An infection similar to thrush may invade the flaky sole in chronic laminitis and destroy all protection of the coffin bone. The sole region also appears convexed.

In the most severe cases, the coffin bone "sinks" within the hoof capsule due to loss of attachments of laminae around the entire circumference of the coffin bone. In these cases, the entire sole, rather than being cupped, will appear dropped.

When trimming the feet of a horse that has been affected with laminitis, it is easy to cause reddening and bleeding of the sole, because the vascularity of these regions increases with laminitis. Additionally, it is common for abscesses to develop in the sole and in the portion of the hoof wall that has rotated. This increased tendency toward hemorrhage abscess formation remains for many months after an attack of laminitis.

Hoof tester examination in the chronic phase rarely causes a painful response. The reason for this is unknown.

Diagnosis

The observable signs make diagnosis of laminitis relatively easy. The typical attitude of the animal, the increased pulsation of the digital arteries, the heat in the foot, and the pain evidenced by hoof testers in the acute phase should furnish adequate proof of laminitis. Chronic laminitis shows characteristic changes in the foot and a typical gait. In some cases, the cause is difficult to determine; occasionally, it is never determined.

Because the signs of laminitis are obvious and the diagnosis is easily made, nerve blocks are used rarely for the diagnosis.

If you suspect a laminitis emergency:

1. Call your veterinarian immediately; do not wait to see how the horse progresses.
2. Remove all feed from the horse's stall or pen; if the horse is on pasture, take it off pasture.
3. Make the horse as comfortable and calm as possible in a stall or small pen with soft footing (preferably sand).
4. Restrict exercise; no handwalking.

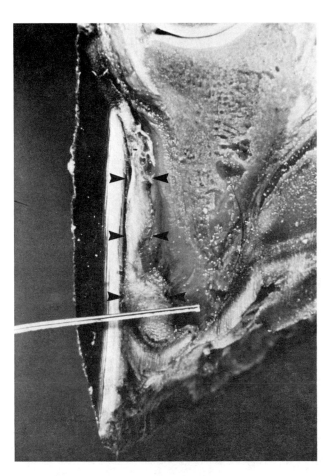

FIG. 5–6. A sagittal section of the hoof wall of a horse with rotation of the coffin bone. The metal probe is pointing to the site of penetration at the sole. Note the wedge of tissue that separates the white line from the dermal laminae (arrows).

X-rays are generally taken from 48 to 72 hours after the acute onset of laminitis, to identify laminar swelling, rotation, and sinking of the coffin bone. Subsequent x-rays will help the veterinarian monitor these changes. In most cases, x-rays should be taken every other day during the acute painful stages of laminitis. Using this information will help the veterinarian decide on the appropriate treatment and predict the outcome. Evidence of rotation of the coffin bone is identified by divergence of the bone in relationship to the hoof wall (Fig. 5–11). A metal object (e.g. wire) can be placed on the dorsal surface of the hoof wall to more clearly identify the hoof wall's relationship to the coffin bone. Additionally a thumbtack can be placed in the apex of the frog. This will give the farrier insight into proper placement of a heart bar shoe.

Generally, a horse's recovery can be predicted from the following guidelines. *Group 1*: Horses that have less than 5.5° of rotation usually return to athletic performance. *Group 2*: Horses that have rotation between 5.5° and 11.5° generally can perform but not up to their previous capabilities. *Group 3*: Horses that have rotation above 11.5° generally remain lame regardless of treatment. Nuclear scintigraphic examination (nuclear scan) can identify increased uptake "hot spots" of the radionuclide, indicating a very early stage of laminitis. The increased uptake is seen before radiographic changes.

Treatment

Laminitis is considered a medical emergency and treatment for complete recovery should begin before the signs of laminitis appear such as in cases as overeating of grain. In others, treatment should begin as soon as possible after the first signs of laminitis are seen. Treatment is aimed at prevention of rotation of the coffin bone because early signs of rotation can be observed on x-rays within a 48-hour period.

Prevention is important in groups of horses that can be considered a high risk (e.g., grain overload, twisted intestine resulting in colic, diarrhea resulting from infection, and mares with retained placenta or metritis). A gram negative vaccine that appears to be effective as a preventive is also available.

Developmental Phase. In grain overload, the treatment is directed at neutralizing the effects of the ingested grain and at controlling the developmental phase of the laminitis. Because the signs of laminitis from this cause often do not appear for 12 to 18 hours after ingestion of the grain, the treatment to clear the intestinal tract is used regardless of whether signs of laminitis have yet appeared. To clear the intestinal tract of the ingested grain, mineral oil is commonly used. Mineral oil acts as a bulk laxative and also coats the wall of the intestine, perhaps inhibiting absorption of toxins. Mineral oil can be repeated at 4- to

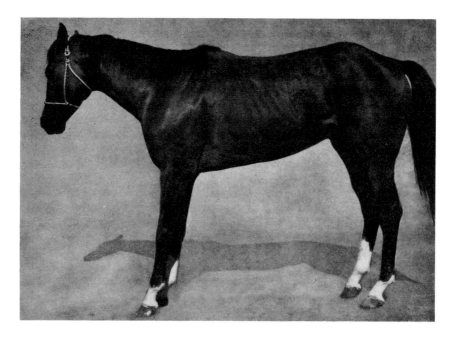

FIG. 5–7. Typical attitude of a horse with laminitis. The hindfeet are carried up farther forward to help take more weight off the forefeet, which are extended forward. This horse had laminitis following a respiratory infection. It was beginning to lose the hoof walls, which was evidenced by cracking at the coronet. Hoof wall changes were minimal, but the sole had dropped and the coffin bones were protruding through the soles of the forefeet.

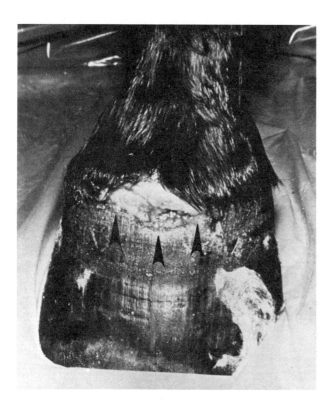

FIG. 5–8. This horse had severe laminitis with rotation of the coffin bone and separation at the coronary band (arrows).

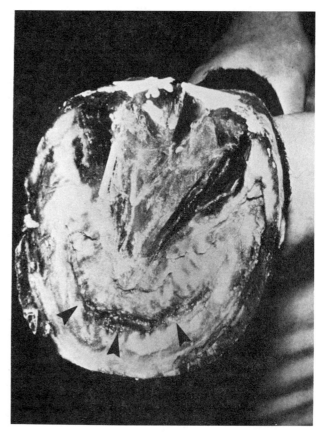

FIG. 5–9. This is the horse shown in Figure 5–8. Note the semicircular separation of the sole just dorsal to the apex of the frog (arrows).

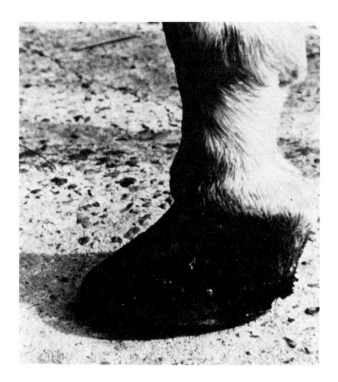

FIG. 5–10. This horse has had chronic laminitis for some time. Note that the spaces between the rings at the heels are wider than those at the toe. The horse has had improper and irregular farrier care.

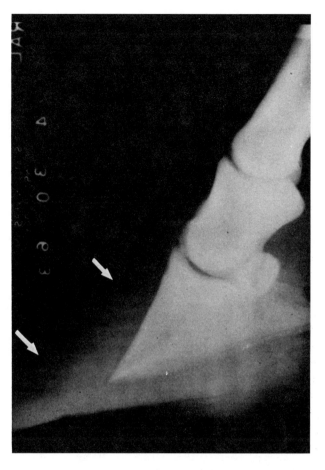

FIG. 5–11. Lateral x-ray of a horse with rotation of the coffin bone. Note that the dorsal part of the coffin bone is not parallel to the dorsal surface of the hoof wall (arrows).

6-hour intervals until all grain has been removed from the intestinal tract.

Even though exercise is known to increase the flow of blood through the foot, it is not recommended because it increases the chances of mechanical separation of the coffin bone from the hoof wall.

Administration of phenylbutazone is helpful because it may prevent the alteration in clotting and may help in dulling the pain and breaking the hypertension cycle that develops in association with the onset of signs of lameness. Banamine may be used because of its antiendotoxic effect.

In cases of infection (e.g., retained placenta, and/or endometritis) antibiotics are often added to the preventative treatment.

Acute Phase. Medical treatment in the acute phase is aimed at the sequence of events happening within the foot, the prevention of progression, and the systemic alterations in the cardiovascular and endocrine systems. Again, analgesics are used to alleviate the pain-induced secretion of catecholamines by the adrenal gland, which causes vessel constriction and systemic hypertension. Presently, the most effective means of breaking the pain-hypertensive cycle appears to be the administration of phenylbutazone intravenously in combination with Acepromazine. Horses should also be placed in stalls with 6 inches of dry soft sand underfoot; this allows the horse to stand in a more comfortable position, and walk more comfortably with reduced tension on the deep digital flexor tendon.

Arguments can be made for the use of hot and cold soaks. Because the foot has a reduced blood flow to the laminae, the decreased temperature obtained with cold soaks should decrease the metabolic requirement for oxygen within the foot. Hot soaks, on the other hand, serve to dilate the vessels within the foot and increase the capillary flow.

Exercise can be a "double-edged sword." It is well known that exercise serves to pump the blood from the foot, which indirectly increases blood flow. The negative side of exercise is twofold: 1) it increases the mechanical forces that are believed to contribute to coffin bone rotation; and 2) walking may increase the pain-related positive feedback cycle that precipitates and perpetuates hypertension and vessel constriction. Because of this, forced exercise is not recommended.

An important part of the treatment is the prevention of coffin bone rotation. Theoretically, soft sand provides good physiologic support for the sole. It also decreases the mechanical forces required to flex and extend the phalangeal joints. Soft sand is more comfortable because it allows the horse to stand in a position of choice. Horses are often found standing with their toes buried in the sand and appear to be quite comfortable. Another benefit may be derived from this: horses appear to walk more comfortably in sand-covered stalls, and this may increase the pumping of blood from the distal region of the foot.

An alternate approach is to eliminate the tension of the deep digital flexor tendon by elevating the heels 18° to 20° with wedge pads. Studies have shown this approach to be effective in preventing rotation of the coffin bone and improving the blood flow to the laminae.

In those cases in which sand stalls or 18° to 20° wedge pads are impractical or cost prohibitive, the sole can be protected with cotton padding or *unvulcanized* rubber, and positive frog support can be achieved with a "lily pad" or a roll of elastic gauze.

It is important to eliminate grain from the diet and offer a good-quality grass hay. Additionally, overweight ponies or horses that have suffered an acute attack should have their feed intake reduced with a long-term commitment by the owner for gradual weight loss.

For mares that develop laminitis accompanied by prolonged diestrus (no signs of estrus), it may be beneficial to bring them in estrus. In some cases, laminitis symptoms disappear with the onset of estrus. For mares that are in heat for prolonged periods with accompanying laminitis, progesterone therapy can be used.

Chronic Laminitis. Treatment of chronic laminitis cases is directed toward preventing further systemic problems and arresting the rotation of the coffin bone.

Systemic hypertension should be controlled because it can lead to secondary complications such as vascular accidents, renal damage, and further foot disease. This is probably best treated with low doses of phenylbutazone to eliminate the pain, Acepromazine, and possibly Lasix. Treatment of hypertension must be done slowly, because many of these horses are chronically hypertensive patients that have accommodated to the elevated pressures. Salt deprivation is recommended. Decreased salt lowers the overall plasma water volume, further reducing the hypertension. When salt is removed from the diet, it should be replaced with 30 grams of potassium chloride administered once a day.

Thyroid therapy, either in the form of iodinated casein or direct oral replacement, has been recommended by some, particularly for horses that are overweight. The direct oral replacement is preferred. The benefit of this treatment is still unproven.

Systemic antibiotics are given to decrease the chances of infection that occurs with separation of the white line (seedy-toe) and separation at the coronary band. Additionally, antiseptic-soaked protective bandages or treatment shoes must be applied to horses that have the corium of the tip of the coffin bone penetrating through the sole. Serious consideration should be given to euthanasia in these cases, because they have a very poor prognosis.

Methionine therapy has been recommended for the reestablishment of the depleted keratin sulfate necessary for generation of healthy horn. Ten grams of methionine are given in the feed for 1 week, after which the dose is decreased to 5 one time a day for 3 to 4 weeks. This will aid in repair of the hard and soft laminar bond.

Elimination of grain from the diet and the offering of a high-quality mixed legume or grass hay is recommended. Overweight horses and ponies should have their food intake decreased gradually to promote weight loss. Exercise is limited to decrease the chances of further rotation of the coffin bone due to mechanical influences.

An important part of the treatment of horses with chronic laminitis is foot care, to prevent further rotation initially, and later to establish a more normal anatomic alignment of the hoof wall and sole with the coffin bone.

Controversy surrounds the best approach for trimming and shoeing the foot that is beginning to rotate, is in the process of rotating, or has rotated. Traditionally, it was recommended to lower the heel to reestablish a normal weight-bearing association of the coffin bone with the sole and ground surface. However, lowering the heel has been shown to increase the tension of the deep digital flexor tendon, which increases the tensile forces that are partially responsible for rotation of the coffin bone. Shortening the toe reduces the tearing forces. Similarly elevating the heel decreases the tension of the deep digital flexor tendon.

In reality, the approach to chronic laminitis in horses depends on the stage of the rotation process. For our purposes, the stages will be separated arbitrarily into impending rotation, rotating, rotated (stable), and rotated and penetrated.

Horses with impending rotation of the coffin bone are usually in the very early stages of chronic laminitis and radiographs may indicate changes on the dorsal surface of the coffin bone. These horses have been treated successfully by putting them in stalls bedded with soft sand. Minimal exercise is given, and medical treatment is instituted. Frequent radiographic monitoring at 48-hour intervals to identify further rotation is important.

Horses that have a severely rotated coffin bone that is painful represent a more challenging situation to both the veterinarian and the farrier. One must realize that with this condition the major suspensory and support structures within the hoof are lost. Correction depends on being able to artificially support these regions until sufficient healing occurs so that the hoof can take over this function. Even though the principles of treatment are simple, there are so many variables, such as the horse's weight, degree of pain, degree of coffin bone rotation, degree of separation of the white line, subsolar infection, amount of hoof wall remaining, thickness of the sole, environment the horse is kept in, and willingness of the owners to treat the horse, that it makes the outcome highly unpredictable. All of these factors are important considerations, because any one of them can determine success or failure of the treatment. It is important for the owner to realize that a severely rotated coffin bone is a life-threatening situation and it is unlikely that treatment will completely correct it. Only rarely will these horses return to previous levels of performance. On the other hand, patients with less damage to the laminae and minimal rotation of the coffin bone may respond quickly to treatment and often completely. However, we have all experienced failure in these areas as well.

The basic principle of foot treatment includes trimming and shoeing to reestablish the normal alignment of the coffin bone and hoof wall and protecting the painful sole from pressure from trauma. To reestablish some normal alignment of the coffin bone for the hoof wall, often excessive hoof wall is removed (Fig. 5–12). Additionally, it is helpful to trim the toe from the ground surface to decrease the pressure on this sensitive region. Trimming of the sole should be done very carefully to avoid the sensitive region. The area just in front of the apex of the frog should not be pared out, for this may expose the dermal laminae associated with the tip of the coffin bone. Therefore, trimming and rasping lines for the heel area should not pass the apex of the frog (Fig. 5–12).

Realistically, the most important thing is to provide good support. Regarding the type of shoe, some prefer a full egg bar, "goose necked" egg bar, or heart bar, whereas others prefer a wide web or wide bar shoe. A shoe placed in a reverse fashion can also be used. Further elevation of the hoof wall can be accomplished by combining a plastic rim pad for those horses that have very flat soles or drop soles. A heart bar pad with an open toe can be applied to protect the subsolar region. A wedge pad can be used to elevate the heels in those horses that are in severe pain after the heels have been lowered. A wedge pad can be used in a reverse fashion in horses that are not in much pain after the heels are trimmed but cannot be sufficiently trimmed to obtain a normal alignment with the coffin bone and the ground surface. In either case, the shoe and pad should not apply direct pressure to the sole in front of the frog. The shoe can be attached by conventional nailing or glue. In extreme cases in which a very thin wall exists, the shoe may have to be glued on or strapped onto the hoof wall. Often, nerve blocking will have to be performed for shoe placement. Horses treated with therapeutic trimming and shoeing will have to be observed closely for signs indicating that further rotation has occurred or that abscesses are developing. In most horses, therapeutic trimming and shoeing is repeated at 4- to 6-week intervals and is continued as long as it is required. In some cases, this may be for the rest of the animal's life.

Surgical Treatments. Surgical treatments are aimed at reducing the tension (pull) of the deep digital flexor tendon and opening the hoof wall and/or sole to allow drainage. Surgeries to reduce the tension of the deep digital flexor tendon include severing the carpal (interior) check ligament (desmotomy) and/or deep digital flexor tendon (tenotomy).

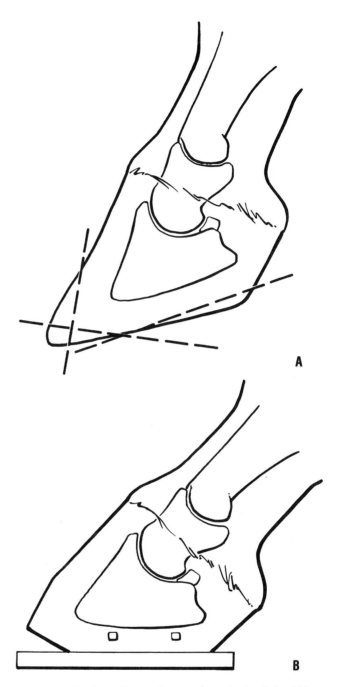

FIG. 5–12. *A*, The dotted line indicates where the hoof should be trimmed to reestablish a more normal alignment of the coffin bone and hoof wall. The toe should also be trimmed slightly to decrease the pressure in this region. *B*, After trimming, a shoe is applied. (From Moyer, W.: Corrective trimming. Vet. Clin. North Am. (Large Anim. Pract.), 2:3, 1980.)

Tenotomy of the deep digital flexor tendon is considered a salvage procedure and is usually done in horses that are valuable for breeding. Generally, positive results of tenotomy only last from 8 to 12 months but in some cases, prolonged benefit is achieved. The hoof wall and sole may be resected (opened) to allow drainage of abscess and blood clots.

Once the hoof wall is resected over the front of the hoof, it takes 7 to 9 months for the hoof wall to completely regrow.

Horses that have rotated and in which the coffin bone has penetrated the sole create a special therapeutic problem. Unless they have great sentimental or breeding value, euthanasia should be considered for humane reasons because of the poor prognosis. In cases that are treated, systemic antibiotics are necessary and the protection of the ground surface of the foot from pressure and contamination is important. Low levels of phenylbutazone or flunixin meglumine (Banamine) are used to reduce the pain. There are two popular methods of protecting the ground surface of the foot. Bulky antiseptic bandages with gauze and cotton held in place with tape can be applied. Additionally, a rubber boot can be fashioned over the top of this to further protect the foot from moisture and contamination. The other treatment commonly used is to apply a metal "treatment plate" to the bottom of the shoe in such a manner that it can be removed so antiseptic packs can be changed. Both of these techniques have been used successfully to manage this type of case for variable periods of time; 2 years is the longest we have experienced.

Successful laminitis treatment involves the cooperative effort of the horse owner, the veterinarian, and the farrier. Although an experienced veterinarian and farrier can set the stage for a horse's recovery, the owner's long-term commitment to the treatment program is paramount. Dealing with laminitis can require emotional strength and a considerable investment of time and money. Besides initial emergency care, a horse suffering from laminitis will need frequent farrier attention and periodic veterinary care for a year or more. Most cases will require daily treatment, specialized management, and close supervision for life. Some horses, despite conscientious treatment and care, will fail to improve or may worsen.

Prognosis

The prognosis is always guarded in any case of laminitis. If the symptoms continue for more than 10 days, the prognosis is unfavorable. However, some cases, such as those that seem to be associated with endocrine imbalances, may continue for prolonged periods without causing excessive changes in the foot, such as rings on the wall and rotation of the coffin bone. Some cases of laminitis continue for a long period and then disappear, leaving the feet distorted. The coffin bone often is rotated when viewed on radiographs (see Fig. 5–11). Whenever rotation of the coffin bone has occurred, the prognosis is unfavorable. Occasionally, infection will enter the corium of the foot as the result of separation at the white line (seedy-toe) caused by disunion of the dermal and epidermal laminae; it may also enter through the sole. Any infection makes the prognosis unfavorable. If cracks appear in

the coronary band, the hoof is likely to slough, making the prognosis more unfavorable.

Although rotation of the coffin bone is a useful prognostic indicator, the control of pain is a major determinant to the outcome.

Navicular Syndrome

Navicular syndrome, first described in 1752, is one of the most common causes of intermittent, often-shifting, forelimb lameness in horses between 4 and 15 years of age. In North America, male Quarter horses and Thoroughbreds, particularly geldings, appear to be at the greatest risk, whereas the syndrome is rarely diagnosed in ponies or Arabian horses. Although the hindlimbs can be affected, for all intents and purposes it is considered a problem of the forelimbs.

The syndrome has been shown to have hereditary predisposition, which is perhaps related to conformation. Factors such as faulty conformation, improper or irregular shoeing, and exercise on hard surfaces are believed to aggravate the condition.

In the past, the condition has been described as a chronic, progressive disease that affects the navicular bone, navicular bursa, and flexor tendons. Recently, this concept has been challenged and new theories regarding the cause and course of the disease have been described.

Anatomy of the Navicular Region

The directional and anatomical terminology used to describe the navicular bone and associated structures has been illustrated earlier in this text. (see Chapter 1). The navicular bone articulates with the coffin joint on its palmar surface and serves as a support to the coffin and short pastern bones. A synovial bursa is interposed between the flexor surface of the navicular bone and the deep digital flexor tendon. This relationship creates a mechanical advantage for the deep digital flexor tendon by allowing it to glide more easily (friction free) over the navicular bone.

The navicular bone is supported in its position by three ligaments. Paired collateral (suspensory) ligaments attach the proximal extremities of the navicular bone to the distal lateral and medial aspects of the long pastern bone. The impar ligament attaches the distal extremity of the navicular bone to the coffin bone. The blood and nerve supply (proximal, distal, medial, lateral) to the navicular bone is distributed through these supportive ligaments. In the mature horse, the distal blood vessels supply almost two-thirds of the navicular bone blood supply.

Causes

Because the term "disease" implies a specific cause, the term "navicular syndrome" better describes the complex factors and mechanisms that produce the clinical signs associated with the navicular region. However, not all lamenesses associated with the heel region of the hoof should be labeled navicular syndrome; this term should be reserved for chronic bilateral forelimb lamenesses that fit a specific set of diagnostic criteria (which will be discussed later).

Possible predisposing factors to navicular syndrome include poor conformation, such as upright pasterns coupled with improper or irregular trimming, and shoeing practices that may create abnormal forces in the foot region. A common error that can lead to the navicular syndrome is associated with the false economy of stretching the intervals between shoeings. As a hoof grows past its optimum reset time, the toe becomes too long and the heel too low, resulting in a broken back axis. Increased pressure between the deep digital flexor tendon and the palmar aspect of the navicular bone may occur with long toe/low under-run heels (those in which the horn tubules are more nearly horizontal than vertical) and sheared heels and/or quarters. This pressure causes the heel pain associated with navicular syndrome. Quarter horses are more likely to develop navicular syndrome than other breeds. This might be because their feet are relatively small compared to their large body mass. Such a conformation increases the force per unit area on the foot, and, in general, predisposes them to more foot problems. In addition, Quarter horses are frequently required to make quick turns and stops, which may increase stress on the feet. Heel problems can also result from applying shoes too narrow and too short for the feet.

In any working horse, concussion and biomechanical forces on the foot within normal limits will cause remodeling of the navicular bone and soft tissue support structures. During the early remodeling phase, the navicular region may be painful from soft tissue sprain and from bone remodeling. As the bone remodels, the flexor surface of the navicular bone increases in density and the horse's heel pain may subside. If excessive loading of the navicular bone occurs during work, the remodeling process results in destructive (degenerative) changes within the navicular bone and continued navicular pain. If noticed early, cases of navicular pain may resolve with treatment, such as corrective trimming and shoeing, both of which reduce abnormal forces on the navicular bone. Table 5–1 summarizes one proposed concept of the course of altered function in navicular syndrome.

It was previously suggested that navicular syndrome was caused by progressive blockage in the arteries, which eventually resulted in reduction in blood flow and oxygen, and nutritional starvation of the navicular bone. The canals along the distal border of the navicular bone were thought to be vascular channels containing the blood supply to the bone. The enlargement and change in shape of these canals (such as "lollipop lesions" seen on x-rays) were said to be the result of the reduced blood supply (ischemia). The severity of the changes seen on x-ray supposedly correlated with the severity of the disease. However, research since then has been unable to substantiate the "ischemia theory" of navicular syndrome.

Recent research has shown that the channels on the distal aspect of the navicular bone do not contain blood vessels. These canals communicate with the coffin joint and are lined by synovium (the type of membrane that lines joints and secretes synovial fluids) and so are more correctly termed "synovial fossae." The blood supply of the navicular bone enters both distally, palmar to the canals, laterally and medially, and proximally, along the border of the navicular bone. While some changes have been seen in the distribution of these vessels in navicular syndrome, the changes do not alter the shape of the synovial fossae. However, enlarged synovial fossae (such as "lollipop lesions") are seen more frequently in horses with navicular syndrome than in normal horses. Because of this, it has been suggested that navicular syndrome results from degeneration of the coffin joint. However, microscopic studies have not supported the concept and no evidence of coffin joint arthrosis has been observed. Presently, it is believed that the enlarged synovial fossae result from aggressive remodeling of the navicular bone's inner cavity and synovial fossa merely fill the available space.

History and Clinical Signs

Horses with navicular syndrome usually have a history of progressive, chronic, unilateral, or bilateral forelimb lameness, which may have had subtle or masked onset. The syndrome is usually bilateral, but the lameness may appear unilateral. The horse may tend to point one forelimb or to alternate pointing of each forelimb. Various abnormalities of the hoof can be associated with navicular syndrome. For example, the heels may be low and underslung with a broken back hoof/pastern axis. This conformation tends to exaggerate deep flexor tendon tension and puts pressure on the navicular bone. One forefoot may also be smaller and more upright than the other, and the heels in one or both feet may be contracted.

While walking or trotting, the horse with navicular syndrome will tend to land on the toe of the foot and may occasionally stumble. At a trot, a horse with bilateral foot pain will tend to have a stiff, shuffling gait and carry its head high and neck rigidly. When these horses are circled in either direction, the lameness will be exaggerated in the limb that is to the inside of the circle. The horse may hold its head and neck to the outside of the circle in an effort to reduce the amount of weight carried on the inside limb. A sharp turn might cause a sudden exaggeration of the lameness on the inside limb, and this might be misinterpreted as shoulder pain.

TABLE 5–1.

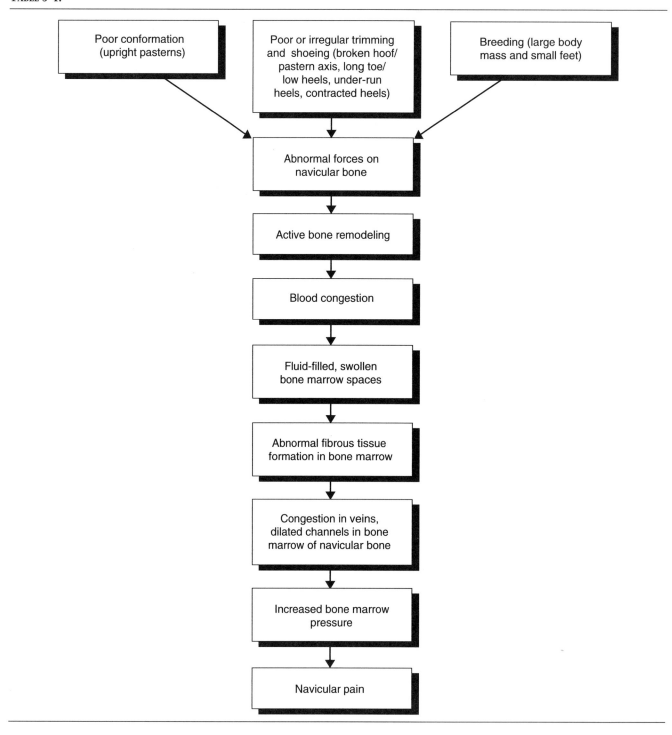

| Poor conformation (upright pasterns) | Poor or irregular trimming and shoeing (broken hoof/ pastern axis, long toe/ low heels, under-run heels, contracted heels) | Breeding (large body mass and small feet) |

Abnormal forces on navicular bone

Active bone remodeling

Blood congestion

Fluid-filled, swollen bone marrow spaces

Abnormal fibrous tissue formation in bone marrow

Congestion in veins, dilated channels in bone marrow of navicular bone

Increased bone marrow pressure

Navicular pain

Occasionally, a horse with severe navicular syndrome coupled with deep flexor tendon damage will land on its heel first, tipping its toe up off the ground as weight is applied to the limb. However, this action is seen more often in cases of laminitis with rotation of the coffin bone and only rarely in cases of navicular syndrome. When this action occurs because of navicular syndrome, it can be assumed that the horse's deep digital flexor tendon is severely damaged, which, if confirmed, is grounds for euthanasia.

A thorough veterinary examination with hoof testers is essential for the clinical diagnosis of navicular syndrome. A hoof tester is used to systematically evaluate pain around the soles and heels. First, the sole is examined. Because horses with heel pain tend to land toe first, they frequently bruise the sole at the toe.

CLINICAL SIGNS ASSOCIATED WITH NAVICULAR SYNDROME
(those in **bold** are the most common classical signs)

---

1. **A history of progressive, chronic, unilateral, or bilateral forelimb lameness**.
2. Pointing of the most severely affected forelimb or alternate pointing if both feet are equally involved.
3. Low underrun heels.
4. Broken back hoof/pastern axis.
5. If unilateral, one forefoot smaller and more upright.
6. Contracted heels in one or both feet and/or sheared heels and quarters.
7. Landing on the toe when walking or trotting to avoid loading the heel region.
8. Occasional stumbling.
9. **Stiff, shuffling gait with shortened, choppy stride**. The stiffness may decrease slightly as the horse warms up, but after rest, it is more pronounced.
10. When circling, lameness of the inside limb more exaggerated and head carried to the outside of circle.
11. A marked lameness after a sharp turn.
12. **Sensitivity to hoof testers with compression of the central one-third of the frog**.
13. A pain response and/or increase in lameness in response to the phalangeal flexion test (flexes coffin, pastern, and fetlock joints) (see Chapter 3).
14. **A positive response to "blocking" (low palmar digital nerve block)** resulting in 70–80% improvement (reduction) in lameness.
15. A pain response and/or increase in lameness from a tendon stress test. The toe is blocked up (elevated) to place extra pressure on the deep flexor tendon and the horse is forced to stand on that limb by holding up the opposite forelimb.
16. A pain response and/or increase in lameness from the frog wedge pressure test. A wedge is placed under the frog to apply pressure to the navicular region, and the horse is forced to stand on that limb by holding up the opposite forelimb.

Even though the primary problem is in the heel region, a hoof tester may elicit pain in the toes of these horses.

After the bottom of the hoof has been tested, the hoof tester is used to evaluate the navicular region. Pressure is applied at an angle to ensure that the navicular bone itself is compressed. Horses that respond to the hoof tester examination (attempt to pull their limb away when pressure is applied) over the navicular region are then closely examined for abnormal hoof conformation, poor trimming, and other causes of pain. Once the hoof abnormalities are corrected, the lameness is reevaluated. It is important to remember that heel pain can occur during remodeling of the navicular bone and may resolve if abnormal stresses are relieved by proper trimming and shoeing. Pain that persists in spite of proper farriery is due to navicular syndrome.

Distinguishing Navicular Syndrome From Other Lamenesses

Navicular syndrome and laminitis are causes of bilateral forelimb lameness. Although both conditions will cause the horse to take short, choppy strides, a horse with navicular pain will land on the toe first. Horses with laminitis tend to land on the heel first. Horses with laminitis also react sharply to tapping over the toe area of the hoof wall and may react painfully to hoof tester examination over the toes. Horses with navicular syndrome will respond more dramatically to hoof tester examination over the central third of the frog. However, it is not always easy to differentiate these two conditions with the hoof tester alone. Nerve blocks and x-rays may be necessary for a diagnosis. These procedures are discussed later.

In addition to navicular syndrome, pain in the heel region of the front feet can be caused by a number of other problems. For example, bruising of the heels may cause heel pain and may be visible after several weeks as red or purple discoloration when the sole is pared with a knife by the veterinarian or farrier. The bruising is due to trauma, and the lameness will usually resolve with 2 to 3 weeks of rest. It is necessary to protect the feet with pads during treatment and to prevent recurrence.

Sheared heels and/or quarters result when one heel and/or quarter of the hoof grows faster, and therefore longer, than the other. They may also result from poor hoof trimming. When examined from behind, one heel bulb and/or quarter is distinctly higher than the other. Ideally, the feet should be balanced so they can achieve even growth.

Horses with fractures of the navicular bone or of the wings of the coffin bone also show heel pain. However, there will usually be a sudden onset of severe lameness. These fractures are differentiated from navicular syndrome by x-raying the foot.

Punctures of the sole resulting in abscesses can also cause heel pain. The pain is usually characterized by sudden onset, with a severe nonweight-bearing lameness in one limb. The specific area of pain is located with hoof testers. Often paring is required to reveal the puncture site and the abscess.

A low, bowed deep digital flexor tendon may cause pain in the heel region and is characterized by soft tissue swelling and warmth between the bulbs of the heel and at the rear portion of the pastern. An ultrasound examination may be required if an injury to the deep digital flexor tendon is suspected.

Other Diagnostic Procedures

Most horses with navicular syndrome will react positively to a phalangeal flexion test (see Chapter 3) because flexion of the phalanges not only increases the compression of the navicular bone between the short pastern bone and the coffin bone but also stresses the soft tissue supporting the navicular bone. The increased lameness after flexion may persist for several minutes in affected horses.

Palmar digital nerve blocks are used to localize the site of pain to the heel region of the hoof. In horses that show lameness primarily in one limb, a unilateral nerve block (blocking only one limb) may eliminate the lameness if it is actually a unilateral problem. However, after a unilateral nerve block, if the lameness shifts to the opposite forelimb, both forelimbs are affected. The lameness only may have appeared unilateral because the pain was more severe in one limb than in the other. In horses with a shuffling, bilateral forelimb lameness, a nerve block in one limb often causes the lameness to appear more severe in the other forelimb. Bilateral nerve blocks usually eliminate the lameness.

Elimination of the lameness by palmar digital nerve blocks suggests pain in the heel region of the hoof. Because the navicular bone is only one of several structures in this region of the hoof, not every horse that improves with palmar digital nerve blocks has navicular syndrome. Therefore, the results of the nerve block are interpreted in light of the horse's history, clinical examination, and findings from x-rays. A coffin joint block may be done to see if there is improvement in lameness. If there is improvement, your veterinarian may recommend treatment of the coffin joint with anti-inflammatory drugs. In some cases, the veterinarian may want to block the navicular bursa. If the lameness improves, treatment of this site may be recommended.

Radiographic Evidence. If navicular syndrome is suspected as the cause of forelimb lameness on the basis of physical examination findings, x-rays are often taken of both navicular bones. X-rays may also be taken in order to rule out other painful conditions of the foot.

It is necessary for the veterinarian to examine several views of the navicular bone; therefore, three to five x-rays may be taken of each hoof. In the past, it was believed that flask- or "lollipop"-shaped fossae were associated with abnormal forces on the navicular bone (Fig. 5–13). However, flask-shaped fossae are seen in the navicular bone of only 40% of horses with navicular syndrome and are also found in 10 to 11% of normal horses. Therefore, enlarged synovial fossae alone are no longer believed to be a reliable x-ray indication of navicular syndrome.

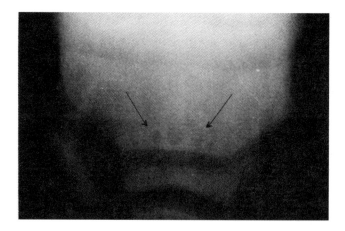

FIG. 5–13. Mushroom- or lollipop-shaped enlarged vascular foramina at the distal border of the navicular bone.

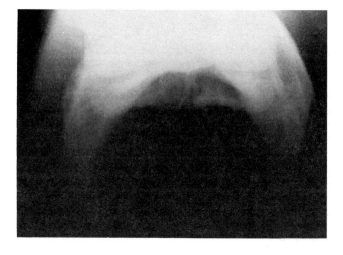

FIG. 5–14. An x-ray view of the navicular bone. Arrows are pointing to the thinning of the central eminence on the flexor surface of the navicular bone.

Loss of the outer layer of bone on the flexor surface of the navicular bone (Fig. 5–14) is associated with degeneration of the bone and possibly with adhesions between the navicular bone and deep digital flexor tendon. Therefore, it is an important indicator of the disorder. Calcified areas along the flexor surface of the navicular bone represent adhesions between the deep digital flexor tendon and the navicular bone.

Loss of the distinct border between the outer surface (flexor cortex) and inner (medullary) cavity of the navicular bone, is an important finding in cases of navicular syndrome (Fig. 5–15). This change may be present in up to 80% of horses with navicular syndrome, but in less than 20% of normal horses (without lameness). Abnormal hardening (sclerosis) of the inner cavity of the navicular bone may also be seen in horses with navicular syndrome.

Bony outgrowths (osteophytes) on the wings of the navicular bone may result from abnormal biomechanical forces on the navicular bone. Although the outgrowths may cause pain while developing, once visible on x-rays, they are of questionable significance.

The veterinarian may find other abnormal changes in a horse's x-rays. The presence of the x-ray changes, in conjunction with physical examination findings, may suggest a diagnosis of navicular syndrome. However, abnormal x-rays alone do not indicate that a horse has navicular syndrome. They are interpreted along with the horse's history, its response to hoof testers and flexion tests, its movement, and its response to palmar digital nerve blocks.

Treatment Strategies

In the past, a diagnosis of navicular syndrome spelled doom for the athletic horse. With early diagnosis and treatment, however, many horses with the syndrome can be returned to full use. Many cases can be resolved simply by adjusting the hoof angles with corrective trimming and regular proper shoeing.

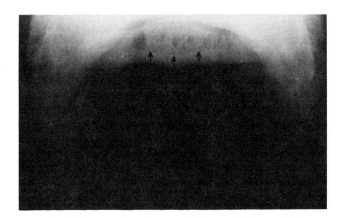

FIG. 5–15. Loss of the distinct border at the corticomedullary junction (arrow). This x-ray change is usually seen in older horses (over 5 years of age).

Other cases require the use of drugs and surgical procedures.

The treatment of navicular syndrome begins with careful examination of conformation and hoof balance. Correction of hoof angles and heel contraction can reduce the pain and slow the progression of navicular syndrome. Drugs are often administered concurrently with corrective trimming and shoeing. As a last resort, surgical treatment can be used to relieve pain and return the horse to work.

CORRECTIVE TRIMMING AND SHOEING
(See Chapter 6)

Many horses with navicular syndrome will respond to corrective trimming and balancing of the feet and will not require medical or surgical therapy. In one study, the clinical signs of navicular syndrome in 36 horses treated only with trimming and shoeing improved within 3 months, and 86% of the horses remained free of lameness after 1 year. Therefore, corrective trimming and shoeing are the cornerstone of navicular syndrome therapy and should be routinely employed. However, in many cases, isoxsuprine treatment is included to promote increased blood flow to the foot.

The primary goal of corrective trimming and shoeing for navicular syndrome is to reduce abnormal biomechanical forces on the navicular region. This is accomplished by restoring the normal hoof/pastern axis and providing maximum support.

The hoof should be trimmed to achieve a normal hoof/pastern axis. The angle of the hoof should be parallel to the angle of the pastern. To attain a parallel axis, excess toe (and in some cases, excess heel) may need to be removed. If the hoof cannot be trimmed to the desirable alignment, special shoes and/or pads must be applied to achieve a parallel axis. Wedge pads or wedge-heel shoes can be used for horses with low heels to raise the heels, which corrects the hoof angle until the heels have grown sufficiently.

For hooves with under-run heels, shoes that provide maximum support should be used. Ideally, a line drawn at the hoof wall at the toe should be parallel to one drawn at the hoof wall at the heels. Many horses with navicular syndrome, however, have under-run heels where the heel angle is much lower than the toe angle. Under-run heels result in an area of support that not only is too small for the horse's weight but the base of support is displaced forward. If the underrun condition is longstanding or severe, there is little chance of restoring normal hoof conformation.

Egg bar shoes will increase the area of weight distribution on the ground, increase protection of the heel area, move the base of support rearward, and provide maximum support for the deep flexor tendon. Egg bar shoes are oval when viewed from the sole. When viewed from the side, the heel of an egg bar shoe should be behind a point that lies below the midpoint of the cannon. For maximum support, a vertical line dropped from the heel bulbs should touch the back of the shoe. The application of egg bar shoes requires a farrier who is knowledgeable in the principles of therapeutic trimming and skilled in making and applying these shoes.

In some cases, shoes with extended heels may be helpful. Extended heels might make a shoe appear too long for the hoof. The extra length of the branches provides more support than a standard-length shoe but not as much support as an egg bar shoe.

To allow heel expansion, nails should not be used past the bend (widest part) in the quarters. The shoe should be wide enough at the heel region so normal expansion and growth of the foot will not cause the hoof to spread beyond the edges of the shoe.

Horses with contracted heels can be shod with slippered pads or shoes, which encourage the heels to expand with each stride. For horses with bruised or flat soles, rim pads may be necessary for the initial shoeing to raise the sole off the ground. Full pads can also be used for bruised soles, offering more positive sole protection than rim pads.

Horses with navicular syndrome tend to land toe first, sometimes stabbing the toe into the ground. Squaring, rocking, or rolling the toe of the shoe may help prevent the stumbling that can result when the toe catches on the ground upon landing. Modifying the toe of the shoe will also help ease "breakover," resulting in less stress on the deep flexor tendon as the hoof leaves the ground.

Although adjustment to a horse's hoof angles can be made rather dramatically, the response might be immediate or gradual. It could take 2 to 3 months before clinical signs improve. It will likely take months to achieve a normal hoof conformation and, in some severe cases, the run-under heels may be past the point of no return.

MEDICAL TREATMENTS

Periodic administration of phenylbutazone ("bute") and other nonsteroidal anti-inflammatory drugs may be necessary to relieve pain if the horse is to continue working. However, continued use of bute without trying to correct the underlying problems will hasten the progression of navicular syndrome and may have toxic systemic side effects, such as alimentary canal ulcers and kidney damage.

Isoxsuprine hydrochloride is another drug that has been used to treat horses with navicular syndrome. Isoxsuprine has been proven useful in treating navicular syndrome, although its mechanism of action is not completely understood. In two separate trials using horses with navicular syndrome, the animals treated with isoxsuprine hydrochloride showed significantly greater improvement than those that received a placebo. The improvement in clinical signs can persist for up to a year after the discontinuation of isoxsuprine, especially when foot problems are also corrected. However, in some cases, isoxsuprine ther-

apy is continued year round but at lower doses. The continued treatment with isoxsuprine is used in horses that perform year round and that become painful when taken off the drug. Isoxsuprine is an orally administered drug with no known adverse side effects when given at the recommended dosage. Horses receiving isoxsuprine usually have palpably warmer extremities than normal because the drug causes the blood vessels to dilate. The drug has not been proven safe for use in pregnant mares.

SURGICAL TREATMENTS

Surgical therapy is usually reserved for cases of navicular syndrome that have not responded to the more conservative treatments already discussed. Two surgical treatments are currently available—palmar digital neurectomy and navicular suspensory desmotomy.

Palmar Digital Neurectomy. Severing the palmar digital nerves in the pastern region desensitizes the caudal one-third to one-half of the foot, relieving the pain associated with this region. Palmar digital neurectomy is done in conjunction with corrective hoof trimming and shoeing to reduce abnormal forces on the foot and to slow the progression of navicular disease. Before considering a neurectomy, the horse owner should check with the breed and performance association regarding their regulations.

In all cases in which palmar digital neurectomy is being considered, a diagnostic nerve block should be performed first. The degree of response to a nerve block will be similar to the response obtained by neurectomy. Some horses have additional nerve branches supplying the navicular region, and if these nerve branches are not identified and cut, the response to neurectomy will be less than optimal. Neurectomy may be delayed for several days after the diagnostic nerve block has been performed in order to reduce inflammation at the surgical site. The surgery may be done while the horse remains standing, using only a local anesthetic agent. However, epineural capping, which may reduce the rate of nerve regrowth and neuroma formation, requires general anesthesia.

Palmar digital neurectomy is not recommended in cases of deep digital flexor tendinitis (as manifest by a heel-toe action while walking, swelling between the heel bulbs, and mineralization of the tendon on radiographs) because the tendon might rupture with normal use of the limb.

High nerving (cutting the palmar nerve at the level of the sesamoid bones) desensitizes the entire foot and because the horse cannot feel its feet, it is prone to stumbling. High nerving, once considered an option, is no longer used for riding horses.

Several complications can occur following palmar digital neurectomy. The most common is regrowth of the nerve and a recurrence of clinical signs of navicular syndrome. This regrowth may occur as soon as 6 months after neurectomy but usually does not occur until more than a year later. Unfortunately, the nerve may regrow more than once. The only treatment is to repeat the neurectomy and special techniques can be used to prevent the regrowth of nerves.

Painful neuromas (firm lumps) can form on the severed nerves in their disorganized attempts to regrow. This makes the neurectomy site extremely sensitive when palpated and causes lameness. The treatment for this complication is to perform a second neurectomy above the neuroma and select a method of neurectomy that has less chance of neuroma formation.

An uncommon complication of palmar digital neurectomy is loss of blood supply and sloughing of the foot. Sloughing occurs when excess fibrous tissue develops at the surgical site (due to tissue trauma) and envelops the palmar digital arteries and strangles them. There is no treatment for this complication and euthanasia should be performed (Figures 5–16 and 5–17).

The deep digital flexor tendon may rupture if degenerative changes were present in the tendon before neurectomy or it may rupture afterward as the navicular syndrome progresses. Normal weightbearing on the affected limb following neurectomy can cause the damaged tendons to degenerate to the point of rupture. Although there is no treatment for this condition, some horses may be salvaged for breeding purposes by fusion (arthrodesis) of the coffin joint.

Although complications can arise after palmar digital neurectomy, this surgery allows many horses with navicular syndrome to return to full use. The period of pain relief after neurectomy varies, but some horses remain pain-free for up to 5 years after surgery.

Navicular Suspensory Desmotomy. In this infrequently used technique, the suspensory ligament of the navicular bone is cut close to its attachments on the long pastern bone. In one report, 13 of 16 horses that underwent the procedure were able to return to their previous level of activity three months after surgery. However, the surgery can be technically difficult because it is not easy to locate the ligament and general anesthesia is required in all cases. Presently it is not widely recommended.

Treatment Summary

After navicular syndrome has been diagnosed, the hoof conformation should be carefully evaluated. The hooves should be properly trimmed and shod by a qualified farrier. It is imperative that the horse be shod at regular intervals to maintain optimum hoof alignment. Medical treatment with concurrent use of isoxsuprine hydrochloride and phenylbutazone may be used if necessary. Surgery should be considered only after corrective trimming and shoeing have been attempted and medical treatment has failed. Of the surgical techniques available, palmar digital neurectomy is the safest and yields the most reliable results.

Prognosis

Generally, the prognosis must be guarded in all cases. This is supported by the fact that only 9 of 38

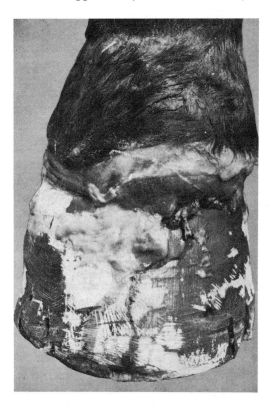

FIG. 5–17. Appearance of a foot that sloughed after two operations for neurectomy. The first one was for palmar digital neurectomy and the second was for removal of neuromas. Several weeks later, the foot presented the above appearance. At necropsy, the vessels and nerves were dissected out, and it was found that neurofibers and scar tissue had completely occluded and even invaded the digital arteries. Water could not be forced through the arteries by syringe.

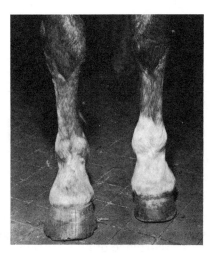

FIG. 5–16. Contracted left foot resulting from chronic navicular disease.

horses became sound after treatment, and no clear-cut advantage between medical and surgical therapy can be established. However, with the advent of new medical therapy such as isoxsuprine hydrochloride a better prognosis may be predicted in the future. Neurectomy should be considered as a last resort and may provide many added years of service.

Palmar digital neurectomy is not legal in all states or in all breed or performance associations. Therefore, if the intent is to race or show the horse after the neurectomy, it is essential to check on the legalities. As long as only the palmar digital nerve is neurectomized, the horse will be as sure-footed as it was before the surgery. Although the heel region is desensitized, nail punctures in this region will cause the inflammation to spread to sensitive areas in a very short time.

Fractures of the Navicular Bone

Fractures of the navicular bone are rare, but they may follow navicular syndrome or result from trauma to the foot.

Generally, three types of fractures affect the navicular bone: chip fractures, simple fractures, and comminuted (multiple break) fractures.

Chip fractures usually involve the distal border of the navicular bone. They are considered uncommon and are frequently associated with other radiographic signs of navicular syndrome. Fracture fragments will range from rectangles to ovals and usually measure from one-twelfth to one-half inch across.

Simple fractures run vertically, slightly oblique (angled), or transversely (across the bone). The vertical and slightly oblique fractures usually occur fairly close to the central ridge of the navicular bone, either lateral or medial to it. Generally, these fractures are not displaced, but they are usually slightly separated so an obvious fracture line exists on the x-ray (Fig. 5–18). The forelimb is most frequently affected with simple fractures, although they have been reported in the hindlimbs as well.

Comminuted fractures are considered to be even more uncommon than simple fractures. With comminuted fractures there may be some displacement of the bone fragments.

Causes

Chip Fractures. On x-rays, chip fractures separate from the margins of the navicular bone at the attachments of the ligaments. The bone surfaces are sharp, with good density in the surrounding bone. Because these fractures are frequently involved with other radiographic signs of navicular syndrome, it is easy to assume that the changes occurring at the distal border of the navicular bone may predispose this type fracture.

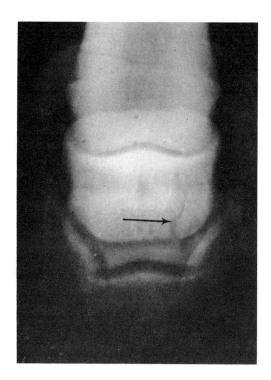

FIG. 5–18. Fracture of the navicular bone (arrow).

Simple and Comminuted Fractures. Violent concussion to the foot may cause fracture of the navicular bone, or the condition may follow a chronic case of navicular disease. In the case of a horse that has received a palmar digital neurectomy, if the navicular bone has become demineralized, adhesions between the deep flexor tendon and the navicular bone may fracture the bone when the horse starts to use the foot normally. The demineralized bone may break because of stress from the adhesions or pressure imparted by the deep digital flexor tendon. Rear limb navicular fractures can occur from kicking solid objects. The navicular bone may also fracture as a result of a penetrating wound (e.g., nail puncture).

Signs

The signs are identical to those caused by navicular syndrome, but they may be more acute. Unilateral contraction of a front foot may be evident, especially if only fracture is present and not a bilateral navicular syndrome. X-ray will reveal the fracture (see Fig. 5–18).

Treatment

Healing of the navicular bone is poor and most of these develop into a nonunion. Chip fractures should be treated in a similar manner described for navicular syndrome. If poor results are obtained from therapeutic shoeing, a palmar digital neurectomy should be considered. Simple fractures that occur from a traumatic incident may be helped by palmar digital neurectomy. Alternatively, bone screws have been used to successfully treat some of these fractures. Comminuted fractures can even be more difficult to treat, but neurectomy can be tried. Nerve blocking is used to evaluate the effectiveness of neurectomy. Prolonged rest should be considered to allow the fracture to heal and prevent further damage to the surrounding structures.

Prognosis

The prognosis is unfavorable, but palmar digital neurectomy will permit limited use of some horses.

Sheared Heels and/or Quarters

Sheared heels and quarters are descriptive terms for the structural breakdown that occurs between the heel bulbs and quarters with a disproportionate use of one heel and/or quarter. Either the lateral or medial heel and/or quarter may be out of balance and result in the overuse of one heel and/or quarter (Fig. 5–19). The degree of damage and lameness is proportional to the duration and degree of the foot imbalance. This shearing of the heel and/or quarter can result in a chronic heel soreness (similar to navicular syndrome), hoof cracks in the heel bar or quarter, and deep thrush in the central sulcus of the frog, and/or it may initiate navicular syndrome.

Causes

Improper trimming and shoeing so that one heel and/or quarter is left longer than the other is one of the most common causes of this condition. A right-handed farrier might tend to remove slightly more heel and quarter off of the lateral side of the left forefoot and the medial side of the right forefoot when rasping. Because the heels and quarters are a different length and height, the foot is said to be out of balance, and a disproportionate force is applied to the longer heel and/or quarters during weight-bearing. This creates an abnormal shearing force between the heel bulbs and structural breakdown occurs. Also, horses with long toes and short heels are believed to be more susceptible to the development of sheared heels and/or quarters. This heel conformation is commonly seen in racing Thoroughbreds in North America. Another situation in which sheared heels and/or quarters may occur is when corrective trimming is used in an attempt to alter conformational defects in young horses. For instance, it is a common error to remove more of the lateral heel and quarter (lower it) and raise the medial (inside) with a shim placed between the shoe and the hoof wall in a base-wide horse that has a tendency

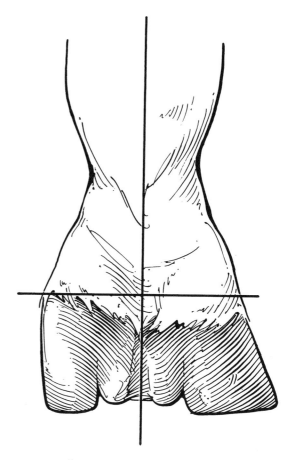

FIG. 5–19. An illustration of a horse with sheared heels. Notice that the left heel bulb is higher than the right. The hoof wall is straighter on the affected side (left side), whereas the hoof wall associated with the lower heel (right side) is flared. At exercise, the left heel will contact the ground first, causing an upward displacement of the heel bulb.

to toe-out. Although the "correction" may result in an aesthetically more pleasing picture, it causes a disproportionate force to the medial quarter of the heel during weight-bearing. This then can result in the upward displacement of the medial heels. Heel caulks ("stickers") can further exaggerate the slightest imbalance in the heels and result in a shearing effect. Additionally, a sprung branch on a shoe that has gone undetected could cause medial/lateral imbalance. This imbalance, if continued, could predispose a horse to shearing of the heels and quarters. Finally, selective weight-bearing on one side of the foot for a lengthy period could result in shearing.

Clinical Signs and Diagnosis

Visually, the heel bulb and/or quarter on the affected side is usually higher, the hoof wall is straighter, and there is often an abnormal flare to the hoof wall opposite the affected side (see Fig. 5–19). The differential height in the heel bulb and/or quarter is best viewed from behind either with a horse standing on a hard, flat surface or when the limb is hand-held and viewed directly. The accentuated flare opposite the affected side is noticed while viewing the horse from the front or from above at the shoulder level. The hoof wall on the affected side can also be rolled under in very severe chronic cases.

In horses viewed from the rear as they are walked on a smooth, hard surface, the heel of the affected side usually contacts the ground surface first and an upward displacement of that heel bulb occurs (see Fig. 5–19). The lameness can be variable and is dependent on the degree of damage from the shearing effect.

On palpation, an important finding is the loss of structural integrity between the heel bulbs. On manipulation, the heel bulbs can be separated more easily and can be displaced in opposite directions (Fig. 5–20). Manipulation can be painful. Because hoof testers frequently indicate pain similar to that observed in navicular syndrome and blocking of the palmar digital nerves will alleviate the lameness, this condition must be differentiated from navicular syndrome. X-rays will help rule out the possibility of any bony structure involvement.

Treatment

Treatment is directed toward bringing the foot, heels, and/or quarters back into balance and alleviating the pain. The selection of treatment depends on the severity of the shearing and the degree of hoof wall deformation. Cases with a mild imbalance usually respond to trimming of the longer heel and/or quarter and the application of an egg bar shoe for stability. Because low heels and long toes are believed to predispose horses to sheared heels and/or quarters, consideration should be given to the removal of the long toe and leaving the heel as long as possible. Some feel that just removing the shoe, trimming the foot, and allowing free exercise will suffice.

More exaggerated cases will require an additional trimming and more resets of the shoe to achieve balance. In these cases, the affected heel and/or quarter is displaced sufficiently upward so that a single trimming cannot restore the foot to balance. For treatment, the affected side is trimmed from the heel through the quarter to create a space when the shoe is applied (Fig. 5–21). Body weight and time will force the heel back into alignment. Because these horses frequently exhibit instability between their heels, an egg bar shoe is recommended, and in some it may be required for the rest of the animal's athletic career.

In very severe cases in which considerable structural damage to the heel bulb and/or quarter cracks has developed, a diagonal bar shoe can be added to the egg bar shoe. This is applied to the affected side to provide more protection and stability.

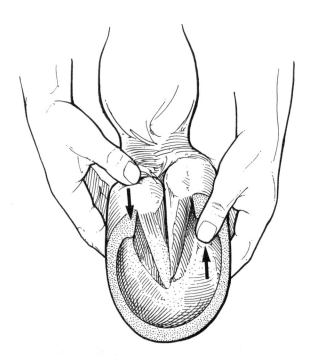

FIG. 5–20. On palpation, the heel bulbs of a horse affected with sheared heels may be separated more easily and displaced in opposite directions. This increased movement is caused by loss of structural integrity between the heel bulbs, and manipulation is often painful.

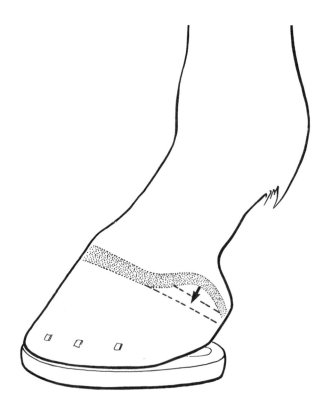

FIG. 5–21. Corrective trimming and shoeing of a horse affected with sheared heels and quarters. The affected side is trimmed from the heel through the quarter to create a space between the hoof wall and the full-bar shoe. The stippled area indicates the level of the coronary band. The arrow is pointing to where the coronary band should be located.

If the hoof wall on the affected side begins to curl under, the horse can be shod full to the affected side in an attempt to encourage hoof wall growth to that side and to a more normal alignment with the limb.

Foals with sheared heels and/or quarters are best treated with corrective trimming of the heels and rounding the toe to encourage proper breakover. This should be done early to prevent possible damage to developing bones. But shoes should probably not be applied before 8 to 9 months of age.

Prognosis

Prognosis is considered good for mildly affected horses. Horses with severely exaggerated sheared heels and quarters will require several resets of the shoe to bring the foot back into balance. In cases with severe structural damage, the heel may require the added support of a full bar shoe for the rest of the animal's life.

Pedal Osteitis

Pedal osteitis is a demineralization of the coffin bone resulting from inflammation. On x-rays, it appears as a roughening of the solar borders of the coffin bone. Although the problem may be found anywhere in the coffin bone, it is usually confined to the toe and wing regions of the front feet.

Causes

Persistent inflammation of the foot, due to numerous factors, may cause the coffin bone to become less dense. Chronic bruising of the sole (as in navicular disease), persistent corns, laminitis (especially from concussion or road founder), puncture wounds, and other inflammations over a long period of time may cause the disease. In some cases of osteitis, there is actually an infection present. Whenever an infected corn or a puncture wound causes damage to the coffin bone, this is the case. Other causes, such as laminitis or persistent sole bruising, are not infectious. Nutritional and heritable causes must also be considered. Lameness leading to disuse osteoporosis has also been implicated.

In some cases, bony outgrowth may be the result of local inflammation of the periosteum due to detachment of a few dermal laminae. However, outgrowths of this type are not uncommon in horses that show no lameness.

Signs and Diagnosis

Lameness is obvious in all gaits, and examination with a hoof tester will reveal pain at the bottom of the foot. This pain may be diffuse or localized. Pedal osteitis may merely be a sign of one of the diseases mentioned in the discussion of causes.

X-rays indicate demineralization at one or more points in the coffin bone (Figs. 5–22 and 5–23), not to be confused with the normal notch of the toe of the coffin bone. Roughened areas along the solar border of the coffin bone may appear anywhere from the toe to the lateral wings. These ridges are not normally smooth because of vascular patterns in the bone.

The vascular channels and roughening of the solar border will vary considerably with the x-ray view that is taken and some of these findings occur in normal horses. The degree of roughening can also vary from the medial to lateral, and the lateral border usually appears to be more roughened when a variation exists. The diagnosis of pedal osteitis is made only when physical signs concur with the radiographic findings.

Treatment

Treatment of this problem depends on the cause. Shoeing may help by keeping the sole away from the ground and preventing pressure on it. Rim pads will elevate the sole from the ground; full pads will protect the sole from ground trauma. For very flat soles, a combination of a rim and a full pad may be necessary: the rim pad will elevate the sole from the flat pad, and the flat pad will provide protection from the ground. See Chapter 6 for information on pads and packing. No matter what type of packing is used, the amount should be minimal to avoid putting pressure on the sole and subsequently the coffin bone. A wide web shoe with the inner edge relieved (to prevent sole pressure) can also be helpful. When pedal osteitis affects

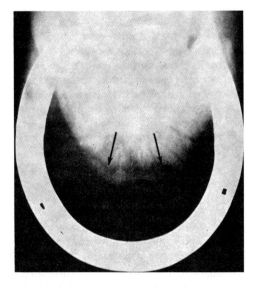

FIG. 5–22. Pedal osteitis. Note the ragged appearance of the tip of the coffin bone indicating osteitis and fragmentation. This was caused by a sole abscess at the toe, and osteitis resulted.

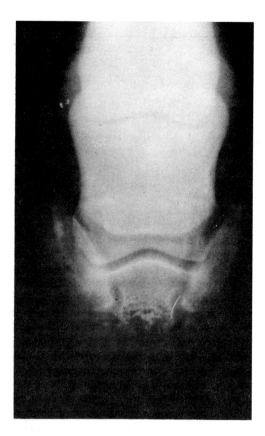

FIG. 5–23. Example of severe pedal osteitis. Notice demineralization of toe portion of the coffin bone. This condition usually results from a chronic inflammatory condition of the foot, such as laminitis, sole bruising, or persistent infection of the foot.

the lateral wings of the solar border of the bone, severing the palmar digital nerves may be helpful, provided soundness occurs after blocking these nerves with a local anesthetic. However, neurectomy is only used in extreme cases. In most, protective shoeing, anti-inflammatory therapy for variable periods, and rest will usually suffice. In cases in which the sole is thin and soft, it can be medicated topically with equal parts of phenol, formalin, and iodine to toughen it. If fracture of the coffin bone is associated with pedal osteitis, a prolonged convalescence will be required. The primary cause should always be treated first.

Prognosis

The prognosis is guarded to unfavorable if the disease is chronic; such a condition is difficult to reverse.

Subchondral Bone Cysts of the Coffin Bone

Subchondral (beneath the cartilage) bone cysts of the coffin bone are uncommon and can affect a wide variety of horse breeds of all ages. Trauma is considered to be the most likely cause.

A history of an acute onset of lameness with a chronic course of intermittent lameness is common. Often lameness subsides with rest and recurs with exercise.

Treatment

Recommended treatments of subchondral bone cysts have included: 1) enforced rest, 2) complete stall rest followed by increasing exercise, and 3) surgical curettage (a scraping or cleaning out of the abnormal tissues). Surgical curettage appears to be the best method; however, local infection can be a complication.

Fractures of the Coffin Bone

Fractures of the coffin bone are not common. The injury is usually associated with exercise on hard surfaces, and the forefeet, particularly the left forefoot, appear to be predisposed in horses racing counterclockwise. Horses turning abruptly (barrel racing, roping) also appear susceptible. Although all breeds and classes of horses are affected, a higher incidence has been identified in racing breeds.

Although fractures of the coffin bone can assume a variety of configurations, there are basically six types of fractures that affect it: 1) Nonarticular (not involving the coffin joint) wing fractures (Fig. 5–24), 2) articular (involving the coffin joint) wing fractures, 3) a central articular fracture that roughly divides the coffin bone into two separate halves (Fig. 5–25), 4) fragmented articular and nonarticular fractures (Fig. 5–26), 5) chip fractures usually at the solar margin. (Fig. 5–27), and 6) extensor process fractures (covered in the next section). Of these, the articular wing fracture appears to be the most common. See also p. 396–7, Figure 6–75.

Causes

Trauma, especially when accompanied by a twisting action as the foot lands, is the predominant cause of fracture of the coffin bone. Occasionally, the coffin bone may be fractured as a result of the penetration of a foreign body through the sole. The coffin bone also may be fractured as the result of trauma to a large sidebone. In such a case, the coffin bone usually breaks through one of the lateral processes.

Although trauma is regarded as the primary cause of fractures of the coffin bone, other factors such as stone bruises, hard surfaces, improper shoeing, infectious conditions, and nutritional deficiencies have been incriminated. It is felt that wing fractures affect the lateral left forelimb and the medial right forelimb because of selective trauma to these regions during counterclockwise racing. On the other hand, central

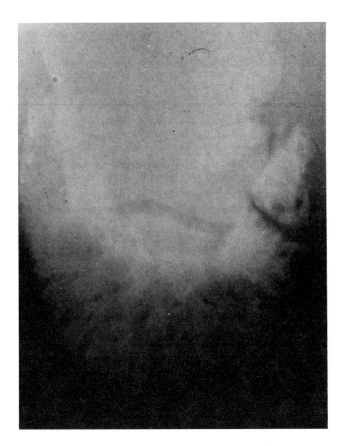

FIG. 5–24. An x-ray illustrating a nonarticular wing fracture.

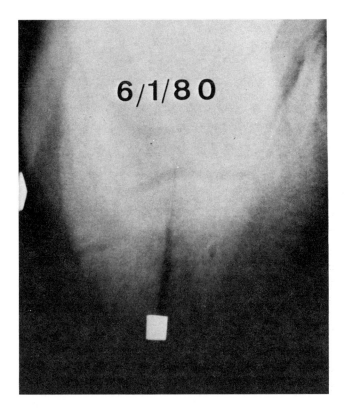

FIG. 5–25. A central articular fracture.

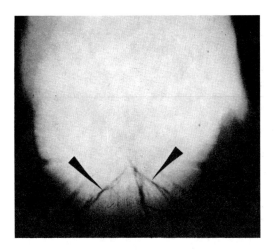

FIG. 5–26. A comminuted (multiple, fragmented) fracture. This fracture occurs in three places (arrows) and extends into the coffin joint.

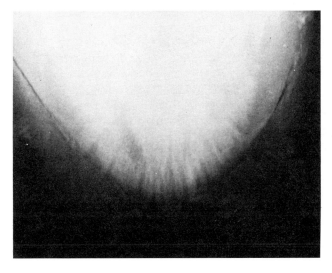

FIG. 5–27. Chip fractures at the solar margin of the coffin bone.

fractures are thought to result from external trauma to the hoof from kicking solid objects or when the foot lands on an unyielding object.

Signs

With articular fractures, the lameness is an acute supporting-limb lameness. In some cases, the horse may refuse to place the affected foot on the ground for as long as 72 hours. The history will often reveal that the lameness occurred suddenly during work and that no known trauma had occurred. There often will be increased digital pulsation and heat in the affected foot, and examination with hoof testers and percussion (tapping) will reveal pain over the entire sole region. With nonarticular fractures, the lameness will not be so severe. Hoof testers will cause selective pain over the affected quarter. If the fracture has been present for some time, signs of lameness will not be as evident, and the history, hoof testers, and x-rays will be necessary to diagnose it.

Fractures of the coffin bone in the rear limb might be overlooked because the attitude of the limb may resemble that in injuries further up the limb. Any acute weight-bearing lameness should be examined for the possibility of coffin bone fracture. Withdrawal of fluid from the coffin joint will reveal blood with an articular fracture.

Diagnosis

The diagnosis can be positively confirmed only by the use of x-rays. These should be taken to determine not only if the fracture is present, but also where it is. In some cases, it may be necessary to take special views in order to find the crack in the coffin bone. The defect in the bone may remain for a long time and, in some cases, may never show clinical union. Horses so affected may be sound even though union is not obvious on the x-rays.

Examination of the foot with hoof testers, along with the history, is often used in establishing a diagnosis before x-rays have been taken.

Treatment

Therapy is aimed at immobilizing the fracture and preventing expansion of the hoof wall. To do this, the coffin bone can be immobilized by the use of a Klimesh contiguous clip shoe (Fig. 6–90, p. 409). The

shoe is shaped to fit close around the entire hoof so no expansion can occur. A bar is used to prevent heel expansion and steel clips (approximately 1 inch long) are welded around the perimeter of the shoe, from heel to heel. The bases of the clips are touching (contiguous) and their angles approximate that of the hoof wall. Generally, 8 to 12 clips are required. Any space between the clips and the hoof wall is filled with a quick-setting hoof acrylic. The foot should be kept in this type of shoe for 6 to 8 months; the shoe should be reset every 4 to 6 weeks. After clinical relief of the symptoms, the horse should be shod with quarter clips and a bar shoe to prevent hoof wall expansion (Figs. 5–28 and 5–29). Some horses require constant use of clips or a bar shoe to ensure working soundness. The affected horse should not be worked for approximately 8 to 10 months and, in some cases, one year of rest may be advisable if symptoms do not disappear. Alternatively, the foot can be placed in a rim shoe or confined in a cast. Both effectively prevent the expansion of the hoof wall during weight-bearing.

If the fracture has been caused by a puncture wound, the wound must be treated as discussed in the Penetrating Wounds of the Foot section in this chapter. A bone abscess or demineralization of the coffin bone may result from such a fracture. A corrective shoe may be necessary.

In some cases of persistent lameness resulting from fracture of the coffin bone, severing the palmar digital nerves may afford enough relief that the horse can be returned to full use. The success of this operation can be determined beforehand by blocking the palmar digital nerves with a suitable local anesthetic.

The surgical application of lag screws is sometimes considered for articular fractures, particularly central fractures in horses over 3 to 4 years of age. Sometimes a bar shoe with quarter clips is applied to the foot prior to surgery to prevent foot expansion immediately

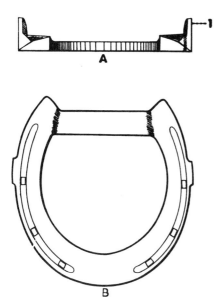

FIG. 5–28. Full bar shoe used in fracture of the coffin bone. *A*, Rear view of shoe showing quarter clips (1). *B*, Ground surface view of the shoe showing full-bar and quarter clips welded to shoe.

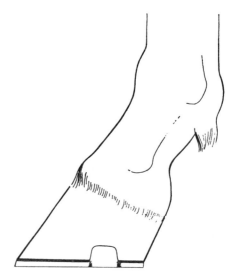

FIG. 5–29. Side view of shoe used for coffin bone fracture showing quarter clip in place.

upon recovery from surgery. A small hole is made in the hoof wall to gain access to the coffin bone. After surgery the piece of hoof wall is either replaced or the hole left open and packed with an antiseptic and protective bandage until it is keratinized and dry; then hoof repair materials can be used. Corrective shoes are applied at this time. Fracture healing can be expected in about 3 months postoperatively, and the screw may have to be removed if infection around the implant is evident.

Because coffin bone fractures that have healed by both conservative treatment and screw fixation have refractured after they return to racing or performance, it is strongly recommended that the performance horse be maintained in corrective shoes to prevent hoof wall expansion while competing.

Fractures of the perimeter of the coffin bone generally only cause lameness for a period of about 2 to 3 weeks, after which the horse may remain sound if shod with pads. If the fracture is at the tip of the distal phalanx, the opposite foot should also be x-rayed as well.

Prognosis

The prognosis for nonarticular and wing fractures treated conservatively appears to be good for all ages of horses if sufficient stall rest is afforded. Variable results have been obtained from screw fixation of central fractures, but the technique does decrease healing time. In all cases, it must be emphasized that it is very important to rest the horse for sufficient periods of time and to use corrective farriery to prevent hoof expansion while the horse is in active competition.

Extensor Process Fractures of the Coffin Bone

Fracture of the extensor process may occur unilaterally or bilaterally in the forefeet of horses. It is seen less frequently in the hindfeet. It may or may not be accompanied by buttress foot, which is produced by periosteal new bone growth; see Pyramidal Disease (Buttress Foot) section in this chapter.

In one review of coffin bone fractures 23 of 79 cases involved the extensor process. In another review, 4 of 65 cases involved fractures of the extensor process. It appears that grade and Quarter Horses between 3 and 17 years of age are the most susceptible.

Cause

The apparent cause is excessive tension on the common digital extensor tendon. This could produce enough force to fracture the process. It can also occur from overextension of the coffin joint. Bilateral cases could be due to congenital fractures (Fig. 5–30). In this

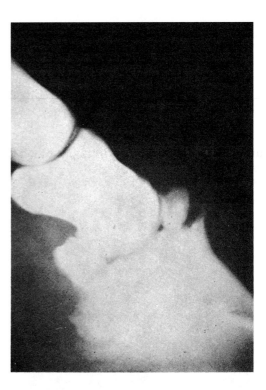

FIG. 5–30. Fracture of the extensor process of the coffin bone. This horse was affected with fracture of the extensor process of both forelimbs. It is possible that such a condition has a congenital origin when bilateral and not accompanied by periosteal new bone growth. Such fragments can be removed surgically.

case, it may be that the process has attempted to ossify from a separate ossification center, weakening the process and allowing it to be separated from the rest of the bone. Cases of this type do not have large amounts of periosteal new bone growth or the appearance of buttress foot.

Signs

On visual observation and palpation, swelling of the coffin joint capsule just proximal to the coronet may be detected. Lameness signs are relatively obscure. The cranial phase of the stride is shortened, and the horse may show a stride similar to that seen in navicular syndrome. However, there is no reaction to the hoof tester over the frog or other parts of the foot. After the condition has been present for some time, there is a change in the shape of the hoof wall, with a tendency for a V-shaped foot. If the condition has been present for a year or longer, this shape will extend the full length of the hoof wall. X-rays of the foot reveal the fracture or a separated extensor process (see Figs. 5–30 and 5–31). If extensive amounts of periosteal new bone growth are present, the foot assumes the typical appearance of buttress foot, which is discussed next as a separate condition. Pain may be shown when pressure is applied over the center of the coronary band.

Diagnosis

Diagnosis is established by the changes in the shape of the hoof wall, pain on pressure over the extensor process (which may or may not be present), and x-rays. Three types of extensor process fractures have been observed (see Figs. 5–30, 5–31, and 5–32).

Treatment

Although conservative treatment consisting of rest for 3 to 10 months has been used successfully in some cases, it would appear that the convalescent period can be markedly shortened with surgery. Small frag-

ments of the extensor process can be removed arthroscopically. Large fragments can be removed by arthrotomy or an attempt can be made to fix large fragments with a bone screw. Only selected cases are appropriate for screw fixation because the fragment must be large and in proper position to make the operation feasible. Convalescence post-op ranges from 3–8 months. Coffin joint treatment may be employed where synovitis persists.

Prognosis

Prognosis is guarded if degenerative joint disease of the coffin joint is present. New bone growth involving the joint makes for an unfavorable prognosis.

Pyramidal Disease (Buttress Foot)

Pyramidal disease, due to new bone growth in the region of the extensor process of the coffin bone, is an advanced form of low ringbone. This new bone growth may be due to fracture or inflammation of the periosteum (periostitis) of the extensor process. Healing of the injury produces new bone growth, causing an enlargement at the coronary band at the center of the hoof (Fig. 5–33). The same bony enlargement occurs in periostitis of the extensor process, making the clinical picture identical to that for fracture of this process.

Causes

Pyramidal disease is caused by excessive strain on the common digital extensor and the extensor branch

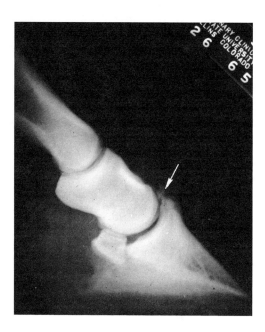

FIG. 5–31. An example of a small fracture of the extensor process of the coffin bone.

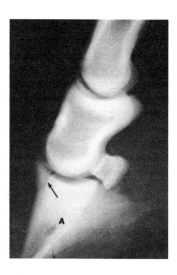

FIG. 5–32. Large fracture (arrow) of extensor process of coffin bone.

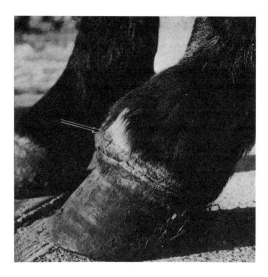

FIG. 5–33. Buttress foot. Note the extensive swelling at the dorsal portion of the coronary band as the result of low ringbone. This foot is also shown in Figure 5–34.

of the suspensory ligament as they insert on the extensor process of the coffin bone. This results in a periostitis that causes new bone growth or in a fracture of the extensor process of the coffin bone that heals with excessive callus (Fig. 5–34).

Horses with high heels and short toes and horses that move with limbs lifted high in a short and rapid manner (a "trappy gait") such as the Paso Fino appear to be predisposed to this disease. It has been suggested that the rapid vertical rise with increased joint flexion of the foot in high-heeled horses may be responsible for tearing the insertions at the extensor process.

Signs

Signs of lameness are not specific, but the horse often will show a tendency to point with the affected foot and the cranial phase of the stride will be shortened. There often is a tendency to land heavily on the heel. In early stages, heat, pain, and some swelling are evident at the coronary band in the center of the wall, and lameness is present in all gaits. The hair shows a

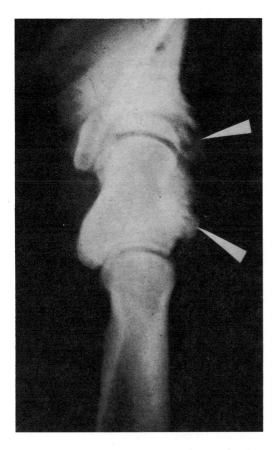

FIG. 5–34. Buttress foot changes on x-ray. The new bone growth is extensive, as shown by the upper arrow on the short pastern bone. The lower arrow shows new bone growth on the extensor process of the coffin bone. This is the same foot as shown in Figure 5–33. Because the proximal end of the short pastern bone is involved, the horse actually has both high and low ringbone.

tendency to stand upright at the center of the coronary band (see Fig. 5–33) and the horse flinches when finger pressure is put on the affected tissues. Arthritis of the coffin joint results and usually becomes chronic (see Fig. 5–34). After some time, a change takes place in the shape of the front of the hoof wall, with a bulging from the coronary band to the bearing surface of the wall. X-rays reveal variable changes in the short pastern bone and coffin bone and in the coffin joint (see Fig. 5–34).

Treatment

No treatment is of particular value in relieving this disease. Firing and blistering have been used but these are of doubtful value. In early cases, injection of anti-inflammatories and immobilization of the part may be of some help. Palmar digital neurectomy may relieve some signs of lameness and allow limited use of the horse. Corrective shoeing consists of using full roller motion shoes (Fig. 6–95) on the affected foot to decrease motion as much as possible in the coffin joint.

It has been suggested that rasping the dorsal hoof wall from just below the coronary band to the toe may relieve pressure and pain temporarily. However, this has very little effect on the progress of the disease process. Radiation therapy has been suggested to reduce the development of the periostitis.

Prognosis

The prognosis is unfavorable in all cases.

Penetrating Wounds of the Foot

Puncture wounds of the foot are quite common in horses. A variety of objects may produce the wounds. Some puncture wounds are extremely difficult to find, especially if they occur in the frog and the foreign body is missing. Puncture wounds in the middle one-third of the frog are most serious because of the possibility of puncture of the navicular bursa. Puncture wounds of the sole may cause inflammation of the coffin bone (pedal osteitis), fracture, and necrosis (tissue death) of the coffin bone or of the digital cushion. Puncture wounds in the white line often cause infection that migrates upward to break out the coronary band.

Signs

In some cases, the foreign body will still be in the foot, making the diagnosis relatively simple. In such a case, the type of foreign object and the damage that has occurred to underlying structures must be determined. The attitude of the gait of the horse often is very helpful in determining the location of the puncture wound if it is not obvious. If the wound is in the toe region of the sole, the horse tends to land too heavily on the heel. If the puncture is in the heel of the sole, the horse attempts to land on the toe. If the wound is on the medial side of the sole, the horse attempts to put most of his weight on the lateral side of the foot. If the wound is on the lateral side of the sole, the horse attempts to load most of his weight on the medial side of the foot. Because of variation in this type of lameness, no characteristic signs can be described. However, once the infection becomes established, horses will assume a nonweight-bearing stance. Hoof testers are used to locate the site of the wound. Puncture wounds (from nails, staples, wires, sticks, etc.) sometimes appear as fissures in the white line or black spots in the white line or sole. However, a correctly driven horseshoe nail can also be surrounded by a black spot. If necessary, the veterinarian will probe the puncture location to determine its depth and proximity to sensitive structures.

Lameness may not be evident until after infection has caused an inflammation of the corium of the hoof. If infection is present in the foot and the puncture wound has no drainage, the infection will force drainage at the coronary band near the heel. Occasionally, drainage will occur slightly forward of the heel and drain near the puncture wound, e.g., toe puncture draining at front of coronary band. Drainage at the coronary band is usually only a result; the bottom of the foot should always be checked for puncture wounds. Supporting-limb lameness is usually evident because of the pain in the foot.

It is not uncommon to find that puncture wounds of the foot cause distention of the flexor tendon sheath just above the fetlock joint. Careful examination of the tendon sheath usually will reveal that there is no pain on pressure, although heat may be evident. Examination of the foot with the hoof testers will reveal a painful spot; this spot may be the position of the puncture wound.

Some cases of puncture wounds in the foot will cause a systemic infection and acute inflammation of the limb accompanied by pus formation with elevation of temperature and severe systemic manifestations. Other conditions that may occur as the result of puncture wounds include infectious laminitis, necrosis (tissue death) of the coffin bone, fracture of the coffin bone, infection of the navicular bursa or digital cushion, fracture of the navicular bone, and tetanus.

Puncture wounds of the hind foot may cause a stringhalt attitude to the gait. The horse will move the limb in a hyperflexed manner, arousing suspicion of lameness involving structures farther up the limb. A lameness in any limb warrants full examination of the foot and sole for pathologic changes.

Diagnosis

The bottom of the hoof should be thoroughly examined. One should always be sure that a shoe nail or separation of the white line (gravel) is not causing the lameness. These conditions cause the same pathologic changes and signs as direct puncture wounds. X-rays might be taken to determine damage, if any, to bony structures. Puncture wounds of the frog are the most difficult to locate, because once the foreign body has been pulled out, the spongy frog closes over the wound, making it difficult to find.

Occasionally, the coffin joint will be involved with infection. Deep penetrating wounds over the navicular bone region that miss the bone are most likely to cause the problem. Also, infection of the coffin joint can result from extension of infection in the navicular bursa. Typically, these horses are nonweight-bearing lame and are reluctant to place any part of the foot on the ground.

Treatment

Treatment of a puncture wound involves establishing drainage of the lesion, keeping the region clean and protected until healing occurs, and preventing tetanus. The entire sole, frog, and sulcus should be cleaned and washed. The area of the puncture wound will be drained so that there is at least a $\frac{1}{4}$-inch opening into the dermal laminae.

Following drainage, the wound will be cleaned with an antiseptic solution. The opening of the wound should be packed with povidone iodine, and the foot bandaged thoroughly. The foot is bandaged to protect it from moisture and dirt, and the horse kept stalled, if possible, or at least in as dry an area as possible. An antiseptic (or sterilized) boot can be used in place of bandaging. A tetanus booster is given, and antibiotics are used as indicated.

When the infection causes drainage from a sinus at the coronary band, the foot should be checked carefully so the original puncture site can be located and drained. The veterinarian may choose to flush the tract from the coronary band with an antiseptic solution. Flushing once a day for 2 to 3 days is usually sufficient. Some veterinarians will request that you soak the foot daily in an Epsom salt antiseptic solution instead of flushing the tract. Following soaking or flushing, povidone iodine can be applied to the hole established in the sole and the foot should be bandaged. Once healing begins, it is not essential that soaking, flushing, and bandaging take place daily; every 3 to 4 days should be sufficient. It is essential to keep the wound clean until healing occurs.

If the puncture wound penetrates the navicular bursa, the bursa may require surgical drainage through the center third of the frog. Although this surgery can be done in the standing horse, it is best done under general anesthesia.

If the penetrating object has entered the coffin bone or infection has extended into that region the bone must be surgically scraped and cleaned down to healthy bleeding tissue and treated in a similar fashion as described previously.

Occasionally, the coffin joint will become involved. This is a very serious situation that requires immediate treatment. Synovial fluid will be removed from the coffin joint so the infection can be diagnosed. The joint may need to be flushed with a sterile salt solution. Most cases are so painful that a nerve block will be required to perform this. Tranquilization may also be necessary. The horse must be put on systemic broad spectrum antibiotics as well. If there is no improvement after 2 to 3 days of flushing, the coffin joint may need to be opened surgically and drained. However, this can be one of the most difficult joints in which to treat infection. If the treatment is successful, progressive increase in weight-bearing will be noted. It is absolutely mandatory to maintain this hoof in an antiseptic environment. Cases that go untreated may progress to this point (Fig. 5–35).

Emergency treatment for puncture wounds when the horse must be used for a time after treatment, such as on a trail ride, consists of removing the foreign object, establishing a small drainage hole with straight walls at the site of the puncture, and packing it tightly with povidone iodine and cotton. Additional treatment can be done after the horse has been moved to a more suitable place.

For cases that require prolonged treatment, a protective boot or a shoe with a removable treatment plate can be used. Both allow direct frequent treatment of the wound without the expense of daily bandaging. Treatment is continued in all cases until the infection is cleared. Some cases may require reopening of the involved site or staging the removal of the sole if a particularly large region is undermined.

After the drainage of pus has subsided, the veterinarian may apply astringents to dry the wound. However, in most cases this is not necessary. The maintenance of a sterile environment appears to be most important, and the lesion dries uneventfully. Once the lesion is completely dried and there is no evidence of drainage, a shoe with a full pad can be applied to protect the ground surface. An antibacterial packing is applied between the pad and the hoof. The decision to reapply a full pad when the shoe is reset depends on the amount of sole growth at that time.

Prognosis

The prognosis is favorable in early cases when the puncture wound has not damaged underlying structures. If the underlying bone or navicular bursa is damaged, the prognosis is guarded to unfavorable.

Quittor (Necrosis of the Collateral Cartilage)

Quittor is a chronic pus-forming inflammation of a collateral cartilage of the coffin bone characterized by necrosis of the cartilage and sinus drainage at or above the coronary band. It is most common in the forelimb (Fig. 5–36).

Causes

Injury near the coronary band over the region of the collateral cartilages may cause quittor by producing a subcoronary abscess. Quittor can be secondary to a penetrating wound through the sole where infection has gained access to the collateral cartilage or to trauma of the cartilage resulting from wire cuts or bruises that damage the cartilage and reduce circulation in the region. Interfering may cause quittor by damaging a medial collateral cartilage.

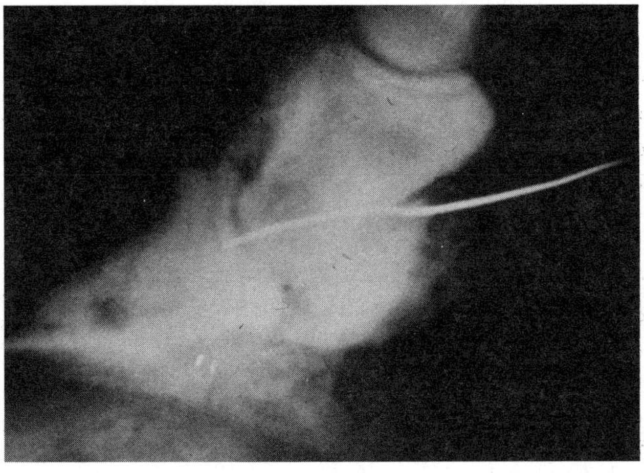

FIG. 5–35. This extensive inflammation of the bone and marrow spread from an infection within the coffin joint. A metal probe was placed in the tract to identify the origin of the infection.

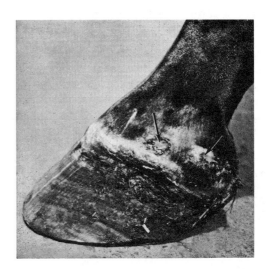

FIG. 5–36. Clinical appearance of typical quittor. Arrows point to two draining tracts. This case was cured by making an elliptical incision above the coronary band.

Signs

The condition may occur over either the medial or lateral collateral cartilage. Swelling, heat, and pain over the coronary band, in the region of the affected collateral cartilage, and chronic pus-filled sinus tracts that tend to heal and then break open at intervals characterize quittor. Lameness occurs in acute stages but may show remission when the lesion appears to be healing. Some sidebone may occur with the lesion, and permanent swelling usually results over the area of the involved collateral cartilage. Permanent damage and deformity of the foot may result, causing persistent lameness.

Diagnosis

Enlargement over the affected collateral cartilage, characterized by one or more sinus tracts that are chronic and recurring is characteristic of quittor. Drainage at the coronary band occurs with "gravel" and other foot infections; these should be differentiated from quittor.

The drainage tract associated with gravel is located at or above the coronary band, and the inflammatory process usually is localized. With quittor there may be multiple sinus tracts, the swelling is usually more diffuse, and it is located over the collateral cartilages.

X-rays might be used to rule out involvement of the middle and distal phalanges. The depth and dimension of the sinus tracts can be elucidated with sinography (using a contrasting medium to highlight the tracts) or the placement of a sterile probe in the tract (Fig. 5–37).

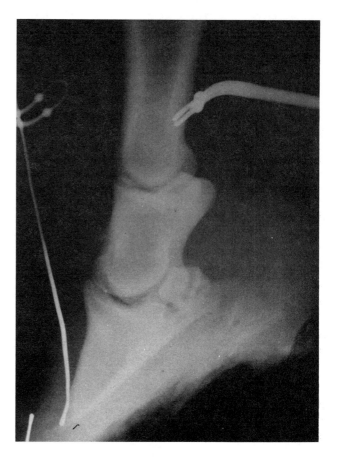

FIG. 5–37. A sterile probe can be used to identify the depth and location of a tract.

Treatment

The treatment of choice is surgical removal of the necrotic tissue and cartilage. Necrotic cartilage is recognized by its dark blue or reddish-blue appearance. If the necrotic cartilage extends to or below the coronary band, a hole is drilled in the hoof wall to provide drainage. A polyethylene tube is placed in the wound and is sutured to the limb. The foot and sole can either be bandaged or placed in a protective boot. In either case, the surgical site is protected with sterile bandages. The following day the bandage is removed and the wound is flushed with a 1% povidone iodine solution. This is continued on a once-a-day basis until all evidence of infection is gone. Antiseptic packing through the hole in the hoof wall is continued until infection is abated. In cases in which the necrotic cartilage does not extend to or below the coronary band and good ventral drainage can be achieved without drilling a hole, a flush system is applied and the remaining drain tract is packed directly. Most cases require drilling the hoof wall either to establish drainage or to remove necrotic cartilage at that depth. Antiseptic flushes are usually continued for 3 to 5 days, after which the flush tube is removed. The packing is continued with smaller volumes of gauze until the veterinarian is assured that no infection remains. Sutures are removed on day 14 and the remaining hole in the hoof wall is filled with hoof repair material as soon as a firm cornified layer develops. If hoof repair material is placed in the hole before this time, the exothermic (heat) reaction results in necrosis of the sensitive laminae and infection. Most frequently hoof repair material can be placed in the hoof wall 4 to 6 weeks after the initial surgery. Exercise can usually begin in about $2\frac{1}{2}$ to 3 months.

Prognosis

The prognosis for acute and subacute cases is good with the treatment described, although some chronic cases can be difficult to treat.

Puncture Wounds of the White Line (Gravel)

Gravel is a common term for what supposedly is a migration of a piece of gravel from the white line upward to the coronary band. This does not occur; what does happen is that an opening in the white line permits infection to invade the sensitive structures. Because there is no drainage, inflammation follows the line of least resistance, and drainage occurs at the coronary band, as it does with puncture wounds that cannot drain through the sole.

Causes

A puncture wound or crack in the white line may occur in feet that are too dry. In addition, chronic laminitis with its associated "seedy toe," causing a poorly defined seal in the toe region of the white line, may cause this condition. The sole and white line should be carefully examined to determine the real cause.

Signs

Lameness will usually appear before drainage at the coronary band occurs, but the condition may go undiagnosed until after drainage takes place. Signs of lameness vary according to severity of the infection and the location of the entry of infection. The horse will modify its gait, as described in the discussion of penetrating wounds of the foot, according to the location of the entry. Careful examination of the white line and sole will reveal black spots, which should be probed to their depth. Veterinary examination with a hoof tester will determine the approximate area of penetration. If the black areas are probed to their depth, one will be found that penetrates into the dermal laminae. After the depth of the crack has been probed, pus will often exude from the wound. When the condition has been present for some time, drainage at the coronary band will be noted (Fig. 5–38). Systemic reaction to the infection varies, but in most cases infection remains localized.

The horse will show a supporting limb lameness.

Diagnosis

Diagnosis is made by careful veterinary examination of the hoof with a hoof tester. All cases of lameness should have this examination. Most cases can be diagnosed before the coronary band region breaks and drains, if the signs are noticed early. Careful observation of the way the horse sets his foot on the ground is helpful in localizing the region of penetration.

Treatment

Treatment consists of establishing proper drainage for the infection, as described in penetrating wounds of the foot. The foot may be soaked in Epsom salt (magnesium sulfate). Applying iodine to the drainage area and bandaging the foot until it is healed may be

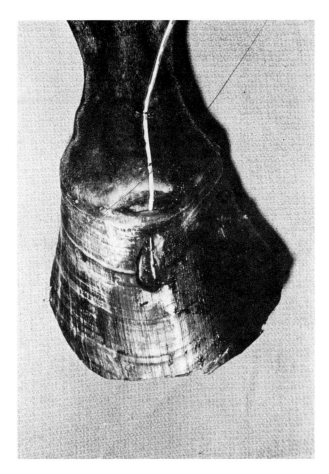

FIG. 5–38. An oblong hole was made in the dorsal surface of the hoof wall to remove the involved tissue and provide good drainage.

necessary. Antiphlogistic (substance that reduces inflammation) pastes may also be used under the bandage. Tetanus toxoid should be given as a booster if the horse has previously been immunized with this product. Otherwise, tetanus antitoxin should be used. After the first week of involvement, bandaging of the foot may be delayed to once every 3 or 4 days if it stays dry.

In more chronic cases with a long-term history of drainage at the coronary band that has resulted in considerable undermining of the hoof wall, it is often helpful to create a circular hole in the hoof wall midway between the solar surface and the coronary band (see Fig. 5–38). This will allow the veterinarian to more thoroughly clear the tract of necrotic and infected material. Bandaging to protect the foot from contamination should follow until all signs of infection have disappeared. Soaking the foot in supersaturated solutions of Epsom salt and antiseptic agents is the traditional approach. Systemic antibiotics may be required if the infection involves the regional soft tissue of the pastern.

In all cases, a shoe with a pad can be applied after the infection is controlled, to protect the solar surface from dirt and manure being packed into the hole. Prosthetic hoof wall material can be applied to the circular hole in the hoof wall after it has become cornified and all signs of infection are gone.

Prognosis

Prognosis is favorable if the condition is diagnosed before drainage at the coronary band occurs, except in cases in which the foot is subject to recurrence of the condition because of chronic laminitis. The prognosis is guarded if drainage at the coronary band already has occurred. Careful treatment, however, will permit many of these horses to be returned to complete soundness. If the condition is long-standing, the prognosis is unfavorable, because permanent changes already may have occurred.

Sidebones

Sidebones, a change into bone (ossification) of the collateral cartilages, are usually found in the forefeet and are most common in horses having poor conformation. The condition is uncommon in Thoroughbreds.

Causes

Excessive concussion of the quarters of the foot causing trauma to cartilages (such as from road work) is probably the cause of most cases. Some believe that there is a hereditary predisposition, but this is probably through poor conformation. Horses that are base-narrow may be prone to develop lateral sidebone, while horses that are basewide may be prone to develop medial sidebone. However, in both of these conformations, sidebone may eventually develop in both cartilages.

Poor shoeing may cause increased concussion, resulting in sidebone. Shoeing with long heel calks for a prolonged period may cause the condition by increasing concussion. Shoeing a horse off level may throw more stress on the inside or outside of the hoof wall, thereby increasing concussion to one of the cartilages. Such trauma may produce sidebone. Some cases of sidebone are produced by traumatic lesions, such as wire cuts that damage the cartilage.

Signs

Lameness may or may not be present. Lameness is often blamed on sidebones when they are not actually the cause. Lameness resulting from sidebones is rare, usually being present only when the cartilages are in the process of becoming ossified and when inflammation is present. Lameness may be evident when the horse turns, but the signs are seldom acute. Massive

bone formation in the collateral cartilages may cause mechanical interference with foot action.

If sidebones are a cause of lameness, there will be heat and pain over one or both of the cartilages. Careful examination of the cartilages will reveal that hardening is present. Firm pressure over the region will cause the horse to flinch if the cartilage is in the active stages of bone formation. In some cases, there will be a visible bulging of the quarters at the coronary band. Sidebone may accompany other lamenesses, such as navicular syndrome, and may be mistaken for the cause. X-rays will reveal that the cartilages have partially or completely ossified (Fig. 5–39). After ossification stops, there are usually no signs of lameness, although the involved cartilages no longer function in the normal physiologic processes of the foot. Occasionally, a sidebone is fractured, resulting in a fragment that can be surgically removed.

Diagnosis

A diagnosis of sidebones as the cause of lameness should not be made unless pain and heat are present over the involved cartilage or cartilages. X-ray examination will reveal bone formation in the cartilages, but this does not necessarily mean that sidebones are the cause of lameness. Most cases of sidebones can be palpated, but again, their presence does not mean they are the cause of lameness. If sidebones are truly the cause of lameness, a palmar digital nerve block at the base of the sesamoid on the affected side should relieve signs of lameness.

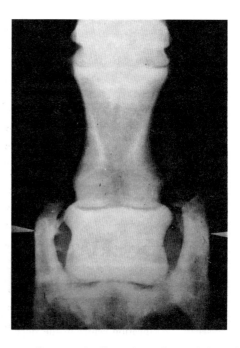

FIG. 5–39. Ossification of collateral cartilages of the coffin bone (sidebones).

Treatment

If the sidebones are definitely the cause of lameness, the foot is shod to promote expansion, which may help relieve the pain. The horse should be shod with full roller motion shoes to decrease the breakover forces in the coffin joint region.

In contrast, when fractured sidebones are the cause of lameness, small proximal chips can be removed surgically. After surgery, a pressure bandage is kept in place for 2 weeks. Proximal fractures are different from sidebones with separate ossification centers (Fig. 5–40). Large proximal fragments and fractures of the coffin bone require the foot to be immobilized in the coffin bone fracture shoe until healing has occurred (see Fractures of the Coffin Bone earlier in this chapter).

Rest should be enforced until the inflammatory process resolves. In some cases in which it is believed that a sidebone causes chronic and persistent lameness, a palmar digital neurectomy can be performed on the affected side or sides.

Prognosis

The prognosis is guarded to favorable unless abnormal bone growth is extensive, in which case it is unfavorable.

White Line Disease

White line disease syndrome, often mistakenly called seedy toe, is due to invasion of the inner horn by a bacteria, yeast, or fungus which results in varying

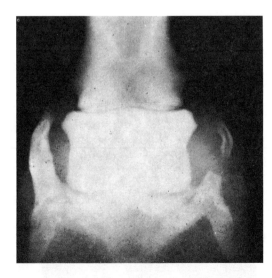

FIG. 5–40. Sidebones. On the left, note the large sidebone. On the right, note the separate ossification center in the sidebone. This should not be confused with fracture of a sidebone, which is sometimes surgically removed. This type of ossification does not require surgical removal.

degrees of damage to the structural integrity of the hoof.

Causes

This disease usually occurs in horses two years of age or older and may affect one or as many as all four hooves. White line disease is rarely seen in barefoot horses on healthy pastures. It is a disease characteristic of over-managed horses, those that have limited turn-out and exercise, that are bedded in damp wood shavings, have a high grain and low roughage ration, are always shod, and have frequent moisture episodes such as daily baths or rinsing, standing in wet stalls, or being turned out in dewy grass. There seems to be a greater occurrence of the condition in hot, humid climates.

Signs

The area of an affected hoof is characteristically filled with a white cheesy material and air pockets that are often packed with debris. Soil, sand, and manure may be able to enter along the sole margin and continue to invade the interlaminar space as the white line deteriorates. The disease starts at ground level and can work its way up to the coronary band.

Most commonly white line disease appears in the dorsal portion of the hoof, from the center of the toe to approximately the last nail position at the quarter but it often occurs at the toe as well. There may be areas of the hoof wall that when tapped give a hollow sound.

Depending on the extent of the damage, it can result in lameness from mechanical loss of horn support. In severe cases, the separation may allow a mechanical rotation to occur. The pull of the deep digital flexor tendon coupled with the forces of the horse's weight on the coffin bone can cause displacement of the coffin bone relative to the hoof capsule. X-rays may help to differentiate between laminitis and white line disease and to locate the areas of diseased horn.

This condition needs to be diagnosed early to prevent extensive damage and to minimize treatment time and costs. An affected horse may show symptoms similar to those of laminitis: lameness, heat, sole tending to be flat, slow horn growth, tenderness when nailing, and pain over the sole when hoof testers are applied.

Treatment

First, all diseased or unsound tissue must be removed by knife, nippers, rasp, motorized burr, and/or sandpaper. It is important that all infected tissue is removed to prevent spread of undesirable organisms, to get down to solid healthy horn for good healing and to provide a good base of attachment for hoof repair materials if used.

The area is then washed and scrubbed with denatured alcohol which is safer for both farrier and horse than is acetone which is also sometimes used. The hoof is completely dried using a heat gun if necessary. The holes and caves are filled with the hoof repair material and let cure. Curing time will vary from 1–30 minutes depending on the hoof repair material used and the environmental temperature. In some cases, a piece of specialized reinforcing cloth is used with the adhesive. Major repairs can require the application of several layers. After the material has completely cured, it can be nipped, rasped, and nailed (if desired) like ordinary hoof material.

Conventional egg bar or full support shoes can often be nailed onto the restored hoof. For severely damaged hooves, special shoes can be glued on.

For cases with extensive hoof wall resected, if hoof rebuilding is not desirable or possible, a type of goose neck shoe can be used where the top of one or more T-shaped hangers is screwed into the solid hoof wall parallel to the coronary band.

Mild cases of white line disease can be treated using the Klimesh CVP gasket pad (see page 410).

The coronary band can be stimulated and kept supple daily with a three to four minute lanolin (Corona) massage. Following the massage, all excess lanolin should be removed. Nutritional supplementation is often recommended for increased hoof horn growth.

Prognosis

The prognosis for horses affected with white line disease is good when discovered early and treated in this fashion.

Corns and Bruised Soles

A corn is an involvement of the sensitive and insensitive tissues of the sole at the angle formed by the wall and the bar (Fig. 5–41). Corns occur most frequently in the front feet and are rarely found in the hind feet. This may be due to the fact that the front feet bear more weight than the hind feet. Flat feet predispose the sole to bruising.

Causes

Corns are usually due to improper or irregular shoeing or neglect. When shoes are left on the feet too long, the heels of the shoe are forced inside the wall and cause pressure on the sole at the angle of the wall and the bar (See Fig. 6–47).

Good farriery consists of proper foot preparation, including optimum paring of the sole at the angle of the bars to relieve possible pressure. If a shoe that is one-

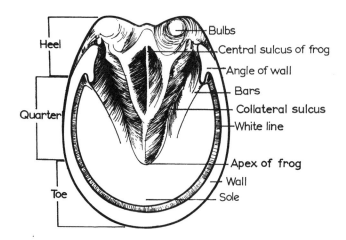

FIG. 5–41. Normal forefoot showing structures.

half to one full size too small for the foot is applied, it will increase the pressure on the sole at the angles. Heel calks will exaggerate this effect. This pressure bruises the sole and causes corns. Improper trimming of the feet, making the heels too low, increases pressure at the angle of the wall and bar and also may cause corns. If a horse is shod too closely at the quarter, corns may result. Another common cause of corns is gravel and sand lodged between the heel of the shoe that has been bent inward and the seat of corn that has not been cleaned out. (Also, any time a sole is trimmed too short, there is increased chance for sole bruising.)

Corns are rare among horses that are used barefooted but sole bruising does occur as a result of trauma to the sole from rocks and other objects. Horses with thin soles are more subject to the disease, as are horses that have been affected previously with laminitis.

Signs

Three types of corn lesions may be evident:

1. *Dry Corn.* In this case, hemorrhage on the inner surface of the horn resulting from bruising of dermal tissue usually causes red stains.
2. *Moist Corn.* This is caused by severe injury that results in serum beneath the injured horn.
3. *Suppurating Corn.* The corn becomes infected, resulting in necrosis of the dermal lamina and the digital cushion.

Pathologic changes due to bruised sole are similar to those caused by corns but occur in the toe or quarter regions of the sole rather than at the angle of the wall and bar. Bruised sole also may be of dry, moist, or suppurating types.

The horse will show varying degrees of lameness depending on the severity of the bruise or corn, while the attitude of the lameness will vary according to the location of the bruise or corn. Hoof testers will reveal the location of the pathologic changes. A cleaning of the flaky sole from the bottom of the foot with a hoof knife will reveal red stains in the sole, indicating a bruised region. In some cases, this region may show a bluish discoloration, especially if a sole abscess is developing.

The horse will tend to favor the heel, especially on the affected side. If the corn is present at the inside heel, the horse will tend to place more weight on the outside of the foot because of the pain. In some cases, the horse will tend to bear most of the weight on the toe and will rest the foot with the knee forward to decrease heel pressure. If the toe region of the sole is bruised, the horse will tend to land on the heel to protect the toe. Although a hoof tester examination will be positive for pain, a varied response will be noted.

Treatment

In cases in which shoeing is the cause, removal of the offending shoe may be all that is necessary. To prevent shoes from causing corns, the heels of the shoe should always extend beyond the heels and should fit full at the quarters and heels. Heel calks increase the chance of corns if a horse is shod too short at the heels or if the shoe is left on too long. Removal of some of the tissue over the corn helps relieve pressure, but sensitive tissue should not be exposed. The horse should be rested and should be properly reshod.

In the case of a suppurating corn, the sole over the region should be removed so that drainage of the sensitive tissues can be established. The foot should be soaked daily in an antiseptic or in a solution of magnesium sulfate (Epsom salt), after which tincture of iodine is applied. The foot should be bandaged and protected from contamination.

If the horse must be used for some reason, the wall and bar in the area of the corn may be removed to prevent pressure by the shoe. A bar shoe can be applied, as for quarter crack. A bar shoe (straight bar, heart bar, or full support shoe) stabilizes the hoof and allows the weight that would be over the corn to be transmitted to other parts of the hoof wall and/or frog via the shoe (see Chapter 6).

Another option is to apply a wide-web shoe that offers protection of the bruised site. In cases in which it is difficult to place the wide-web shoe, a $\frac{1}{8}$-inch plastic rim can be applied and cut out over the region of the affected sole.

In cases of sole bruising, the horse should be rested from heavy work, especially if his soles are abnormally thin. When possible, the environment of the horse should be changed so that he is not worked on rough ground. If the horse must be used, the sole can be covered with a suitable hoof packing and a full pad applied between the shoe and the hoof.

If the bruised region becomes a sole abscess, it should be drained by cutting away a portion of the diseased sole and exposing the dermal corium. The foot then should be soaked daily in antiseptic solution and bandaged with an antiseptic ointment until healing can occur. In some cases, a treatment plate shoe may prove more time and cost effective.

Prognosis

The prognosis is always guarded, because some such cases tend to become chronic, which eventually may cause inflammation of the coffin bone (pedal osteitis).

Canker

Canker is a chronic moist pus-forming inflammatory enlargement of the horn-producing tissues of the foot, which may involve any one or all of the feet; it most often is found in the hind feet. Although it is a rare condition, the disease is most commonly diagnosed in horses in tropical climates similar to that of the southern United States.

Causes

The main cause is presumed to be unhygienic stabling, where horses stand in mud or in bedding that is soaked with urine and feces and whose feet do not receive regular attention. Horses raised in a warm humid climate that are out on moist, wet pasture year-round are also at a higher risk of developing canker. The specific cause is believed to be an infectious process, and the most likely microorganisms involved are *Fusobacterium necrophorum* and one or more of the *Bacteroides Spp.*

Signs

Lameness is usually present. When the foot is examined, it usually has a fetid odor and the frog, which may appear intact, has a ragged appearance. The horn tissue of the frog loosens easily, and when removed, reveals a foul-smelling, swollen corium covered with a cheese-like white exudate. The swollen horn appears as filamentous fronds instead of the normal uniform flat keratinized surface.

Diagnosis

A presumptive diagnosis can be made by the appearance of the foot and by the offensive odor, but it must be differentiated from thrush. The definitive diagnosis is made by looking at samples of affected horn under the microscope.

Treatment

Treatment often is lengthy and improvement, if it occurs, is slow. All loose horn and affected tissues is removed surgically and an antiseptic, astringent dressing applied. Various astringents and caustic agents are sometimes used. Canker has been treated successfully with penicillin injected intramuscularly and applied topically as an ointment. Duration of treatment varied from 10 days to 6 weeks. Bandages should be kept on the foot to protect it from further infection and to keep it dry. Daily bandage changes are often required until normal horn appears. The horse should be kept in a clean, dry stall until the wound is covered with normal horn.

Prognosis

The most common problem is recurrence, usually within 4 to 7 days. With proper treatment and care, most can be treated successfully but may require further surgical removal of affected tissue.

Thrush

Thrush, a degenerative condition of the frog involving the central and lateral sulci, is characterized by the presence of a fetid gray/black necrotic material in the affected areas. The infection may penetrate the horny tissues and involve the sensitive structures.

Causes

The predisposing causes of thrush are unhygienic conditions (especially when horses are kept in poorly managed stalls or filthy surroundings), dirty, uncleaned feet, and lack of proper frog trimming. During hoof preparation for shoeing, the clefts of the frog often need to be pared so they are self-cleaning. Otherwise, flaps of frog tissue can seal debris and bacteria in the clefts and make it impossible for the owner to clean the clefts with a hoof pick. Many organisms are probably involved, but *Spherophorus necrophorus* appears to be the most important of these.

Signs

There is an increased amount of moisture and a black discharge in the sulci of the frog. This discharge, which varies in quantity, has a very offensive odor. When the affected sulci are cleaned, it will be found that they are deeper than normal and may extend into the sensitive tissues of the foot, causing the horse to flinch when they are cleaned. The frog will be undermined, and large areas of it may require removal because of the loss of continuity with the underlying frog. In severe cases that have penetrated the sensitive

structure of the foot, the horse may be lame, and the foot may show the same signs of infection that would be encountered in a puncture wound of the foot. Swelling of the limbs may be seen (stocking-up). Generally, the rear limbs are more frequently affected.

Diagnosis

Diagnosis is based on the odor and physical characteristics of the black discharge in the sulci of the frog.

Treatment

Treatment is cleanliness, removal of the cause, and return of the frog and hoof to normal conformation and condition. The foot should be cleaned daily and the cleft of the frog packed with a proper medication. The treatment should be repeated until the infection is controlled.

The cause can be removed by placing the horse in cleaner surroundings or by daily cleansing of the frog after removal of the debris. Degenerated frog tissues should be removed, and an effort should be made to return the frog to normal by cleaning up all infection.

Prognosis

The prognosis is favorable if the disease is diagnosed before the foot has suffered extensive damage. It is guarded if the sensitive structures are involved.

Keratoma

A keratoma is a rare tumor that develops in the deep aspect of the hoof wall, most commonly at the toe. It may or may not cause lameness, but when lameness is present, it usually results from pressure of the growing keratoma on the dermal laminae.

Causes

A keratoma can occur without a history of previous injury, in which case it is conceivably a *tumor* from the keratin-producing cells of the hoof. However, it can also result from an abnormal development of hoof horn (keratinization) in response to injury (e.g., binding nail, hoof crack, or chronic corn) or infection (e.g., sole abscess).

Clinical Signs and Diagnosis

The hoof wall and sole are often abnormally shaped. Most of the keratoma growth appears at the toe but it has been reported to involve the quarters and sole as well. Signs of lameness are usually moderate to severe. Close examination of the foot is required to identify the abnormality. A deviation in the white line toward the center of the foot is suspicious of keratoma. In some cases, pus-forming tracts may also be present. X-rays usually indicate an increased tissue density of the hoof wall and bone deterioration of the coffin bone.

Treatment

Treatment involves surgical removal of the abnormal growth. After surgery, and initially, the foot is protected by bandaging, after which a protective shoe with toe clips strategically placed to prevent hoof expansion is applied. Prosthetic material can be used to repair the hoof wall defect after a firm, dry cuticle has formed. These tumors may recur after surgical removal.

Prognosis

The prognosis appears good but it is somewhat dependent on the size and location of the lesion and the degree of damage to the surrounding structures. In one case series involving seven horses treated surgically for keratoma, six of seven were completely sound after a 1-year follow-up.

Selenium Poisoning (Toxicosis)

Poisoning from ingestion of selenium is classically divided into three categories: acute, subacute, and chronic. The acute form occurs when large amounts are ingested and it usually results in death of the horse. The subacute form is characterized by blind staggers and depressive mania, which is believed to be caused by selenium's effect on the liver and brain. Presently, blind staggers is believed to be the result of an alkaloid in selenium accumulator plants rather than ingestion of high levels of selenium. Brittle hair, abnormal hoof wall growth, and lameness are characteristic of the chronic form (alkali disease), which reflects selenium's ability to bind sulfur-containing compounds. The following discussion refers to the chronic form of this disease.

Causes

Selenium poisoning usually develops when horses ingest secondary accumulator plants while grazing. There are three major plant groups that extract selenium from the soil. *Obligate accumulators* (indicator plants) require high selenium soil to survive, and they can accumulate up to 100 times the selenium levels found in other plants (Fig. 5–42). *Facultative accu-mulators* do not require high-selenium soil to live, but when selenium is present they build up 10 times the level of selenium as compared to other plants in the same area. *Passive accumulators* passively accumulate selenium if it is present. Cereal grains from selenium soil may contain above 5 ppm of selenium, which is above the tolerance limits. Areas of high selenium soils in the United States are Colorado, Utah, Kansas, New Mexico, Wyoming, Montana, South Dakota, and Nebraska. The selenium concentration in the soils of these regions range from 2 to 10 ppm compared to soils in other regions of the United States, which have selenium concentrations of less than 2 ppm. Chronic poisonings from selenium salts have also been reported in animals or drinking water containing 0.5 to 2.0 ppm of selenium. Concerns regarding drinking water should be addressed to the county extension agent.

Signs

Horses with chronic selenium poisoning will have histories of hair loss and lameness of variable duration. The hair coat usually appears dull, short, and brittle, whereas the tail hairs and mane may be short (Fig. 5–43). The hoof walls on all four feet will usually have uniform transverse grooves or cracks in the hoof wall that may extend down to the sensitive lamina (Fig. 5–44). Subsolar abscesses may also be present. X-rays usually indicate no changes in the deep hoof wall structures.

Diagnosis

Although the diagnosis can be made from the clinical signs alone, hoof, hair, and blood samples should be taken to make a definitive diagnosis. Diagnostic levels of selenium in the hooves (8 to 20 ppm), hair (11 to 45 ppm), and blood (1 to 4 ppm) are indicative of chronic selenium poisoning.

Treatment

The treatment of chronic selenium poisoning is based on local therapy of the feet and systemic treatment for prevention. If abscesses are present, they must be opened, drained, and the feet placed in antiseptic bandages until they are healed. Horses that have lost their hoof walls distal to the transverse cracks will also have to be maintained in antiseptic hoof bandages or treatment boots until the keratinized layer forms. After this, the hoof wall defects can be replaced with hoof repair materials. Treatment and prevention of chronic exposure to selenium can be accomplished by using organic or inorganic arsenic or naphthalene. The horse should be fed a balanced, high-protein, low-selenium diet. Linseed oil in the ra-

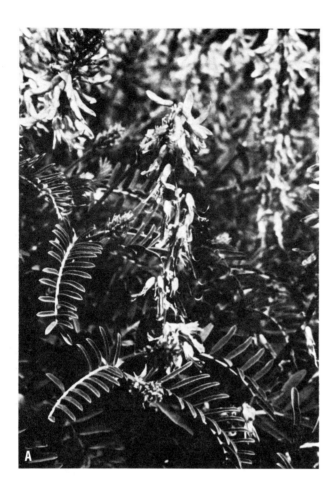

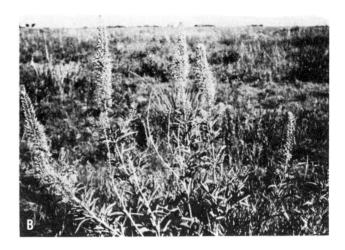

FIG. 5–42. Two examples of selenium indicator plants. *A*, Prince's plume (*Stanleya pinnata*). *B*, Two grooved milk vetches (*Astragalus bisulcatus*). (Courtesy of Dr. A.P. Knight.)

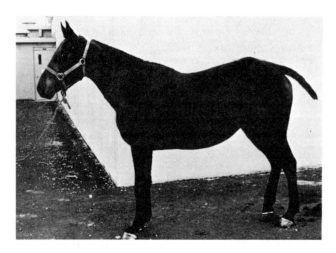

FIG. 5–43. This horse had progressive hair loss and lameness. On physical examination, a dull, dry hair coat, loss of tail and mane hairs, and lameness were present. Transverse hoof wall cracks were evident on all four feet. These signs are consistent with selenium poisoning.

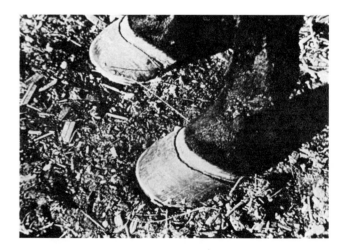

FIG. 5–44. Transverse cracks in the hoof walls are often seen with chronic selenium poisoning. If these cracks extend down to the dermal lamina, horses often become lame.

tion improves the efficacy of arsenic salts protective effect.

Prognosis

The prognosis for the chronic form of the disease appears good if the treatment of the feet is successful. In some cases, 8 to 10 months will pass before the affected horse can be ridden.

Separation (Avulsion) of the Hoof Wall at the Heel (Heel Avulsion)

Separation of the hoof wall at the heel is an uncommon injury that can seriously limit the athletic function of the horse. As the name implies, there is a disruption in the horny wall at the heel. It may start as a small separation at the heel and gradually progress until the hoof wall at the quarter becomes separated from the underlying dermal laminae. In the chronic state, infection often accompanies this condition.

Causes

Although this can be a natural progression of a vertical tear of the hoof wall, the most common cause appears to be trauma. The causes for heel avulsion include: 1) infection and subsequent separation, 2) kicking or stepping on sharp objects, 3) entrapment injuries, 4) continual foot imbalance, and 5) improper removal of shoes where the nails are torn out of the heel and quarter.

Clinical Signs and Diagnosis

Lameness usually ranges from mild to severe. Visually varying amounts of the heel and quarter will be separated (Fig. 5–45). Hoof tester pressure over the region results in a painful response. Initially, the dermal laminae will be exposed and hemorrhage is present. With time, infection will also become a prominent feature.

Treatment

Attempts to repair such injuries are usually futile, and it is often best to simply remove the separated portion (Fig. 5–46). This can be done with the horse standing after a local anesthesia has been administered, or it can be done under general anesthesia if the disruption is excessive. After the avulsion of the hoof wall is removed, it is bandaged in an antiseptic solution and protected from contamination. Bandages are changed every 2 to 4 days and topical antiseptics are applied until a cornified epithelial layer forms. After this, the hoof wall stability can be ensured by appli-

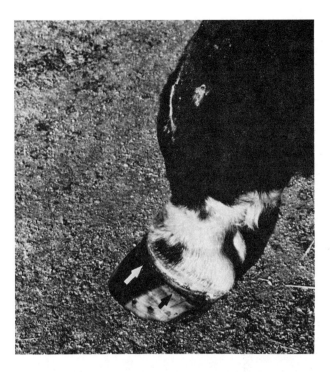

FIG. 5–45. This horse had a history of a small separation at the heel bulb region that progressed to involve the entire lateral half of the hoof wall (arrow). The horse was exhibiting mild lameness.

cation of a full bar support shoe and a prosthetic hoof repair material can be applied until the hoof wall grows down.

If the coronary band is involved, the hoof wall distal to it is removed and the coronary band is sutured (Fig. 5–47). After application of an antiseptic bandage, a cast is applied and maintained for at least $2\frac{1}{2}$ to 3 weeks. After this, sutures are removed and the coronary band is bandaged for another 2 to 3 weeks. A corrective full-bar shoe and prosthetic hoof repair material can be applied when a dry cuticle forms.

In some cases, a full support shoe can be put on before the removal of the separated hoof wall and before cornification takes place to support one frog and take weight off the "walls."

Prognosis

The prognosis is usually good for normal hoof wall growth if the coronary band is not involved. If the tear in the coronary band is acute and repaired soon after injury, the prognosis is still good as long as there is no deficit in the coronary band and the epithelial cells necessary for hoof wall growth are present. The prognosis is guarded to poor for chronic cases with coronary band involvement for obtaining normal hoof wall growth.

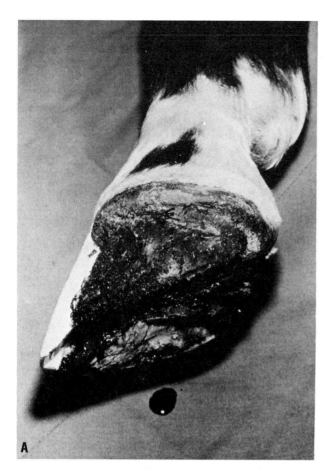

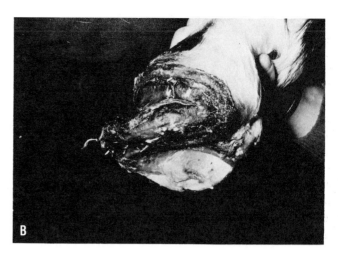

Fig. 5–46. Treatment of the horse illustrated in Figure 5–44 included removing the separated portion of the hoof wall, cleaning the hoof, and maintaining it in an antiseptic bandage protected by a rubber boot. *A,* Hoof immediately after removal of the separated portion of hoof wall. *B,* Three-week follow-up. A dry, keratinized epithelial layer has formed over the exposed dermal laminae. Because of the extensive loss of hoof wall, a shoe could not be applied to the foot. Also at this stage, it would have been difficult to use hoof repair material.

Toe Cracks, Quarter Cracks, Heel Cracks (Sand Cracks)

These are cracks in the wall of the hoof, starting at the bearing surface of the wall and extending a variable distance up the hoof wall, or cracks originating at the coronary band, as the result of a defect in the band, and extending downward. These cracks are identified as toe, quarter, or heel, depending on their location in the hoof wall, and may occur in either the front or hind feet.

Quarter cracks and heel cracks are usually the most severe because they often involve the dermal laminae. Affected horses are usually lame and hemorrhage after exercise may be noticed. Infection is commonly observed.

Causes

Excessive growth of the hoof wall, causing a splitting of the wall, from lack of trimming of the feet, is a common cause. Injury to the coronary band, producing a weak and deformed hoof wall, will lead to cracks originating at the coronary band. Weakening of the wall due to repeated episodes of moisture and drying also causes hoof cracks.

Moisture is the key to flexibility and health of the hoof wall and sole. The normal hoof wall contains about 15% to 20% moisture content in the dense tough outer layer and about 45% in the inner layer. The two layers are held together by interlocking sheaves of epidermal (outer layer) and dermal (blood-rich inner layer) laminae. Moisture from the inner layer diffuses outward toward the dry hard outer hoof wall. A spring-like action exists in the normal hoof but is dependent on a balance in moisture between the outer and inner layers of one hoof wall. With weight-bearing, the inner wall expands and pushes the outer wall, which resists with a curling contracting force. This allows the normal hoof to absorb shock. When the hoof is off the ground or when the horse is standing still, the spring-like recoil of the outer hoof will cause the hoof to return to its original shape. Repeated episodes of excessive moisture and dryness of the outer hoof wall can result in hoof cracks by altering the normal spring-like action. While excessive moisture results in lack of resistance to expansion, exces-

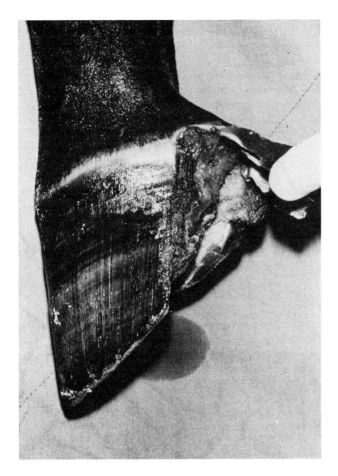

FIG. 5–47. An example of separation of the hoof wall involving the coronary band. Treatment includes removal of the hoof wall distal to the coronary band. Then the coronary band is sutured. A cast should be applied and left in place for at least 17 to 21 days.

sive dryness makes the outer hoof wall susceptible to splitting from expansion pressure.

Signs

The presence of the split in the wall will be obvious. Lameness may not be present, but it will become evident if the crack extends into the dermal tissues, allowing infection to gain access to these structures. A discharge under the cracks or pus-forming inflammation of the laminae may be present, depending on the size of the opening into the dermal tissues. The location of the crack will be obvious. Variable lesions will be found above the coronary band in those cases in which the crack is due to injury of the band. Lesions may result from lacerated wounds or from other causes, such as over-reaching and interfering.

Diagnosis

The diagnosis is based on the presence of the crack, which is easily identified, and is classified according to its location.

Hoof testers verify that the lameness is associated with the crack in the hoof wall. Nerve blocking can also be helpful in some cases to gain a better appreciation of the percent contribution the hoof crack has to the lameness picture. Bleeding from the crack after exercise indicates that the crack has extended down to the dermal laminae. Pus will exude from an infected hoof when pressure is applied.

Treatment

The goals of crack treatment are to stabilize the crack and keep it clean and dry. Hoof repair materials often help accomplish both of these goals. Treatment of cracks often requires a trimming of the bearing surface of the hoof wall so it will not bear weight (see Toe Crack and Quarter Crack).

Whenever this is done, the space between the shoe and the wall should be cleaned daily to ensure that dirt does not fill the space and cause pressure. An unshod hoof with a crack will seldom heal because of the constant presence of debris forced into the crack.

In all cases in which it is believed that the crack has permitted infection to enter the dermal tissues, tetanus toxoid should be administered (assuming the horse is up to date on permanent immunization). Hard, dry areas on the coronary band should be rubbed daily with products containing lanolin, fish oil, or olive oil to keep them soft.

Most dry hoof cracks or hoof defects can be treated by the use of hoof-repair material. The crack must be thoroughly cleaned and undermined to hold the repair material in place. There are numerous ways to aid binding of the repair material, and one is to undermine, drill, and lace or suture the crack (Figs. 5–48 and 5–49). The main goals are to give the repair material an anchor to keep it in place and stabilize the crack. Alternative methods for stabilizing the crack without drilling the hoof wall and lacing or suturing are to use a glue-on patch or Equilox (Fig. 5–50). Both bond to the hoof wall surface sufficiently to stabilize the crack.

Repair materials are an excellent way to deal with dry hoof cracks because they seal the crack and prevent infection of the dermal tissues. Defects in the hoof wall can also be filled with such materials. One serious problem with some repair material is the heat generated by hardening, which can destroy tissue beneath it, causing abscess formation.

In the event that the hoof wall crack is infected, it is best to allow the region to remain open for drainage and topical treatment. Covering it with repair material will only serve to entrap the infection and worsen the outcome. For cases that must continue to perform where instability of the hoof wall exists, they can be treated by applying the sutures alone or a polyethylene tubing under the repair material. Because the repair material does not adhere to the polyethylene, the tubing can be removed so that adequate drainage can occur through the tunnel left behind.

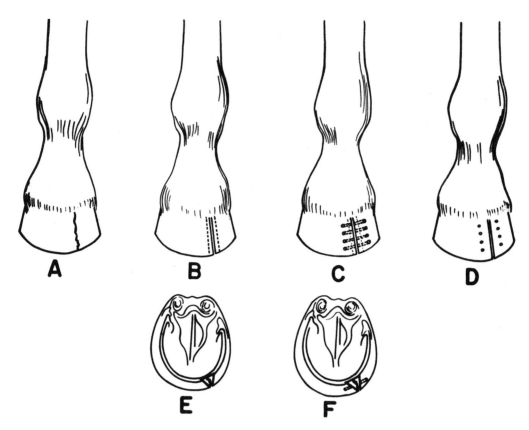

FIG. 5–48. Summary of preparation of hoof crack for hoof repair materials. *A,* Hoof crack. *B,* Crack has been undermined in triangular fashion; compare with *E. C,* Crack undermined and drilled (dotted lines); compare with *F. D,* Crack ready for application of umbilical tape or wire lacing and hoof repair material. *E,* Ground surface view of triangular undermining of crack. *F,* Ground surface view of undermining and drilling (dotted lines).

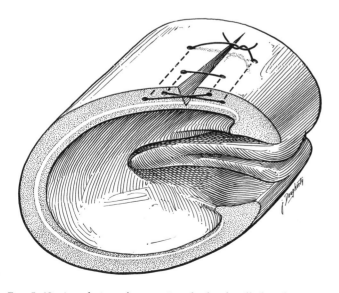

FIG. 5–49. A technique for suturing the hoof wall that does not weaken it because the holes are placed at different levels and depths within the hoof wall.

Treatment varies somewhat depending on the location of the crack.

Toe Crack. If the crack extends only part of the way up the hoof wall, a groove can be filed or burned above the crack (as shown in Fig. 5–51) to limit its upward progress. The horse should be shod with a toe clip on either side of the crack to prevent expansion of the wall (see Fig. 5–51). In addition, a squared-toe shoe will decrease stress on the hoof wall at the toe. The crack should be thoroughly cleaned and povidone iodine should be applied if it is determined that infection is present, after which the foot should be protected with bandaging until the infection is under control. Alternative methods of treatment include glue-on patches, drilling, and lacing the crack (Fig. 5–48) and/or using hoof repair materials.

Quarter Crack. For quarter cracks, either the bearing surface of the hoof wall should be trimmed (floated) in back of the crack or the bearing surface 1 inch on either side of the crack should be relieved allowing the heel on the affected side to still bear weight

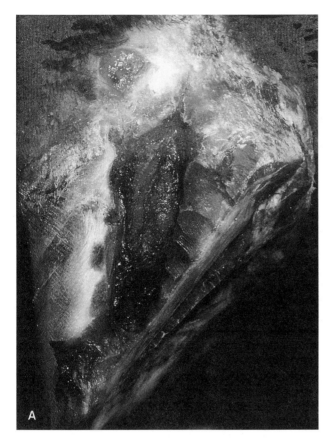
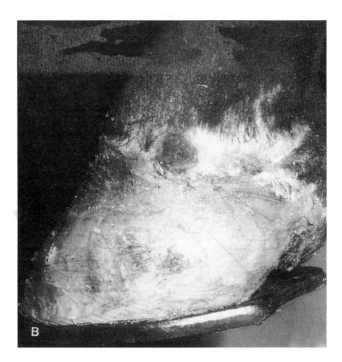

FIG. 5–50. *A*, An extreme quarter crack that involved the dermal laminae. The tissue within the hoof wall defect is completely keratinized and ready for the repair material. *B*, The hoof wall crack in *A* has been filled with repair material (Equilox) and a shoe has been applied.

(see Fig. 6–71). The determining factors are the location of the crack and the overall configuration of the hoof. A heart-bar or full support shoe (heart bar/egg bar) should be applied. The frog-support portion of the shoe should contact the frog evenly and should press against the frog with $\frac{1}{8}$ to $\frac{1}{4}$ of an inch of pressure when the shoe is applied. This allows the frog to bear the weight that normally would be taken by the hoof wall, which has already been floated. The corrective shoe also may have a quarter clip on either side of the crack to help prevent expansion of the crack. Dry quarter cracks may be stripped to a $\frac{1}{4}$-inch width down to the dermal laminae and filled with hoof repair material.

Resection of the entire hoof wall defect, including a superficial portion of the coronary band may be considered for cracks that are not responding to the treatment described above.

Prognosis

The prognosis is favorable if the crack originates at the bearing surface of the wall and if infection has not entered the foot. The prognosis is guarded if infection is present. In cases in which the crack originates in defects of the coronary band, the cause will be persistent, so corrective shoeing may be necessary for the life of the horse. This makes the prognosis guarded to unfavorable. A considerable period may be necessary for the crack to grow out, because the wall grows approximately one-quarter inch per month.

Infection of cracks may cause foot abscesses that break and drain at the coronary band; this situation is similar to that seen in "gravel."

Vertical Tears of the Hoof Wall

Vertical tears of the hoof wall occur most frequently at the medial quarter and heel of young Thoroughbreds. There is a loss of the normal attachment between the laminae.

Hemorrhage can often be seen through the hoof wall in white-footed horses. The degree of lameness can range from mild to severe.

Treatment is aimed at correcting any shoeing disorder that exists (poorly placed shoe or a shoe that is too small), using steel training plates with quarter clips to provide hoof wall stability, and eliminating calks and toe grabs.

The prognosis should be good if the proper corrective trimming and shoeing are afforded and the owner-trainer continues to treat the problem.

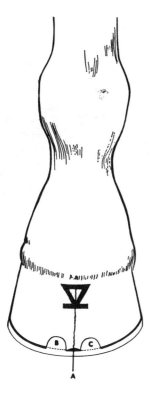

FIG. 5–51. Correction for toe crack. Triangle and bar design below the coronary band is burned or cut in, as shown, to limit the extension of the crack. The hoof wall is trimmed away below the crack so that it will not bear weight on the shoe, as shown by *A. B,* and *C* are the toe clips used on the shoe to support the wall so that the crack cannot expand under pressure.

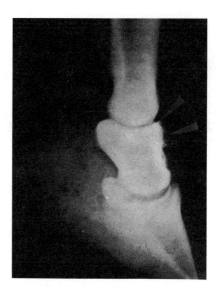

FIG. 5–52. High ringbone. The top arrow indicates new bone growth at the edge of the pastern joint. The lower arrow indicates new bone growth on the dorsal surface of the proximal end of the short pastern bone. These growths resulted from a pulling of the fibrous portion of the joint capsule or from a pulling of the attachment of the common digital extensor tendon.

The Pastern

Ringbone

Ringbone is new bone growth that occurs on the long pastern bone, short pastern bone, or coffin bone. It is the result of an inflammation of the periosteum (bone skin) and may lead to an arthritis or fusion of the pastern or coffin joints. This condition is seldom found in Thoroughbreds but is relatively common in other breeds.

Ringbone is classified in two ways:

High or Low Ringbone

High Ringbone. This is new bone growth occurring on the distal end of the long pastern bone and/or the proximal end of the short pastern bone (Fig. 5–52 and 5–53).

Low Ringbone. This is new bone growth occurring on the distal end of the short pastern bone and/or the proximal end of the coffin bone, especially at the extensor process of the coffin bone (see Fig. 5–54).

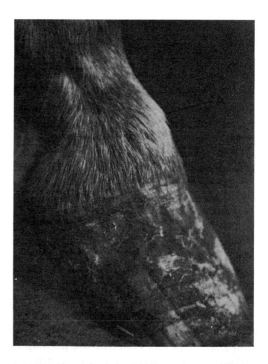

FIG. 5–53. Clinical appearance of high ringbone on the distal end of the long pastern bone and the proximal end of the short pastern bone. Notice the bulging effect approximately 1 inch above the coronary band (*A*).

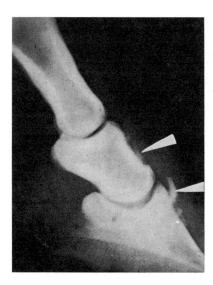

FIG. 5–54. Low ringbone. The upper arrow points to new bone growth on the distal end of the short pastern bone; the lower arrow shows proliferation of a portion of the extensor process of the coffin bone. These changes are caused by tension on the common digital extensor tendon.

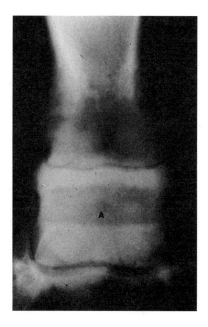

FIG. 5–55. Severe osteoarthritis (ringbone) of the pastern joint.

Articular or Nonarticular Ringbone

Articular Ringbone. Articular ringbone means that the new bone growth involves the joint surface at the pastern or coffin joints (Fig. 5–55).

Nonarticular Ringbone. Nonarticular ringbone means that the new bone growth is around the joint but does not involve a joint surface. It is most common in high ringbone (Fig. 5–56).

In describing ringbone, the following terminology is used: nonarticular high ringbone; articular high ringbone; nonarticular low ringbone; or articular low ringbone.

Causes

Nonarticular ringbone results from a inflammation of the periosteum (bone skin) produced by pulling of the collateral ligaments of the joints involved, pulling of the joint capsule attachments to the bone, pulling of the attachment of the extensor tendon to the long pastern bone, short pastern bone, or coffin bone, and direct blows to these bones. Pulling of these structures disturbs the periosteum, and inflammation and new bone growth result.

Nonarticular high ringbone is most common in horses that do not perform at speeds (e.g., stable hacks, draft horses) and have coarse, boxy-appearing pasterns. Horses with high heels and short toes that work with a trappy gait like the Pasofino are predisposed to low nonarticular ringbone. Wire cuts in the pastern region may cause inflammation that will cause ringbone, if the cut extends into the periosteum (Fig. 5–57).

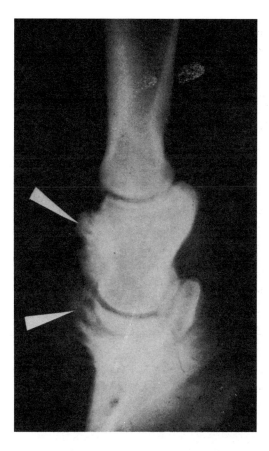

FIG. 5–56. Buttress foot changes on x-ray. The new bone growth is extensive, as shown by the upper arrow on the short pastern bone. The lower arrow shows new bone growth on the extensor process of the coffin bone. This is the same foot as shown in Figure 5–58. Because the proximal end of the short pastern bone is involved, the horse actually has both high and low ringbone.

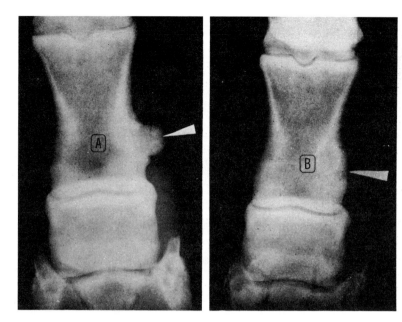

FIG. 5–57. *A*, High ringbone on the medial aspect of the distal end of the long pastern bone resulting from an old wire cut. Inflammation of the periosteum produced by external trauma will produce ringbone, as shown. This growth was successfully removed surgically, as shown in *B*. Removal was necessary because the growth caused chronic lameness as the result of interference to the tendon of the superficial digital flexor.

Articular ringbone (osteoarthrosis), particularly high ringbone, occurs most frequently in horses used for high speed (other than racing) that make quick stops, short turns, and rapid twisting movements (western performance, polo ponies, and some show horses). Uneven spacing of the articular surfaces of the pastern joint and insufficient height of the ridge dividing the articular surfaces on the proximal surface of the short pastern bone may also be a cause. Another cause of articular high ringbone (degenerative joint disease of pastern joint) in young horses (3 years or younger) is described as an osteochondrosis-like lesion (see Chapter 4) that appears to be most severe in the distal aspect of the long pastern bone. This lesion is most frequently observed in the hindlimbs and may be bilateral.

In some cases, one of the bones will fracture in the region of the pastern, and this may lead to osteoarthritis of the pastern joint and to severe ringbone. Fracture of the extensor process of the coffin bone results from tension on the extensor tendon (see Fig. 5–31). Healing of this fracture may result in a large, low ringbone. If the insertion of the common digital extensor tendon is strained, but the extensor process of the coffin bone does not break, an inflammation of the periostium still can result, causing new bone growth and low ringbone. This type of damage is commonly termed "buttress foot" (See Fig. 5–56).

Poor conformation may predispose to pulling of the collateral ligaments, joint capsule, and tendon insertions. Pasterns that are overly upright will result in increased concussion to the pastern joint. Poor conformation increases stress on ligaments and tendons and may cause ringbone resulting from an osteoarthritis caused by uneven pressures on the articular surfaces.

Signs

Ringbone may occur in either the fore- or hindlimb, but it is more common in the forelimb. The exceptions to this are ringbone resulting from fracture of the coffin bone, and pastern bones, and degenerative joint disease of the pastern joint associated with osteochondrosis of the distal end of the long pastern bone, which occurs most frequently in the hindlimb.

Signs of lameness are not specific. Lameness is usually evident in all gaits and upon turning. Heat and swelling will be present over the involved regions, and the horse will sometimes flinch when finger pressure is applied to the region of the active ringbone. In a case of low ringbone, in which the distal end of the short pastern bone or the extensor process of the coffin bone is involved, the hair on the coronary band will stand erect at the front of the foot. There also will be heat and pain present in this region, and after the condition becomes chronic, there will be a change in shape of the toe of the hoof wall (Fig. 5–58). When there is bilateral degenerative joint disease of the coffin joints the horse may point the feet and shorten the cranial phase of the stride much as in navicular syndrome, but more often the gait is characterized by excessive landing on the heel.

Some cases of ringbone do not show lameness especially if they are periarticular. Those cases of ring-

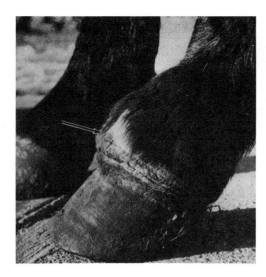

FIG. 5–58. Buttress foot. Note the extensive swelling at the dorsal portion of the coronary band as the result of low ringbone. This is the foot shown in Figure 5–56.

bone that are nonarticular may have little if any lameness, and no heat or pain is present after they are healed. Articular ringbone is accompanied by arthritis (usually osteoarthritis) of the affected joint, but fusion of the pastern joint may occur. X-rays of ringbone will show minor to extreme bony changes on the long pastern bone, short pastern bone, and coffin bone.

Early cases of high ringbone, especially those involving the proximal end of the short pastern bone, may show periodic swelling and lameness that will disappear with rest. This will reappear after the horse is put back to work until the firm swellings of ringbone are recognized. Radiographic changes showing periosteal new bone growth will then be present. The gait in these cases often resembles that of laminitis, with the heel landing long before the toe.

On palpation, heat and firm swelling will be evident in acute and subacute cases. Occasionally, firm finger pressure will elicit pain. As the disease becomes chronic, the swelling will feel firm and cool to the touch. Flexion and rotation of the pastern joint results in a painful response, and reduced flexion is usually present.

Nerve blocking may be required in some cases to identify the percentage of contribution that ringbone has to the total lameness picture.

Diagnosis

A definite diagnosis of ringbone cannot be made without x-rays. In early cases, when swelling is not marked, the diagnosis is based on finding heat and pain in the involved regions. Careful comparison with the opposite limb should be made.

In early cases of articular and nonarticular ringbone, soft tissue swelling may be present, but x-rays will be negative; 3 to 4 weeks later evidence may be present.

The opposite pastern region should be x-rayed for comparison.

Treatment

If a case is diagnosed in the very early stages before new bone growth begins, limiting motion of the joints from the hoof wall to just below the carpus may be tried. This can be accomplished by bandage splinting or by cast application.

When the pastern joint has become fused, signs of lameness may not be present. This is especially true in the hindlimb, where fractures may heal by fusion of the pastern joint. If high ringbone is articular in nature, the horse will be lame until the pastern joint is fused. Too often, the joint does not fuse; this results in massive deposits of new bone growth around the joint with a hairline articular space shown on radiographs.

The treatment of subacute or chronic cases of ringbone involves surgically created joint fusion. Fusion relieves pain by preventing joint movement. Of the techniques described, internal fixation with or without bone grafting gives the best results when degenerative joint disease of the pastern joint is present. Good results have been reported with three parallel-placed screws that cross the pastern joint and compress it when the screws are tightened (Fig. 5–59).

After surgery the limb is immobilized to just below the hock or knee in a cast. The foot must be included in the cast.

The cast is removed if needed, but may be left in place for a period of 6 to 7 weeks if a good fit exists. Most frequently, however, the cast is removed once, and in a few cases two times, during the 6- to 7-week period required for casting. The cast is removed and replaced by bandage support when x-rays show that fusion exists. This usually occurs between the fifth and seventh week postoperatively. Stall confinement is recommended for another 8 weeks. Hand-walking exercise can begin when satisfactory x-rays are obtained after this time. Free exercise can usually begin after 16 weeks, but each case is assessed individually. Contrary to other reports, a year of convalescence may be required before horses can be returned to full serviceability.

If the coffin joint is involved, there is little hope of ever obtaining a sound horse for riding (see Fig. 5–56). A neurectomy is sometimes performed to reduce the pain. If a bilateral neurectomy at the base of the proximal sesamoid bones is done, the same precautions should be used as described for palmar digital neurectomy for navicular syndrome. Loss of the hoof wall can be a complication. It is probably caused by the loss of blood supply rather than nerve supply; this loss of blood supply results from connective tissue and nerve regeneration that surround and occlude the palmar arteries. In some cases, the dorsal or palmar branch of the digital nerve may be cut to relieve pain. Surgical fusion of the coffin joint has been used successfully in a few cases.

Horses with ringbone are usually shod with full roller motion shoes (Fig. 6–95), which aid in reducing some of the action from the fused or involved joints.

In some cases of nonarticular ringbone, removal of the new bone growth is indicated because it is causing lameness by encroaching on adjacent structures (see Fig. 5–57). However, this is uncommon.

Prognosis

Prognosis is good for serviceability (return to intended work) for the acute nonarticular form of ringbone, provided that it is treated early. Cases of articular high ringbone invariably progress to degenerative joint disease if not treated, and the prognosis is unfavorable. With the advent of lag screw fixation or T-plate application, the prognosis is greatly improved. In general, fewer complications and a better outcome can be expected for treatment by surgically created joint fusion of the hindlimb versus that of the forelimb.

Prognosis for low nonarticular ringbone is usually guarded and, frequently, a mechanical alteration in the gait exists after the pain is gone. Low articular ringbone carries a very unfavorable prognosis for serviceability. In some cases a neurectomy may be helpful.

Dislocation of the Pastern Joint

Partial dislocation (subluxation) and complete dislocation (luxation) of the pastern joint are rare. A partial dislocation is often referred to as "Thoroughbred ringbone," because it most commonly affects the racehorse that has sustained previous injury to the support structures. Complete dislocations usually occur in a lateral to medial direction, as a result of traumatic tearing of the collateral ligaments (e.g., when a horse gets its foot caught and then attempts to escape or falls). Partial dislocations usually occur in a dorsal palmar or dorsal plantar direction and are thought to result from injury to the stabilizing structures of the fetlock. Palmar subluxation has been observed most frequently in young foals that have jumped from heights (i.e., out of trailers or the back of a truck) (Fig. 5–60).

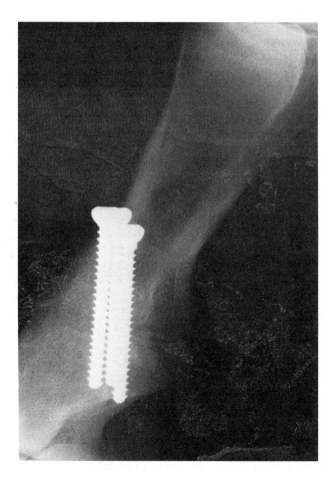

FIG. 5–59. Fusion of the pastern joint was accomplished with three screws placed across the joint to compress it. The cartilage from the pastern joint was removed before screw placement. Good healing occurred.

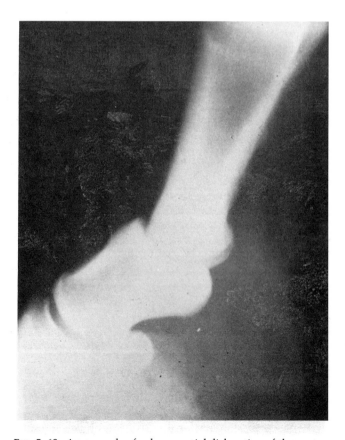

FIG. 5–60. An example of palmar partial dislocation of the pastern joint.

Horses with a dislocation are usually nonweight-bearing, and a limb deformity associated with the pastern region is present.

Treatment depends on the cause and the duration since injury. Early cases may be treated with casting and/or internal fixation.

Horses treated early have a reasonable chance to return to light work and breeding services. Internal fixation may provide a good prognosis for return to serviceable use if it is performed early.

Fractures of the Short Pastern Bone

Fractures of the short pastern bone occur most commonly in the hindlimbs of middle-aged (4 to 10 years) western performance horses used for cutting, roping, barrel racing, pole bending, and reining.

A wide range of fractures can affect the short pastern bone. Chip fractures can involve either the pastern or coffin joint surfaces, whereas wing fractures involve the pastern joint (Fig. 5–61). Comminuted (fragmented) fractures most frequently involve the pastern joint, but they may extend into the coffin joint as well.

Causes

Chip fractures probably result either from direct trauma or tearing of insertional attachments. Wing and fragmented fractures are thought to result from compression trauma, and the torque and twist that occurs with sudden stops, starts, and short turns. Horses shod with heel calks appear to be more prone to such fractures because the calks tend to fix the foot to the ground, preventing the normal swivel of the hoof or shoe on the ground surface when the horse is rapidly changing directions. Such fractures have also occurred during unrestrained paddock exercise.

Signs

The history of acute onset of severe lameness, painful withdrawal, and a crackling on manipulation of the pastern is diagnostic. Often a "pop" was heard just prior to the onset of severe lameness.

On gross observation, swelling is usually present just above the coronary band in cases of fragmented fractures. With wing fractures and chip fractures the swelling is less evident and may not be apparent. Lameness is obvious for a fragmented fracture, and a horse will be reluctant to place its foot on the ground. Wing fractures initially present with severe lameness, but with rest it is less evident. Chip fractures may require circling at a trot to identify if lameness is present.

On palpation varying degrees of swelling will be detected. Flexion and rotation of the pastern region will result in a crackling feeling, instability, and painful withdrawal with wing fractures and fragmented fractures. In some cases direct palpation of a wing fracture will cause movement of the fracture and pain. Physical diagnosis of chip fractures of the pastern can be difficult and usually requires nerve blocking to localize the problem. A definitive diagnosis requires x-rays.

Treatment

Chip fractures associated with the pastern joint may be treated conservatively or by surgical removal. The choice depends on the horse's intended use, the amount of articular surface affected, the duration of fracture, and the amount of pain identified on physical examination. In some cases joint blocking will be required to make a final decision as to the contribution the fracture may have to the lameness picture.

Fractures of either the lateral, medial, or both wings of the short pastern bone that involve the pastern joint can be treated by casting, compression screw fixation, and/or fusion of the joint. Casting can be used for periods of 8 to 12 weeks in selected cases in which only pasture or breeding soundness is desired. After cast removal, a pressure support bandage is applied and continued for an additional 3 weeks. Exercise is permitted according to the horse's capabilities.

Internal fixation of wing fractures has been successful in returning horses to athletic performance. After application of screws and suture closure a cast is applied to protect the limb during recovery. The cast is

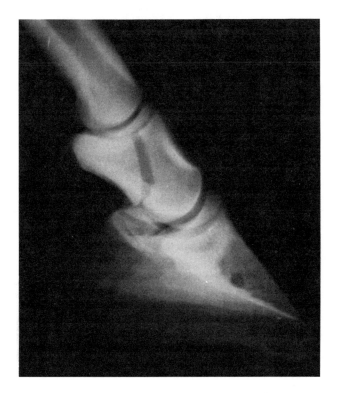

FIG. 5–61. A large wing fracture of the short pastern bone.

removed in 14 to 21 days, depending on the degree of stability achieved. Horses are stalled for 6 weeks and controlled hand-walking exercise is begun after that time. A total rest period of approximately 12 to 16 weeks is recommended before free exercise is begun. Riding exercise may begin in 9 to 12 months.

Surgical fusion of the pastern joint is another option for treatment of the wing fracture (see Ringbone section in this chapter).

Severely fragmented fractures are usually best treated with casting similar to that previously described or by casting over metal pins that have been placed through holes made in the cannon bone. Usually three pins are placed from lateral to medial, after which cast material is applied around and over the pins. This transfixation pin technique effectively reduces the pressure on the fractured bone while the horse bears on the pins. The prognosis for these fractures is decreased if the fracture extends into the coffin joint. In most cases the initial damage to the joint surface is sufficient to create fusion with time. However, surgical fusion has been used successfully in a limited number of cases. Generally, pasture soundness can be achieved, and in a small percentage of cases, varying degrees of athletic performance can be afforded.

Prognosis

The prognosis for a limited number of cases treated for chip fracture appears to be good for return to full serviceability. The prognosis for fragmented fractures is good for pasture and breeding soundness when conservative treatment is used and guarded for return to athletic function. When surgery, either fracture fixation using the lag screw principle or fusion, is used, a good prognosis can be expected for return to athletic function.

For fragmented fractures involving the pastern joint surface only, a good prognosis can be given for pasture soundness and a very guarded to poor prognosis for return to athletic performance. Conversely, horses that have sustained fractures of both the pastern and coffin joint surfaces are reported to have a 50% survival rate and slightly greater than a 1 to 10 chance of return to athletic performance with casting alone. Surgical intervention in these cases did not improve the survival rate but increased the chance of return to athletic function by a 1 to 4 margin.

In general, the prognosis for hindlimb fractures is better, no matter what treatment is used. If protracted pain results in lameness after healing has occurred, fusion of the pastern joint can be performed or neurectomy considered. A slightly higher percentage of cases with short pastern bone fractures (71%) will return to partial or full function when surgery and casting are used compared to 67% when casting is used alone.

Longitudinal and Fragmented Fractures of the Long Pastern Bone

Longitudinal and fragmented fractures of the long pastern bone are relatively common in horses. Fracture configurations of the long pastern bone may range from small fissures that enter the fetlock joint to severe fragmented fractures that affect both the proximal and distal joint surfaces. (Figs. 5–62 and 5–63). The fissure fracture (so-called "split" pastern) is more commonly seen in Thoroughbreds, Standardbreds, and hunter jumpers; whereas the severely fragmented fracture is most common in the western performance horse (cutting and barrel racing horses). The fissure fracture may present a diagnostic challenge because horses frequently do not appear fracture-lame, particularly after they have had a few days' rest. Long pastern bone fractures are rarely open.

Causes

A combination of longitudinal compression in conjunction with twisting of the long pastern bone in relation to the cannon bone, appear to be the cause. Probably two situations exist. During the weight-bearing phase, the convex sagittal ridge of the distal end of the cannon bone comes to fit in congruity with

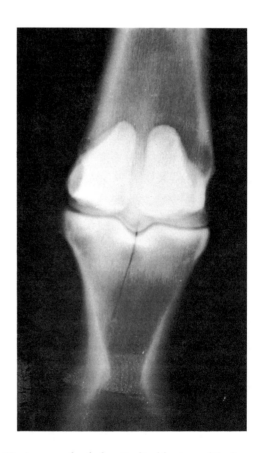

FIG. 5–62. An example of a longitudinal fracture of the long pastern bone, a candidate for compression using the lag screw principle.

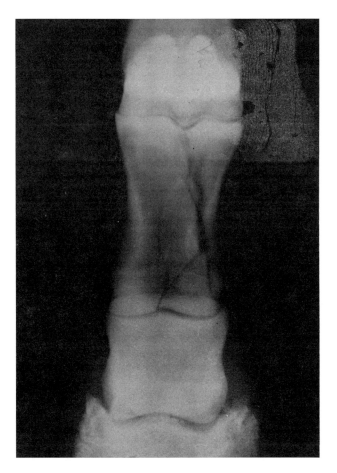

FIG. 5–63. An example of a fragmented articular fracture of the long pastern bone. Note that the fracture extends into the fetlock and pastern joints. This type of fracture is very difficult to treat.

the concave grove in the proximal surface of the long pastern bone. If the alignment is not perfect, the convex sagittal ridge acts as a wedge to cleave a fracture slab off the long pastern bone. This would occur when the horse is required to make quick turns. Also, as the limb goes to the flexed position, there is a lateral-to-medial rotation of the long pastern bone around its long axis. In this case, if the rotary movement is accelerated, as it would be if the foot slips, a fracture may result. Procedures such as shoeing the horse with heel calks tend to fix the position of the foot, allowing the cannon bone to twist in relation to the structures below it, resulting in a fracture from the torque.

Signs

The clinical signs of long pastern bone fracture are variable and depend on the type of fracture that has been sustained. Whereas the fissure fracture may be quite subtle, particularly after a period of rest, the fragmented fracture will cause non-weight-bearing lameness. However, in either case there is usually an acute onset of lameness. On visual observation the pastern will be obviously swollen with fragmented fractures because of the hemorrhage and edema associated with the soft tissues. The swelling associated with the fissure fracture, on the other hand, is usually less pronounced. On palpation and manipulation a painful response will be elicited with flexion and rotation of the foot in cases of fissure fracture. For fragmented fracture, an obvious crackling feeling and loss of upright stability and alignment will be obvious. If a fissure fracture is suspected, x-rays will need to be taken immediately. Nerve blocking and/or excessive exercise to establish lameness is counterproductive because it may result in complete disruption of the fracture and lessen the prognosis for athletic performance in the future.

Diagnosis

X-rays are taken to characterize the type of fracture sustained and to indicate if internal fixation is required. If the horse has to be transported a short distance, a large tight-fitting bandage splint or a commercially available splint should be applied. Although most horses protect their limbs quite well because of the extreme pain, casts are recommended for horses that must be transported for long distances.

Treatment

Although longitudinal and fissure fractures have been treated successfully with prolonged casting alone, internal fixation with lag screws is preferred for the best outcome. If the fissure fracture is treated conservatively, excess bone growth associated with the healing process may be sufficient to cause residual painful lameness. Because conservative treatment of longitudinal fractures usually results in the crippling effect of degenerative joint disease of the fetlock, joint surgical fixation is recommended.

After surgery, a cast is applied to prevent refracture during recovery. The cast can be removed in 7 to 14 days for fissure fractures, whereas longer periods are required for more unstable fractures. The horse is confined to a box stall for 6 weeks, followed by 6 weeks of hand-walking exercise. Followup x-rays will need to be taken about 12 weeks after surgery to evaluate healing.

Fragmented fractures of the long pastern bone are best treated with screw compression and casting. Frequently, casting alone results in the cannon bone wedging the fragments of the long pastern bone apart, and a painful slow union results. With internal fixation an attempt is made to reconstruct the articular surfaces of the proximal and distal joint surfaces and the center is bridged with a bone plate. If considerable damage is present at either or both joint surfaces, joint fusion may be performed. A cast is applied from the ground surface of the hoof to the cannon and maintained until radiographic healing is present. In most cases casts are required for at least 8 to 12 weeks.

An alternative to lag screws is the transfixation pinning technique (refer to the section on short pastern fractures), which allows the pins to bear the weight, thus removing it from the fracture site. This approach is generally selected when performance is not required and pasture soundness is acceptable. Transfixation can also be used in conjunction with lag screws in the most severely fragmented fractures.

Prognosis

The prognosis for fractures of the long pastern bone depends on the configuration of the fracture sustained, the severity of injury, the stability achieved with internal fixation, and the expectations of the outcome by the owner. Acute fissure fractures and longitudinal fractures that are treated promptly by internal fixation have a good to guarded prognosis for athletic function in the future. Fragmented fractures, on the other hand, have a poor prognosis for return to athletic function, but have a good prognosis for pasture soundness if treated surgically by internal fixation.

Inflammation of the Distal Sesamoidean Ligaments

Sprain of the distal sesamoidean ligaments (see Figs. 1–10 and 1–11) may also include fracture of the sesamoid bone and/or excessive bone production at the site of the sprain. It is generally a secondary disorder that is rarely the primary cause of lameness.

Horses with acute inflammation present with lameness of sudden onset. Direct digital palpation over the region, lateral or medial to the flexor tendons and midway between the heel bulbs and the sesamoid bones, may result in pain (Fig. 5–64). Generally, the clinical findings alone lead to this diagnosis; however, nerve blocking may also need to be performed. A definitive diagnosis is made with ultrasound, with which the severity of the inflammation can be visualized and documented.

For the acute case, rest, support, antiinflammatory therapy (i.e., cold and phenylbutazone), and very gradual return to work are indicated. If the inflammation is severe, casting for 2 to 3 weeks along with administration of phenylbutazone may be helpful. After cast removal, support bandages are applied and maintained with stall confinement for another 6 weeks. Gradual hand-walking exercise is begun. The region of injury should be monitored closely by palpation for heat and pain. Less severe cases are treated with support bandaging in conjunction with phenylbutazone. In most cases a minimum of 6 to 8 weeks of stall rest is required and ultrasound examination is used to document healing. If the inflammation is not treated, considerable scar tissue formation and calcification

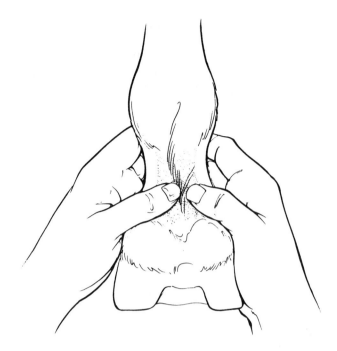

FIG. 5–64. Direct digital palpation of the palmar (or plantar) surface of the pastern, midway between the proximal sesamoid bones and the heel bulb, may cause a painful response in horses that have sustained a sprain to the distal sesamoidean ligaments.

within the distal sesamoidean ligaments can occur. Occasionally these horses may require a year or more convalescence before they become serviceable. As with any musculoskeletal disorder, an informed thoughtful owner usually successfully manages these problems, whereas an anxious owner or trainer may push the horse too fast, resulting in recurrence of the problem.

Prognosis is guarded because of the high probability of reinjury. Also, when inflammation of the distal sesamoidean ligament is combined with other skeletal problems (ringbone, navicular disease, proximal sesamoidean ligament desmitis), the prognosis is worse.

The Fetlock

Chip Fractures (Osteochondral Fragments) of the Fetlock Joint

Chip fractures of the proximal dorsal end of the long pastern bone are relatively common. Most proximal dorsal fractures involve the forelimbs. On the medial side of the long pastern bone, chip fractures from the distal end of the cannon bone also occur but are less common. Other less frequently occurring fractures of the long pastern bone include proximal wing fractures (Type I and II) and articular margin fractures (Type III) just below the sesamoid bone.

Lameness associated with chip fractures of the proximal dorsal border of the long pastern bone is generally observed in horses racing at speed on hard surfaces (i.e., hard-surfaced race tracks), and lameness associated with chip fractures of the distal cannon bone is usually seen when training begins. Lameness associated with wing fragments is often seen in horses pushed to maximum performance.

Cause

Trauma is the cause of chip fractures of the proximal dorsal margin in the horse. From the appearance of the fractures, it seems that overextension of the joint is probably involved (Fig. 5–65). Overextension places stress on the dorsal aspect of the proximal end of the long pastern bone as it is pressed against the cannon bone. Limb fatigue is a factor in overextension of the fetlock joint. Why the fracture most frequently occurs medial to the midline is not fully understood (Fig. 5–66).

Type I and II fragments from the wings of the long pastern bone and fragments from the distal cannon bone appear to be caused by osteochondrosis, whereas Type III fractures are felt to be true avulsion (pulled-away) fractures.

Signs

Synovitis (inflammation of the synovial membrane) of the fetlock joint indicated by distention of the joint capsule is commonly found.

Lameness is often most obvious at the trot. It is primarily a concussion lameness. Some horses have only a small amount of swelling or lameness to indicate that there is a chip fracture. There may be enlarge-ment on the dorsal surface of the fetlock joint that is easily palpated. Lameness will usually increase after exercise, and a workout or a race may cause the horse to be markedly lame. It is difficult to produce pain in the affected region by digital pressure, but some heat can usually be detected over the dorsal surface of the joint. Flexion of the affected fetlock will often elicit pain as compared to the opposite fetlock. A flexion test can be performed by holding the fetlock flexed for 30–60 seconds after which the horse is trotted off and the degree of lameness documented. After prolonged rest, the horse may seem to be sound, only to go lame again when returned to training. Occasionally, there may be acute lameness followed by dramatic relief when a chip that was caught in the joint is dislodged.

Diagnosis

Diagnosis cannot be made without x-rays (Fig. 5–67).

It is important to x-ray the opposite fetlock, since bilateral fractures are common, and clinical signs may not appear until the horse is back in training.

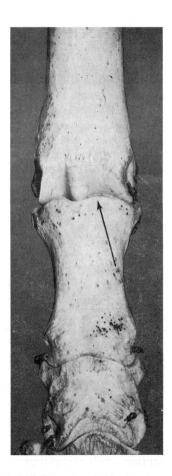

FIG. 5–66. The fetlock joint reveals the most common region of occurrence for fractures of the long pastern bone medial to the midline (arrow). (From Adams, O.R.: Chip fractures into the metacarpophalangeal (fetlock) joint. J. Am. Vet. Med. Assoc., *148*:360, 1966.)

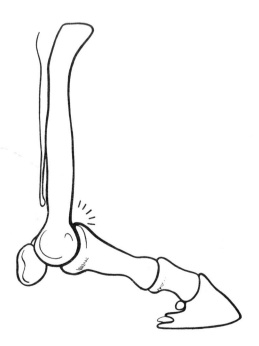

FIG. 5–65. Mechanism of chip fracture of the long pastern bone. (Courtesy of Dr. W. Berkeley.)

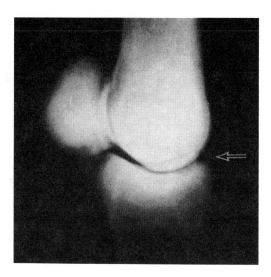

FIG. 5–67. Lateral x-ray of the fetlock joint revealing a chip fracture (arrow) of the long pastern bone. (From Adams, O.R.: Chip fractures into the metacarpophalangeal (fetlock) joint. J. Am. Vet. Med. Assoc., *148*:360, 1966.)

Treatment

Proximal Dorsal Chips of the Long Pastern Bone. Many small, nondisplaced fractures can be treated successfully with adequate rest for 120 days. However surgery is indicated if larger displaced fragments are present or in cases in which recurrent lameness is attributable to the presence of the chip. When surgery is selected, arthroscopic removal of the chip is the preferred approach. Three to four months' rest is recommended before training is resumed.

Fragments from the Distal Cannon Bone. Usually multiple limbs (two to three) are involved and removal by arthroscopic surgery is recommended. Postoperative rest is recommended for 3 to 4 months.

Type I Fracture. Type I fracture originates from the proximal wing of the long pastern bone. Usually the hindlimbs are affected. Removal by arthroscopic surgery is advised, and generally 3 to 5 months of rest are recommended before training resumes.

Type II Fracture. Originate Proximal Wing of the Long Pastern Bone. Nonarticular fractures of the medial and lateral proximal wing of the long pastern bone will frequently respond to stall rest of approximately 120 days. Articular fractures that continue to be a source of pain are removed surgically (Fig. 5–68). Although internal fixation, with bone screws has been performed the outcome has been less rewarding than surgical removal. Six months of rest are recommended in these cases. Bandaging alone can be used for postoperative cases in which chip fractures have been removed.

Type III Fractures. These fractures originate from the base of the sesamoid bones. They are felt to be true avulsion (pulled-away) fractures. They are seen in both fore- and hindlimbs and are often associated with prominent joint swelling. Although rest alone has

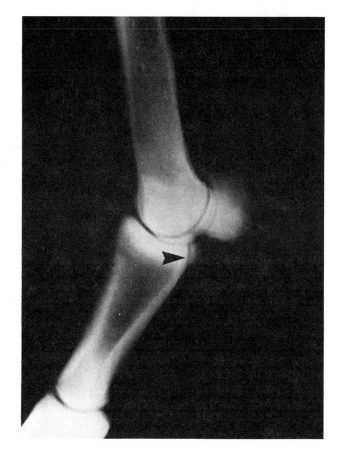

FIG. 5–68. An articular fracture off the proximal palmar wing of the long pastern bone.

been tried, the outcome is greatly improved if the fragment is removed arthroscopically.

Prognosis

The prognosis is usually good after arthroscopic removal of proximal dorsal chip fractures, but it is somewhat dependent on the size and number of chip fractures, their duration, and the degree of degenerative joint disease.

The prognosis for return to performance for distal cannon bone and proximal palmar/plantar fractures of the fetlock joint is considered good for all three types when surgery is used to remove the fragment. The exception to this is that nonarticular type II wing fractures have a good prognosis for return to performance with rest.

Fractures of the Sesamoid Bones

Fractures of the sesamoid bones are common injuries in racing Thoroughbreds, Standardbreds, and Quarter horses. The forelimbs are most frequently affected in the Thoroughbred and Quarter horse, whereas the hindlimbs are more frequently affected in the Standardbred. Most of these fractures separate as a result of the pull of the suspensory ligament and the distal sesamoidean ligaments.

Fractures of the apex (point) of the sesamoid bone are by far the most common. They are frequently articular, singular, rarely fragmented, and usually involve less than one third of the bone (Fig. 5–69 A and B). They occur most frequently on the lateral sesamoid bones of the right hindlimb in Standardbreds, whereas a more equal distribution is observed in the forelimbs of Thoroughbreds and Quarter Horses.

Fractures at the base are less common than at the apex. They are frequently multiple and can be small articular (Fig. 5–70), transverse articular (Fig. 5–71), or nonarticular. The treatment and surgical approach depend on an accurate identification of the type of fracture.

The abaxial (away from center) fracture is the least common of the four types. These fractures can be either articular or nonarticular. They can be difficult to diagnose and may require additional x-rays to identify their exact location.

The midbody horizontal fracture is seen most frequently in Thoroughbreds and in young foals under 2 months of age. It roughly separates the bone into equal portions and invariably enters the fetlock joint. Because of the forces of the suspensory ligament and the distal sesamoidean ligament, most of these tend to separate.

In general, sesamoid fractures are considered an occupational disease of racing horses. An exception to this is the fracture seen in foals under 2 months of age. As a group sesamoid fractures represent a structural failure of bone in response to stresses applied through one or more of the many ligaments that attach to the surface of the bone. Factors such as muscular fatigue, unequal tension applied to the sesamoid bones, and direct trauma have also been implicated in the development of sesamoid fractures.

Causes

The causes of sesamoid bone fractures are varied. It is felt that the cyclical forces to which the sesamoid bone is subjected during continuous strenuous exer-

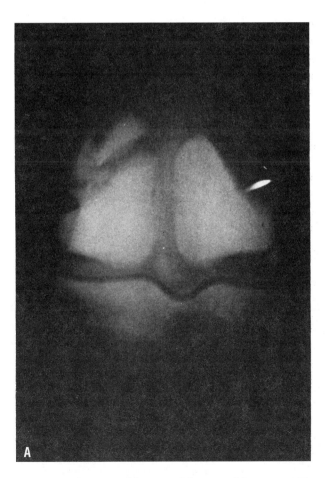
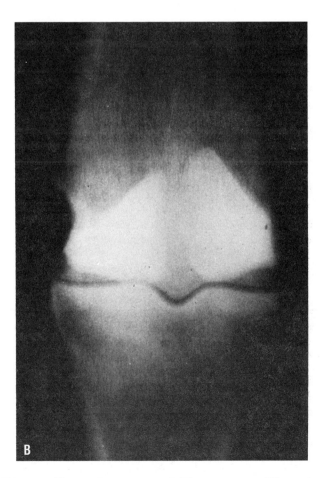

FIG. 5–69. *A*, A fragmented fracture of the apex of the sesamoid bone. This type of fracture is uncommon. *B*, The same sesamoid bone after the fragment was removed.

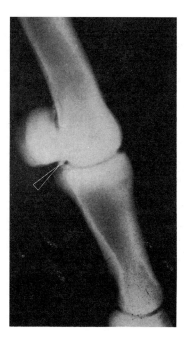

FIG. 5–70. Small distal fracture from the sesamoid bone (arrow).

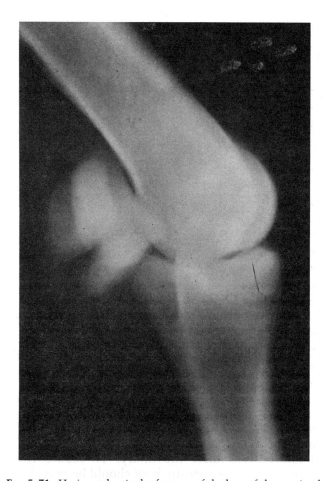

FIG. 5–71. Horizontal articular fracture of the base of the proximal sesamoid bone.

cise actually decrease the strength of the bone, making it more susceptible to failure. Additionally, the enlargement of the vascular canal that is observed in chronic sesamoiditis represents a weak point in the bone which may predispose it to fracture.

Muscular fatigue that frequently develops toward the end of long races is also an important factor. As muscles tire, more weight is supported by the suspensory apparatus and hyperextension of the fetlock occurs. When the sesamoid bone can no longer withstand the pulling forces applied to it by the suspensory ligament and distal sesamoidian ligaments, the bone fails. Other factors such as poor conditioning, improper or irregular trimming and shoeing, and poor conformation create additional stresses on this bone. This muscle-fatigue factor is most clearly illustrated when young foals that are placed on pasture fracture their sesamoid bones while running to keep up with their mothers.

Unequal tension applied to the sesamoid bone as the foot strikes the ground in an unbalanced position may also cause these fractures. Sesamoid bone fractures have been reported with a simple injury such as stepping on a golf ball or stepping into a hole.

Direct trauma to the sesamoid bone has also been implicated. The medial sesamoid bone is reported to be the most frequently involved when interference is the cause. However, it is interesting that there is rarely any evidence of external trauma (wound) associated with sesamoid fractures. Lack of coordination between the body and the limbs has also been implicated as a cause of fractures of the base of the sesamoid.

Some fractured sesamoids appear to be congenital. In these cases the proximal portion of the sesamoid bones show fracture lines through both of the sesamoids on both forelimbs. These are not accompanied by any detectable heat, pain, swelling, or history of lameness. It is possible that these represent a congenital imperfection in the bone, termed bipartite sesamoids, or that these are old fractures that have healed by fibrous union.

Signs

The medial or lateral sesamoid bones, or both, may be fractured. Lameness is very pronounced in acute stages: The horse may be reluctant to bear weight on the limb and will not permit the fetlock to descend to a normal position during weight bearing. Swelling, heat, and pain are marked in the fetlock region. Tendosynovitis (inflammation of the tendon and its sheath), which also may be present, may confuse the diagnosis if x-rays are not taken. The horse evidences pain when pressure is applied to the affected bone or bones. Descent of the fetlock during weight bearing causes pain. Observation of the gait will reveal that the fetlock is held rigid so that it cannot descend as much as the opposite normal fetlock. The fracture in the bone may occur in any area of the sesamoids, but proximal fractures are more common than distal fractures; proximal fractures also are more amenable to treatment (see Fig. 5–69). Inflammation of the suspensory and distal sesamoidean ligaments may occur concurrently with fractured sesamoids.

A history of galloping to exhaustion in an attempt to keep up with the dam is common cause for foals under 2 months of age to sustain fractures of their sesamoid bones. These fractures often occur in foals that have been confined to a boxstall for several days and then turned out for free exercise with their mothers.

Diagnosis

Diagnosis is based on x-ray examination of the affected fetlock and the physical changes described.

Because the density and contrast may be poor in radiographs taken in very young foals (as a result of limited ossification), good-quality radiographs and close scrutiny are required for the diagnosis. In some cases the fracture cannot be diagnosed immediately and may require a few weeks before it becomes apparent. This is also true for hairline nondisplaced fractures that occur in adults. If an incomplete sesamoid bone fracture is suspected, a repeat x-ray should be taken after 2 to 4 weeks of stall rest. This will permit better evaluation of the fracture line because it allows sufficient time for lysis (breakdown) of the bone to occur. If a horse with an incomplete fracture is allowed to exercise, there is a great risk of separating the fracture and worsening the prognosis. Special x-ray views are required for some abaxial (outer surface) articular fractures. Additionally ultrasound is done to rule out damage to the suspensory ligament.

Treatment

The selection of treatment of sesamoid bone fractures is based on the location of the fracture and the intended use of the animal. Treatments include cast or splint application, surgical removal, lag screw fixation, or placement of an encircling loop of surgical wire, and bone grafting.

In general, most horses that are not intended for performance and will be relegated to breeding will not require surgery, and simple support, bandaging, splinting, or casting with stall rest is sufficient.

Casting or splinting the limb for a period of 12 to 16 weeks has proved successful in those cases in which nondisplaced sesamoid fractures have occurred in the young horse. This prolonged period of time is needed because the sesamoid bones heal very slowly. It is thought that the poor healing capabilities of this bone may result from its relatively poor blood supply, limited periosteal (bone skin) covering, the absence of a marrow cavity, and the extensive ligamentous attachments that cause separation and movement. Most fractures that are treated conservatively heal by a weak fibrous union, and the fracture line will be ob-

served on x-rays for prolonged periods of time. Also, some of these fractures that have apparently healed will separate at a later date. Generally, the conservative approach should be used for those cases that are not going to be used for performance in the future and for young foals that do not show displaced fracture fragments.

Surgical treatment of sesamoid bone fractures in the horse intended for performance appears to be beneficial because it reduces the chances of secondary degenerative joint disease developing within the fetlock joint.

Apex fractures involving less than one third of the sesamoid bone and small base fractures are best treated by arthroscopic surgical removal of the fragment. Nonarticular abaxial fractures may require removal, but horses will often perform successfully without surgery. On the other hand, abaxial articular fractures should be removed to prevent secondary degenerative joint disease within the fetlock. Midbody horizontal fractures affecting the middle third and transverse base fractures have been treated with lag screw fixation (or with surgical wire). Thin, horizontal fractures involving the entire base are very difficult to treat. Surgical removal of these fractures not only disrupts the support of the distal sesamoidean ligaments, but it frequently interrupts the collateral sesamoidean ligament support as well. These thin fractures are usually not large enough to support compression screw fixation without risking the chance of splitting them into two smaller fragments. When a base fracture is too thin to support compression screw fixation but is too large to remove, an encircling surgical wire and/or bone grafting is recommended. Good bone healing can be expected between 20 and 40 weeks after bone grafting.

Fractures through the bodies of both sesamoid bones are a common cause of breakdown in the racing horse. Because the suspensory apparatus is lost, these horses are frequently humanely euthanized. However, animals with breeding potential or great sentimental value can be salvaged but early treatment is required for a successful outcome. Even with early treatment the initial soft tissue trauma may be severe enough that the blood supply to the foot is lost. Management of such injuries is directed toward the support and immobilization of the fetlock joint for a sufficient time to allow soft tissues to heal by fibrosis and to prevent further injury to the vascular supply. Various treatments have been recommended and include casting, joint fusion, and bandage splinting.

A major complication can be laminitis in the opposite weight-bearing limb. This will often be first recognized as increased weight bearing on the affected limb and can be erroneously recorded as a good sign. In most cases the laminitis occurs between the third and fourth week after the injury. To reduce the chances of this, the opposite hoof should be provided with support from a heart bar shoe and/or a frog support pad. Analgesics might need to be administered to increase the weight bearing on the injured limb and to decrease the stress to the weight-bearing limb.

Prognosis

The prognosis is guarded if more than one third of the bone has been fractured, as it is for long-standing fractures that have not been cast or treated surgically. Small fragments of long duration may be removed successfully, but the sooner after acute inflammation subsides the better, as far as the outcome for the patient is concerned. Small articular fragments off the apex or abaxial surface may be removed with a favorable prognosis. Fractures involving the base of the sesamoid bone generally have a guarded prognosis for return to performance and a good prognosis for pasture soundness. If both sesamoids are fractured, the prognosis is less favorable.

The prognosis for treatment of fractures of the sesamoid bones that result in loss of the suspensory apparatus is poor and only should be considered for salvage of valuable breeding stock and horses of great sentimental value.

In all cases, however, the prognosis can only be made after thorough x-ray evaluation of the fetlock joints for signs of degenerative joint disease and evaluation of the suspensory ligament as a source of pain from desmitis can be made.

Sesamoiditis

Sesamoiditis, or inflammation of the sesamoid bones usually involves an inflammation of the bone skin (periosteum) as well as the bone itself. The suspensory ligament and the distal sesamoidean ligaments are also affected and may show calcified areas. Demineralization of the sesamoid bone(s) may result from inflammation and impaired blood supply (Fig. 5–72).

Sesamoiditis can be articular or nonarticular. The articular form is characterized by bony outgrowth at the apex (point) and base of the sesamoid bone and is usually secondary to disease within the fetlock joint cavity. The nonarticular form is associated with primary diseases involving the suspensory apparatus and is characterized by enlarged canals and/or coarseness of the bone and increased bone production on the abaxial (away from center) base of the sesamoid bone. Comments will be confined to the nonarticular form.

Sesamoiditis is observed frequently in racing horses and hunters and jumpers between 2 and 5 years of age. Primary disease of the suspensory ligament or distal sesamoidean ligament can also accompany this disease.

Causes

Any unusual strain or sprain to the fetlock region may produce sesamoiditis. It can affect any type of horse. It is caused by injury to the attachment of the suspensory ligament to the sesamoid bones. This injury to the suspensory ligament attachment may impair blood supply to the sesamoid bone(s). Injury to the distal sesamoidean ligaments may also occur at their attachment to the base of the sesamoid bones.

Signs

Symptoms of this disease are similar to those caused by fracture of the sesamoid bone. In the early stage, minimal swelling will be observed, but increased heat can be felt over the abaxial surface of the sesamoid bone. As the disease progresses, a visible enlargement of the soft tissues overlying the palmar surface of the fetlock can be seen.

At exercise the lameness varies considerably and depends on the acuteness and degree of the injury. In general, the lameness is most evident during the first part of exercise and is more exaggerated when the horse is exercised on hard surfaces. On close observation, a reduction in extension of the fetlock will be noticed.

On palpation, pain withdrawal can be elicited by placing pressure over the abaxial surface of the sesamoid bone. In more advanced cases, pain can usually be elicited by applying pressure over the branches of the suspensory ligament and distal sesamoidean ligament as well. Flexion of the fetlock is also painful, and flexion tests usually exacerbate the lameness.

Diagnosis

Diagnosis usually can be made by careful examination of the limb. X-rays may have to be taken approximately 3 weeks after onset of the condition to determine if bony changes will occur on the sesamoid bones. Significant radiographic findings include bone growth (Fig. 5–72) and linear canals greater than 1 mm in width. The condition may occur with, fracture of the sesamoid bones and injury to the suspensory ligament from which it must be differentiated. Ultrasound examination of the suspensory ligament is often recommended.

Treatment

Efforts should be made to reduce the inflammation. Cold packs, as well as antiphlogistic packs, can be used. One of the best methods of therapy of early acute cases appears to be cold therapy followed by support bandaging the limb, from the hoof wall to just below the carpus. Alternatively, a cast can be applied and left in place for 2 to 3 weeks and then removed, after

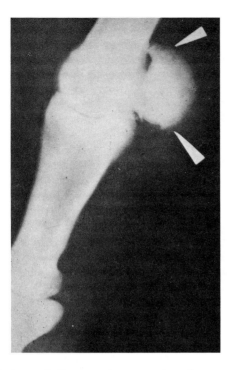

FIG. 5–72. Arrows indicate new bone growth on the sesamoid bone in sesamoiditis. This bone growth resulted from irritation caused by tearing the suspensory ligament (at the top) and the distal sesamoidean ligaments (below).

which a support bandage is applied. Prolonged rest for several months is recommended, after which a gradual increase in exercise is begun. Nonsteroidal antiinflammatory drugs are also used.

Prognosis

The prognosis is guarded to unfavorable, depending on the amount of new bone growth that occurs on the sesamoid bones and the extent of injury to the suspensory ligament and to the distal sesamoidean ligaments.

Traumatic Arthritis of the Fetlock Joint (Osselets)

Refer to Chapter 4.

Traumatic Rupture of the Suspensory Apparatus

Traumatic rupture of the suspensory apparatus with or without fractures of both proximal sesamoid bones is a common cause of acute breakdown in the racing Thoroughbred and often results in humane destruction of the animal. Proximal dislocations of the sesamoid bone without fracture can occur with traumatic

rupture of the distal sesamoidean ligament. Besides the severe trauma sustained by the supporting soft tissues and bone, the adjacent digital arteries are frequently damaged sufficiently to result in blood deprivation and death to the hoof tissues.

Causes

The extreme overextension of the fetlock is the likely cause for disruption of the suspensory apparatus. It is also logical to assume that preexisting disease within the sesamoid bones and distal sesamoid ligaments can also contribute to rupture. The bony projections associated with tearing of the distal sesamoidean ligament at the bone-ligament interface are also considered weak points that may predispose to rupture.

Signs

On gross observation the affected fetlock will be very swollen, and the horse is usually bearing its entire weight on the unaffected limb. The lameness will be obvious, and if the animal transfers its weight to the affected limb, the fetlock will sink to the ground. Palpation will often reveal the proximal displacement of either the intact sesamoid bone or its fractured point. In some cases the ends of the fractured fragments can be felt.

Diagnosis

X-rays usually reveal either the proximal displacement of the intact sesamoid bone or proximal displacement of the apex (point) of the fractured sesamoid bone. Associated swelling of the soft tissues is also quite evident, and preexisting degenerative lesions within the sesamoid bones and fetlock joint may also be present.

Treatment

Treatment should be considered only for salvage of horses considered valuable for breeding or of great sentimental value. For treatment to be successful, immediate immobilization of the affected limb is required to decrease the chances of further injury to the soft tissue as well as the vascular supply. Immobilization should be done as soon as the injury is noticed and before the animal is transported. The application of a bandage splint or cast for a 4- to 5-day period prior to the selection of the final treatment will allow the horse to acclimate to the immobilization and recover from the trauma. This will also provide the veterinarian with a better appreciation for the status of the vascular supply to the foot. Treatments include casting, bandage splinting, and joint fusion. Casting and bandage splinting are aimed at supporting and immobilizing the fetlock until soft tissues have healed sufficiently to support it. Joint fusion is used to achieve a pain-free stable fusion of the fetlock joint in those cases that have not responded to more conservative measures. Since laminitis of the unaffected limb is a common consequence of this injury, a heart-bar shoe or pad should be applied to the opposite unaffected foot as soon as it is practical. Alternatively, the horse can be placed in a stall bedded with dry sand.

Cast immobilization for a period of 4 to 6 weeks is usually required. After this period the limb is supported in a bulky bandage and a special shoe is applied to elevate the heel (Figs. 5–73 and 5–74). The height of the support at the heel is gradually lowered in increments over the next 4 weeks until finally only a wedge is required. The support bandages are usually required for at least an additional 3 weeks after the cast is removed, but they also may be needed for longer periods if pressure sores are persistent.

An alternative to casting is the application of a bandage splint (Fig. 5–75) or Hitchcock splint (Fig. 5–76). The splint is maintained for 4 to 6 weeks, after which elevated heel shoes are applied. A heavy support bandage will be needed for an additional month. The advantage of the splint is that it can be applied to the horse while it is standing. Commercially made splints are also available.

Joint fusion of the fetlock should be considered in those cases in which a chronic dislocation of the fetlock exists or a painful arthritis has developed as an extension of the original injury.

Prognosis

The prognosis appears to be guarded to good for pasture soundness and breeding. With joint fusion, a majority of the cases are successful and pasture soundness can be achieved.

Fetlock Dislocation

Fetlock joint dislocation is uncommon and affects all ages and breeds of horses. Usually, either the lateral or medial collateral ligament is ruptured, creating a varus (outward deviation of the cannon bone) or valgus (inward deviation of the cannon bone) deformity of the limb. Occasionally, a fracture associated with the insertion of these ligaments or joint capsule may occur. Both forelimbs and hindlimbs can be affected with dislocation, but the joint is rarely open. The diagnosis is quite obvious because an angular deviation of the fetlock joint will be present. Occasionally the dislocation will reduce spontaneously and only a lateral or medial swelling will be noticed.

Partial dislocations of the fetlock joint resulting from flexure deformity of the limb is covered in the Flexural Deformities section in Chapter 4. Fetlock dislocation resulting from traumatic rupture of the suspensory apparatus is covered in the Traumatic Rupture of the Suspensory Apparatus section in this chapter.

Causes

This injury frequently occurs when the horse steps in a hole or gets the foot caught fast between the par-

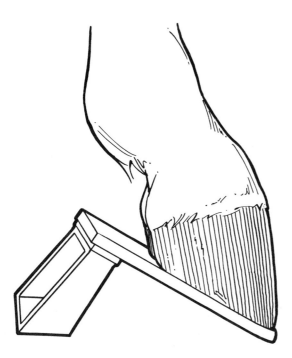

FIG. 5–73. An example of an extended heel shoe. Ideally, this shoe should be adjustable so that the height can be changed with time.

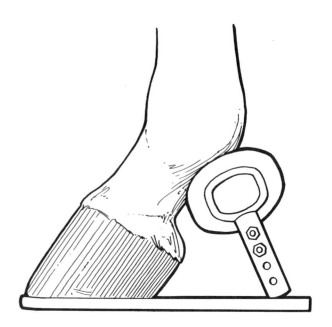

FIG. 5–74. An illustration of a "Roberts" or fetlock sling shoe. The height of the fetlock support can be adjusted.

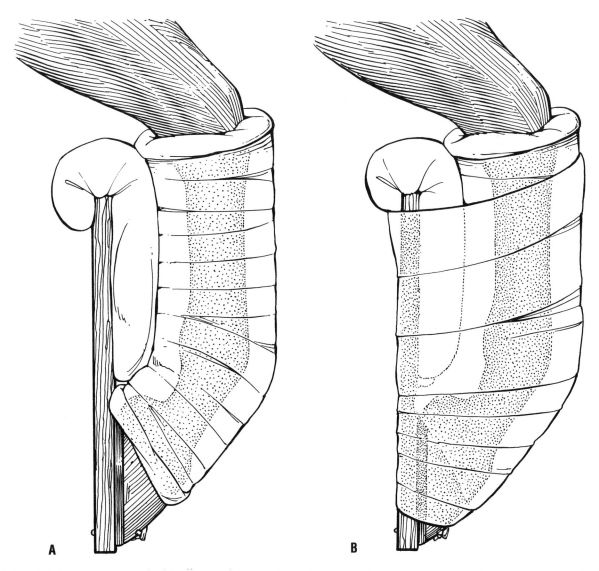

FIG. 5–75. *A,* A heavily bandaged limb is illustrated. The padded splint is brought up to approximate the palmar aspect of the limb. *B,* Bandage splint is complete. (From Wheat, J.D., et al.: A technique for management of traumatic rupture of the equine suspensory apparatus. J. Am. Vet. Med. Assoc., *176*:205, 1980.)

allel pipes of a cattleguard. The dislocation results while the horse attempts to gain freedom. Owners frequently relate the history of finding the horse caught in this situation. Occasionally horses spontaneously dislocate their fetlock during high speed activities (e.g., racing, rodeo eventing).

Signs

The clinical signs are usually obvious, and a varus or valgus angular deformity is often present. Occasionally, the dislocation will reduce spontaneously and the remaining evidence of its occurrence will be lameness and swelling over the torn collateral ligament.

On palpation, the fetlock can be realigned and then dislocated without the degree of pain, or evidence of crackling associated with fracture. Most frequently, the swelling that is present is less than that observed with fracture, also the swelling is located selectively over the lateral or medial surface.

Diagnosis

Generally, the diagnosis can be made by physical examination alone. However, x-rays should be taken to identify a fracture or damage to the articular surface. (Fig. 5–77 A and B). X-rays are particularly important in young foals.

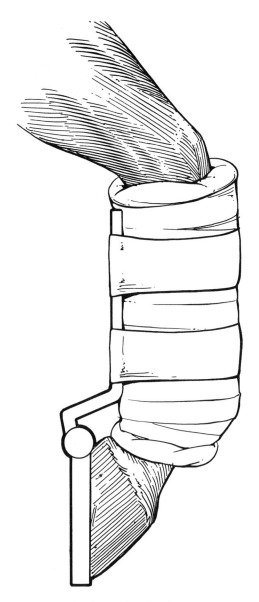

FIG. 5–76. An example of a Hitchcock splint.

Treatment

Treatment of simple dislocation of the fetlock can be rewarding. In most cases, the injury is limited to the supporting soft tissues, and after the dislocation is repositioned under anesthesia, good axial alignment can be maintained by casting or splinting the limb until healing occurs. In young foals, a bandage splint will usually suffice. Alternatively, a cast that does not encase the foot can be used. Casts or splints are maintained for 6 weeks. After cast or splint removal, bandage support and limited exercise are recommended. Initially, horses will appear stiff but soon feel free to flex their fetlocks. Only slight swelling (thickening) will be noticed over the area of collateral ligament rupture and a cosmetic blemish will remain. If the joint surface has been damaged seriously and arthritis develops, range of motion will be limited.

Chronic severe injuries such as traumatic rupture of the suspensory apparatus or dislocation combined with extensive fracture can best be managed with surgical joint fusion (see Traumatic Rupture of the Suspensory Apparatus section in this chapter).

Prognosis

The prognosis for simple dislocation of the fetlock is good for breeding soundness and guarded for athletic performance. However, the final decision should be made regarding the outcome after follow-up x-rays are taken at 2 months. Acute open luxations exposing the fetlock joint also respond well to early therapy. However, joint infection and degenerative joint disease from direct trauma must be ruled out as complications. The long-term outlook for return to serviceability depends on the degree of initial trauma sustained by the bone and joint surface. Follow-up x-rays in 3 to 4 months can be helpful in forming a realistic prognosis.

Angular Limb Deformities Associated With Fetlock Joint

An angular deformity refers to a lateral or medial deviation of the limb. The terms varus and valgus are used to identify the type and direction of the deviation. Fetlock varus refers to an outward deviation of the distal part of the cannon bone and an inward deviation of the coffin bone and pastern bones. (Fig. 5–78). Valgus refers to the opposite situation in which there is an inward deviation of the cannon bone and outward deviation of the coffin bone and pastern bones. Of the two, the varus deformity is most common. Varus deformities of the fetlock are often associated with carpus valgus.

At the present time, angular limb deformities are being seen with increased frequency in foals of all breeds. However, a slightly higher incidence has been reported in Quarter Horse foals. There appears to be an equal sex distribution. Foals can either be born with crooked limbs (congenital) or develop the angular deformity shortly after birth (acquired).

The crooked limbs of many foals will straighten on their own in a short period of time and will not require treatment. In others, the angular deformity either remains static or worsens, and these usually require treatment. Those foals that are born with straight limbs and acquire an angular limb deformity as they mature most often require the assistance of a veterinarian. Some cases can present with multiple limb and joint involvement such as carpus valgus with tarsus valgus or carpus valgus with fetlock varus.

Regardless of the situation, *it is most important to correct the angular limb deformity well in advance of growth plate closure*, and early enough to prevent secondary changes to the joints and bones distal to it.

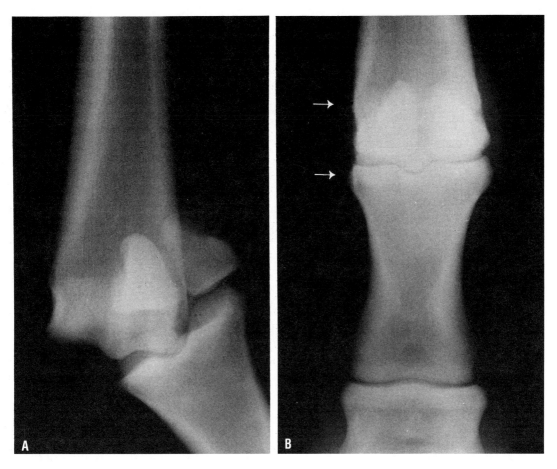

FIG. 5–77. *A*, Subluxation of the fetlock joint with rupture of the lateral and medial collateral ligaments. *B*, Six-week follow-up x-ray examination after cast removal. At this time, minimal bony outgrowths associated with tearing of the collateral ligaments are present (arrows).

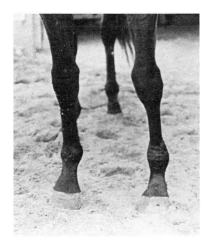

FIG. 5–78. Fetlock varus of the left forelimb.

Early treatment is particularly important for the fetlock, for unlike the carpus, treatment within the first 3 to 5 weeks of life is necessary for a successful outcome. The reason for this is twofold: 1) The growth of the distal end of the cannon bone rapidly slows at 90 days and it virtually stops at 120 days, and 2) the distal growth plate of the cannon bone accounts for only 5% of growth in the total length of the bone. In general, the ideal time for treatment is within the first 30 days of life, because after 60 to 80 days the deviation will be virtually uncorrectable by conventional means.

Causes

The causes of angular limb deformity appear to be complex and multifactorial. The structural changes associated with angular deformity of the fetlock include: 1) Asymmetric growth of the metaphysis (growth center) of the cannon bone, 2) wedging of the epiphysis (ends of the cannon), 3) asymmetric longitudinal growth of the coffin bone and pastern bones, and 4) a degree of joint laxity, which may be present particularly in very young foals. Accompanying this asymmetric growth may be varying degrees of defective endochondral ossification (bone formation in cartilage). Since many of the factors for this entity are the same as those observed with angular limb deformity associated with the carpus, the reader is referred to the

Angular Limb Deformities Associated with the Carpus section in this chapter.

Signs

The signs of angular limb deformity are quite obvious; however, the determination of the exact entity causing the angular limb deformity requires some discussion. A thorough history and physical examination are essential. The history should provide answers to the following questions: 1) Was the foal premature? 2) Was the angular deformity present at birth or was it acquired? 3) Was the mare markedly overweight during the last half of gestation? 4) Has the angular limb deformity improved, stayed the same, or worsened? 5) Were there any signs of lameness in the limb opposite the angular deformity? 6) Did the angular deformity develop acutely or was it slowly progressive? 7) What has been the foal's diet?

On visual observation, the degree of deviation and the pivotal point (center of deviation) can be roughly estimated. The foal should be exercised to gain an appreciation for any lameness and joint laxity. This can be difficult to appreciate with very active foals. In most cases it is best to walk the mare slowly away from the foal and attempt to make this observation as the foal trots toward her. If a unilateral angular limb deformity of the fetlock is present, pay close attention to the limb opposite the angular deformity. The affected limb should be palpated for heat and pain on pressure as well as swelling. Manipulation by flexion, extension, and rotation is important to evaluate pain and joint laxity.

Diagnosis

X-rays are important to characterize the angular deformity and to identify structural changes within the bones and soft tissues. The pivot point (axis of deviation) is determined by placing an overlay of acetate on the appropriate x-ray. A line is drawn to bisect the cannon bone and another to bisect the long pastern bone. Where these lines intersect (axis of deviation) is referred to as the pivot point. The pivot point is important to determine because it will help identify the underlying cause of the angular deformity. If the pivot point is located close to the growth plate (metaphyseal or epiphyseal side), the probable cause of the angular limb deformity is asynchronous growth in the distal cannon metaphysis. If the pivot point is closer to the fetlock, then there may be wedging of the epiphysis or asymmetric growth of the proximal end of the long pastern bone (Fig. 5–79). The angle of deviation can also be calculated or measured with a protractor from this pivotal point.

The structural changes commonly observed on the x-rays and the identification of the pivot point are important in deciding what course of treatment should

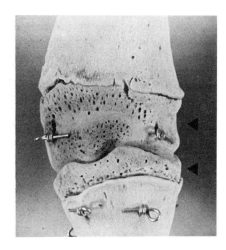

FIG. 5–79. A dried bone specimen of the fetlock of a 3-month-old foal. Note the wedging of the epiphysis of the distal end of the cannon (upper arrow) and the proximal end of the long pastern bone (lower arrow).

be selected as well as in helping to predict the eventual outcome.

Treatment

Early correction of the angular deformity associated with the fetlock region is important because of the relatively short period of time with which rapid longitudinal growth from the growth plate occurs. There is also a limited gain in total length. Treatment after 60 to 80 days yields virtually no improvement in the angular deformity. This is contrary to what has been thought in the past. Studies have shown that a maximum of 12° correction could be expected if the treatment (by transphyseal bridging) was performed at 14 days of age. Therefore foals with deviations greater than 12° will not have angular limb deformities fully corrected by the technique of transphyseal bridging. Therefore, it is of utmost importance to have foals examined by a veterinarian as soon as the angular deformity is recognized.

Treatment is directed toward two approaches, conservative and surgical. Because many foals born with angular deformities spontaneously straighten on their own, the conservative approach is worth a try for a short period of time. This treatment consists of stall confinement, corrective trimming, altering the mare's nutrition and, in some cases, bandage splinting or casting. Stall confinement is recommended to decrease the axial compressive forces (trauma) to the growth plate. To a certain point, the stress from compressive forces stimulates growth. When the level of stress passes a certain physiological limit, it retards growth.

With a varus deformity, increased compressive forces become focused on the medial aspect of the growth plate. If these forces become excessive, as in the case of foals running on pasture, the compression trauma to the medial side may be sufficient to arrest or delay the growth of the growth plate. This would result in perpetuation or worsening of the angular deformity. On the other hand, normal physiologic axial compression forces focused on the medial aspect of the growth plate result in stimulation in long bone growth, with eventual straightening. Therefore, stall confinement serves to shift the potential pathologic compressive forces into the physiologic range (see Angular Limb Deformities Associated with the Carpus section in this chapter).

Corrective trimming serves to balance the foot and assist in proper alignment of the limb. With a varus deformity of the fetlock, increased wear will be noted on the lateral side (outside) of the hoof wall as compared to the medial side. If this is allowed to remain, the compressive forces continue to be increased on the medial (inside) side of the growth plate. Trimming the foot to base level (balancing the foot) will serve to distribute the pressure more equally across the growth plate and joint surfaces. Lateral glue-on extension shoes can further help to distribute weight bearing more evenly and place the support more directly underneath the cannon bone. Overtrimming in an attempt to "crank" the coffin and pastern bones into alignment can cause serious problems later in life and therefore is discouraged.

Nutritional management should include restriction of concentrates, offering good quality alfalfa, high phosphorus, and free choice balanced minerals. If the foal responds favorably by exhibiting rapid straightening of the limb, the conservative treatment should be continued until the limb straightens. However, if the angular deformity remains static for a week or more or worsens, a veterinarian should be contacted immediately.

If the examination reveals that joint laxity is the problem, application of tube (sleeve) casts or bandage splints for 10-day intervals are often helpful. A full-limb cast encasing the entire foot is not recommended. This 10-day period is usually sufficient to allow maturity of the support structures. On the other hand, if joint laxity is not evident and the angular limb deformity results from asynchronous growth in the distal metaphysis of the cannon bone, and epiphyseal wedging is present, temporary transphyseal bridging with or without periosteal stripping is indicated.

Transphyseal bridging can be achieved with either staples or screws and wires (see Angular Limb Deformities Associated with the Carpus section in this chapter for a complete discussion and comparison of the surgical technique). At this time the screw and wire technique is preferred over the stapling procedures. In either case, the growth plate on the convex side is temporarily bridged to arrest its growth. Because the growth continues on the concave side, the limb will eventually straighten, if sufficient potential for long bone growth is present. Once the limb is straight, the implants are removed. In most cases, it is ideal to treat these angular limb deformities associated with the fetlock surgically within the first 30 days of life. If the angulation is greater than 12°, the earlier the treatment the better, and even then complete straightening may not be achieved. During the time when the implants are in place, it is absolutely necessary that these foals be confined to the stall environment. If they are allowed to run free, the chance of damaging the growth plate to the point where it will close prematurely is increased.

It appears that horizontal transection of the periosteum proximal to the growth plate will stimulate longitudinal bone growth. If the periosteum is transected horizontally on the concave side, proximal to the growth plate, straightening of the limb is expected.

It is theorized that the periosteum represents a restrictive fibroelastic tube that not only surrounds the diaphysis of the longbone but also serves to connect the proximal and distal epiphysis which places it under tension. For longitudinal bone growth to occur, the fibroelastic tube must stretch and grow in synchrony with the longitudinal bone growth. When the periosteum is transected horizontally arround part of the bone's circumference, it serves to reduce the tension at the growth plate and rapid longitudinal bone growth will occur. This tension theory is substantiated by the fact that when the periosteum is transected horizontally to the long axis just up above the growth plate, a 5-mm gap appears as the periosteal edges separate.

After surgery, a light bandage is applied over the surgical site, changed about the third day postoperatively, and removed in about 10 to 14 days. Stall rest is recommended for at least 1 month to decrease the stress on the crooked limb, after which the foal can be placed in a small run until straightening has been achieved. During this rest period, corrective trimming of the foot should be continued. In most cases, rapid straightening occurs within 2 months after surgery. If a considerable angular deviation still exists, another periosteal transection can be performed.

The advantages of this technique over that of implantation of staples or screws and wires include: 1) simplicity of approach, 2) orthopedic implants are not required, 3) minimal instrumentation is needed, 4) only one surgery is required in most cases because there are no orthopedic implants to remove, 5) rapid straightening can be achieved within 2 months, 6) a good cosmetic end result is achieved, and 7) there is a decreased chance of infection as compared to operations associated with the techniques of orthopedic implantation.

For foals with severe angular deformity, greater than 12° of deviation, it is probably safest to use the temporary transphyseal bridging technique. We have incorporated periosteal transection in conjunction with temporary transphyseal bridging in very severe cases of angular limb deformity in the hope that better correction could be realized.

In cases in which an angular deformity of the fetlock is present but the growth plate is already closed, a wedge osteotomy can be considered to straighten the limb. Wedge osteotomy of the distal end of the cannon bone was reported to be successful in the treatment of varus deformity of the fetlock region in 5 foals that had greater than an 8° deviation remaining in their fetlocks after the growth plate had closed. The following criteria are used to select foals for surgery: 1) The foals were older than 120 days, 2) a greater than 8° deviation of the limb existed, 3) no lameness or degenerative joint disease of the fetlock was observed.

Prognosis

In general, the prognosis is good for straightening of the limbs in those cases in which the angular limb deformity is mild (under 12°) and caused by asymmetric growth of the distal metaphysis of the cannon bone that is treated early. The prognosis is guarded to poor, on the other hand, for complete straightening of the angular deviation if it is severe (greater than 12°) or the growth plate of the long pastern bone is severely affected or osteochondrosis lesions are present. An improved prognosis may be forthcoming with the advent of the wedge osteotomy technique for those foals that have angular limb deformities associated with a closed growth plate. However, more cases are needed before this statement can be generalized.

Constriction of or by the Fetlock Anular Ligament

Anular ligaments are tough, fibrous, thickened parts of the fascial sheath. They are lined with synovia and act to prevent displacement of the tendon, thereby preserving their mechanical efficiency. Tendons lying within anular ligaments can suffer great damage due to loss of blood supply.

Constriction of the anular ligament of the fetlock occurs from trauma and/or infection resulting in thickening (desmitis) of the anular ligament. It may occur with a low bowed tendon, or as a result of a wire cut or puncture wound in the region of the palmar or plantar aspect of the limb. As the injury heals, the anular ligament thickens, which in turn exerts constricting pressure on the flexor tendons. In other cases the structures within the confines of the anular ligament swell and the tendon becomes constricted by the anular ligament. In both cases, lameness will persist until the ligament is surgically severed to relieve the pressure. Adhesions often form between the superficial flexor tendon and the anular ligament.

Causes

The inflammation and scar tissue formation that occur in the anular ligament during the healing process, result in thickening (desmitis) of the anular ligament and pressure on the flexor tendons.

Because anular ligaments are not elastic, swelling of the superficial digital flexor caused by tenosynovitis (bowed tendon) can cause the same signs as constriction of the anular ligament, but the tendon becomes constricted by it. In some cases, wire cuts or nail punctures occur in the region of the palmar or plantar aspect of the fetlock. As a result, the anular ligament is injured, and in the healing process, it may constrict from scar tissue formation.

Signs

In nearly all cases there will be distention of the digital sheath (tenosynovitis) proximal to the anular ligament. There may be thickening of the flexor tendons, and one may mistakenly assume that the primary problem is low bowed tendon. Viewing the fetlock from the side, one can usually see "notching" at the proximal part of the anular ligament (Fig. 5–80). This notching is caused by anular ligament constriction. The lameness is characterized by its persistence; it does not improve with time and usually becomes worse with exercise because of inflammation. Lameness is characterized by a decreased extension (dorsiflexion) of the fetlock during weight bearing and a shortened caudal phase to the stride. In the most severe cases the horse will be reluctant to place the heel on the ground and will accentuate the cranial phase of the stride to compensate for this. A fetlock flexion test invariably worsens the lameness. Continued pres-

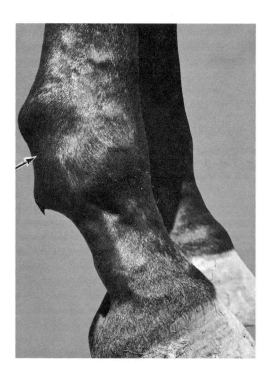

FIG. 5–80. Constriction of the anular ligament. Notice the "notched" appearance on the palmar aspect of the fetlock above the ergot. The upper swelling is caused by fluid distention of the flexor tendon sheath.

sure may produce changes in the superficial digital flexor tendon in the form of inflammation. Careful palpation of the region will usually reveal thickening and fibrosis at the junction of the superficial flexor tendon and the anular ligament, leading one to suspect involvement of the ligament. Injection of a local anesthetic into the digital sheath will often improve lameness by 50 to 70%.

Diagnosis

Persistent lameness accompanied by a notching at the proximal part of the fetlock anular ligament, combined with palpation of the region and a positive fetlock flexion test is the basis for diagnosis. Ultrasound examination will confirm the diagnosis, and thickening of the anular ligament can be identified. If tendinitis is also present, the tendon will appear larger than normal and exhibit evidence of tearing with blood within the tendon. The anular ligament will often appear thickened as well. Following ultrasound examination, injection of a local anesthetic into the digital sheath can be used to confirm that pain is coming from the anular ligament and the structure within the digital sheath.

Treatment

Severing the anular ligament surgically is the only effective treatment (Fig. 5–81). The horse is put in a

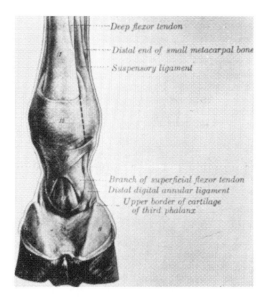

Fig. 5–81. Anatomy specimen showing anular ligament. Dotted line indicates line of incision on either medial or lateral edge of the superficial digital flexor tendon through the anular ligament. 14, Deep digital flexor tendon; 15, superficial digital flexor tendon; 16, anular ligament; 17, proximal digital anular ligament; 11, cartilage of coffin bone; 24, digital cushion. (From Sisson, S.: Myology. *In* Anatomy of Domestic Animals (Grossman, J.D., ed.). 4th Ed. Philadelphia, W.B. Saunders Co., 1953.)

snug-fitting support wrap of elastic gauze and tape or medicated gauze bandage. Exercise is begun in 3 days, by hand-walking the horse and gradually increasing exercise so that adhesions will not unite the freshly cut edges of the anular ligament. Antibiotics and nonsteroidal anti-inflammatory agents are usually administered.

Prognosis

If the primary involvement is that of constriction of the anular ligament and is not accompanied by extensive changes in the tendon (bowed tendon), the prognosis is favorable. All cases show much improvement, and if tendon changes are not extensive, the horse may be freed of lameness by use of the techniques described above.

The Cannon

Bucked Shins and Stress Fracture of the Dorsal Cannon Bone

Bucked shins and stress fracture of the dorsal cannon bone are commonly observed in young (2 to 3 years of age) racing Thoroughbreds and Quarter horses. The incidence is very high in the United States where 70% of 2-year-old racing Thoroughbreds buck their shins compared to an incidence of less than 17% in racing Thoroughbreds in England. Training methods and consistency of the racing surface are felt to be important factors. Shorter training periods at higher speeds on hard surfaces makes the horse more susceptible to bucked shins.

Causes

During fast-gaited exercise as the foot impacts the ground it slides forward, and if it is not allowed to rotate because of toe grabs, hard footing or excessively sticky footing, the dorsal cortex (the outer dense bone) of the cannon bone is put under greater compression than the palmar cortex. As a result of compression, the dorsal cortex of the cannon bone begins to remodel and gradually increases in thickness in response to this stress. During the remaining process, the dorsal cortex becomes less dense and thus weaker for a short period. After the initial weakening, the bone becomes stronger and thicker to withstand stress. The outer surface of the bone gets thicker from the development of new bone underneath the periosteum (subperiosteal callus) (Fig. 5–82). If the remodeling cannot keep pace with the repeated compression stresses then bone failure results. Simply stated, the damage to the dorsal cortex occurs more rapidly than the repair process can counteract it, resulting in microfracture and hemorrhage beneath the periosteum. The greater the load

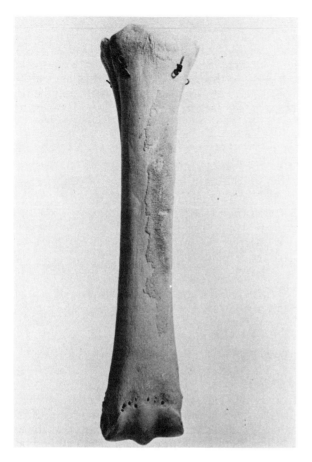

FIG. 5–82. A macerated specimen of the right cannon bone illustrating a subperiosteal callus on the dorsal medial surface of this bone.

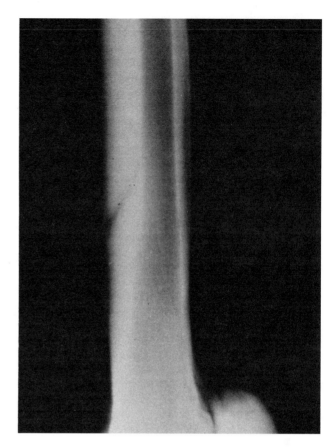

FIG. 5–83. An x-ray of the cannon bone. The fracture enters the dorsal cortex and courses proximally.

(weight), the faster the speed, and the harder the surface, the greater will be the deformation (bending) of the cannon bone which makes the horse more susceptible to bucked shins. Of interest is the fact that horses that jog produce principal strain directions in their cannon bones that are 40° out of alignment with the principal strain that occurs during high-speed work. Thus the recommendation by some is to train as you race with short-distance high-speed work.

Occasionally a stress fracture will develop in the dorsolateral cortex of the cannon bone at the junction of the distal and middle third (Fig. 5–83). This is most commonly observed in race horses above 2 years of age and most frequently involves the left forelimb 5 × more frequently. It is believed that the fracture is an acute manifestation of the chronic "dorsal metacarpal disease" that has led to remodeling of the dorsomedial cortex. As the dorsomedial cortex remodels and becomes thicker, the dorsolateral cortex remains somewhat less affected and remains thinner and weaker, making it more susceptible to acute stress fracture. Also, excessive compression develops on the dorsolateral surface of the left fore metacarpus in horses raced and trained in a counterclockwise direction. This increased compression compiled with a theoretic

decrease in elasticity of the remodeled third metacarpal bone may also contribute to the location of the fracture.

Signs

Clinical signs are separated into three categories, Types 1, 2, and 3, respectively.

Type 1 acute is usually observed in young Thoroughbred racehorses (8 to 36 months of age), and occasionally in older horses that have not been strenuously trained or raced as 2-year-olds. The disease has an acute onset and is most obvious after intense exercise. There is usually minimal alteration of the horse's gait, particularly after short periods of rest. Digital pressure often elicits a painful response. X-rays taken at this time are usually negative.

Type 2 is considered subacute or chronic. It develops as a result of acute Type 1 disease that is unresponsive to therapy or has gone unrecognized. It is most frequently seen in horses 26 to 42 months of age. At exercise only mild degrees of gait deficit may be noticed. Digital pressure elicits varying degrees of pain, but a more obvious swelling is felt on the dorsomedial cortex. The pain response is typically more profound after strenuous exercise. The left limb is usually more severely affected. On x-rays a bone proliferation is usually observed (Fig. 5–84).

Type 3 results from a fissure fracture in the cortex of the cannon bone. It is usually observed in older horses 3 to 5 years of age. As with Types 1 and 2, the lameness may not be prominent while the horse is rested. However, it is usually prominent after strenuous exercise. Painful area can be palpated on the dorsolateral surface of the left cannon bone at the junction of its middle and distal third. Only rarely will the right cannon bone be involved. X-rays usually point to a cortical fracture (see Fig. 5–83).

Diagnosis

A tentative diagnosis of bucked shins or stress fracture can be made from the clinical findings and the age relationship. Only with x-rays can a definitive diagnosis be made.

With Type 1 disease it is rare to see anything on x-ray. With Type 2 disease subperiosteal lysis (bone loss) may be observed early, and later a thickening of the dorsomedial cortex with associated subperiosteal callus new bone formation is seen (see Fig. 5–84). With Type 3 the cortical fissure fracture usually enters the

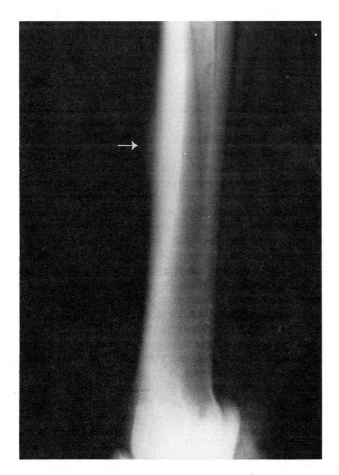

FIG. 5–84. Bone proliferation on the dorsal cannon.

cortex distally and progresses proximal at a 35 to 45° angle. Most frequently the fracture appears on x-ray as a straight or slightly concave fracture line (tongue fracture) (see Fig. 5–83). Occasionally it will proceed proximal to exit through the dorsal cortex (saucer fracture). Repeating at 7- to 10-day intervals may be necessary in those cases in which a fracture is suspected but is not observed on initial x-rays examination. This period of time usually allows for sufficient demineralization bone resorption to occur so the fracture becomes more obvious. Nuclear scintigraphic examination (nuclear scan) can identify increased uptake ("hot spots") in the dorsal cortex of the cannon bone, indicating a high probability of a stress fracture. These "hot spots" are seen before x-rays can identify a fracture. The nuclear scan is also used to document healing of the fracture.

Treatment

Type 1 usually responds to varying periods of rest. Daily hand-walking exercise is permitted and can be increased when the cannon is no longer painful. Periods of convalescence vary from 30 to 90 days, but depend totally on the extent of the injury. A controlled exercise program should be employed when the horse is returned to work. The idea behind this is to gradually increase the stress to the dorsal surface of the cannon bone at such a rate that it can remodel according to compressive demands. At first the horse should be ponied, after which the intensity of workouts can be increased as long as the cannon remains nonpainful. During this controlled exercise period the horse should be shod without toe grabs. Periods of controlled exercise programs vary and are dependent on the severity of the disease. Because the bone strains occur at different locations on the dorsal surface of the cannon bone depending on the speed of the workout, it has been recommended that horses be trained as they race with short distance high speed. At least in the northeastern United States, this approach has proved beneficial.

Type 2 cannon stress fractures can be difficult to treat. Some never resolve, whereas others require a year or more to resolve. Presumably the delay in healing of the multiple microfractures is a result of poor blood supply to the dorsal cannon region. The controlled exercise program previously described is also recommended here. Drilling small holes through the cortex (osteostixis) may help improve the blood supply and thus hasten healing.

Type 3 dorsal fissure fractures in young horses may resolve with the conservative approach outlined above. Convalescent periods may extend from 4 to 6 months. However, older horses often do not respond to conservative treatment and surgery is required. Surgery may consist of fixation with bonescrews or drilling and electromagnetic pulsation therapy.

Postoperative management includes limiting the exercise until the surgical site is no longer painful. In most cases 6 weeks of rest are recommended. After the second week of stall rest, however, hand-walking exercise is begun and continued for the next 4 weeks. At 6 weeks the horse can be turned out and/or light exercise begun alongside a lead pony. Close physical monitoring of the fracture site should occur during the exercise period. At 12 weeks, radiographs are taken to assess healing and determine time for screw removal. Horses can resume training approximately 2 weeks after screw removal.

The cortical drilling approach is popular because it does not require a second surgery for removal of the screw and it is technically less demanding. A combination of drilling and internal screw fixation also might be used.

In all cases, no matter what the treatment, an adequate period of rest combined with a controlled exercise program is required for cannon remodeling to occur.

Prognosis

The prognosis is good to guarded depending on the degree of involvement.

It is worthwhile implementing some preventive measures. Young horses should be put on deliberate controlled exercise programs that will afford them the best opportunity for remodeling. It has been recommended that adequate galloping of young horses for a 90-day period before speed work commences will prevent most cases of bucked shins. The proper interval of rest should also be afforded between heavy workouts. Horses should be examined daily for pain in the dorsal cannon region. If inflammation is present, training exercise should be discontinued until the inflammation subsides. Then controlled exercise should be resumed. Even though total rest allows the microfractures to heal, little stress remodeling of the dorsal surface occurs; therefore, controlled exercise should be continued for the best end result. The intensity of this exercise should be adjusted according to the horse's response. Horses that start to get sore shins can often benefit from changing the exercise programs to include short-distance high-speed works with decrease in their jogging routine.

Horses should be trained and run on surfaces with adequate cushioning that allow the foot to grab and rotate properly rather than slide. Where cushioned surfaces will decrease the compression of the dorsal surface of the cannon bone, hard surfaces that result in sliding lead to increased compression. Horses that run on turf rarely develop this disease, whereas horses that are run on hard surfaces have a high incidence (estimated 90%).

The use of toe grabs and the practice of lowering the heels both delay breakover and result in increased compression on the dorsal aspect of the cannon bone. Avoiding these trimming and shoeing practices may also be helpful in preventing this disease.

Fractures of the Condyles of the Cannon Bone

Fractures of the condyles of the cannon bones occur frequently in racing Thoroughbreds, infrequently in Standardbreds, and occasionally in Quarter horses and Polo ponies. The lateral condyle of the cannon bone is the most frequently affected.

The configuration of these fractures can range from an incomplete fissure entering the fetlock joint to a displacement with complete separation from the cannon bone (Fig. 5–85). When the fracture fragment displaces, it is invariably in a proximal (upward) direction. These fractures can be difficult to identify as a cause of lameness, particularly if they are the fissure type, because the lameness may be only subtle. Little if any crepitation (crackling feeling) may be present, and the diagnosis can be missed entirely unless x-rays are taken.

Causes

The cause is trauma from uncoordinated, longitudinal rotation of the cannon bone and from exercise on uneven surfaces. There is normally a regular, coordinated lateral-to-medial rotary motion of the cannon bone and the long pastern bone along their long axis at the end of the weight bearing phase of the stride. If this rotary motion becomes out of sync, and either the long pastern bone does not rotate or is delayed in the rotary action, a condylar fracture can result. It is proposed that this fracture occurs when the cannon bone and the long pastern bone are in the maximal extended position, during full weight bearing at the end of the stride. In this position, there is a delay in breaking over of the phalanges in relationship to the cannon bone. This delay may result from: 1) The foot slipping backwards, 2) fatigued flexor tendons, 3) overload of one limb (i.e., turns) and, 4) a long toe and low heel. As the cannon bone begins to rotate independently of the long pastern bone, the lateral condyle contacts the proximal lateral border of the long pastern bone and becomes fractured. Theoretically, for a condylar fracture to occur, the foot must also be fixed and not allowed to rotate. Therefore, anything that prevents rotation of the coffin bone, such as shoe calks, branch shoes, and other factors, can contribute to development of this type of fracture.

Other considerations can include the possibility that, if there is continual uncoordinated rotary movement of the cannon bone in relation to the long pastern bone, there may be a gradual structural failure, beginning at the cellular level which progresses to a clinical fracture. Also, horses that have galloped on uneven terrain may place abnormal axial compressive forces over the lateral condyles resulting in this fracture.

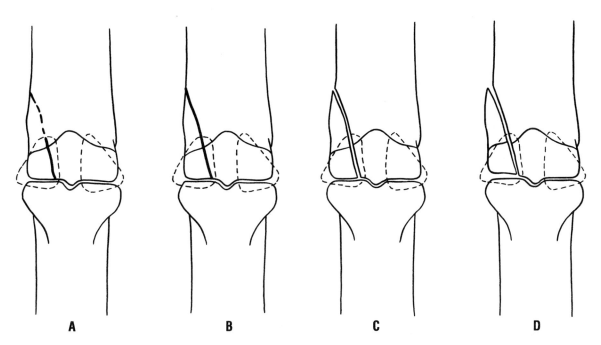

FIG. 5–85. *A*, An incomplete condylar fracture. *B*, A complete nondisplaced condylar fracture. *C*, A complete separated condylar fracture. *D*, A complete displaced condylar fracture.

Signs

The clinical signs may vary from a mild lameness that is worsened by exercise, with little heat or swelling being present with fissure fractures, to severe lameness with heat, pain, and swelling in the acute displaced fracture. The fissure fractures are often so subtle they are missed. However, in all cases in which the fracture has extended into the fetlock joint, there will be increased synovial filling. This is best seen in the palmar or plantar recess of the fetlock joint capsule. The external swelling of the lateral side of the cannon bone depends on the degree of separation of the proximal end of the fragment. More swelling will be observed with greater separation of the fracture fragment. The degree of pain associated with the palpation and the amount of heat that is felt depends on the acuteness of the fracture. More heat will be palpated with the acute displaced fracture. Fracture movement and a crackling may also be felt.

Increased lameness can be observed in a horse after it has been exercised and when the horse is circled to the affected side. Flexion and rotation of the fetlock usually result in sufficient pain to cause withdrawal of the limb. In the acute displaced fracture, a crackling may be felt with rotation of the fetlock. When flexion tests are used in cases in which there is a fissure fracture, increased lameness can be observed.

Diagnosis

If a condylar fracture is suspected, it is advisable to have x-rays taken. Nuclear scintigraphic examination ("nuclear scan") can identify "hot" areas in the bone which are highly suspicious of a nondisplaced fracture. The "hot" areas are seen before the fracture is apparent on x-rays.

Treatment

In general, the treatment depends on the degree of displacement of the fracture and the intended use. If the fracture is of the fissure type (see Fig. 5–85A) (nondisplaced and incomplete) and the horse is to be used for breeding or light exercise, placing the limb in a cast or bandage with sufficient stall rest may suffice. On the other hand, if the fracture is complete, nondisplaced or displaced, (see Fig. 5–85B, C, and D) and the horse is intended for athletic performance, internal fixation with cortical bone screws is recommended. Without internal fixation, there may be continued and further separation of the condylar fracture with increased cartilage damage and resultant degenerative joint disease occurring within the fetlock joint. The advantages of screw fixation include the insurance that the original fracture will not become further displaced, shorter convalescence, a reduced incidence of refracture at the same site, and primary bone healing which decreases the chances of degenerative joint disease of the fetlock. Articular alignment and minimal cartilage gap are maintained best when compression is used.

Incomplete fractures that are treated with cast or support bandages should be confined to box stalls and observed closely over 2 to 3 weeks for signs of increased pain. If there are signs of increased pain in the affected limb, the cast should be removed. X-rays will need to be taken to establish whether displacement has occurred and internal fixation is required. If bandages are used, they should be reset every third or fourth day, at first. The limb is then assessed for increased pain or swelling or heat that may indicate separation or displacement of the fracture. Casts are usually applied for 3 to 6 weeks, but this also depends on the type of fracture and the rate of healing that occurs. After the cast is removed, bandage support is continued until healing is observed on x-rays, usually between 2 and 4 months. Hand-walking exercises can be begun after about 6 to 8 weeks, but stall confinement is continued until the fracture is totally healed. Then the horse is allowed free exercise in a small confined paddock. After another 3 months, free exercise is allowed on pasture. Riding should not be allowed for 6 to 8 months, at which time the cartilage should be healed.

When internal screw fixation is used, the horse may emerge from surgery with a cast that might remain in place for 2 days to 2 weeks. In some cases, only bandage support is used. In either case heavy support wraps are applied after cast removal and maintained until evidence of healing has occurred. Phenylbutazone can be administered in low doses if the horse shows marked pain. Where low doses of phenylbutazone are beneficial to dull the pain, high doses may be counterproductive in that they will allow too much weight bearing. Antibiotics started just before surgery are usually administered for 3 to 5 days postoperatively.

Postoperative exercise should be limited for at least 90 days. Stall rest confinement is recommended for this period, and after 4 to 6 weeks hand-walking exercise can begin. Followup x-rays should be taken at this time, and if the healing is progressing normally, the horse can be turned out into a small paddock for an additional 90 days. If the x-ray followup shows good healing, the horse can be placed on pasture or in a large paddock. Training should not be begun before 6 to 8 months and until followup x-rays are taken. Although the x-rays show healing of the bone is present, it will take cartilage from 6 to 8 months to bridge the defect. The average time from the date of surgery to the first racing start is about 10 months and ranges 5 to 24 months.

Screws are generally not removed after healing has occurred unless residual lameness results that can be directly attributed to their presence. Horses that appear sore during initial training periods and have screws remaining often go sound within a short period of time after training begins. Those that continue to be sore should have the screws removed. Some surgeons prefer to remove the screws, and if a plate is used, around 4 or 5 months after surgery. If the screws are to be removed, it is easily done under general anesthesia.

Prognosis

Generally, prognosis for future athletic performance appears good following internal fixation of acute non-displaced condylar fractures that are operated on within 48 hours. In cases of complete displaced fractures or where there has been a delay in diagnosis and treatment and/or improper immobilization has been selected, a guarded to poor prognosis can be expected. This prognosis is altered because of increased damage to the articular surface that is likely to result in degenerative joint disease of the fetlock and irritation to the periosteum resulting in increased callus formation. The prognosis for return to racing is considered guarded when there is fragmented fractures or lesions in the cannon bone.

Fractures of the Cannon Bone

Fractures of the cannon bone occur commonly in all ages and breeds of horses. These bones appear to be particularly susceptible to fracture because of their distal location and the fact that there is very little soft tissue covering the bone.

Although fractures of the cannon bone can assume a variety of configurations, ranging from a incomplete simple fissure to severe fragmentation, younger horses seem to sustain simpler fractures than adults. The fracture can occur anywhere along the bone length and can enter either the proximal or distal joint. Incomplete palmar fracture of the proximal cannon bone generally enters the lower (carpometacarpal) joint of the knee (carpus). Frequently, distal fractures will involve the growth plate in young animals (Fig. 5–86). Also, because of the minimal soft tissue covering, the complete fractures are commonly open or become open soon after the injury occurs. Concurrent fractures of the splint bones are common. Fractures of the splint bones and those associated with bucked-shins are covered separately in the Fractures of the Splint Bones and Bucked Shins sections in this chapter. One important consideration worth mentioning is that the saucer-shaped dorsal cortical fractures associated with the "bucked shin" complex can be worsened to a transverse fracture if exercise is continued. This is particularly important in racing Thoroughbreds.

Although these fractures can be difficult to treat as a group, they have the best prognosis for a good outcome when compared to other longbone fractures.

Causes

External trauma in any form can cause this fracture. Injuries that are frequently mentioned include kicks, halter-breaking injuries, injuries associated with ground holes or fences, or cattleguards, slipping accidents, slipping on ice, and accidents associated with moving vehicles. When foals are affected, the mother has invariably stepped on the limb, and this led to the fracture. In contrast, it is reasonable to assume that

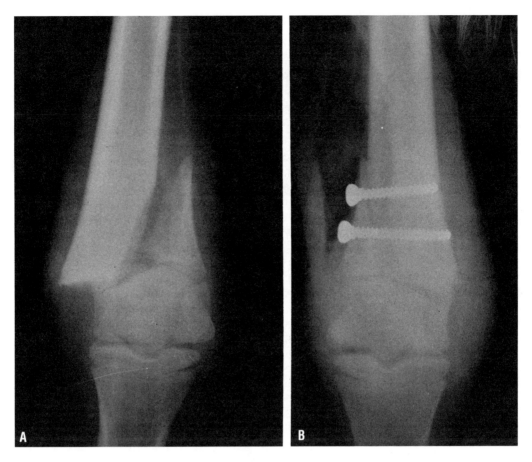

FIG. 5–86. *A*, An example of a Salter II type fracture in the cannon. *B*, Two bone screws were used to repair this fracture. (Courtesy of Dr. A.S. Turner.)

fissure fractures and transverse fractures resulting from saucer fractures of the dorsal cannon region result from internal rather than external trauma. This is also true for incomplete proximal cannon bone fracture.

Signs and Diagnosis

Fissure fractures may be difficult to diagnose. The lameness associated is often nonspecific and may be variable. On gross observation the cannon bone may be enlarged slightly, and on palpation heat, swelling of the soft tissues overlying the fracture, and pain on deep digital palpation will usually be present. Because these signs are similar to those observed with bucked shins, the diagnosis may not be made. One clue is that the swelling is usually more diffuse than that associated with bucked shins, and the lameness and palpable pain last longer than 5 days.

In the other cases, except for nondisplaced condylar fractures (see Fractures of the Condyles of the Cannon Bones section in this chapter), and incomplete proximal cannon bone fracture, the diagnosis of fractures of the cannon bone is obvious. An angular limb deformity is usually present, along with a nonweight-bearing lameness. In all cases, these fractures should be x-rayed to identify the type (simple versus fragmented) and their location in relation to joint surfaces. The limb should not be manipulated excessively during physical examination because this may lead to penetration of bone fragments through the skin. If the horse has to be transported for x-rays or there will be a delay before they can be taken, it is advisable to apply cither a bandage splint or cast to support this limb. This decreases the chances of opening the fracture to the outside.

Nuclear scintigraphic examination (nuclear scan) can be used to identify fissure fractures that are not seen on x rays. Increased uptake "hot spots" are highly suggestive of these types of fractures. Nuclear scanning is also very useful for documenting healing of the fracture.

Treatment

The treatment of cannon bone fractures depends on the type of fracture (open versus closed, simple versus fragmented), the location of the fracture (articular versus nonarticular, proximal versus distal), the animal's age, its intended use, and the economics.

External fixation has been used successfully to treat many cases of cannon bone fractures. This technique is probably most suitable for horses that have a fissure fracture or young horses or ponies with a gentle nature that have sustained a simple transverse fracture. Support bandaging of the limb has been used successfully for fissure fractures. If a cast is selected, it should incorporate the entire foot and extend upward to the proximal third of the radius or tibia. The purposes of the cast are to maintain good axial alignment of the long bones and decrease the rotational forces brought to bear on the fracture site. In cases in which the fracture is easily repositioned and the axial alignment can be maintained, the limb can be cast in slight flexion. This technique will further decrease the axial and rotational forces on the fracture site. In many cases, however, traction will be required to reposition the fracture as well as maintain its alignment.

Casts in conjunction with transfixation pinning have been used successfully in a limited number of cases in foals and adults that have sustained proximal fragmented fractures of the cannon bone. These fractures are so proximal that they are not amenable to routine techniques of internal fixation (e.g., bone plating). In most cases, two to three large-diameter pins are placed transversely from lateral to medial through the distal end of the radius, and the other two to three pins are placed in a similar fashion below the fracture site in the cannon bone. A cast is then applied over and around the pins. With the new fiberglass casting materials presently available, a very strong lightweight external support can be applied. The pins are used to further stabilize the very unstable fragmented fracture. Foals can be maintained in stall confinement, whereas adults may require slinging.

Temporary casts might be applied prior to internal fixation in cases in which a contaminated open fracture exists and/or severe trauma to the soft tissue has been sustained. The cast serves to support the fracture until the soft tissues have sufficient time to heal and the host defenses are sufficient to decrease the chance of spreading the infection.

Other forms of external fixation, such as leg braces in many forms and splints, have been used to successfully treat cannon bone fractures in a limited number of cases.

Internal fixation is used in cases in which the fracture line is at a steep angle (oblique), or a marked displacement has occurred or an articular component is evident.

Open fractures with moderate to severe contamination and increased soft tissue inflammation may need to be treated by temporary casting for periods of 7 to 10 days after which internal fixation can be applied. This delayed approach is only recommended if reasonable stabilization of the fracture can be achieved. Depending on the state of the wound, the cast is removed in 3 to 10 days and a decision is made regarding the application of internal fixation. If the wound is clean, internal fixation can be attempted. If, on the other hand, the wound is obviously infected, euthanasia may be advised. This delay provides sufficient time to identify if infection will be a problem before committing to the expense of internal fixation. Any contaminated open fracture has a markedly poor prognosis.

In young foals sustaining fractures that have extended into the growth plate, it may be necessary to bridge the growth plate with an implant to achieve stability of the fracture. In very young foals, from birth to 6 weeks, this may alter limb growth sufficiently to cause shortening or an angular limb deformity may develop. Because most of the growth from the physis (growth plate) occurs prior to two and a half or three months of age, there is little chance of altering or arresting growth after this age.

Bone grafting is recommended in all cases in which a bone defect is present (Fig. 5–87). This is especially important for adults because the defect usually requires a long time to repair and represents a weak point. Bone grafting is also used in cases in which internal fixation has been used and localized infection exists in the fracture site. Bone for grafting can be retrieved from the pelvis or sternum.

In most cases it is safest to apply a full-limb cast that includes the foot and extends to the proximal third of the radius or tibia in those cases that have sustained midshaft or proximal fractures. This will reduce the chances of implant failure during recovery from anesthesia. A splint bandage may suffice in horses that have sustained fissure fractures, and distal limb casts are frequently used in young foals with fractures involving the growth plate. The casts are left in place for variable periods of time depending on the type of fracture, the age of the animal, and the stability of the fracture following internal fixation. Foals with a plate or plates that have sustained midshaft transverse fractures that have been rigidly immobilized may have their casts removed in a period of 2 to 3 weeks. This decreases the amount of osteoporosis bone absorption and atrophy of the flexor muscles associated with longer casting periods. Others, especially adults, may require casting for up to 4 months. If the mother is particularly clumsy and both are confined to a small area, a full limb cast should be left in place on the foal until x-ray evidence of healing is present. In adults, casts are left in place until the signs of x-ray healing are evident. Again, this is dependent on the circumstances. Casting periods of up to 4 months are required in some instances.

Whether bone plates are removed depends on the animal's age, its intended use, and whether draining fistulae are present. In general, young animals that still have considerable potential for growth and horses that are to be used in athletic eventing should have their plates removed.

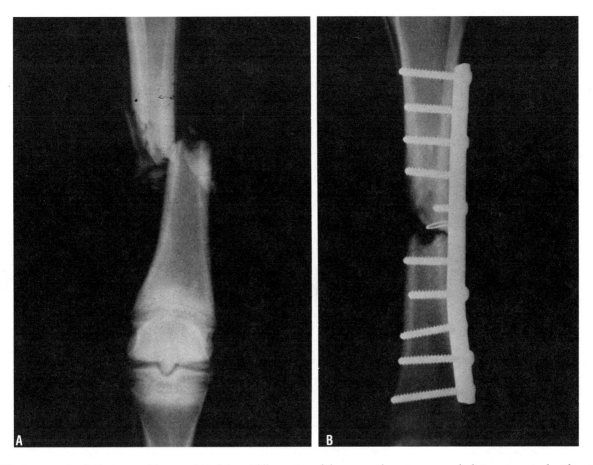

FIG. 5–87. An example of a fragmented fracture (*A*) of the middle portion of the cannon bone in a young foal. It was repaired with a standard bone plate placed on the medial surface (*B*). Cancellous bone grafts were placed in this fracture gap and the limb was supported with a cast for 6 weeks postoperatively.

Prognosis

The prognosis for successful treatment of cannon bone fractures is dependent on the nature of the injury, the type of fracture, where the fracture has occurred, and whether it is opened or closed. The horse's disposition and intended use are also important. Forelimb fractures tend to respond more favorably than hind-limb fractures. Transverse simple fractures in the midcannon bone region in foals under 7 months of age have a good prognosis. Older horses have a guarded prognosis. Horses with open, fragmented fractures have a guarded to poor prognosis for recovery. The final prognosis should be withheld until the effectiveness of early treatment has been evaluated.

Angular Limb Deformities Associated With the Shaft of the Cannon Bone

Angular limb deformities associated with the shaft of the cannon bones are a congenital deviation that rarely affects foals. In most cases the angular deformity is noticed shortly after birth. Although the deviation is centered in the mid to proximal portion of the cannon bone rather than the distal extremity, the fetlock joint may also be involved secondarily. Both varus (outward bowing of the cannon), and valgus (inward deviation of the cannon) have been seen.

Cause

The cause is unknown. However, it has been suggested that it is a result of abnormal positioning of the fetus in the uterus.

Signs

At first glance, the angular deformity may appear similar to the angular deformity associated with the fetlock joint. However, on closer observation it will become obvious that the pivotal point (axis of deviation) is located more proximal in the shaft of the bone. Observing the limb from above the shoulder and/or hip and looking downward is most informative. The fetlock joint may also be secondarily involved, making the diagnosis more difficult. Most foals appear quite vigorous and do not show any signs of lameness.

On palpation, mild pain may be elicited from rotation and flexion of the fetlock. On direct palpation of the cannon bone, no heat, swelling, or pain with pressure are elicited.

Diagnosis

A definitive diagnosis is made from an x-ray examination. Lines are drawn to bisect the cannon bone and fetlock joint. Where these lines intersect is the pivot point (axis of deviation). The degrees of deviation can be recorded with a protractor. This information is particularly important if surgery is contemplated.

Treatment

Although stall confinement and hoof trimming may be tried, they do not appear to be of any benefit in these cases. A few cases have been treated successfully by wedge ostectomy removal of a wedge-shaped piece of bone from the convex side and internal fixation with bone plates.

Prognosis

Realistically, not enough horses have been treated surgically or long-term followups obtained to make a valid comment regarding the prognosis.

"Splints"

"Splints," a disease of young horses, most often affect the forelimbs. Splints most commonly are found on the medial aspect of the limb between the medial splint bone and cannon bone. This disease is associated with hard training, poor conformation, improper hoof care, and possibly imbalanced or over-nutrition of a young horse.

A brief review of the anatomy should clarify any questions regarding the location and proposed function of the splint bones. The second and fourth metacarpal bones and metatarsal bones are commonly called splint bones. Each is attached intimately to the respective cannon bone by an interosseous ligament, thus splinting the large bone. If one views a cross section of the cannon, it becomes obvious that the splint bones provide considerable support to the cannon bone, since the dorsal cortex of the cannon bone is much thicker than its palmar surface (Fig. 5–88).

The terminology used to identify diseases of the splint bones is variable. A true splint refers to a sprain or tear of the interosseous ligament. The resultant enlargement is most frequently observed $2\frac{1}{2}$–3 in. below the knee on the medial side at the junction of the splint and cannon bones (Fig. 5–89). The term blind

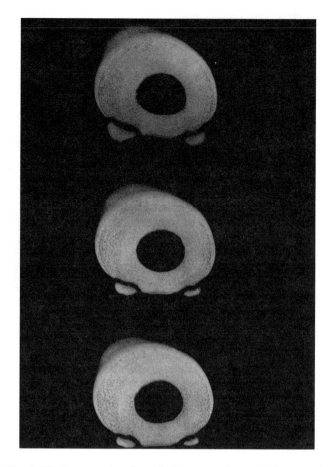

FIG. 5–88. Cross section through the cannon bone of a horse with bucked shins. Notice that the dorsal cortex is thicker than the palmar cortex. (Courtesy of Dr. P.F. Haynes.)

splint refers to an inflammatory process of the interosseous ligament that is difficult to detect on physical examination because the swelling occurs on the axial (inner) side of the splint, between the splint bone and the suspensory ligament. On x-ray examination a destruction of bone between the splint and cannon bones may be observed. Periostitis (an inflammation of the periosteum, bone skin) of the splint bones results from superficial trauma to the periosteum which, in turn, causes a proliferative (an overgrowth of tissue) periostitis (Fig. 5–90). Although a residual blemish remains, the horse is usually not lame. A knee splint refers to the enlargement of the proximal portion of the splint bone that may lead to osteoarthritis within the knee joint.

Causes

The enlargement of the splint bones associated with this disease results from proliferation of fibrous tissue and osteoperiostitis (inflammation of the periosteum and the underlying bone). Either tearing of the interosseous ligament that binds a splint bone to the cannon bone, external trauma, or healing of a transverse

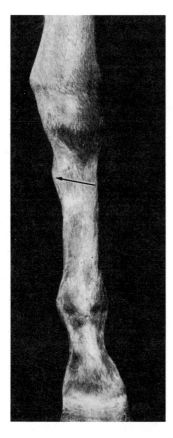

FIG. 5–89. Medial "splint." This horse was also affected by bench knees.

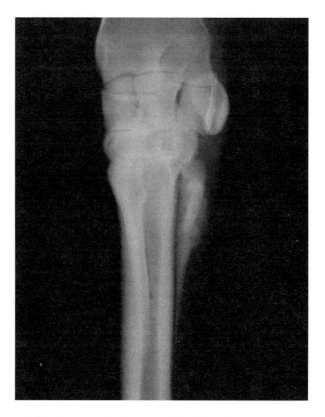

FIG. 5–90. An example of a periostitis of the splint bone.

or longitudinal fracture are the causes. If the inflammation associated with the periosteum is sufficient, with time, it will result in ossification (a change to bone). The size of the "splint" usually depends on the degree of inflammation and the surface area involved. In any case, the "splint" usually assumes an elongated form lying parallel to the bone.

The medial splint bone is more frequently involved because of the difference in its articulation with the knee. If one examines the medial splint bone, it becomes obvious that it articulates with the knee over its entire surface and its articulation is flatter than that of the lateral splint bone.

Conformation abnormalities that increase the stress on the splint bones also increase the incidence of this disease. "Bench knees" is an example of a conformational abnormality that predisposes to splints on the medial splint bones. Also, horses that have a base-narrow, toe-out conformation may cause external trauma to the splint bone by hitting it with the opposite limb (interference). Improper shoeing and trimming can cause enough alteration in the foot flight that the horse may interfere as well. All can cause either a tearing of the interosseous ligament or a proliferative periostitis of the medial splint bone and/or cannon bone. The lateral splint bone may be affected by external blows (hitting objects or being kicked). A higher incidence of this type of injury has been observed in the lateral splint bone of the hind limb.

Imbalanced nutrition or overnutrition in young horses has also been implicated in the development of splints. Imbalances in calcium and phosphorus as well as deficiencies in these minerals have been associated with an increased incidence of splints. However, no well documented studies have proven this to be true. In many cases horses that are suspected of having a calcium and phosphorus imbalance are also growing rapidly. It may be that their increased weight causes sufficient compressive forces so that splints develop as a result of this rather than the imbalance.

Young horses that are poorly conformed, overweight, and vigorously overexercised have a greater chance of tearing the interosseous ligament before it naturally ossifies.

Signs

Lameness is most common in 2-year-old horses undergoing heavy training, but occasionally occurs among 3- or 4-year-olds. Splints most often are found on the medial aspect of the limb, because the medial splint bone normally bears more weight than the lateral splint bone; therefore, it is more subject to stress. Lameness is usually most obvious at the trot. Heat, pain, and swelling over the affected region may occur anywhere along the length of the splint bone. Splints most commonly occur about 3 inches below the knee joint (see Fig. 5–89). One large swelling or a number of smaller enlargements may occur along the length of the splint bone at its junction with the cannon bone.

If new bone growth occurs near the knee joint, it may cause carpal arthritis (knee splints). Extensive new bone formation on a splint bone may encroach on the suspensory ligament and cause chronic lameness unless it is removed. The existence of growths of this kind can be determined by palpation and x-ray examination. Splint lameness becomes more marked with exercise on hard ground. In mild cases, no lameness may be evident in the walk, but is exhibited during the trot. After the inflammation subsides, the enlargements usually become smaller but firmer as a result of the ossification. The reduction in swelling is usually the result of resolution of fibrous tissue and not a decrease in size of the actual bone formation. In the early stages, the greatest bulk of the swelling is from inflammation, and this normally resolves to a much smaller size. This often misleads one into thinking that a certain method of treatment has reduced bony swelling. This is not true, and in many cases the actual new bone growth is larger than when originally treated. Some cases of splints may not cause lameness.

Diagnosis

If the affected limb is examined carefully, the obvious signs will lead to a diagnosis. Heat, pain, and swelling over the regions mentioned, plus lameness, are enough for diagnosis. Fracture of the splint bone is commonly confused with splints. With a fractured splint bone, the edema of the limb usually is distributed over a larger area and the animal remains chronically lame for a longer period. In any case, x-rays should be taken. An important part of the diagnosis is to determine whether the knee joint is involved or not and whether the new bone growth has extended palmarly so that the suspensory ligament is involved.

New bone growth resulting from trauma may occur on the cannon bones and may be mistaken for splints. Palpation and x-rays, however, will show that these swellings are dorsal to the junction with the splint bones. This type of new bone growth on the cannon is most often caused by interference. X-rays reveal that the splint bone is not primarily involved and the bony growth is almost entirely on the cannon bone. When doubt exists a video with high speed shutter freeze frame and slow motion capabilities can be very helpful.

Treatment

There are many recommended methods of treating "splints," but all basically rely on the use of antiinflammatory agents and rest for the acute phase, and counterirritation and occasionally surgery in the more chronic stages.

In the acute phase, inflammation and swelling are the hallmark of this disease. The administration of phenylbutazone coupled with the application of cold therapy and the application of pressure support wraps appears to be most beneficial to decrease the heat, pain, and swelling. Cold therapy can be attained with either ice packs or whirlpool boots. They should be applied for at least 30 minutes 2 times a day for 5 to 7 days. Some veterinarians recommend hand massage for 10 minutes after each treatment, after which a support bandage is applied. Others prefer to apply DMSO/Furacin or DMSO/Steroid sweats. After 10 days, when the inflammation is gone, a mild liniment may be applied underneath the support wraps. Affected horses should be confined to a stall for at least 30 to 45 days, and handwalking exercise for 15 to 20 minutes 2 times a day should be begun after the acute inflammation subsides.

Another method of treatment is to inject the splint region with a corticoid. This treatment reduces inflammation and may help prevent excessive bone growth. Corticoid therapy should be accompanied by counterpressure bandaging. In this case, the horse must be rested longer than 30 days and should not be returned to training as rapidly as when counterirritation is used. However, the swelling may be considerably less. It is also true that a case of splints will heal without therapy, provided adequate rest is given.

If the "splint" results from interference, splint or shin boots (guards) may help prevent further trauma. If the reason the horse interferes is because of improper or irregular trimming and shoeing, this should be corrected. Injecting the swelling with steroids may be helpful along with systemic administration of phenylbutazone to decrease the acute inflammation. Support wraps and stall rest may be required in acutely affected cases. If the proliferative bone is excessive, surgery may be appropriate in a very small percentage of the cases.

Counterirritation in the form of pin firing, local injection of hardening agents, topical applications of blisters, and radiation are used occasionally in subacute or chronic cases. The rationale for this treatment is that it converts a low level inflammatory process into an acute one which may accelerate the healing process. Unfortunately, this form of treatment results in a larger blemish.

In some cases it is necessary to surgically remove a bony growth that interferes with the action of the suspensory ligament or the knee joint or one is so large that it is being hit repeatedly by the opposite foot. In other cases, it is done because the horse is a halter-class horse and the owner feels that the blemish will lessen his chances of winning in the ring. "Splints," however, should not be regarded by judges as a serious blemish, provided they are not accompanied by base-narrow, toe-out, or bench-knee conformation. Successful removal of the bone growth can be accomplished in most cases. If the bone growth has been caused by trauma from interference, the surgery will not be successful unless preventive or corrective shoeing can stop the interference. In some cases of conformation-related interference, aggressive corrective shoeing may not only fail to stop the interference, but it may introduce balance and stress problems in another portion of the limb.

Prognosis

Prognosis is favorable in all cases except those in which the bony growth is large and encroaches on the suspensory ligament or the knee joint or when it is due to interference.

Fractures of the Splint Bones

Fractures of the splint bones can occur anywhere along their length but are most commonly located at the distal third. In most cases, fractures located at the distal third are simple fractures (Fig. 5–91), in contrast to fractures of the middle and proximal portion which are often complicated by fragmentation, osteomyelitis (bone infection), and bone sequestration (diseased or dead bone tissue separated from the healthy bone) (Fig. 5–92).

Fractures of the distal part of a splint bone usually occur in older horses (5 to 7 years of age) and only rarely occur in horses under 2 years of age. This is thought to occur as a result of decreased pliability in the interosseous ligament and more strenuous training programs in older horses. In contrast, younger

horses tend to sustain damage to the interosseous ligament supporting the splint bones resulting in the condition referred to as "splints." Generally, the forelimbs are more frequently involved than the hindlimbs, with the left forelimb more commonly affected than the right. The relationship between suspensory ligament inflammation, fractured splints, sesamoiditis, and fetlock arthritis or arthrosis is more than casual. It would appear that the enlarged fibrotic suspensory ligament decreases the absorptive capacity of the fetlock and creates a space-occupying mass that may cause the fracture and further displacement of that fractured splint bone. It is assumed that the decreased ability to extend the fetlock contributes to the arthrosis.

Fractures of the proximal half of the splint bone are often fragmented, and osteomyelitis with or without sequestrum is a complicating feature. The lateral surface of these bones is most frequently involved and it is thought to result from direct trauma.

Causes

Fractures of the distal part of the splint bone result from external as well as internal trauma. External trauma can result from a kick from another horse, interference, direct blows from hitting an object, or puncture wounds. Internal trauma occurs from in-

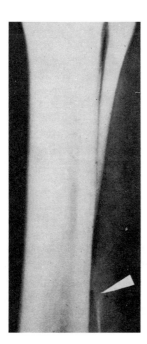

FIG. 5–91. Fracture of the distal end of the medial splint bone (arrow).

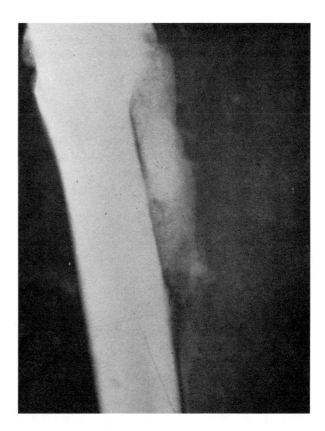

FIG. 5–92. Fracture of the middle third of the medial splint bone that is complicated by osteomyelitis.

creased axial compression forces on these bones during races or from pressure from the suspensory ligament or increased tension from the fascial attachments. It is conjectured that the increased incidence in the front limbs of left lateral splint bone and right medial splint bone fractures observed in Thoroughbreds may be the result of increased weight bearing on the bones when they are racing in a counterclockwise direction. In contrast, the suspensory ligament and supporting fascia may put these bones under tension sufficient enough to cause fracture in the hindlimbs. Since there is an increase in incidence in the hind limbs of left medial splint bone and right lateral splint bone, which is the tension side of the hindlimb in horses that run counterclockwise, it is logical to assume that tension created by the bow-string effect of the suspensory ligament or increased tension developed by the internal fascia may lead to fracture.

It is difficult to decide whether the incidence of suspensory ligament inflammation is a result of fractured splint bones that may cause irritation to this structure or, conversely, that the swollen suspensory ligament becomes space-occupying enough to cause these fractures. Whichever the case, a higher incidence of suspensory ligament inflammation is noted in the forelimb in association with these fractures.

More complicated fractures of the proximal part of the splint bones result from direct trauma, either from interference or direct blows to the surface. These fractures are often open initially, which frequently results in bone infection. In some cases there is not a break in the skin initially, but the fragmented fractures become separated from the healthy bone and result in recurrent draining tracts.

Signs

Swelling is usually a prominent feature of the proximal splint fracture, but it may or may not be present with the distal splint fracture. In general, the degree of swelling associated with the distal splint fracture depends on the acuteness of the fracture. The more acute the fracture, the more swelling. Associated swelling in the suspensory ligament as well as the fetlock joint may also be observed.

In the acute case, in both instances, horses frequently point their foot. Trotting exercises may or may not cause lameness, but this depends on the acuteness and type of fracture that has resulted. Circling or fast work may be required to cause sufficient lameness to be observed.

On palpation heat, pain, and swelling will be obvious features of the acute fracture and in some cases draining tracts will also be present. The pain and heat will decrease with time. However, since callus formation is a frequent result of the nonsurgically treated fracture, as time passes the fracture site will become enlarged. In cases in which only mild pain is evidenced with palpation but the horse is quite lame, the limiting features of this horse returning to perform-

ance may be associated with suspensory ligament inflammation or fetlock arthrosis. To gain an appreciation as to the involvement of the splint bone, the limb is flexed so that the full extent of this bone can be palpated. A thorough physical examination of the suspensory ligament should follow. Direct pressure can be applied for one minute over the painful region of the bone, after which the horse is exercised and lameness recorded. A marked increase in lameness usually indicates primary involvement of the splint bone, a mild increase in lameness may indicate that other structures are contributing to the lameness.

Diagnosis

A persistent swelling over the affected splint bone, exhibiting heat and pain when pressure is applied, should lead one to suspect fractured splint bone. Some fractured splint bones closely resemble the disease called "splints." Some such fractures heal, but the bony swelling is confused with "splints." X-rays are necessary for a positive diagnosis of a fractured splint bone and to differentiate between a fracture of the splint bone and the disease called "splints" (see Fig. 5–89).

X-rays should be taken in all cases to identify the fracture, its limits, and if sequestration and osteomyelitis exist in association with a complicated fracture (Fig. 5–93). In some cases the proximal fracture may extend toward the knee joint (Fig. 5–94).

Treatment

Traditionally, removal of the distal fragment of the fractured splint is recommended. However, this may be unnecessary when healing is progressing and minimal callus formation and lameness are present. Some proximal fragmented fractures may also be treated successfully with full-limb cast application for a period of 4 to 6 weeks, after which bandage support may be needed (Fig. 5–95). After healing is complete, horses should be returned to work and an assessment is made at this time if surgery is needed. Surgery is indicated for nonunion of the distal fractured splint bone or if a proximal fracture has healed with a large callus. In the latter case, it is sometimes better to remove the fractured bone as soon as practical to shorten the convalescent period and to decrease the chances of increased callus formation leading to impingement on the suspensory ligament. When more than two thirds of the splint bone is to be removed, internal fixation may be used to stabilize the remaining proximal fragment. If the proximal fragment is not anchored, excessive movement of this fragment may occur and result in interosseous ligament inflammation, degenerative arthritis of the knee or hock joint, or avulsion of the proximal fragment.

After surgery, a sterile pressure bandage is applied and changed as needed. For an optimal cosmetic end

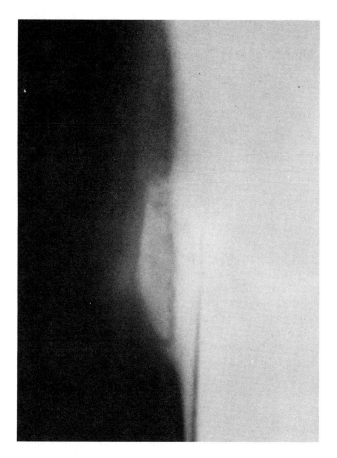

FIG. 5–93. A sequestrum of the medial splint bone is present. This can be treated by surgical removal of the sequestered piece of bone alone, without removal of the remaining distal segment of the splint bone.

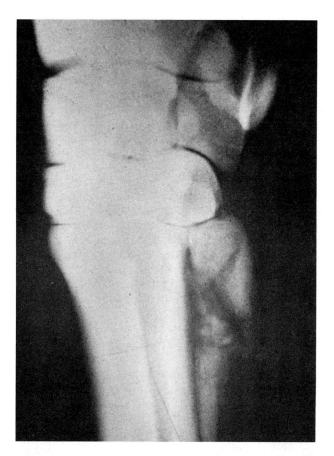

FIG. 5–94. A fragmented fracture of the proximal end of the lateral splint bone. This type of fracture usually requires internal fixation with a bone screw to hold it in place.

result, bandages are maintained for a minimum of 6 weeks postoperatively. Phenylbutazone is usually administered 3 to 7 days postoperatively and sutures are removed around the fourteenth day after surgery. The horse should be maintained in a boxstall for at least a total of 6 weeks. Hand-walking exercise can begin at about the second week after surgery and free exercise can begin after 6 weeks. Training is usually initiated after 2 to 3 months of rest and is totally dependent on the degree of soft tissue damage associated with the fracture site.

Prognosis

The prognosis for return to previous performance of horses sustaining fractures of the distal part of the splint bone which have been treated surgically appears to depend on whether the suspensory ligament inflammation is present or not. In a study of distal splint fractures without suspensory ligament inflammation, 75% of the horses returned to previous levels of performance. Only 25 to 50% of the cases returned to previous levels of performance if suspensory ligament inflammation accompanied the fractured splint.

The prognosis for complicated cases of splint fractures appears to be good, particularly if the horse is used for performances other than racing. For racehorses, a guarded prognosis is given for return to previous levels of performance.

Lameness Associated with the Proximal Palmar/Plantar Cannon Bone Region

Lameness associated with the proximal palmar/ plantar cannon bone region can be caused by a proximal suspensory ligament inflammation of the attachment, an avulsion fracture of the origin of the suspensory ligament, an inflammation of the radial (inferior) check ligament, and incomplete stress fractures of the proximal cannon bone. Both fore and hindlimbs may be involved. All may present with similar signs as those described for "blind splints" inflammation. In chronic cases of tearing of the origin of the suspensory ligament a periostitis is observed on x-ray. Proximal suspensory ligament inflammation lameness is most frequently seen in Standardbreds, hunters and jumpers, polo ponies, Thoroughbreds, and occasionally endurance horses.

Causes

Overloading of the suspensory ligament or carpal check ligament may cause sprain trauma. It is possible that hyperextension of the knee in conjunction with severe overextension of the fetlock joint may be a factor in the forelimbs, and overextension of the fetlock may be the cause of inflammation of the proximal suspensory ligament inflammation when it is seen in the hindlimbs. The fracture that occurs at the proximal attachment of the suspensory ligament probably results from the bone being torn away (avulsion). Obviously, the more severe the sprain trauma, the more severe the lesion. Deep, soft arenas and eventing where there is excessive rotational movement of the limbs have both been implicated as causes.

Incomplete stress fractures of the proximal cannon bone are probably the result of repeated stress from compression at this site. Why the medial side of the cannon bone is affected more frequently is unknown.

Signs

Most horses with inflammation of the proximal suspensory ligament have a history of intermittent lameness of several days' or weeks' duration that is worsened by strenuous exercise. Horses with inflammation of the carpal check ligament or avulsion fractures most frequently have a history of acute onset of moderate to severe lameness. Horses sustaining a fracture of the origin of the suspensory ligament and incomplete fractures of the proximal cannon bone have often attained racing speeds in their workouts.

Visual observation of the affected limb is usually not informative. However, mild proximal swelling may be felt between the suspensory ligament and the deep digital flexor tendon. On palpation heat is rarely felt, but with pinpoint digital palpation of the origin of the suspensory ligament and carpal check ligament, pain can be elicited, which often results in increased lameness with exercise. To adequately palpate this region, the limb should be flexed at the carpus. In this position the flexor tendons are loose and can be displaced either laterally or medially (Fig. 5–96). While the horse is at a trot the lameness may be most prominent when the affected limb is on the outside of the circle. Flexion of the knee and fetlock (forelimb) and hock (hindlimb) may cause pain and worsen the lameness.

Diagnosis

The diagnosis can be difficult. Pain withdrawal after selective digital palpation should make the examiner suspicious that these regions may be involved with lameness. If local anesthetic injections below the knee or hock eliminate the lameness, one of these entities is the probable cause, and can only be differentiated with ultrasound and x-ray examinations. Nuclear scintigraphic examination (nuclear scan) may be needed to identify the stress fractures on the palmar cortex of the cannon bone.

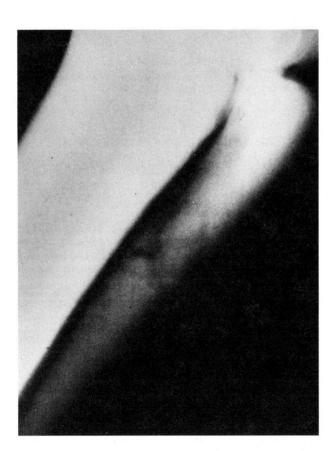

FIG. 5–95. This proximal fragmented fracture of the lateral splint bone was managed successfully with the application of a full limb cast for 4 weeks. After the 4 weeks, the limb was placed in a support wrap for another 2 weeks. Free exercise was begun at 3 months.

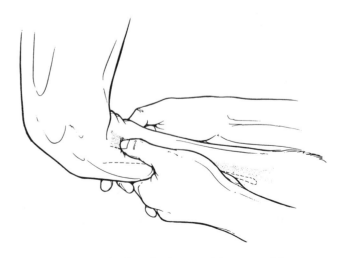

FIG. 5–96. Location for digital palpation of the origin of the suspensory ligament.

Treatment

The treatment for all these entities involves variable periods of rest extending anywhere from 3 to 6 months in duration. Absolute rest is recommended until the acute pain subsides. Avulsion fractures do not appear to separate appreciably and because a good blood supply exists they quite often will heal rapidly. Phenylbutazone is recommended for its antiinflammatory effect. If pain returns after exercise has begun a more prolonged convalescent period will be required. Repeated ultrasound examinations (6 weeks to 3 months) are most helpful in documenting healing of the ligaments. Repeated x rays and or nuclear scans are beneficial in deciding when fracture healing is complete. In both cases, these examinations will ultimately tell your veterinarian when your horse is ready to return to work.

Prognosis

The prognosis of returning to previous performance is good for all cases treated with a sufficient rest period. The prognosis for forelimb involvement is slightly better than that for involvement of the hind limb.

Traumatic Division of Tendons

Tendons are composed of dense, white, fibrous connective tissue arranged in parallel, densely packed bundles. Peritendon surrounds these bundles and epitendon surrounds the entire tendon unit (Fig. 5–97). Both of these connective tissue elements carry the intrinsic (inherent) blood supply to the internal structures of the tendon. Tendon sheaths are present where tendons glide over joints. They are composed of two layers: 1) The outer parietal layer, and 2) the inner visceral layer. These sheaths secrete synovial fluid to aid gliding of the tendon (Fig. 5–97). The mesotendon carries the extrinsic (external) blood supply (Fig. 5–97) to the tendon. Nonsheathed tendons are covered by paratendon; it allows the tendon to glide and supplies the extrinsic blood supply (Fig. 5–98).

Tendon healing occurs intrinsically as well as extrinsically. Intrinsic healing is supported by a sparse intrinsic blood supply that nourishes approximately one fourth of the tendon volume. Extrinsic healing is a result of stimulation of the peritendinous tissue to proliferate and supply cells and capillaries needed for healing. This process is responsible for the formation of adhesions of the tendons to all adjacent structures. This is known as the one-wound/one-scar concept. It has been shown experimentally that the intrinsic blood supply is not sufficient to support primary healing of the tendon.

The sequence of healing is as follows: The inflammatory phase (0 to 10 days). The biological sequence of this is the same as the healing of any wound except in this case it is slower. At 5 to 7 days postwounding the tendon is weaker than at the time of original repair. The proliferative phase (4 to 21 days). A fibrovascular callus is formed surrounding the tendon and attaching all structures of the wound together. The maturation phase (28 to 120 days). The longitudinal orientation of the fibroblasts (specialized collagen-forming cells) and fibers begin. At 45 days, collagenolysis (breakdown of collagen) and collagen formation reach an equilibrium. At 90 days, early collagen bundle formation is seen; and at 120 days, these bundles appear much like those seen in normal tendon.

Traumatic Division of the Digital Extensor Tendons of the Fore- and Hindlimb

Traumatic division of the common and/or lateral extensors of the forelimb and the long and/or lateral extensor in the hindlimb is relatively common. In the hindlimb, the tendon or tendons are usually severed just below the hock as a result of wire lacerations. In the forelimb, the common digital extensor or lateral digital extensor is often severed between the fetlock and the knee, again as a result of wire lacerations. If the laceration is below the middle of the cannon in the hindlimb, where the lateral and long extensor are combined, only one tendon is cut.

Cause

Trauma is the cause in all cases. Wire cuts account for most cases.

Signs

The horse is unable to extend the toe of the foot. When its foot is put down, the toe may catch and force the dorsal surface of the fetlock to the ground. However, when the limb is set under the horse properly, it can bear weight normally. The lateral digital extensor may be cut without any accompanying signs in either the fore- or the hindlimb, because division of the common digital extensor and of the long digital extensor cause most of the signs.

Diagnosis

The diagnosis is obvious in most cases, but the veterinarian may need to determine what structures are involved by sterile palpation and probing of the wound.

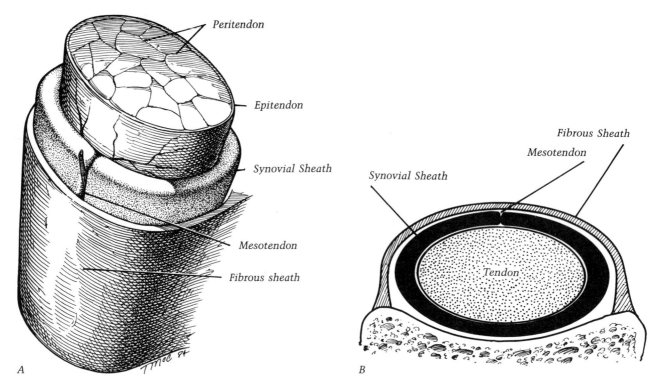

Peritendon

Epitendon

Synovial Sheath

Mesotendon

Fibrous sheath

A

Fibrous Sheath

Mesotendon

Synovial Sheath

Tendon

B

FIG. 5–97. *A*, Illustration of a section of a tendon within a tendon sheath. *B*, Illustration of a cross section of a tendon within a tendon sheath.

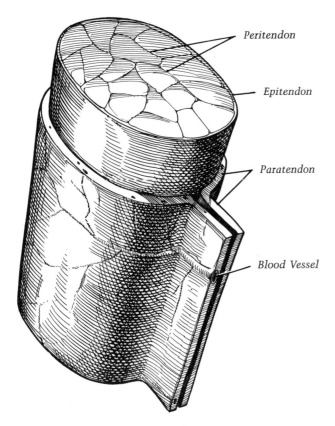

Peritendon

Epitendon

Paratendon

Blood Vessel

FIG. 5–98. Illustration of a section of a tendon within a paratendon.

Treatment

After proper preparation, the wound is sutured. Usually no attempt is made to bring the tendon edges together with tendon sutures, unless a clean sharp laceration exists or the tendon is lacerated over the dorsal surface of the fetlock. The extensor tendons have a better chance to rejoin than the flexor tendons, and with time, most horses will regain normal function of the limb. However, if a clean sharp laceration exists in the tendon or the laceration is over the dorsal surface of the fetlock, it is sutured.

Bandage splints can be used to immobilize the limb postoperatively when the tendon is not sutured, and casts are preferred if the tendon is sutured.

The foot can be placed in a corrective shoe when the bandage splint or cast has been removed. This shoe has an extended toe of approximately 3 inches. A metal bar can be welded to the toe extension so that it conforms to the shape of the dorsal surface of the cannon. The front of the limb should be padded and the bar at the front of the limb bound to the limb by adhesive tape or elastic bandages. This helps keep the toe in extension. With further improvement, the bar on the dorsal surface of the limb may be discontinued, and only the toe extension left on the shoe, until the limb appears to assume nearly normal function. Complete healing usually occurs in about 4 to 6 months, and the horse will again use the extensor tendons normally.

Prognosis

The prognosis is guarded to favorable, depending upon the location and extent of the wound. In some cases, wire may cut into the hock joint, which may make euthanasia advisable if infectious arthritis is present. In other cases, the bone may be badly damaged, so the prognosis must be withheld until the case has been evaluated.

In two studies evolving the outcome of extensor tendon lacerations, 73 to 80% returned to athletic soundness.

Traumatic Division of the Digital Flexor Tendons of the Fore- and Hindlimb

Traumatic division of the digital flexor tendons usually occurs between the carpus and the fetlock or between the tarsus and the fetlock. The greatest difficulty in tendon repair is to reestablish a smooth gliding surface. Division of the flexor tendons within their sheaths presents a special problem with regard to healing.

Cause

Trauma is the cause in all cases. Numerous types of accidents may be the cause; they are not all listed here. Injury may occur as a result of backing into or kicking a sharp object or being cut down in a race by a horse coming from behind. In such a case, the hindlimb would be involved. A horse may cut his own flexor tendons by overreaching and cutting the tendon region of the forelimb with a toe grab of the shoe on the hind foot of the same side.

Signs

All degrees of laceration have been found. The superficial digital flexor tendon alone may be severed, while in other cases the deep digital flexor may also be severed. In some cases, both flexor tendons and the suspensory ligament may be cut. If the flexors are cut above the middle of the cannon, the check ligament may also be severed. If only the superficial flexor tendon is cut, the fetlock joint will drop, but it will not touch the ground. If the superficial and deep flexor tendons are cut, the fetlock will drop and the toe will come up in the air when weight is applied to the affected limb. If both flexors and the suspensory ligament are cut, the fetlock will rest on the ground. When the laceration is below the distal end of the long postern bone, only the deep flexor and the associated digital sheath are cut.

If the wound has been present for some time, there may be infection of the tendon sheath, (septic tendosynovitis) and varying amounts of swelling in the limb may result. Infection increases the amount of scar tissue formation and decreases the chance of a full recovery. Lameness, which is severe, will vary according to the severity and duration of the wound.

Diagnosis

The veterinarian will determine what structures have been severed by observing the clinical attitude of the foot and by sterile palpation and probing of the wound.

Treatment

The general result of flexor tendon lacerations is less satisfactory than lacerations involving the extensor tendons. If the laceration involves both flexor tendons and the suspensory ligament, euthanasia may be indicated unless the owners are interested in salvaging a valuable animal for breeding. In general, if the laceration in the flexor tendon is fresh, clean, and sharp, primary suturing is recommended.

Postoperatively, the limb is placed in a cast. A cast is superior to most types of braces and shoeing. Extended heelshoes are useful when the cast is removed. The opposite limb should be kept in a supporting bandage to prevent it from breaking down.

Prognosis

The prognosis is guarded to unfavorable, depending on the number of structures that are severed. If both flexors and the suspensory ligament are cut, the prognosis is unfavorable. The presence of septic tendonitis makes the prognosis more unfavorable. If the vascular supply is cut, necrosis may result. When a tendon is partially severed or is crushed or bruised from a closed injury, it swells and softens and may rupture from ordinary pull several days to 3 weeks later.

The prognosis for suture repair of clean lacerated flexor tendons within the paratendon is good, but a year's convalescence will be required before full function is returned. A guarded to poor prognosis is expected for lacerated flexor tendons within their sheaths that are repaired. A good prognosis can be given in most cases, however, for return to breeding soundness. In one case study of the outcome of treated flexor tendon lacerations, 18% of the horses returned to their original level of performance and 41% returned to limited riding.

Idiopathic Synovitis
Windpuffs (Windgalls)

This is distention of a joint capsule, tendon sheath, or bursa, with excess synovial fluid, not accompanied by lameness. See Chapter 4 for more details.

The Carpus (Knee)

Angular Limb Deformities Associated with the Carpus (Knee) (Carpus Valgus and Carpus Varus, Medial Deviation of the Carpus and Lateral Deviation of the Carpus)

An angular limb deformity refers to a lateral or medial deviation of the limb. (This is apposed to flexure deformities associated with tendon contracture or rupture that results in a cranial-to-caudal deviation of the limb.) The terms valgus and varus are commonly used to describe the manner of the angular deformity in foals. Carpus valgus (knock-kneed) refers to a deformity in which the cannon deviates laterally (outward) and the distal radius (forearm bone) deviates medially (inward) (Fig. 5–99). Carpus varus (bowlegged) refers to the opposite situation in which the cannon deviates medially and the distal radius deviates laterally (Fig. 5–100). These deformities can result from asymmetric growth of the distal radial metaphysis, the distal radial epiphysis, or incomplete development of the cuboidal (knee) bones and splint bones, or joint laxity.

Angular limb deformities are seen with increased frequency in foals of all breeds. However, a slightly higher incidence has been reported in the Quarter horse foal. There appears to be an equal sex distribution. The concept of natural or normal crookedness of the forelimbs of foals is important, for incorrect diagnosis can be made. It is not uncommon for foals to be slightly knock-kneed (less than 7% at 4 months of age) and have both forelimbs rotated outward from the chest to the toes. Outward forelimb rotation is common in narrow-chested foals. As the foal matures to a yearling, there is a growth spurt on the lateral side of his growth plate that strengthens the limbs, and as the chest gets wider, the forelimbs rotate inward to fur-

ther strengthen the limbs. All in all, a foal's limbs are not expected to be straight until he is a long yearling (see p. 418–422). Further discussion will address angular limb deformities that are not considered normal crookedness.

Foals can either be born with deviated limbs (congenital) (Fig. 5–101) or develop the angular deformity within several weeks to months after birth (acquired). The deviated limbs of many foals born with an angular deformity will straighten in a short period of time on their own, and will not require treatment. In others, the angular deformity either remains static or worsens and these usually require treatment. Foals born with straight limbs that acquire the angular deformity of the carpus as they mature will most often require the assistance of a veterinarian. Some cases can have multiple limb and joint involvement (e.g., carpus valgus plus tarsus valgus or carpus valgus with fetlock varus). Regardless of the situation, it is most important to correct the angular limb deformity well in advance of growth plate closure and early enough to prevent secondary damage to the carpal bones and the other joints distal to the carpus.

Causes

The causes of angular limb deformities appear to be complex and multifactorial. The basic problem with angular deformities associated with the carpus ap-

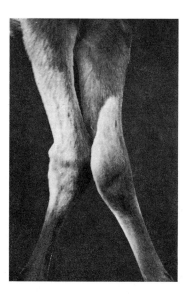

FIG. 5–99. Knock knees in a foal (carpus valgus).

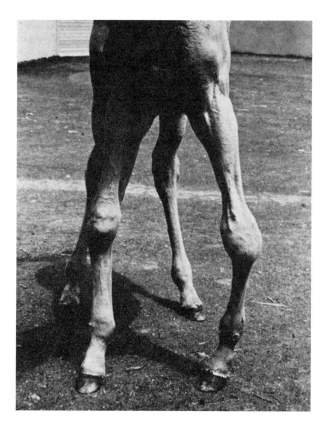

FIG. 5–100. A foal with carpus varus.

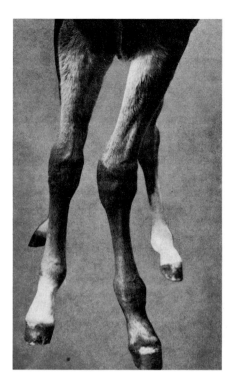

FIG. 5–101. An example of congenital limb deviation caused by uterine positioning. The right forelimb has slight lateral deviation (varus) of the knee, and the left forelimb has severe medial deviation (valgus) of the knee. Both limbs are bowed in the same direction.

pears to be an asymmetric growth of the long bones, carpal bones, and to a lesser degree, the splint bones associated with the carpus. Accompanying this asymmetric growth are varying degrees of defective endochondral ossification (cartilage to bone formation).

Before a thorough discussion of the causes can occur, a brief review of developmental anatomy is in order. The physis (growth plate) is responsible for the longitudinal growth of the metaphysis of the longbones, and to a lesser degree, the epiphysis adjacent to it. The subarticular epiphyseal cartilage plays an important role in the development and maturation of the epiphysis of longbones and the cuboidal bones of the carpus. As the cartilage grows from these regions, it dies and undergoes endochondral ossification to form bone.

There appear to be a number of factors that can alter or arrest endochondral ossification. Of the many factors that can influence endochondral ossification, compression trauma appears to play a major role in the development of congenital and acquired angular limb deformities in foals.

Briefly, axial compression forces can be physiologic (within normal limits) or nonphysiologic (greater than normal limits). Physiologic compression stimulates the growth and transformation of cartilage models into bone in the growth plate, articular cartilage associated with the distal radial epiphysis, and in the carpal cuboidal bones. Nonphysiologic (excessive) compression forces, on the other hand, suppress or arrest the development of cartilage models to bone, which in turn causes a reduction in longitudinal bone growth. It is proposed that nonphysiologic compressive forces not only cause microfractures of the newly formed bone but also alter the blood supply sufficiently at the zone of provisional calcification (transition zone between cartilage and bone) to result in defective endochondral ossification. The excess cartilage that builds up creates enough pressure to arrest further cartilage cell development. Many feel that the development of defective endochondral ossification is one of the manifestations of osteochondrosis.

If we apply these principles to a valgus deformity of the carpus resulting from asymmetric growth in the distal radial metaphysis, the concave side (lateral) will be under greater axial compression than the convex side (medial). In this case we have an asymmetric axial compressive loading of the lateral aspect of the growth plate. If it is within physiologic limits, the lateral side of the growth plate will be stimulated to grow more rapidly than the medial side and the limb will straighten on its own. However, if the compressive forces are nonphysiologic (excessive), the growth on the lateral side (concave) will be reduced or arrested and the angular deformity will remain static or worsen. The more asymmetric the nonphysiologic compressive forces become, the worse the angular deformity. This brings about confusion in some cases as to which comes first, the alteration in endochondral ossification leading to asymmetric compressive forces, or the asymmetric compressive forces resulting in defective endochondral ossification. Both appear reasonable. With congenital angular limb deformities, it could be postulated that incomplete ossification of the cuboidal bones and/or splint bones occurring from altered endochondral ossification can cause asymmetric loading during weight bearing. On the other hand, for the developmental angular deformity, asymmetric compressive forces cause the defective endochondral ossification on the lateral side of the distal radial metaphysis with carpal valgus. Asymmetric loading leading to compression can be exacerbated by severe angular deformity from carpal bone hypoplasia (underdevelopment) and joint laxity.

Congenital Angular Limb Deformity

When a foal is born with an angular deformity of the carpus (congenital angular limb deformity) the cause may be due to intrauterine malposition, overnutrition of the mare in the latter half of pregnancy, joint laxity, defective endochondral ossification (hypoplasia) of the cuboidal bones, or maldevelopment of the splint bones. Toxic chemicals and other poorly understood mechanical and endocrine influences are also included.

With intrauterine malposition, the angular limb deformity associated with the carpus may occur as a result of the limb being placed in an abnormal position. This malposition can lead to asymmetric growth of the metaphysis and epiphysis, the carpal bones and splint bones, and result in joint laxity. If the angular deformity is severe and/or excessive joint instability is present, asymmetric loading during weight bearing can further alter the development of these regions.

Overnutrition in the latter half of pregnancy can result in a high incidence of unilateral angular limb deformity. It is proposed that mares that are overfed in the latter half of gestation and become fat develop a sufficient intraabdominal mass of adipose tissue to compress the uterus, leading to malposition of at least one limb. Seventeen out of 30 foals born on one farm had unilateral angular deformities. The only common denominator appeared to be overnutrition of a previously poorly fed mare in the latter half of pregnancy.

Varying degrees of carpal joint laxity are particularly evident in newborn foals. The surrounding soft tissues are simply not strong enough to support the carpus, and a valgus angular deformity of the carpus usually results. In most cases, exercise on pasture increases muscle tone and sufficiently tightens the adjacent soft tissue support to bring about correction. However, if no improvement is seen within the first 5 to 7 days of life, or if the deviation is greater than 15°, veterinary attention is warranted. Varying degrees of cuboidal bone and splint bone hypoplasia may accompany this entity. However, joint laxity alone can result in asymmetric nonphysiologic (excessive) compressive forces and result in progression of an angular limb deformity.

Defective ossification of the cuboidal carpal bones involves the third, fourth, and ulnar carpal bones most frequently, and to a lesser degree, the radial carpal and second carpal bones. Because the lateral portion of the third, fourth, and ulnar carpal bones are most commonly affected, a valgus deformity of the carpus results. The exact cause of this entity can only be conjectured, but at least initially, trauma appears to play a secondary role. Basically, two types of changes are observed: 1) the cuboidal bones have an abnormal size and shape, and 2) the articular cartilage associated with these bones is hypertrophied (enlarged). The alteration in size and contour of the cuboidal bones represents a true hypoplasia and not degeneration. The reduced height of the hypoplastic bone creates an angular limb deformity. The x-ray and structural features of these bones closely resemble those of fetal carpal bones; the ossified nucleus is rounded and is surrounded by cartilage that is thicker than normal. Clefts in the hypertrophied cartilage have also been noted that are very similar to those observed with osteochondritis dessicans. It is suggested that this may represent a manifestation of osteochondrosis because there appears to be a disturbance in the normal differentiation of these cartilage cells and an alteration in normal endochondral ossification which has resulted in cartilage retention. This may represent a normal variation in bone formation, a relative immaturity, or a defect in endochondral ossification.

Incomplete development of the proximal part of the splint bones appears to fall into the category of incomplete ossification similar to that described for the carpal bones. Affected splint bones appear shorter than the larger cannon bone and, as a result, a wider joint space is formed between the proximal articulation with these bones and the adjacent carpal bones. The lateral splint bone appears to be involved more frequently resulting in a valgus deformity. If the medial is involved, a varus deformity would be expected.

To summarize the congenital angular limb deformity associated with the carpus, it is reasonable that all of these conditions could be brought about by abnormal intrauterine positioning, placing abnormal stresses on the developing cartilage and stretching ligamentous support. It is also logical that the asymmetric compressive forces brought to bear on this developing cartilage in premature foals may deform it and alter the pattern of endochondral ossification which would result in perpetual worsening of the condition. These concepts may be oversimplified and a true developmental problem may exist that is influenced by hereditary, nutritional, and hormonal factors.

Acquired Angular Limb Deformity

With acquired angular limb deformity, the foal is born with relatively straight limbs that begin to deviate within the first few weeks or months of life. The cause may be an unrecognized subtle congenital angular limb deformity, a growth plate injury, excessive contralateral (opposite) limb weight bearing, overnutrition, improper trimming, excessive exercise, asymmetric growth of the distal radial metaphysis or distal radial epiphysis, and poor conformation.

It is reasonable to assume that some foals are born with subtle angular limb deformities of the carpus, resulting from joint laxity, hypoplasia of the carpal bones or small metacarpal bones, or alteration of the epiphysis. These go unrecognized, and with increased growth, active exercise, and overnutrition, asymmetric nonphysiologic compressive forces are brought to bear on the developing cartilage, which results in defective endochondral ossification and cartilage deformation. With time, the tension side (convex side) continues to grow and the angular deformity worsens. The nonphysiologic compression forces can further influence the development of distal radial metaphysis, distal radial epiphysis, cuboidal bones, and proximal splint bones. In some cases of hypoplasia of the cuboidal bones, nonphysiologic compressive forces can result in fracture and collapse of the affected bones.

Direct trauma to the distal radial physis (growth plate) can result in angular limb deformity and produce an asynchronous longitudinal growth. If the damage is severe, premature closure may occur on one side or progress across the entire growth plate. This can lead to an irreversible angular limb deformity if the closure is asymmetric, or a total loss in limb length if the entire growth plate is involved. The degree of alteration depends on when the trauma occurred. The average time for complete closure of the distal radial physis in the horse is 22 to 36 months. If the injury occurs close to the time of plate closure, minimal alteration in limb conformation will result. On the other hand, direct traumatic insults leading to early closure of the growth plate can result in a devastating end-result.

Excessive contralateral limb weight bearing can occur in the foal after sustaining trauma to either limb; because the affected limb is painful it will bear most of the weight on the opposite limb. This increased weight bearing is often sufficient to create a unilateral angular deformity opposite to the lame limb. It is commonly seen in foals that sustain injuries severe enough to warrant a full-limb cast application. It is also observed frequently in foals that have exhibited a chronic unilateral lameness that has not been treated.

Overnutrition and imbalanced nutrition may result in developmental angular limb deformities of the carpus in two ways. First, the increased body weight from overnutrition results in an increased compressive force and, if an angular deformity is present, this may lead to nonphysiologic (excessive) asymmetric compressive forces. Second, imbalances in nutrition may alter endochondral ossification. The role of imbalanced nutrition as cause of an angular limb deformity complex is unclear. Previously, deficiencies and excesses of calcium and phosphorus, vitamin A, and vitamin D were incriminated, and the condition was erroneously called ricketts. Ricketts results from a vitamin D deficiency, and although some of the features of angular limb deformity are there, a likening of the two conditions is an oversimplification. Certainly, the genetic ability to grow rapidly with a degree of overnutrition is implicated in shifting the compressive forces into the nonphysiologic (excessive) range. Deficiencies in trace minerals, copper in particular, have been implicated in the angular limb deformities of cattle. The role of zinc, manganese, molybdenum, and other trace minerals is unclear and requires further investigation.

Asymmetric growth in the distal radial metaphysis may result from trauma or a deformity in the distal radius epiphysis, or be produced by incomplete ossification of the cuboidal and small metacarpal bones, ligament laxity, or improper trimming. Trauma can simply be the result of an overweight foal actively exercising on hard ground. Whatever the cause, the asymmetric growth in the distal radial metaphysis results in a "vicious cycle" of asymmetric loading with nonphysiologic (excessive) compressive forces that decrease the endochondral ossification and growth on that side. In carpus valgus, the lateral side is most affected by compression and the medial side continues to grow resulting in an even greater asynchronous longitudinal growth.

Abnormal development of the distal radial epiphysis can result from congenital or developmental problems. It can also be worsened by asymmetric nonphysiologic compressive forces, which in turn alter its further development and delay endochondral ossification.

Signs

The signs of angular limb deformity are quite clear, but the diagnosis of the exact entity resulting in the angular deformity requires discussion.

Obviously, a thorough history and physical exam are required. The history should provide answers to the following questions: 1) Was the foal premature? 2) Was the angular deformity of the carpus present at birth or was it acquired? 3) Was the mare markedly overweight during the last half of gestation? 4) Has the angular deformity improved, stayed the same or worsened? 5) Were there any signs of lameness in the limb opposite the angular deformity? 6) Did the angular deformity of the carpus develop acutely or was it slowly progressive? 7) What has been the mare's and foal's diet?

On visual observation, the degree of angular limb deformity should be estimated and recorded. Any angular deformities greater than 15° involving hypoplasia of the cuboidal bones or altered endochondral ossification of the epiphysis will usually require the veterinarian's immediate attention. An estimation of where the deviation is centered (pivot point) should also be made. This is particularly important in foals seen for the first time. If the deviation appears to be centered around the distal radial physis or epiphysis, asymmetric growth of the distal radial metaphysis or an abnormally shaped distal radial epiphysis is likely (Fig. 5–102*A* and *B*). If the deviation is centered over the knee joints (midcarpal joint) one should be suspicious of hypoplasia of the cuboidal bones, joint laxity, or incomplete development of small metacarpal bones (Fig. 5–102*C* and *D*). It is important to remember that this is only an estimation and radiographs are required to obtain a more definitive answer. If the angular deformity affects only one limb, a contralateral limb lameness leading to increased weight bearing on the affected limb or intrauterine malposition may be the cause. If joint swelling is present and the pivot point is centered over the midcarpal (intercarpal) joint, hypoplasia and/or collapse of the carpal bones or ligament laxity should be suspected. If the foal is lame on the limb with the angular deformity, the examiner should be suspicious of direct trauma to the growth plate or epiphysis or carpal bones, or joint infection (septic arthritis or osteomyelitis).

The foal should be exercised to evaluate the change in the degree of angular deformity and to observe any signs of lameness. Young foals with an angular limb deformity of the carpus resulting from hypoplasia of the carpal bones, ligament laxity, and incomplete development of the metacarpal bones frequently exhibit an increased angular deformity during weight bearing and a relative straightening of the limb when it is not

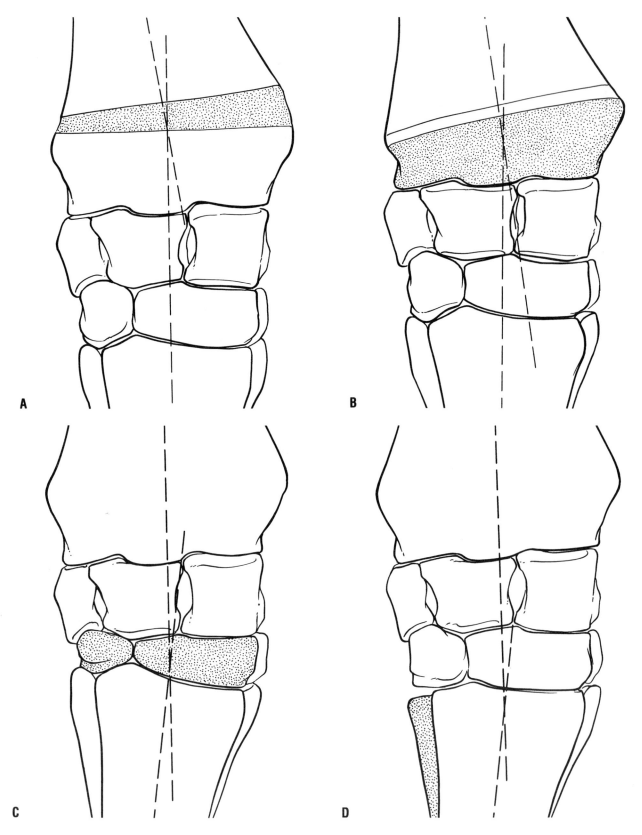

Fig. 5–102. Front view of distal radius and carpus. In each example, one line bisects the cannon bone, the other line bisects the radius. The intersection of the lines indicates the pivot point. Stippled areas indicate the location of the problem. *A,* The pivot point is centered over the physis. Asynchronous growth of the distal radial metaphysis is the cause. *B,* The pivot point is centered over the distal epiphysis of the radius. Wedging of the epiphysis is illustrated (stippled area). *C,* The pivot point is centered over the carpal joints. Wedging of the third carpal bone and hypoplasia of the fourth carpal bone is illustrated (stippled area). *D,* The pivot point is centered over the distal carpal joints. Incomplete development of the lateral splint bone is illustrated (stippled area).

bearing any weight. In most cases lameness is not a feature of an angular limb deformity. If it is present, it may be the limb opposite the unilateral angular limb deformity that is affected. A thorough evaluation of the lame limb in this situation is required.

On palpation, the affected limb or limbs should be examined for heat, pain and swelling, and laxity of the limb distal to the carpus. Heat, pain, and swelling associated with lameness may indicate recent trauma or infection from a navel ill or other systemic infectious disease. Swelling of the carpal joint associated with the angular limb deformity may indicate hypoplasia or collapse of the carpal bones. Swelling associated with the distal growth plate of the radius may indicate infection, trauma, or physitis.

Manipulation of the distal limb can be very helpful in defining where the center of deviation of the angular deformity is located. Typically, a looseness or instability of the carpus in a lateral-to-medial direction is felt with ligament laxity, hypoplasia of the carpal bones, collapse of the carpal bones, and incomplete development of the small metacarpal bones. A cranial-to-caudal laxity can be appreciated with collapsed or subluxated carpal bones. Conversely, the distal limb will feel fairly stable with asymmetric growth of the distal radial metaphysis and alterations of the distal radial epiphysis. In all cases, x-rays of the affected limb should be taken.

An X-ray Examination. An x-ray examination of the carpus is extremely important in identifying the structural changes associated with soft tissue and bone as well as identifying the center of deviation (pivot point). Only with this information can a logical course of therapy be developed.

The identification of the center of deviation (pivot point) and the degree of deviation can be determined by placing an overlay of acetate, or an unexposed x-ray film over the cranial-caudal view. Two lines are drawn; one bisects the center of the radius, and the other bisects the center of the third metacarpal bone. Where these two lines intersect is considered the pivot point or center of deviation (see Fig. 5-102A–D). The acute angle formed by this intersection is measured with a protractor and represents the degree of angular deformity. To monitor progress between x-ray examinations, a goniometer (an instrument for measuring angles) can be used to make external measurements on the foal's limbs. Holding the upper arm of the instrument centered on the radius and the lower arm centered on the cannon bone will allow documentation of angle change. When the pivot point is difficult to identify, more than one site may be contributing to the angular limb deformity (e.g., wedging of the distal radial physis plus cuboidal bone hypoplasia).

If the pivot point is located over or near the distal radial physis, asynchronous longitudal growth of the metaphysis should be suspected (see Fig. 5-102A). A pivot point located just distal to the growth plate would indicate an abnormality in the distal radial epiphysis that is contributing to the angular deformity

(see Fig. 5-102B). In most cases, asynchronous growth across the distal radial epiphysis is usually associated with asynchronous growth of the metaphysis. This causes the magnitude of the angular limb deformity to be greater than if the distal radial metaphysis was singularly involved. Hypoplasia of the cuboidal bones shifts the pivot point distal into the radiocarpal or intercarpal joint (see Fig. 5-102C). Alterations in the development of the splint bones results in a further shifting of the pivot point distal (see Fig. 5-102D). It must be remembered that evaluation of the pivot point may be influenced by multiple levels of structural involvement and may only serve as a guide.

Treatment

Correction of angular limb deformity is desirable to improve the conformational defect as well as to prevent secondary degenerative changes that may result from abnormal biomechanical stresses on the deviated limb. Correction of as much of the outward rotation of the limb distal to the carpus is also desirable.

Essentially, there are four therapeutic options that can be considered for an angular deformity associated with the carpus. The treatments include: 1) Stall rest with altered nutrition, 2) the application of a tube (sleeve) cast for conditions that result in joint instability, 3) temporary transphyseal bridging with screws and wires or staples ("stapling") to arrest the growth on the convex side of the growth plate, 4) periosteal stripping ("stripping") to stimulate the growth on the concave side. The rationale for selection of any one treatment is dependent on whether the angular deformity is congenital or acquired, is improving, staying the same or worsening, and what structural changes are present.

Many foals born with minor angular deformities of the carpus progressively improve during the first few weeks of life and require no therapy at all. One must assume that in these cases the compressive forces fell within physiologic limits and the appropriate growth changes occurred to straighten the limb. Many foals born with joint laxity due to inadequate soft tissue support and foals with natural crookedness (carpus valgus) (Fig. 5-103) respond in this manner. Other foals may improve more slowly; for these animals, stall confinement, corrective hoof trimming, and nutritional management often work well.

Confinement is recommended because foals make every attempt to stay with the mares while they are on pasture. This active exercise increases the axial compressive forces to the growth plate, or remodeling epiphysis, or cuboidal bones which may result in delayed or asynchronous growth. Stall confinement will help decrease the trauma to these regions.

Corrective hoof trimming (shortening the long side of the hoof wall) may be necessary to bring the foot back into balance. With carpus valgus, the medial side of the hoof wall is often worn excessively (shorter) and the lateral side of the hoof wall may require rasping.

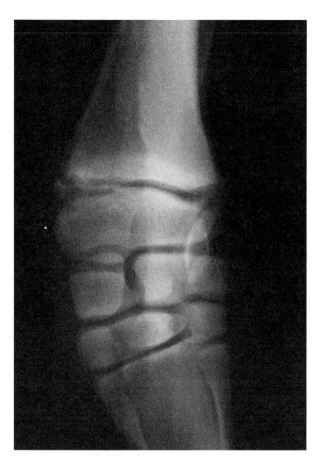

FIG. 5–103. X-ray of left front leg of foal with valgus deformity. Note the irregular width of the growth plate, the wedging of the epiphysis and the third carpal bone, and the hypoplasia of the fourth carpal bone and lateral splint bone.

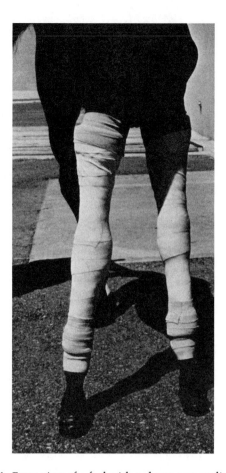

FIG. 5–104. Front view of a foal with a sleeve cast applied to both forelimbs.

Typically, these foals also have a tendency to break over on the inside of the toe. To get the hoof to break over more centrally, it is often helpful to square the hoof wall with a rasp at the center of the toe.

Nutritional management should include good quality alfalfa, with free choice balanced mineral supplements and restriction of concentrates. Foals that do not respond to this conservative management in 2 to 3 weeks, and in which the angular limb deformity remains static or worsens, should be examined immediately by a veterinarian. In cases in which the angular limb deformity is worsening rapidly with conservative management, the foals should be seen sooner. Most of them will require one of the forms of therapy discussed below. Any acquired or congenital angular limb deformity that does not respond to conservative management usually requires casting (Fig. 5–104) or surgical treatment.

Cast and splint applications are used in situations in which the physical examination has pointed to a carpal joint instability (usually in a lateral to medial direction) as the cause of the angular deformity and the limb can be straightened by manipulation. Usually x-rays identify structural changes in the cuboidal

bones (hypoplasia or collapse), proximal splint bones, and/or joint laxity from lack of soft tissue support. The pivot point may be anywhere in the carpal joint region. In some cases a multilevel structural involvement will be identified, and surgery plus casting may be necessary. Cases of cuboidal bone hypoplasia and beginning collapse should be treated early because the cuboidal bones ossify at 3 to 4 weeks of age. If such cases are left untreated, the cuboidal malformation may be permanent. However, with early treatment the problem is usually reversible. In most cases general anesthesia is used and a fiberglass cast is applied from the proximal radius to the distal cannon. The fetlock and foot are left exposed so that normal axial weight bearing can occur. This casting technique provides rigid support to the carpus without promoting osteoporosis, muscle atrophy, and tendon laxity which is associated with full-limb casting techniques. Alternatively, braces can be used (Fig. 5–105). Some prefer braces because they can be adjusted as the angular limb deformity improves. However, daily resetting of the braces is a drawback.

The foal and mare should be kept in stall confinement. The cast will be removed in about 10 to 14 days, and a thorough physical, x-ray examination of the

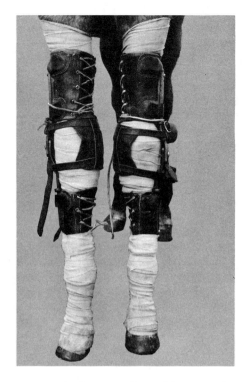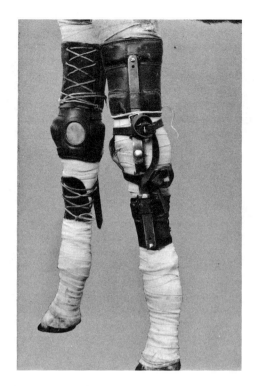

FIG. 5–105. Front and side views of hinged braces used to straighten mild medial deviation of the carpi. These braces can be reversed for lateral deviation. They must be adjusted daily to avoid pressure necrosis. Because the brace is hinged, there is very little muscle atrophy.

limb is performed at this time. If the laxity is still very obvious (rare), another sleeve cast is applied. Two to 4 weeks are usually sufficient to allow maturation of hypoplastic carpal bones and the stabilization of soft tissues, and only rarely will another cast have to be applied.

Surgical Techniques

Temporary Transphyseal (Across the Physis) Bridging with Staples or Screws and Wires. Temporary transphyseal bridging of the distal radial physis with screws and wires, (preferred approach) staples placed on the convex side is used in cases in which asynchronous longitudinal growth occurs at the distal radial metaphysis and/or the distal radial epiphysis. The theory behind temporary transphyseal bridging is that, when the physis is bridged on the convex side, it effectively arrests longitudinal growth until the opposite (concave) side catches up. The less the change in the structure of the distal radial epiphysis the better the final outcome.

Both stapling and screw and wiring are effective methods in straightening an angular deformity if sufficient growth potential is left in the distal radial physis and articular cartilage of the epiphysis. Timing is an important consideration for either procedure. Although the distal radial growth plate does not close on x-ray until 22 to 36 months, it has been shown that active growth continues only until 18 months of age.

Approximately 71% of the longitudinal growth takes place within 12 months, and the most rapid longitudinal growth occurs between 0 and 8 months of age. Surgery should be performed before 2 to 3 months of age. Also, the severity of the deformity must be considered. Foals that have a severe angular deformity that is progressively worsening are definitely candidates for temporary transphyseal bridging at that time. Most carpal deviation emanating from asynchronous growth of the distal radial metaphysis or epiphysis that is greater than 15° should be considered for temporary transphyseal bridging immediately. This technique has been used successfully in foals as early as 2 weeks of age.

Postoperative care for temporary transphyseal bridging with screws and wires (Fig. 5–107) is the same for stapling. It should consist of stall confinement and maintenance of pressure support wraps for two-weeks duration. It is absolutely imperative to maintain the mare and foal in stall confinement during convalescence and until the angular deformity is corrected and the staples are removed (Fig. 5–106). The staples and/ or screws and wires are removed when the limb is straight. If two limbs have been bridged temporarily and one limb straightens before the other, it will have to be removed at the time and the other removed later. The decision as to whether the limb is straight or not requires an informed, cooperative effort between the owner and the veterinarian. Sometimes it is difficult to assess limb straightening. To do this properly requires visual observation while the foal is standing, at

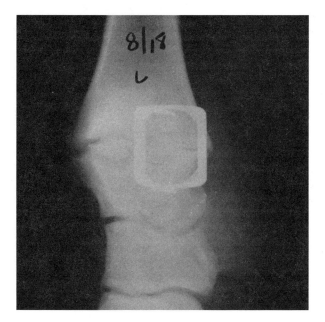

FIG. 5–106. An example of two staples that were inserted properly.

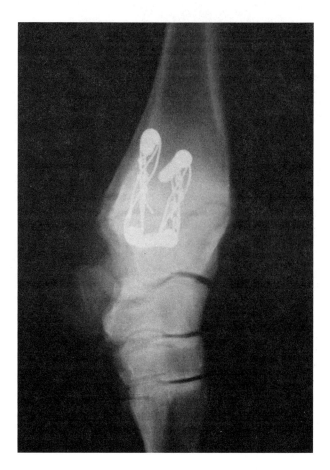

FIG. 5–107. An example of an older foal treated with two sets of screws and wires.

exercise, and during physical manipulation of the limb. It is important that during convalescence the foot of the affected limb or limbs be rasped if necessary about every 2 weeks to compensate for the change in the angular deformity.

A limiting factor to the successful outcome of temporary transphyseal bridging is when the angular deviation is greater than the potential for correcting the ability of the long bone growth. Younger foals are obviously more responsive to temporary transphyseal bridging. This is an important consideration in the selection of surgical candidates. Average correction times in relation to the age at which surgery is performed is listed in Table 5–2.

Both screw and wire and stapling are effective in straightening angular limb deformities. However, the screw and wire technique is less complicated, the screws and wires are easier to remove, and for these reasons this method is recommended as the treatment of choice.

Periosteal Elevation Stripping. Periosteal stripping is a highly successful, commonly used surgical technique. The periosteal connective tissue fibers on the concave side (too short side) of the metaphysis of the radius are cut to relieve the restrictive tension and thus accelerate growth. Following periosteal stripping there is stimulation of the endochondral ossification on that side also.

The surgery is relatively simple and requires minimal instrumentation. The growth plate on the concave side (opposite the side that temporary transphyseal bridging would be done) is approached through a longitudinal incision. An incision is created to form an inverted T (Fig. 5–108). Once the incision is complete, the periosteum is undermined and lifted up. The incision is sutured. Pressure wraps are applied and

TABLE 5–2. *Average Correction Times After Transphyseal Bridging With Staples*

Age and Month	Average Correction in Weeks
0–3	$5\frac{1}{2}$
6–9	$8\frac{1}{2}$
9+	12 and over

maintained for 2 weeks, and stall rest is recommended until the limb is straight. This technique has been used successfully alone or in combination with screw and wire temporary transphyseal bridging.

A combination of temporary transphyseal bridging and periosteal stripping is used in foals that have a combination of problems that lead to angular deformity and in foals with a severe angular deformity.

Prognosis

Generally, the more abnormalities observed distal to the distal radial physis and the more distal the pivot point, the poorer the prognosis. Achievement of complete straightening of the limb is not possible with temporary transphyseal bridging if there is a severe wedging of the epiphysis, but the limb can be straightened considerably. Collapse of the carpal bones and fracture plus injuries to the growth plate carry a poor prognosis. In general, a high degree of success can be expected with the treatments described if these foals are examined and treated early in the course of this condition.

Bucked Knees

Bucked knees is a deformity consisting of a dorsal deviation of the carpus (knee) that causes an alteration in the articulations of the bones forming the joint and results in constant partial flexion of the carpus.

Causes

Several factors are involved in the cause of bucked knees. Many horses exhibit a mild dorsal deviation of both carpi, but this may not be serious, as it is often the result of a congenital condition. Congenital types may be the result of positioning of the limbs in the uterus or of a mineral or vitamin deficiency in the mare.

Some cases of bucked knees are caused by trauma, when certain lamenesses cause inactivity of the extensor group of muscles, allowing the flexors to establish supremacy. Injury to the suspensory ligament, to the deep and/or superficial flexor tendons, or to the heel of the foot often causes a horse to rest the carpus in a flexed position. If the pain persists, the muscle/tendon units contract to such a degree that the carpus cannot be straightened. In some cases carpal injury, such as carpitis, may also cause dorsal deviation of the joint to relieve pain, which will cause contraction of the flexor muscles and tendons. Bucked knee caused by trauma is usually unilateral.

Dorsal deviation of the carpus can also occur secondary to rupture of the common digital extensor tendon within its carpal sheath. In some the opposite sequence is probably true and the carpal flexure deformity contributes to the rupture of the common digital extensor tendon.

Signs and Diagnosis

The severity of bucked knees varies considerably. In some cases the condition is very mild, while in others it is extreme. When the affected horse is in the normal standing position, one or both carpi will be flexed forward at varying degrees. This inhibits normal movement and gait, as there is a shortening of the cranial phase of the stride. The condition may be so pronounced that the horse falls to its knees while standing or walking. The carpus or carpi may be unable to support their share of weight, so damage may occur to other regions of the limb. Knuckling of the fetlock may also be present in this condition as a re-

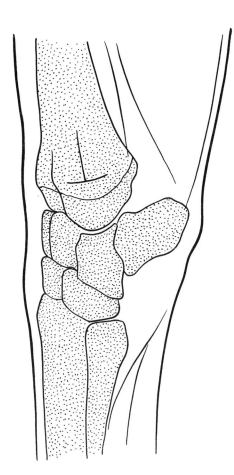

FIG. 5–108. The position for periosteal incision.

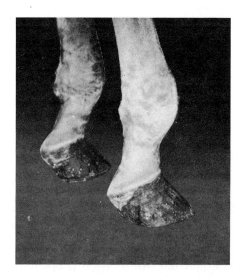

FIG. 5–109. "Cocked" ankles, caused by the shortening of the musculotendinous unit of the flexor tendons, can accompany bucked knees.

sult of the shortening of the muscle/tendon unit of the digital flexor tendon (Fig. 5–109).

Treatment

Bucked Knees in the Foal. If the condition is not severe, meaning that the foal can put its feet flat on the ground without knuckling over to the carpus, and if nutrition has been corrected, treatment often is not necessary. Many foals straighten up remarkably well by the time they are 6 months old. However, if lateral (varus) or medial (valgus) deviation of the carpal joints is present, in addition to bucked knees, corrective procedures may be necessary. If the condition is considered severe, the limbs may be put into a cast or a bandage splint is applied.

The foal should be left in the cast for approximately 10 days to 2 weeks. In many cases it will not be necessary to reapply the cast, but if a new cast is necessary, it should not be applied until 10 to 14 days after the first cast is removed. This interval will allow the foal to partially overcome the effects of disuse atrophy in the musculature. A second cast should be applied in the same manner as the first and removed after 10 to 14 days. An alternative to applying a cast is to use a bandage splint incorporating polyvinyl chloride (PVC).

A complete check of the horse's diet should be made, and the diet fortified, if necessary, with those elements considered deficient. Foals that develop bucked knees after birth should be checked for imbalanced or excess nutrition.

Bucked Knees Due to Injury. When a bucked-knee condition is caused by injury to the carpus or other structures, it is necessary to direct treatment at correction of the original pathologic changes. The bucked-knee condition will usually then take care of itself. Pathologic changes in the flexor tendons, suspensory ligament, foot, extensor tendons, or carpus are most often responsible for this type of bucked knee. If the condition is not of long duration and is corrected promptly, the muscle/tendon unit will gradually stretch, and the carpus will again assume a normal position.

Surgical Correction. When bucked knees are so severe in a foal that the condition cannot be properly corrected with casts, or when the condition persists in a mature horse after injury to some structure, so that there is little hope of natural correction, a tenotomy (tendon division) of the ulnaris lateralis and the flexor carpi ulnaris tendons may be necessary. This operation is most successful for bucked knees that result from trauma and is less successful for those that are congenital. Frequently the carpal bones are deformed in congenital bucked knees, whereas in an acquired condition, the carpal bones are relatively normal. In addition, congenital bucked knees show contraction of the deep and superficial flexor muscle/tendon units, as well as the ulnaris lateralis and flexor

carpi ulnaris. The suspensory ligament can also be involved.

Surgical correction can be performed with the horse in standing position if it is tractable, but general anesthesia is usually used. Tranquilization and sedation will be necessary if the operation is to be done while the horse is standing. The operative region is 1 to $1\frac{1}{2}$-inches above the accessory carpal bone on the caudal aspect of the limb.

The region is kept bandaged for at least 10 days. The patient should not be worked for 6 to 8 weeks. If the limb cannot be fully straightened following tenotomy, it is beneficial to place the limb in a cast from elbow to fetlock joint. This cast should be left in place 10 to 14 days.

Prognosis

The prognosis is guarded in all acquired cases of bucked knees, and it is to be expected that some horses will never be returned to full use. However, most conditions of this kind can be improved so that the horse can serve as a useful breeding animal. The prognosis is favorable in mild, congenital types if the nutrition of the foal has been good or is corrected. Severe congenital types result in an unfavorable prognosis.

Rupture of the Extensor Carpi Radialis Tendon

Rupture of the extensor carpi radialis tendon is comparatively rare. The signs of lameness are distinctive, making it easy to diagnose.

Cause

The cause is trauma. The logical conclusion is that overflexion of the limb would be most apt to cause rupture of this tendon. In most cases, the actual cause is not known.

Signs

With the resistance of the extensor carpi radialis tendon gone, the flexor tendons are able to overflex the limb. Careful observation of the gait will show that in the affected limb the carpus flexes considerably more than the carpus of the normal limb. The tendon sheath of the extensor carpi radialis will be distended. Extension is accomplished by means of the common digital extensor and the lateral digital extensor. After the rupture has been present for a short time, atrophy of the muscular portion of the extensor carpi radialis begins. Palpation over the carpus will reveal the absence of the tendon on the dorsal surface of the carpus.

Treatment

If the rupture is complete and found soon after it occurs, it may be possible to bring the ends of the tendon together surgically. In this case, the limb would be kept in a cast for approximately 6 weeks. In cases of longer duration, it is impossible to bring the tendon ends together. One may be able to substitute the tendon of the extensor carpi obliquus by using tendon suturing. With partial rupture of the extensor carpi radialis tendon, debridement of the adhesion, suturing of longitudinal splits in the tendon and suturing of a torn tendon sheath has proven beneficial.

Prognosis

Prognosis is unfavorable for complete rupture. In horses valuable enough to warrant surgery, either tendon suturing or substitution with extensor carpi obliquus may be used.

The prognosis is favorable for partial tears and longitudinal splitting of the extensor carpi radialis tendon and its sheath if surgery is performed.

Rupture of the Common Digital Extensor Tendon

This condition most frequently affects both forelimbs in young foals and is generally present at birth or develops soon after. Affected foals may have accompanying multiple birth defects, including hypoplasia (underdevelopment) of the carpal bones, underdeveloped pectoral muscles, and also may have a misalignment of the jaw bones. This implies that the extensor rupture may be part of a complex congenital defect. A flexure deformity of the carpus or fetlock may also accompany the rupture. A higher incidence of this disease has been reported in Arabians, Quarter Horses, and Arabian-Quarter Horse crosses.

Causes

This condition may be inheritable and may be part of a complex congenital defect in development. However, it is difficult to decide in some cases whether the flexure deformity of the carpus results in the rupture of the common digital extensor tendon or, in fact, develops secondary to the rupture of the common digital extensor. It is also postulated that rupture of the common digital extensor tendon could result from a single or repeated forced extension of the carpus against resistance.

Signs

A distinguishing characteristic for this problem is the presence of swelling over the dorsolateral surface of the carpus near the level of the distal carpal joint (Fig. 5–110). Foals may be able to stand normally but frequently knuckle forward at the fetlock during progression. In foals that are exhibiting varying degrees of flexure deformities, the diagnosis of rupture of the common digital extensor tendon may go unrecognized and a primary diagnosis of the carpal flexure deformity may be made.

On palpation, fluid distention of the common digital extensor flexor tendon sheath is detected. The blunted ends of the extensor tendon may or may not be felt, and this is totally dependent on the amount of synovial fluid present in the sheath. In those cases in which an excessive amount of fluid is present, aseptic needle aspiration of the synovial fluid might be necessary to allow a more definitive palpation of these tendons. Flexion of the carpal joints usually does not cause a painful response.

Diagnosis

The diagnosis is made from the physical examination. The palpation of the blunted ends of the sepa-

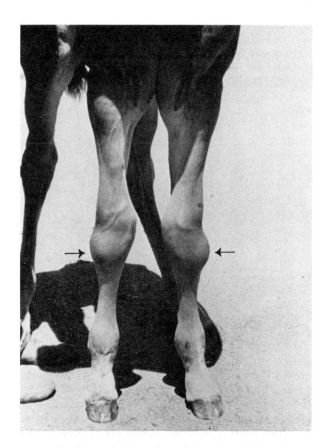

FIG. 5–110. A foal with bilateral rupture of the common digital extensor tendon. Arrows point to the swellings on the dorsal lateral surfaces overlying both carpi.

rated extensor tendon and ultrasound examination provides a definitive diagnosis. Radiographs may need to be taken of the carpus to rule out hypoplasia (abnormal development) of the carpal bones.

Treatment

In general, those foals that do not have a severe flexure deformity of the carpus are treated conservatively with stall rest. The application of bandages to support the carpus and protect the front of the fetlock from abrasions is recommended. Return to function usually occurs without surgery. It is unlikely that the ruptured tendon ends reunite, but rather they adhere to the sheath and, with time, the lateral digital extensor tendon takes over most of the function of the common digital extensor.

Tube casts or polyvinyl chloride (PVC) bandage splints can be used in foals exhibiting flexure deformities of the carpus, but careful monitoring of these must follow. If the flexure deformity involves the fetlock joint and is severe, carpal (inferior) check ligament desmotomy surgically (severing a tendon) may be required to straighten the limb. After surgery PVC bandage splints are used to support the limb in forced extension.

Prognosis

The prognosis for uncomplicated cases of rupture of the common digital extensor tendon appears to be good, and healing usually results with minimal blemish.

The prognosis is guarded for those cases exhibiting severe carpal flexure deformity in association with rupture of the extensor tendon.

Contracted Tendons and Flexure Deformities

Refer to Chapter 4.

Hygroma of the Carpus

A hygroma is a synovial swelling over the dorsal surface of the carpus. Most commonly, it is an acquired bursitis (inflammation of a bursa) resulting from trauma. Normally there is no bursa in this region, but through trauma a bursa may form. The tendon sheath of the extensor carpi radialis or the common digital extensor muscles may also be involved. A synovial hernia of the knee joint capsule can occur. This causes a swelling that is almost indistinguishable from that caused by an acquired bursitis. However, careful examination will reveal that the swelling on the dorsal surface of the carpus is irregular in out-

line and does not uniformly cover the carpus when a synovial hernia has occurred. Acquired bursitis shows an evenly distributed swelling over the surface of the carpus.

Causes

Trauma is the cause in all cases. Horses that get up and down on hard ground most commonly are involved. Hygroma also can be produced as a result of a horse pawing and hitting the carpus on a hard surface such as a wall.

Signs

Signs are swellings of varying shapes over the dorsal surface of the carpus. The swellings vary with the structure or structures involved (Fig. 5–111).

Diagnosis

The diagnosis is made by needle drainage and submission of the fluid for cell analysis. Acute hygroma will result in the formation of a fluid more like serum or water. In chronic cases the fluid becomes thicker and stickier like synovial fluid. If the veterinarian is suspicious of a synovial fistula emanating from a car-

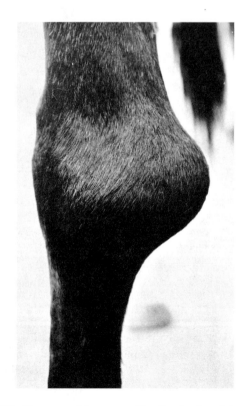

FIG. 5–111. Hygroma of the carpus. The distribution of the swelling indicates a primary involvement of the midcarpal joint capsule.

pal joint or tendon sheath, either of these structures can be injected with contrast material and then x-rayed to identify the communication (Fig. 5–112).

Treatment

Injection of corticoids, followed by counterpressure with elastic bandage, appears to be an effective method of treatment. Injections should be repeated 3 to 5 times at intervals of a week. Continued pressure of the elastic bandage is used to promote adhesions between the distended skin and underlying tissues. The distended skin will thicken, producing a permanent blemish.

Acute cases that have not responded to previously described treatment can be treated by incisional drainage. After sterile bandaging, a polyvinyl chloride (PVC) pipe extension splint is applied to the palmar surface of the carpus. The extension splint is maintained for 10 to 14 days. This is usually a sufficient period to allow adhesions between the two surfaces to occur. Because it is imperative to maintain a drain under the splint in an antiseptic environment (including the application of sterile bandages) the patient may need to be maintained in a veterinary clinic. Drains are a two-way street, and the risk of ascending infection is ever present. In most cases this procedure will result in cosmetic healing.

A hygroma of long standing with a thickened synovial lining can be surgically removed under general anesthesia.

The operative site is handled and maintained in a manner similar to that described for more acute cases.

Prognosis

Prognosis is guarded to favorable. Old cases will retain considerable swelling because of fibrous tissue that has been laid down in the inflamed region. Such cases usually have an unfavorable prognosis because adhesions may not form following corticoid therapy, and the lesion may require surgical drainage or removal.

Intraarticular Fractures of the Carpus (Knee)

Intraarticular fractures (fractures within the joint cavity) associated with the carpal bones and the distal end of the radius are common injuries in racing horses, hunters, jumpers, and actively performing horses in other breeds. An increased incidence of this lesion has been observed in young Thoroughbred horses between 2 and 4 years of age that train and race on dirt. Factors such as speed, immaturity, longer limb length, position of the jockey, and distances run and firm surfaces tend to generate tremendous concussive forces that focus on the dorsal surface of the carpal bones. The fracture can be a simple chip fracture (the most common), slab fracture, or fragmented (comminuted) fracture. The latter occurs rarely.

Chip fractures (osteochondral fragments) involve only one articular surface. They vary in size and location and can be firmly attached, moderately loose, or free floating as joint mice (Fig. 5–113). The radial,

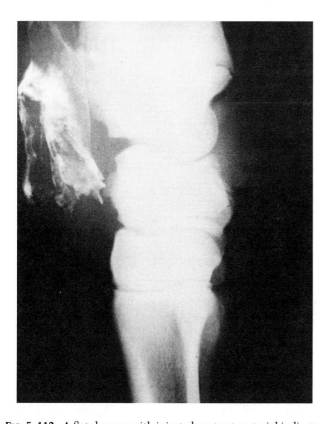

FIG. 5–112. A fistulogram with injected contrast material indicates involvement of a tendon sheath.

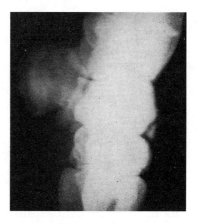

FIG. 5–113. Fracture of the radial carpal bone, viewed on a lateral x-ray of the carpus. In this case, oblique views were necessary to determine whether the intermediate or the radial carpal bone was fractured.

third, and intermediate carpal bones and the distal end of the radius are most commonly affected with chip fractures (Fig. 5–114). Only rarely do carpal chip fractures involve the carpometacarpal (junction with the cannon) joint. Most chip fractures occur on the dorsomedial borders of the carpal bones and the dorsolateral surface of the distal end of the radius. It is not uncommon to have multiple small chip fractures within the same joint or adjacent joints or to find intraarticular fractures in the opposite limb. In cases in which both right and left carpal joints are involved, a fracture probably occurs in one, causing increased weight bearing on the other leading to a fracture.

The direction in which these horses are raced appears to play a role as to which forelimb is affected. Horses raced in a counterclockwise direction have an increased incidence of chip fractures in the right forelimb, whereas the reverse is true for horses raced in a clockwise direction in which the left forelimb is more frequently involved. This could be considered unusual since it would appear logical that the greatest force is being absorbed by the inside limb. However, two factors are important to consider with the horse racing around turns. When the stresses are analyzed, increased concussive forces occur on the lateral surface of the inside limb (left limb) and the medial surface of the outside limb (right limb) in the turn and, of course,

this is where the majority of carpal fractures occur. It also may be that when racing around turns the horse counteracts the centrifugal force by bearing more weight on the outside limb. Also, race horses frequently shift to the right lead on the straightaways and are in the right lead at the end of races which places a greater stress on this limb as the horse becomes fatigued.

Slab fractures, unlike chip fractures, extend through the full thickness of the bone to involve both proximal and distal joint surfaces (Fig. 5–115). They can involve any of the carpal bones but the most commonly affected are the third, followed by the intermediate and radial carpal bones. Slab fractures usually involve the dorsal surface of the bone and are of variable thickness. There appears to be a higher incidence of slab fracture of the third carpal bone of the right forelimb which is contrasted with the increased incidence of chip fractures of the left third carpal bone.

Fragmented fractures can involve any or all of the carpal bones, but they most frequently affect the radial, intermediate, and fourth carpal bones. Fragmentation can accompany chip and slab fractures as well. A great degree of instability results with these fractures which must be counteracted for treatment to be successful.

Oblique fractures of the distal end of the radius are rare, and the reader is referred to the Fractures of the Radius section in this chapter for further discussion.

Anatomy and Biomechanics

The carpus is made up of three joint spaces and six weight-bearing bones which are supported (held together) by intercarpal ligaments (see Fig. 5–114). It is the only joint in the horse through which vertical axial forces are thrust through one long bone (the radius) to the other (the cannon). This arrangement makes the carpus more susceptible to compressive trauma. Although there are six weight-bearing carpal bones, they

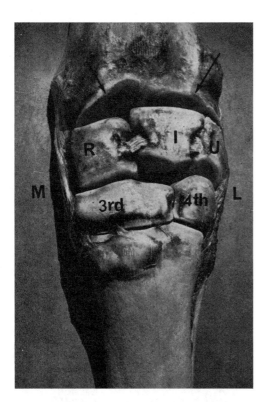

FIG. 5–114. Normal left bony carpus. Arrows indicate areas where chip fractures may occur on radius. The joints from proximal to distal are the antebrachiocarpal (radiocarpal), the midcarpal (intercarpal), and the carpometacarpal. U, ulnar carpal bone; I, intermediate carpal bone; R, radial carpal bone; 3rd, third carpal bone; 4th, fourth carpal bone; L, lateral side; M, medial side.

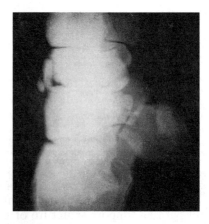

FIG. 5–115. Lateral view showing a fracture of the third carpal bone. Note that two pieces of the third carpal bone have broken off. The large piece is a typical "slab" fracture.

do not share equally in the weight bearing, and the radial, intermediate, and third carpal bones bear most of the weight. Because of this, they are more susceptible to trauma and fracture.

The antebrachial and middle carpal joints allow flexion and extension of the carpus while the carpometacarpal joint remains relatively immobile. During flexion, the antebrachial and middle carpal joints open dorsally and the carpal bones begin to move out of their weight-bearing alignment as much as their intercarpal ligaments will allow. As the foot contacts the ground, these joint spaces begin to close, and at the same time the carpal bones begin to shift back to their weight-bearing position. As the weight-bearing load is accepted, the carpal bones begin to separate laterally and medially from each other, which allows some dissipation of forces. The intercarpal ligaments between the carpal bones become stretched, which transmits some of the axial load to these ligaments. Unfortunately, the medial aspect of the middle carpal joint is unable to attenuate weight-bearing stress by interosseous displacement of the carpal bone, and therefore is more susceptible to load trauma.

Because the antebrachiocarpal joint is a rotating joint, overextension during weight bearing is resisted by palmar soft tissue support structures (joint capsule and flexor tendons). Unlike the antebrachiocarpal joint, the middle carpal joint is a hinged joint that cannot overextend because of the palmar location of the collateral ligaments and the configuration of the joint surface. Because of these differences, it is felt that proper training is very important to strengthen the palmar soft tissue support structures of the antebrachiocarpal joint to resist overextension and to condition the carpal bones in the middle carpal joint to withstand these load stresses.

Cause

Trauma from repeated concussion (internal axial compression) and shear forces or external blows appears to be the cause. Because of the differences in dynamics of the antebrachiocarpal joint and the middle carpal joint, acute injury from overextension is more likely to injure the antebrachiocarpal joint, whereas chronic repeated overload is more apt to injure the middle carpal joint. However, both joints are susceptible to injury from supraphysiologic loads, of which fatigue is probably the most important cause. Proper training should stimulate gradual adaptation of the carpal bones, intercarpal ligaments, and palmar support structures of the antebrachiocarpal joint. If training proceeds faster than these structures can adapt, injury will occur.

Initially, clinical signs of inflammation in the carpus are often caused by soft tissue trauma (intercarpal ligaments and palmar support structure of the antebrachiocarpal joint), and this is referred to as carpitis. This is usually seen in young horses put into training. With the appropriate treatment, the inflammation re-

solves, but the bones continue to adapt to increasing stresses. If training increases and exceeds the ability of these bones to remodel and strengthen, fatigue damage results in microcracking of the subchondral (below the articular cartilage) bone, which weakens the bone and makes it softer and more susceptible to fracture. If this softening occurs on the dorsal margins of the carpal bones, it results in chip fractures. If the bone softening occurs palmar to the dorsal margin, a slab fracture results. Slab fractures are thought to develop as a result of a change in shape of the bone above it, which further focuses stress in a small area, eventually causing bone weakening, softening, and fracture.

Although chronic accumulation of stress causes many of these fractures, acute marginal fracture and crush fractures (fragmented) occur in short distance sprinters (e.g., racing Quarter Horses) following a single acute overloading of the bone. Because many sprinters approach racing fitness without sufficient conditioning exercise to allow the carpal bones to adapt, the threshold of resistance to fracture is lowered and fracture may result.

Contributing factors such as fatigue, extreme speed, poor racing surfaces, an improper angle of the race track, and improper or irregular trimming can result in an asynchronous distribution of the internal forces within the carpus, resulting in trauma.

Fatigue creates abnormal compression on the dorsal surface of the carpal bones in two ways. First, as fatigue progresses, the soft tissue structures supporting the carpus (muscles, tendons, and ligaments) become weakened and an uncoordinated, compensatory overstriding results. More specifically, as the extensor muscle groups begin to fatigue, the foot begins to impact before the limb is in full extension. This results in a backward, snapping, or slamming effect of the carpus rather than a smooth, interlocking of the carpal bones. As the flexor muscles begin to fatigue, the caudal support to the carpus (primarily the antebrachiocarpal joint) is reduced during maximal loading and an overextension can occur (Fig. 5–116). Both result in increased trauma to the dorsal surfaces of the carpal bones.

Faulty conformation plays a significant role when dealing with high speed performance. Horses that are "back in the knees" (calf kneed) are particularly predisposed to carpal fracture. During maximal loading stresses become concentrated on the dorsal surface of the carpal bones. Continued repeated uneven loading leads to progressive weakening of the bone and damage to the articular surface, and an articular fracture results. Most European-bred race-horses are slightly over in the knees. They also race as 3-year-olds rather than 2-year-olds, they run on turf, their turns are very subtle, and they race in both counterclockwise and clockwise directions. These differences result in a decreased incidence of carpal chip fractures in European race horses vs US racehorses.

Improper or irregular trimming and shoeing resulting in an imbalanced foot can cause unequal distri-

FIG. 5–116. Mechanism of carpal fractures. Notice severe extension of the left carpus. (Courtesy of Dr. W. Berkley.)

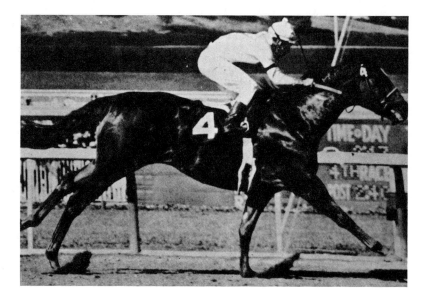

bution of forces up the entire limb to affect the carpus as well. The common practice of lowering the heel and leaving the toe long will lead to abnormal uneven stresses on the carpus. So will extending the period between shoeings to the point that the hoof has grown out of dorsal/palmar balance.

Signs

Signs of carpitis are primarily seen in young horses that have starting into training and include varying degrees of heat, pain, joint distention, and lameness. With an acute chip fracture, the synovitis maybe relatively diffuse (involving the whole joint) at first, eventually becoming more localized in the soft tissue over the chip fracture. This point swelling is usually over the dorsomedial surface of the carpal joints, an area of the joint capsule not covered by ligaments or tendons. With slab fractures, the swelling tends to remain as diffuse swelling that later results in an organized diffuse thickening of the joint capsule. This swelling is usually associated with the midcarpal joint and results from a slab fracture of the third carpal bone.

The degree of lameness depends on the extent, location, and duration of the fracture and the amount of degenerative joint disease that is present. In general, most horses with acute small articular fractures of the carpus exhibit minimal signs of lameness. Horses that have sustained acute large chip fractures or slab fractures usually stand with the carpus partially flexed. At exercise, varying degrees of shortening of the cranial phase of the stride and decreased height of the foot flight arc will be noted. The horse's gait no longer appears free moving, and he exhibits circumduction of the limb, resulting in a characteristic stiff-legged paddling motion indicative of the fact that carpal flexion causes pain. This stiff-gaited appearance is also seen in young horses with carpitis, and the condition is usually bilateral. Circling to the affected side usually increases the signs of lameness. Horses with more chronic fractures may exhibit minimal to moderate signs of lameness at exercise. As a rule, the earlier the problem is recognized, the easier it is to elicit pain and observe lameness.

The assessment of the degree of carpal flexion and the carpal flexion test can be valuable tools in the diagnosis of carpal lameness. Reduced, painful flexion is usually associated with acute intraarticular fractures and slab fractures. Frequently, horses with slab fractures violently resist flexion and rear up to avoid it. Nonpainful, reduced flexion, on the other hand, can result from chronic carpitis and old healed slab fractures. Rarely will chronic intraarticular chip fractures lead to decreased flexion. The carpal flexion test is performed by holding the carpus in a flexed position for 30–60 seconds after which the horse is exercised at a trot. Two or three abnormal steps are normally observed. However, if more are present it may indicate a problem within the carpus, particularly if there is a nodding-head lameness associated with it (see Chapter 3).

Palpation of the dorsal border of each carpal bone in both joints is also an important diagnostic tool. The extensor carpi radialis tendon provides a good landmark. Carpal bones medial to it include the radial and third carpal bones. Lateral to it are the intermediate carpal bone, ulnar carpal bone in the proximal row, and the lateral edge of the third carpal bone and fourth carpal bone in the distal row. All the dorsal surfaces of the carpal bones are palpated as well as the distal end of the radius to determine the fracture location (see Chapter 3, Fig. 3–26).

Diagnosis

Carpal lameness can be confirmed by a joint block. Twenty to 30 minutes after the injection the lameness is reevaluated. If there is any question regarding whether a fracture exists, it is recommended that x-rays be taken prior to injection. The sky line x-ray view of the carpal bones can be very helpful in some cases.

Treatment

Carpitis. Signs of inflammation within the carpus indicate that training is proceeding too rapidly for proper adaption of soft tissue and bone. Therefore treatment involves reducing the stress on the carpus by reducing the exercise for 2 to 3 weeks. Anti-inflammatory medication in the joint as well as systemic medication is often helpful in reducing the clinical signs, but remember, this is not curative, and the appropriate time must pass to allow adaption. If a rest period is not allowed, intra-articular fracture is common.

Chip Fractures. In cases of intra-articular chip fractures, there are essentially two treatments to select from, conservative management and surgical removal. The selection of treatment depends on the physical findings, the size and shape of the chip, and its location. Other factors that should be considered are the animal's age, its sex, and its intended future use. Whether a chip fracture is painful or not depends largely on the duration since injury, its size and location, and the degree of displacement from the parent bone. In general, small chip fractures firmly attached to the parent bone can be handled conservatively with variable periods of rest. This approach however is not recommended for horses used for racing. In these, surgical removal is generally the approach of choice. On physical examination, these horses may exhibit mild lameness or no lameness at exercise and exhibit minimal pain with limb manipulation and direct palpation over the chip fracture. On the other hand, large acute chip fractures with displacement that affects the weight bearing surface or that are floating free within the joint are best treated by surgery. Most of these horses will exhibit increased signs of lameness and increased pain on flexion and palpation when compared to those sustaining smaller chip fractures. These chip fractures should be removed as early as practical (within 10 to 14 days). During this period, the horse should be placed in stall confinement. The use of the arthroscope allows removal of these chips earlier without the complications attendant with arthrotomy (cutting into a joint). It is recommended that acute displaced chip fractures be removed to prevent further degenerative changes in the form of cartilage erosion, adjacent osteolysis (softening of bone), the formation of osteophytosis (bony outgrowths) and "kissing" lesions on the opposite joint surface. Although some of these chip fractures may heal with prolonged rest, considerable degenerative signs usually accompany these lesions, and not too infrequently these chips refracture when the horse is put back into training. Generally a free unattached or markedly displaced chip fracture is thought to create more problems than those that are intimately attached.

Conservative treatment of horses sustaining non-displaced chip fractures usually consists of stall confinement for 6 to 12 weeks with daily hand-walking beginning after 6 weeks. Free exercise can begin around the third and fourth month, and training can begin about the sixth to eighth month after the injury has occurred. This period is usually sufficient to allow adequate healing of the fracture. Nonsteroidal anti-inflammatory drugs can be used initially to reduce the acute inflammatory process. Intrasynovial injections of anti-inflammatory agents may be beneficial in reducing the synovitis, the progressive cartilage destruction, and the formation of osteophytes.

Removal of these chip fractures from the carpus using an arthroscope to visualize the fracture while it is being removed is now the method of choice. The benefits are a shorter surgery time, reduced requirement of bandaging, shorter convalescence to return to performance, and a more cosmetic end result. Large chip fractures can be successfully removed.

Sutures are removed in 12 to 14 days. Phenylbutazone is usually administered for 3 days postoperatively; however, this is optional and depends on the case. Antibiotics are continued for only 48 hours postoperatively.

Surgeons vary in their assessment of the necessary duration of rest after surgery is performed, from several weeks to a year. However, a rest period after arthroscopic surgery of 3 to 6 months is generally considered appropriate. Because of this, the following postoperative rest period is recommended. Box stall rest for a period of 6 weeks, after which the horse can be placed in a small run or paddock for another 6 to 8 weeks. High-spirited horses should be hand-walked or tranquilized before putting them outside. This is usually required for only the first few turnouts. After 3 to 4 months, the horse can be placed on pasture and slow training can begin at the recommended time postoperatively. Daily passive flexion of the carpus for variable periods postoperatively have been recommended by some.

Slab Fractures. Horses with slab fractures of the carpal bone should be surgically treated as soon as practical after the injury has occurred even if corticosteroids have been injected recently. The fracture must be stabilized to minimize the chance of further articular damage and degenerative joint disease.

If the slab fracture is small and thin or is in multiple pieces or degenerative changes have progressed to the point that reduction and stabilization cannot be achieved, they should be removed completely.

Larger acute slab fractures can be reattached to parent bone by interfragmentary compression using the lag screw principle. Slab fractures of the third carpal bone occur most frequently (Fig. 5–117).

A sterile nonadherent dressing is placed over the wound, and the limb is bandaged from the hoof to above the middle of the forearm. The bandage is intended to protect the joint while the animal recovers from anesthesia, and for the first 5 to 7 days after the surgery, it will aid in keeping swelling to a minimum. The bandage is removed in 5 to 7 days, and often the joint is the same size it was before surgery. At this time, the joint is usually cared for by applying snug elastic bandages, and the horse is confined to a box stall for at least 30 days. Counterpressure is maintained by the use of an elastic bandage and elastic tape for at least 4 weeks following surgery. Antibiotics may be given for 5 to 7 days after surgery. Phenylbutazone is administered to minimize pain and swelling after surgery.

Boxstall rest should be continued for 6 weeks postoperatively, after which the horse is maintained in confinement but hand-walked for 20 to 30 minutes 1 or 2 times a day. The handler should be prepared to restrain the horse because it may attempt to run and buck, which may reinjure the joint. After 3 months, x-rays should be taken to check for good screw fixation and bone healing. If healing is progressing normally, these horses can be placed on pasture and allowed free exercise. Light training can be started at 6 to 7 months postoperatively.

Slab fractures of the carpal bones that course in a dorsopalmar direction (sagittal fractures) are difficult to treat surgically. If they are not widely displaced, they can be treated conservatively following much the same regimen as described for lag screw fixation except the convalescence period may be prolonged.

Multiple Fragmented Fractures. Multiple fragmented carpal bone fractures occur infrequently, most commonly in racing and jumping horses. Because there is a loss of internal support, a valgus or varus angulation to the limb usually occurs. Treatment should be considered only for those horses with obvious breeding potential and/or great sentimental value, because only a few of these horses can be treated successfully. The limb should be immediately stabilized until x-rays can be taken to assess the degree of damage. In cases in which a single bone has been affected with fragmentation, internal fixation with screws can be used (Fig. 5–118). If several carpal bones are affected and a large number of fragments are present, an attempt should be made to provide some internal support with screw fixation. In selected cases, the carpus may have to be supported by bridging the carpus with two bone plates.

Prognosis

The prognosis for carpitis (generalized inflammation of the carpus) is generally good as long as an appropriate rest period is afforded and anti-inflammatory treatment is given. The prognosis for chip fractures that are treated by orthoscopic removal of the fragment depends on the degree of articular damage. Loss of articular cartilage up to 30% of the joint surface allows approximately 75% of horses to return to racing. If up to 50% of the articular cartilage is lost, only 50% of these horses are expected to return to racing. Large fractures, multiple fractures, and those cases that have excessive periosteal new bone growth, especially when near the articular surfaces, should be considered unfavorable surgical risks.

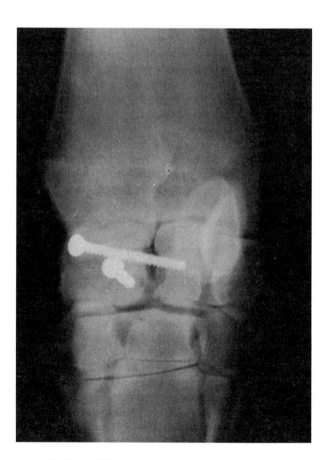

Fig. 5–118. Two ASIF bone screws were used to repair this fragmented fracture of the radial carpal bone.

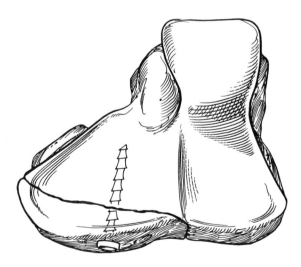

Fig. 5–117. Illustration of screw placement for repair of slab fracture of the third carpal bone to create interfragmentary compression.

The prognosis for cases that have sustained slab fracture of the third carpal bone that are treated by surgical removal or screw fixation is considered to be guarded for return to previous performance levels. In one case study of 155 race horses (Standardbreds and Thoroughbreds) that had sustained a slab fracture of the third carpal bone, 77% of the Standardbreds and 65% of the Thoroughbreds raced after surgery. The average time from admission to the hospital for treatment to their first race was 11.5 months. A good prognosis can be given for those animals that are retired for pleasure riding or breeding.

For fragmented fractures, the prognosis has to be guarded to poor but depends somewhat on the number of carpal bones involved, the degree of displacement, and the amount of anatomic deformity. Horses sustaining multiple comminuted fractures of the carpal bone should be treated only if they have obvious breeding potential or are of great sentimental value.

Luxations of the Carpal Joints

Luxations of the carpal joints with disruption of either the lateral or medial collateral ligament are rare in the horse. They can involve any one of the three carpal joints, but rupture of the medial collateral ligament appears to occur more frequently. The dislocation can be either complete or partial. In most cases, the joint surfaces are spared, but in a small percentage of these, fragmentation of the carpal bones also occurs.

Cause

Any form of severe trauma directed toward the lateral or medial surface of the carpus can result in dislocation. This trauma can occur from applying too much leverage to the tool's limbs during delivery, jumping, falling, and slipping. Occasionally an avulsion fracture associated with one of the attachments of the collateral ligaments may accompany the dislocation. (Fig. 5–119). Alterations to the vascular supply of the distal limb have also been reported with complete dislocation of the carpus.

Signs

In most cases, the horse presents with a swelling and angular deformity of the affected limb and is reluctant to bear weight on it. A history of severe trauma may or may not be revealed. During movement the horse appears obviously painful, and the distal limb is abnormally mobile. This is particularly true with complete dislocations and dislocations associated with fragmented fractures of the carpal bones. On palpation, heat, pain, and swelling are present and varying degrees of instability of the distal limb are evident. If the carpal bones are fractured, a crackling

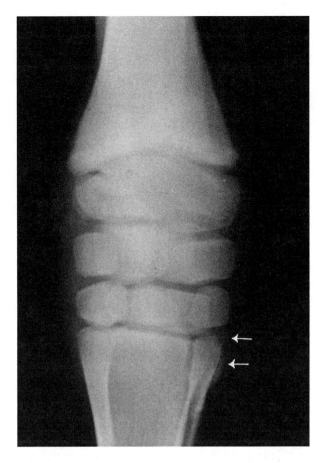

FIG. 5–119. An x-ray of the right front carpus of a foal with a history of subluxation of the carpometacarpal joint that was noticed shortly after birth. A sleeve cast was used to treat this injury. Note the periosteitis associated with the proximal end of the medial splint bone (arrows), indicating previous trauma to the attachment of the collateral ligament.

may be felt. Horses may react quite violently to manipulation of the limb, so the examiner should be careful. Some of the carpal bones may be felt displaced from their normal position.

Diagnosis

An obvious angular limb deformity coupled with an abnormal alignment of carpal bones will identify the dislocated carpus. However, X-ray examination is required to definitively define the amount of bony damage associated with the dislocation. Fractured carpal bones and avulsion fractures may accompany these dislocations.

Treatment

Realignment of the dislocation without surgery but with the horse under general anesthesia can be attempted. Once the limb is realigned, if good rotational stability is present, a tube or sleeve cast that extends from the proximal radius to the distal end of the cannon bone may be all that is needed. If, on rotation, the carpus appears to be unstable, the application of a full-limb cast will be necessary. In most cases, immobilization of the carpus will be required for a period of around 4 weeks in foals and 6 weeks in mature horses. With foals, tube casts (from upper radius to just above the fetlock) can be applied and left in place for the entire treatment period. On the other hand, if a full-limb cast is used, it should be removed and replaced at 10- to 12-day intervals. With the adult horse, however, the full-limb cast can be applied and left in place for the duration of treatment. The period of 4 to 6 weeks is selected because it usually provides sufficient time for the disrupted support tissues to heal in by scarring.

If fragmented fractures of carpal bones accompany the dislocation, euthanasia should be considered unless the horse has great sentimental value or is considered to be a valuable breeding animal. In the latter case, an attempt should be made to realign and repair the fractured carpal bones with bone screws. A full-limb cast should be applied. The cast will have to be maintained for a period of 45 to 90 days in most cases or until there is x-ray evidence of bone healing and joint fusion has occurred.

Prognosis

The prognosis for luxation without fragmented fracture of the carpal bones appears to be good for healing of the support structures but is guarded to poor for return to previous performance. The prognosis is poor for any horse that has sustained a fragmented fracture of the carpal bones in conjunction with rupture of the collateral ligaments.

Carpal Canal (Tunnel) Syndrome

The carpal canal syndrome has been infrequently reported in the horse. It results from trauma or space-occupying lesions (i.e. protruding bone) within the carpal (canal). These lesions in turn compress the soft tissue structures within the carpal canal and result in lameness. With continued irritation to the carpal flexor retinaculum (fascia surrounding the back of the knee), it becomes thickened, causing further compression of the soft tissue structures within the carpal canal.

Cause

Hyperextension of the knee and trauma to the flexor tendons resulting in tendinitis, or fractures of the accessory carpal bone, or inflammation of the radial check ligament, or osteochondroma (abnormal bone/cartilage growth) at the distal radius can result in compression and irritation of the soft tissue structures within the carpal canal. The resultant compression chokes the nerves and vessels at either extremity of the canal during motion, which causes a reduction in blood flow to the distal limb and results in pain leading to lameness.

Signs

Horses usually have a history of moderate, chronic, and sometimes intermittent lameness. Intermittent lameness is usually present in those horses that are rested in between exercise and in cases in which an accessory carpal bone fracture has healed.

On visual observation, varying degrees of synovial fluid distention of the carpal canal can be seen bulging on the medial side of the back of the knee.

With palpation, varying degrees of tenseness of the distended carpal canal can be detected. A reduced angle of flexion of the carpus is usually noted, and rapid flexion of the carpus usually results in extreme pain, with the horse rearing to avoid manipulation. In some cases, a reduction in pulse pressure within the digital artery can be palpated at the base of the sesamoid. Deep palpation over the carpal canal region with the carpus held in moderate flexion will allow the examiner to identify accessory carpal bone fractures and osteochondromas of the distal radius. A crackling can be felt with acute fractures of the accessory carpal bone, whereas in chronic cases an increased lateral-to-medial movement of the fracture accessory carpal bone can be perceived. When the bony prominence of osteochondroma is palpated, it results in considerable pain, and increased lameness is observed with exercise.

Diagnosis

A tentative diagnosis of the carpal canal syndrome can be made with physical findings of a distended carpal canal with a decreased ability to flex the limb, painful carpal flexion and decreased pulse pressure in the palmar digital artery. Anesthesia of the carpal canal with 5 ml of anesthetic can confirm the examiner's suspicion that the carpal canal syndrome is the origin of the lameness. X-rays are required to identify osteochondromas and fractures of the accessory carpal bone as the cause and ultrasound examination is used to identify enlargement and damage to the check ligaments, flexor tendons, and carpal flexor retinaculum.

Treatment

The use of corticosteroids injected into the carpal canal will only provide temporary relief from signs of lameness.

In cases in which an acute fracture of the accessory carpal bone has been sustained, the use of internal fixation may preclude the development of the carpal canal syndrome. In a high percentage of accessory carpal bone fractures that go untreated, however, the carpal canal syndrome will develop and result in chronic lameness. Because the pain is resulting primarily from compression of soft tissue structures within the canal, removal of that pressure by sectioning the carpal flexor ligament will provide relief.

Osteochondromas located at the distal radius that are large and pointed should be handled by surgical removal. However, for smaller osteochondromas in which the carpal flexor retinaculum has become thickened due to chronic irritation, resection of a portion of the carpal flexor retinaculum will provide relief from pain. After resection a pressure bandage is applied and maintained for 3 weeks and sutures are removed in about 2 weeks. These horses should be confined for 6 weeks, after which light exercise can be begun. Rest periods of up to 6 to 8 months may be required if the carpal canal syndrome has been associated with fracture of the accessory carpal bone. Typically, all of these horses exhibit an immediate relief in pain with a free range of nonpainful carpal flexion shortly after surgery is performed.

Prognosis

The prognosis for horses affected with carpal canal syndrome that have been treated by resecting the flexor carpal retinaculum appears to be good. A small percentage of the cases exhibiting the carpal canal syndrome as a result of osteochondroma formation at the distal radius may require both surgical removal of the osteochondroma and resection of the flexor carpal retinaculum. These cases also carry with them a good prognosis.

Fractures of the Accessory Carpal Bone

Fractures of the accessory carpal bone are most commonly seen in Thoroughbreds, cross country steeple chase horses, and hunter-jumpers. Although these fractures can occur in many different planes within the accessory carpal bone, they most commonly fracture in a vertical plane through the lateral groove formed by the long tendon of the ulnaris lateralis muscle (Fig. 5–120). The pull of the flexor muscles results in a constant displacement, and the instability with movement results in a nonunion. This nonunion may be painless, and some horses have been serviceably sound. In most, however, a moderate to severe prolonged lameness is present which may be complicated by the carpal canal (tunnel) syndrome.

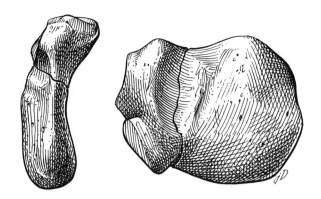

FIG. 5–120. Illustration of the common location for fracture of the accessory carpal bone.

Cause

The exact cause is unclear, and several hypotheses have been proposed. Certainly external direct trauma from a kick or high interference is a reasonable assumption. However, most cases do not show signs of exterior trauma on the skin or hair. The possibility that an asynchronous contraction of the flexor carpi ulnaris and ulnaris lateralis muscles can cause this fracture has been proposed. Also, the bow-string effect of the flexor carpi ulnaris, ulnaris lateralis, and flexor tendons, which is created when the horse lands on a partially flexed forelimb, has been incriminated. The fracture may also occur as a result of the bone being caught between the cannon bone and the radius in a nutcracker fashion. To support this, contact lesions on the caudal aspect of the radius have been identified. Whatever the cause of fractures of the accessory carpal bone, the end result can be a carpal tunnel (canal) syndrome, which usually results in a moderate chronic lameness.

Signs

Signs of lameness are usually not acute. The horse may not put full weight on the limb soon after the injury, and if extensive swelling is not present, a crackling may be found in the early stages. Soon after the fracture, however, the ends are separated so that it is almost impossible to produce crackling. The most prominent signs of the lameness are distention of the carpal sheath (Fig. 5–121) and marked pain with rapid flexion of the carpus.

Pain can be severe enough to cause the horse to rear. The pain results from the fracture of the accessory carpal bone as well as the increased pressure applied to the structures within the carpal canal. Palpation of the accessory carpal bone with the limb partially flexed to reduce the tension of the ulnaris lateralis and flexor carpi ulnaris will allow the examiner to perceive an abnormal lateral medial movement of the accessory carpal bone. In the chronic case, the pain resulting in lameness may be emanating entirely from the carpal

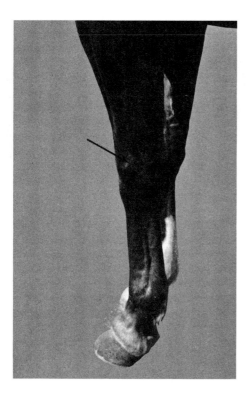

FIG. 5–121. Swelling of carpal sheath (arrow) caused by fracture of the accessory carpal bone.

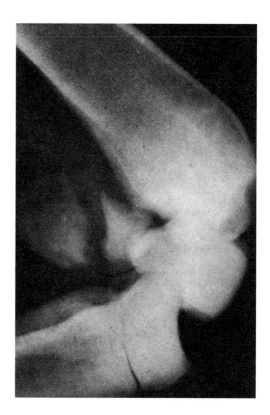

FIG. 5–122. Fracture of the accessory carpal bone. Notice the wide separation of the fragments caused by the pull of the carpal flexor tendons.

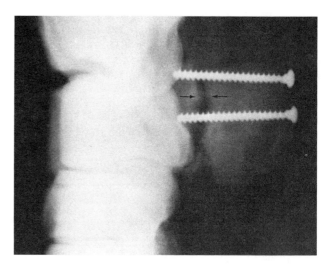

FIG. 5–123. Two bone screws were used to repair a fracture of the accessory carpal bone. Arrows point to the separated fracture.

canal syndrome (see Carpal Canal (Tunnel) Syndrome section in this chapter). A diagnostic feature of this syndrome is a reduced pulse pressure felt in the digital arteries with flexion of the carpus and a very painful response with rapid flexion of the carpus. To determine whether the carpal canal syndrome is a problem, anesthesia of the carpal sheath can be performed.

Diagnosis

Whenever a carpal sheath is distended and pain on flexion is evident, x-rays should be taken. (Fig. 5–122).

Treatment

Basically, there are two forms of treatment that may be considered when dealing with a fracture of the accessory carpal bone. Conservative treatment consists of confining the horse to a box stall for 3 to 6 months. Eventually a fibrocartilaginous union forms. Horses have returned to mild and moderate work with this approach. However, a certain percentage develop the carpal canal syndrome and require surgical resection of a portion of the flexor ligament for treatment (see Carpal Canal (Tunnel) Syndrome).

For the acute vertical fracture of the accessory carpal bone associated with the lateral grooves of the ulnaris lateralis tendon, internal fixation using the lag screw principle should provide the best end-result

(Fig. 5–123). However, this is a technically very difficult surgery to perform and in some cases it is not recommended.

Prognosis

The prognosis would have to be considered guarded but somewhat dependent on the type of fracture, the duration and the method of repair, the intended use of the horse. Good success has been reported for interfragmentary compression. Rest alone may suffice in some cases in which the perceived activity for the future is light to moderate work or breeding status.

The Forearm

Osteochondroma Formation at the Distal Radius

Osteochondroma (abnormal bone/cartilage growth) formation at the distal end of the radius is a rarely reported condition causing lameness in the horse. These new bone growths appear much like those reported for hereditary multiple exostosis (see Chapter 4). However, unlike in hereditary multiple exostosis, they occur as singular lesions or affect only a few other long bones. Hereditary multiple exostosis on the other hand is reported to affect numerous growing bones.

Cause

Although a single dominant autosomal gene is responsible for the development of multiple exostosis in humans and horses, the genetic implications for single osteochondroma remains unclear. In humans, solitary osteochondromas are not considered to be inherited.

Clinical Signs

There is usually an obvious swelling of the carpal canal sheath (Fig. 5–124). At exercise, these horses usually exhibit a moderate swinging limb lameness. Palpation of the caudomedial aspect of the radius with the limb held flexed at the carpus will often allow the examiner to feel the bony protuberance on the caudomedial aspect of the radius. Deep palpation is painful and usually results in withdrawal and an obvious increased lameness. The flexion angle of the carpal joints is often reduced, and considerable pain is elicited with rapid flexion.

Diagnosis

X-rays are necessary to diagnose the extent of this entity. In most cases, these osteochondromas are located on the caudomedial aspect of the distal radius; however, smaller osteochondromas have been observed on the caudolateral aspect of the distal radius as well (Fig. 5–125).

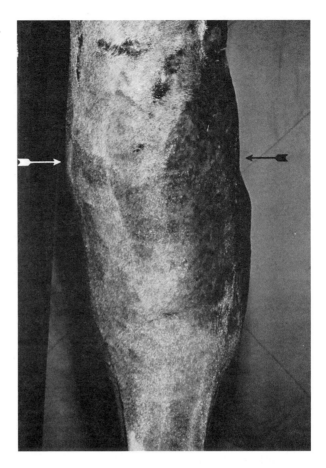

Fig. 5–124. Caudal view of the forelimb. This swelling associated with the carpal canal (arrows) may be observed with osteochondroma formation located in the distal end of the radius.

Treatment

Two surgical treatments have been successfully used. For smaller rounded bony lesions associated with swelling of the carpal canal, removing a part of the carpal flexor retinaculum will usually suffice. For larger bony lesions, the osteochondroma is removed surgically (Fig. 5–126). Support pressure bandages are applied and maintained for 2 to 3 weeks. Stall rest is recommended for 6 weeks.

Prognosis

Long-term followup on these cases has shown the prognosis to be good.

Sprain of the Accessory Ligament (Radial or Superior Check Ligament) of the Superficial Digital Flexor Tendon

The accessory ligament of the superficial digital flexor tendon is a strong, fibrous band that originates from the distal caudomedial surface of the radius and

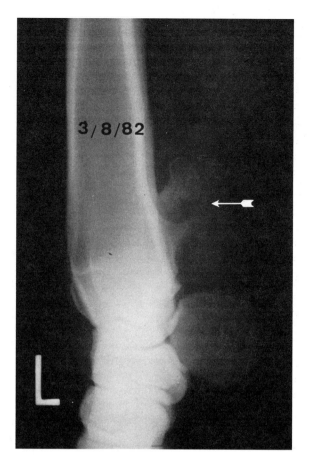

FIG. 5–125. A lateral x-ray of the horse illustrated in Figure 5–124. Two osteochondromas are located at the distal end of the radius (arrow). The larger osteochondroma is located medially and the smaller one is located laterally.

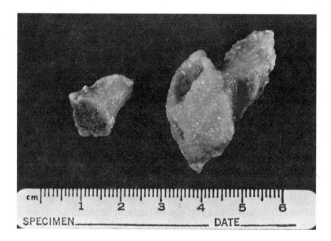

FIG. 5–126. Two osteochondromas after they have been surgically removed. On the left is the smaller fragment illustrated in Figure 5–125 and on the right is the larger fragment.

joins the superficial digital flexor tendon at the level of the carpus. Sprain to this structure is a rather poorly defined entity, for many conditions associated with the caudal aspect of the radius and carpus have similar clinical signs.

Cause

Presumably, extreme hyperextension of the fetlock in conjunction with hyperextension of the carpus can cause a sprain trauma to the accessory ligament of the superficial digital flexor tendon.

Clinical Signs

Typically, these horses have a history of starting races and workouts doing quite well but being reluctant to really sprint out. Rarely do they attain their previous performance levels. A visible swelling of the carpal sheath is observed in some cases. At a walk, a gait impediment characterized by a lateral floating placement of the foot just before it contacts the ground may be observed. Also, with foot placement, the toe and heel are placed on the ground at the same time, much like a horse walking down an incline. In acute cases, the carpal sheath is distended and variably painful to digital palpation. Simultaneous trauma to the superficial digital flexor tendon may also occur, resulting in a painful swelling proximally.

Diagnosis

In acute cases, the physical signs may identify this problem. X-rays are usually negative. However, some changes in the angulation of the accessory carpal bone may be observed (Fig. 5–127). In chronic cases, x-rays of the distal radius reveal an active periostitis associated with the attachment of the accessory ligament of the superficial digital flexor tendon (Fig. 5–128). Ultrasound examination may be used to identify sprain trauma to the accessory ligaments and confirm the diagnosis.

Treatment

In acute cases exhibiting carpal sheath distention, needle drainage and injection of an anti-inflammatory agent. Confinement for up to 4 to 6 weeks in a stall is recommended. Systemic nonsteroidal anti-inflammatory drugs are administered as needed. Pressure support wraps are applied and maintained for 3 weeks. Following stall rest, the horse should be confined to a small run for another month. Rest from exercise for 2 to 3 months appears to be sufficient but this depends on the severity of the injury. Ultrasound examination should be used to confirm healing of the accessory lig-

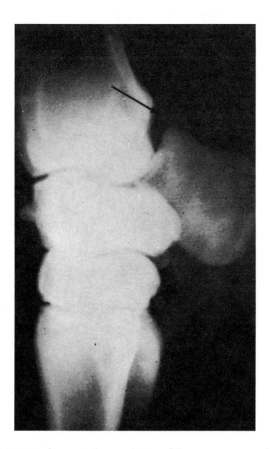

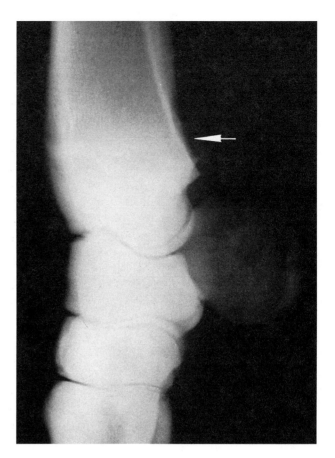

FIG. 5–127. A change in the angulation of the accessory carpal bone that may be associated with sprain trauma to the accessory ligament of the superficial digital flexor tendon.

FIG. 5–128. A periosteitis of the distal radius (arrow) associated with sprain trauma to the attachment of the accessory ligament of the superficial digital flexor.

ament. This examination is usually done at 6 weeks and at 3 months.

Prognosis

The prognosis is usually good for all cases but depends somewhat on the severity of the sprain trauma and whether the superficial digital flexor tendon is involved or not.

Fractures of the Radius

Fractures of the radius are relatively common in the horse. These fractures can be either transverse (horizontal), oblique (most common), incomplete (nondisplaced) stress fractures; complete (generally displaced); and fragmented (comminuted). They can be open or closed, and occur anywhere along the shaft of the radius. An increased incidence of proximal and distal physeal (growth plate) fractures of the radius is noted in young horses. The ulna is also frequently involved in fractures of the proximal end of the radius (Fig. 5–129). Open fractures are not common, but when they do occur, they usually penetrate the medial

surface of the forearm. Either the humeroradial elbow or antebrachiocarpal (radiocarpal) joint can be involved with oblique longitudinal fractures.

Cause

Trauma resulting from the stress of racing, a kick, entanglement in farm machinery or debris, and accidents involving motorized vehicles are reported. Whenever external trauma is the cause, a tremendous impact force is required to fracture the radius. Occasionally a history of slipping on ice will be related to this fracture as well.

Signs

Horses with nondisplaced stress fractures of the radius usually exhibit obvious lameness at exercise that abates with rest and returns when exercise is resumed. Localized swelling on the medial side of the forearm may be present, and carpal flexion can be painful.

Horses with a complete displaced fracture have a nonweight-bearing lameness, varying degrees of swelling, and instability associated with the fracture.

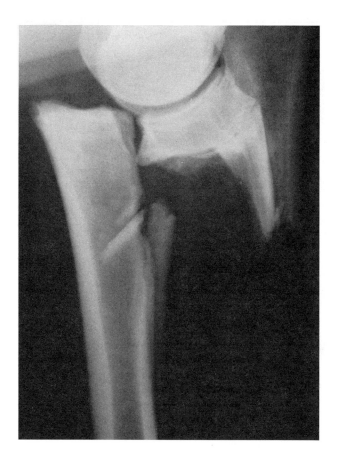

FIG. 5–129. A proximal fracture through the physis of the radius. The ulna is also involved. This type of fracture can be difficult to realign and repair (see Fig. 5–132).

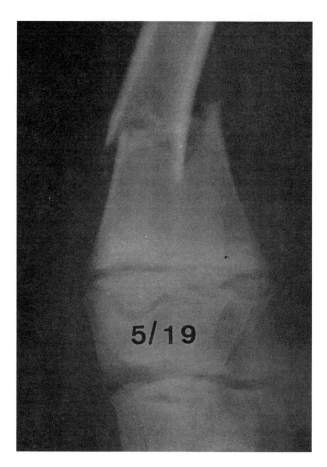

FIG. 5–130. A 3-month-old male Quarter horse was treated for a transverse fracture of the distal diaphysis of the radius.

On palpation, crackling can frequently be felt and pain elicited when the distal limb is manipulated. Open fractures do occur on the medial aspect, so close attention is paid to this region. The use of a proximally placed bandaged splint that incorporates as much of the elbow as possible may be helpful for transport to a hospital. However, the more proximal the fracture, the more difficult it is to immobilize by this method. In fact, in some cases, the application of casts or splints may increase the instability at the fracture site by creating a fulcrum effect. In foals, the incorporation of a Thomas splint with casting is often effective in stabilizing horses with these fractures for transport.

Diagnosis

The diagnosis of incomplete nondisplaced stress fractures may be made with x-rays, but in some cases nuclear scintigraphic examination is required. The fracture will show up as "hot spots" located in the radius.

Diagnosis of complete displaced fractures is not usually difficult. However, to gain a full appreciation of the extent of involvement and type of fracture, x-rays should be taken (Fig. 5–130).

Treatment

Confinement for 3 to 5 months is generally all that is required for incomplete fracture. Initially, a stall (12 × 12) is recommended for at least 6 to 10 weeks. After this, x-rays should be taken or a nuclear scintigraphic examination should be performed to document healing. If healing has progressed, access to a small run may be allowed and hand-walking exercise begun.

Various methods of treatment of complete fractures are recommended and the rationale for selection is based on the horse's size, weight, value, temperament, and the type of fracture and its location.

The application of a full-limb cast alone is not acceptable in most cases because the joint above the fracture (humeroradial "elbow" joint) cannot be adequately immobilized. If a cast is applied, it frequently results in increased rotational forces on the fracture site.

Rigid internal fixation with bone plates alone or in combination with casting can be used for many radial fractures. In most cases, the application of two compression plates is best (Fig. 5–131).

Fractures through to proximal growth plate that also involve the ulna may be managed with a bone plate (Fig. 5–132).

Prognosis

The prognosis for healing of nondisplaced stress fractures is good as long as an adequate rest period is given.

The prognosis for successful repair of fractures of the radius in horses over 600 lbs is guarded to poor. However, a lot depends on the age of the horse, its temperament, and the type of fracture. Mild-mannered foals, or light-weight young horses (under 2 years of age) that have sustained uncomplicated fractures of the midshaft transverse of the radius generally have the best chance for repair and recovery. In one case study of 28 horses that sustained fractures of the radius and were treated surgically, 65% were successfully treated, and all of these were under 2 years of age. Importantly, only 9 of 28 were sound enough to perform athletically. The remaining cases were pasture-sound and could be used for breeding. The prognosis for adult horses was poor. Horses with severely fragmented open fractures or proximal fractures involving the ulna and elbow joint generally do not respond favorably to any form of treatment.

The Elbow

Fractures of the Ulna

Fractures of the ulna are fairly common in horses. They can involve the growth plate in young horses, the olecranon or the distal ulna, or be severely fragmented with a cranial dislocation of the radius. Fractures can extend into the joint (articular) or miss it entirely (nonarticular). The proximal fragment is frequently separated proximally by the pull of the triceps brachii muscle (Fig. 5–133).

Fractures of the growth plate of the olecranon tuberosity are most commonly seen in young horses under 12 months of age, but they have been reported in horses up to 36 months of age which is the upper limit of physeal closure (Fig. 5–134).

Fractures of the olecranon are seen at any age and are usually transverse (most common) or oblique and frequently extend into the elbow (humeroradial) joint. Most of these fractures are extensively displaced and horses show an inability to extend the elbow joint appearing much like radial nerve paralysis.

Fractures of the ulna involving the joint usually originate from the articular surface and emerge in the caudal surface of the ulna.

Cause

Trauma is the cause, and a direct kick by another horse over the elbow region is the most common. Other causes include the horse's being hit by a motorized vehicle or hitting a solid object with the olecranon, or penetrating wounds or a fall. Stress and fa-

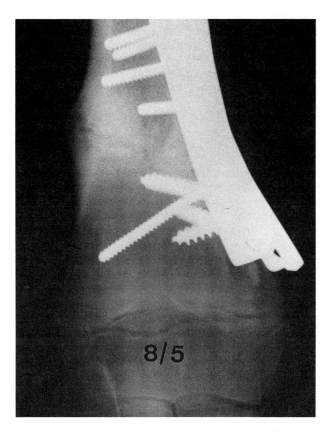

FIG. 5–131. Two bone plates were used to repair the transverse fracture of the radius. This 10-week follow-up indicates that the fracture is healing with minimal callus formation. (Courtesy of Dr. W.A. Aanes.)

tigue may also result in a nondisplaced fracture of the ulna.

Signs

The signs are acute disability of the limb; some degree of radial-nervelike paralysis is nearly always seen. The horse appears to be unable to extend the elbow joint and usually will not or cannot bear full weight on the affected limb. The elbow joint appears to be "dropped." Manipulation of the limb usually causes bone crackling and pain. Cases that have a fracture of the ulna or olecranon process through the articulation usually show more pain than those that have fracture through the proximal end of the olecranon. Heat, pain, and swelling are present to varying degrees.

Diagnosis

Diagnosis is based on appearance of the limb, manipulation, and x-rays (Fig. 5–134).

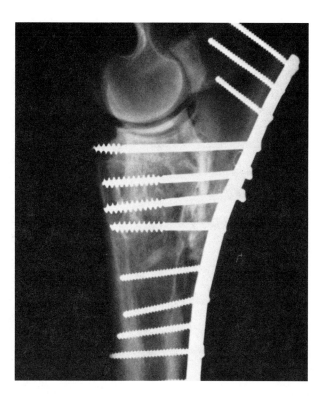

FIG. 5–132. Repair of the fracture illustrated in Figure 5–129 through the proximal physis of the radius. The ulna is also fractured. This type of fracture is difficult to realign and stabilize with internal fixation.

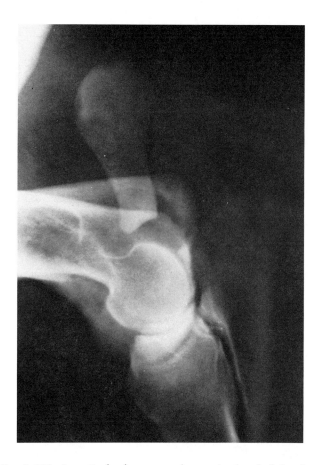

FIG. 5–133. An articular fracture at the proximal end of the olecranon tuberosity.

Treatment

The selection of treatment varies and depends on the type of fracture (articular versus nonarticular), its location, displaced versus nondisplaced, and the age of the horse.

Generally, horses with nondisplaced, nonarticular fractures of the ulna can be treated conservatively with absolute stall rest for 6 weeks to 2 months. Certain nondisplaced articular fractures will also respond well to this approach. Some complications associated with conservative management include contralateral (opposite) limb angular deformity in young horses, flexure deformity of the affected limb, ankylosis (stiffening of the joint), stiffness, permanent pain from the elbow joint, and nonunion due to displacement of the fracture fragments. The addition of a Thomas splint or a PVC pipe bandage splint applied to the caudal aspect of the limb may help prevent further displacement of the fracture by preventing extension and flexion of the elbow joint. A sling may also be helpful if the horse's temperament is suitable. The affected limb should be x-rayed periodically to check for further separation or displacement of the fracture fragments. If the fracture fragments become separated, internal fixation should be considered.

Horses that have sustained fragmented, articular, or displaced fractures of the ulna and olecranon process respond best to bone plate fixation (Fig. 5–135). In most cases, horses respond remarkably well to this treatment and frequently bear weight when returning to their stalls. Further improvement in weight bearing is usually observed over a 7- to 10-day period. However, stall confinement is recommended until x-ray evidence of complete healing has occurred. Return to full exercise usually requires a 4- to 6-month period.

Distal ulnar fractures that are displaced minimally can be repaired with compression screws alone.

Growth plate fractures of the olecranon tuberosity pose a special surgical problem, because they do not respond well to conservative treatment and are difficult to treat surgically. Attempts at conservative treatment have resulted in contralateral (opposite limb) angular limb deformity before weight bearing occurs in the affected limb. Internal fixation that relies on bone plates and screws are not felt to be as applicable in this situation due to the small size of the proximal fragment. However, bone plates that are bent to cover the dorsal aspect of the olecranon tuberosity have been used successfully to repair this type fracture in 5- to 8-month-old horses. Bone screws used for interfragmental compression in combination with figure eight tension band wiring have been used successfully as well.

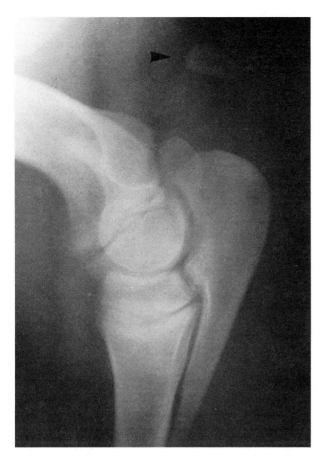

FIG. 5–134. A physeal Salter I fracture of the olecranon tuberosity. Arrow points to separated epiphysis.

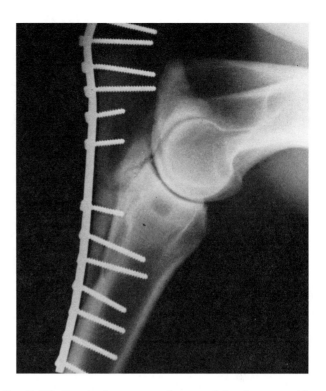

FIG. 5–135. Repair of a transverse fracture of the olecranon with a bone plate.

Prognosis

The prognosis is considered good to guarded for nondisplaced, nonarticular fractures of the ulna. In one case study of nondisplaced/nondistracted fractures of the olecranon process, 70% of the horses treated with stall rest and splinting returned to soundness. Nondisplaced articular fractures that are treated conservatively generally have a poor prognosis because it is difficult to predict the degree of cartilage damage, and some fractures will separate at a later time. When internal fixation is used, the prognosis must be guarded and the final comments regarding prognosis should be made after the degree of postoperative elbow function is realized. In two separate case studies of articular olecranon fractures treated with internal fixation, 68% and 76% returned to complete soundness.

For growth plate fractures of the olecranon tuberosity, the prognosis is based on two factors: the time interval between the injury and the repair, and the degree of damage to the articular surface and soft tissues. If the time interval between injury and repair is more than 5 days, problems with reduction may be encountered. In most cases a good to guarded prognosis can be given if the fracture is a simple physeal fracture. Fractures involving the physis that extend into the elbow joint are given a guarded prognosis. Growth plate fractures in young foals (under 3 months of age) are most difficult to deal with, and a very guarded to poor prognosis is given.

Osteochondrosis of the Elbow Joint

Osteochondrosis-type lesions affecting the elbow joint include subchondral cystic lesions of the proximal radius and OCD of the anconeal process and lateral trochlea. Defective bone formation, as with osteochondrosis elsewhere, is thought to be the cause. However, in one case, a fissure fracture of the proximal radius resulted in the development of a cyst-like lesion.

Intermittent acute onset of lameness that responds to rest is often given as a history. Elbow manipulation, extension as well as flexion, generally results in pain. Intrasynovial anesthesia is often helpful in localizing the lameness to the elbow regions. Cysts that do not communicate with the elbow joint, however, will not be desensitized. Radiographs are required for the definitive diagnosis.

Nonsurgical treatment of the cystic lesions has proven beneficial. Intrasynovial treatment with sodium hyaluronate has also been useful. Rest periods of at least 90 days are required and, in one study, 6 of 7 horses treated conservatively became sound with no evidence of DJD. Surgical treatment is indicated in those cases that do not respond favorably to the rest period as well as OCD lesions. The OCD lesions can be removed arthroscopically and cyst-like lesions can be treated by drilling and enucleation. Postoperative care includes 2 weeks stall confinement, hand walking exercise for 2 months, after which free exercise is given. Training begins at 5–6 months. The prognosis for both the conservative treatment and surgical treatment appears good if DJD has not developed.

Rupture of the Medial Collateral Ligament of the Elbow Joint

Uncommon lameness, occurs when severe abduction (movement away from the midline) of a forelimb occurs, as when a foot is caught in a rope or other restraint. Rupture can also occur if the limb gets caught under a fence. Immediately after the rupture, the horse exhibits considerable pain in the limb, but usually the pain diminishes within 24 hours. Watching the affected forelimb from in front and behind during progression may reveal an outward movement of the limb from the elbow down. The most characteristic sign is the "opening" of the joint on the medial side when the foot is abducted and the elbow joint is pushed medially. This opening of the joint can be detected by palpation. X-rays should be taken to rule out a fracture.

Stall rest and confinement for 4 to 6 weeks are required. In some of the cases, the ligament will heal if the horse will cooperate. A sling is indicated for horses whose temperaments are suitable.

The prognosis is guarded to unfavorable.

Bursitis at the Point of the Elbow (Shoe Boil, Capped Elbow)

Bursitis at the point of the elbow is most frequently observed in draft breeds. The characteristic swelling over the point of the elbow develops from trauma which, in turn, creates an acquired (false) subcutaneous bursa.

It is due to trauma caused by the shoe on the affected limb hitting the point of the olecranon tuberosity while the horse is lying down. Most trauma probably occurs while the horse is down with the foot under the point of the elbow.

The disease is characterized by a prominent swelling over the point of the elbow that may contain fluid, or that may be composed primarily of fibrous tissue in the chronic stage. Lameness is usually mild if present at all.

The use of a shoe boil roll or a boot may help in prevent further trauma. In some instances, the injection of steroids may be beneficial after the fluid has been removed. Chronic bursitis treatment is more problematic.

The prognosis is difficult to predict because the outcome is variable and depends on each case.

The Humerus

Fractures of the Humerus

Fractures of the humerus are relatively uncommon because this bone is short, thick, and well covered by surrounding musculature. Most fractures involve the middle third of the shaft and are either oblique or spiral and almost never open. Because of the strong muscular attachments, there is considerable displacement of the fragments. Occasionally, a fracture of the lateral epicondyle or fragmentation of the condyles will occur. Other fractures that occur occasionally include fractures of the greater tubercle and deltoid tuberosity. Additionally, stress fractures (nondisplaced) have been identified, particularly in race horses.

Because the radial nerve courses in the musculospiral groove of the humerus, it is not surprising that it may be traumatized to varying degrees as a result of fractures involving the shaft or proximal and distal extremities. The damage may range from a minor neuropraxia (alteration in nerve conduction without direct damage to the nerve) to a complete severance of the nerve. Because of the profound effect in prognosis, the veterinarian must be able to evaluate the degree of nerve dysfunction early in the convalescent period.

Causes

A tremendous force is required to fracture the humerus. Frequently a fall in which the horse lands on the lateral shoulder surface area is implicated. Untrained foals that are tied fast or are being led for the first time will often attempt to rear, only to fall sideways, resulting in direct impact trauma to the lateral surface of the humerus. Horses running and then slipping on ice sometimes sustain this type of fracture. Although fractures involving the deltoid tuberosity and greater tubercle can be caused by falling, external blows, from either hitting a solid object or being kicked by another horse, have also resulted in these fractures. Stress fractures most likely occur as a result of a culmination of repeated forces which cause weakening of the bone along lines of stress.

Signs and Diagnosis

The region overlying the displaced fracture of the shaft of the humerus may appear somewhat swollen and shortened as compared to the opposite side. Most cases present as a nonweight-bearing lameness with varying degrees of a dropped-elbow appearance as well as varying degrees of instability associated with the fracture. The dropped elbow appearance is due to displacement (overriding) of the fracture fragments as well as damage to the radial nerve. On manipulation of the distal limb, an increased ability to adduct (move toward midline) and abduct (move away from midline) the limb will be realized. Crackling is often difficult to detect because of the degree of displacement of the fragments and the muffling effect of the swollen musculature. Excessive manipulation of the limb may lead to further trauma to the radial nerve. Varying degrees of swelling and lameness are seen with fractures of the deltoid tuberosity and the great tubercle. Varying degrees of lameness, particularly after galloping, are characteristic of stress fractures.

A definitive diagnosis can usually be made with x-rays. However, stress fractures are difficult to see on conventional x-rays, and nuclear scintigraphic examination is often required. The stress fracture will show up as a hot spot.

Treatment

The selection of treatment is based on the type of fracture, the age of the horse, its size, and its intended use. Because there is a large surface area for callus formation associated with spiral and oblique fractures, and the surrounding muscle mass can immobilize the fracture, spontaneous healing can occur. For foals under 6 months of age, stall confinement for 6 weeks with the application of bandages to bind the forearm to the thoracic wall will be sufficient. However, a dropped-elbow appearance may remain and an angular limb deformity may develop in the opposite limb. Older horses cannot be managed this way and require confinement within a sling for about 6 weeks to 2 months. The application of a light-weight PVC pipe bandage splint to the caudal aspect of the limb can be used to prevent contracture of the flexor muscle/tendon units of the knee. Mature horses that have not been splinted usually develop a flexor contracture that makes weight bearing difficult after fracture healing has occurred. Most can only rest the limb by placing the toe of the foot on the ground because of an inability to extend it into a normal weight-bearing position. Another complication that may occur during the convalescent period in the sling is a rotation of the coffin bone of the unaffected limb. This is thought to result from the excessive weight-bearing requirement by the opposite limb. It is most frequently observed between the third and sixth week of convalescence. It is recognized by the horse being reluctant to bear weight on the good limb and attempting to bear increasing amounts of weight on the fractured limb. Initially this is mistaken as a good sign because the horse shifts its weight intermittently from the good side to the fractured side, appearing as though healing is occurring. A throbbing pulse in the palmar digital arteries can usually be palpated in horses developing support limb laminitis. Because of this, it is recommended that frequent examinations of the opposite limb be performed. If any question exists regarding the status of

the foot of the unaffected limb, x-rays should be taken. The application of a heart-bar shoe or a full support shoe (egg bar with frog support) to the foot of the weight-bearing limb early in the convalescent period may prevent rotation of the coffin bone. Bedding the horse in sand or soft dirt floor may also decrease the chances of support limb laminitis. Horses are often treated with nonsteroidal antiinflammatory drugs as well as drugs that improve the blood flow to the foot.

Intermedullary pinning, ASIF nailing, and bone plating have been used successfully in foals and ponies. Bone screws may be used to repair deltoid tuberosity and greater tubercle fractures. Stress fractures usually require varying periods of rest followed by controlled exercise for successful treatment.

Prognosis

The prognosis for fractures of the shaft and condyles will be postponed until the fracture is healed, because of the many complications that can occur (radial nerve paralysis, rotation of the coffin bone in older horses, carpal flexure deformities, angular limb deformities, failure of internal fixation devices, and pin migration). Clinically, the return of radial nerve function may be evident in 6 weeks. Early return of nerve function is obviously considered a good sign. However, in some cases, return of nerve function may take anywhere from 9 to 12 months. The prognosis for greater tubercle and deltoid tuberosity fractures appears good if they are treated early and the fracture can be adequately stabilized with screws. Stress fractures generally heal without complications if an adequate rest period is afforded.

Paralysis of the Radial Nerve

The radial nerve, often the largest branch of the brachial plexus, (see Fig. 1–27), derives its origin chiefly from the eighth cervical and first thoracic root of the plexus. The radial nerve serves the extensor muscles of the elbow, carpal, and digital joints and also supplies the lateral flexor of the carpus (ulnaris lateralis). It also gives off a superficial sensory branch to the lateral cutaneous brachial nerve. Paralysis of the radial nerve inactivates these muscles and results in loss of sensation to the craniolateral aspect of the forearm.

Causes

In most cases, paralysis of the radial nerve is caused by trauma of the nerve as it crosses the musculospiral groove of the humerus; such trauma often accompanies fracture of the humerus. The nerve is traumatized by a fracture, and in some cases is completely severed by a bone fragment. A kick or a fall on the lateral surface of the humerus may produce enough trauma to cause paralysis of the nerve. Prolonged lateral recumbency on an operating table or on the ground may produce a radial-paralysis-like syndrome in the forelimb that was next to a hard surface.

It is difficult to say whether the paralysis following lateral recumbency is from direct pressure or tension trauma to the radial nerve or a result of compression of the vascular supply leading to ischemia (local anemia due to mechanical blockage of the blood supply) and anoxia (absence of oxygen) of the muscles.

Another possible cause is that overstretching this nerve may result in paralysis. The radial nerve can be put under considerable tension by hyperextending the forelimb and adducting the shoulder. While the horse is in this position, it is conceivable that trauma to the shoulder region could compress the nerve between the shoulder and the chest wall. This condition has also been observed with fractures of the first rib and compression of the nerve by enlargement of the axillary lymph nodes.

Signs and Diagnosis

The signs vary somewhat, depending on the extent or degree and location of paralysis. When that portion of the radial nerve supplying the extensors of the digit is affected, the signs are characteristic. The horse cannot advance the limb to place weight on the foot. If the foot is placed under the horse, it can bear weight with no difficulty. In most cases the branch of the nerve to the triceps muscle also is involved, so the elbow is dropped and extended while the digits are flexed (Fig. 5–136). The muscles of the elbow are relaxed, as are the extensors of the digit, and the limb appears longer than normal. In severe paralysis, dragging of the limb may damage the dorsal surface of the fetlock. If the injury occurs at the point of the shoulder when the humerus fractures, the suprascapular nerve may be paralyzed, causing atrophy of the supra- and infraspinatus muscles. Sensation to the craniolateral aspect of the forearm skin will be lost.

Occasionally, radial-nerve paralysis is accompanied by paralysis of the entire brachial plexus. In this case, the limb shows paralysis of the flexor and extensor muscles and is unable to bear weight. The elbow is dropped, and the affected limb appears to be longer than the opposite limb. The humerus, radius, and ulna are examined for fracture when radial paralysis is present, because many cases of radial paralysis are caused by external trauma from kicks.

Milder cases of radial-nerve paralysis may cause little lameness in a slow walk. Then, as the foot encounters an obstacle, the horse may stumble if the toe catches and the foot does not land flat. More difficulty is experienced on uneven ground.

The diagnosis is made from the clinical signs. If a question exists, electromyography (EMG) can be performed on the extensor muscles of the carpus and digits 5 days after injury.

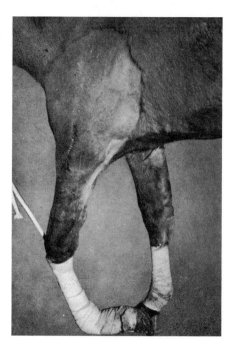

FIG. 5–136. Paralysis of the radial nerve. Note the "dropped" appearance of the elbow and the foal's inability to extend the limb and digits. This filly was later returned to a nearly normal condition by surgery to free the nerve from adhesions and to correct trauma resulting from a fragment of the fractured humerus.

Treatment

Treatment in most cases is of no value, and the horse should be stalled to prevent further injury. The limb may be placed in a light cast or bandage splint to prevent contraction of the flexors of the carpus and digits or protected with heavy bandages so that the dorsal surface of the fetlock is not damaged. The cast can be changed every 2 to 3 weeks. Bandages are replaced as needed.

Limited experience with humeral fracture suggests that surgical correction may be beneficial in repairing the nerve as it crosses the fracture site.

Prognosis

The prognosis is guarded in mild cases and unfavorable in severe ones. Six months should be allowed for recovery after injury or corrective surgery before any final decision is made. If surgery is used in an attempt to correct the paralysis, it should be done no sooner than 8 and no later than 12 weeks after injury.

The Shoulder

Inflammation of the Bicipital Bursa (Bicipital Bursitis)

The bicipital bursa, which is quite extensive, is found between the biceps brachii tendon and bicipital groove of the humerus. Movement of the biceps brachii tendon over the groove in the humerus is cushioned by this bursa. The bursa, along with the biceps tendon, is sometimes affected by acute or chronic inflammation, which is often diagnosed as "shoulder lameness." Although it is often blamed for the lameness, the shoulder is seldom at fault. The incidence of lameness associated with inflammation of the bicipital bursa appears to be very low.

Causes

The most common cause of inflammation of this bursa is severe trauma at the point of the shoulder. Another cause may be a fall or slip that flexes the shoulder and extends the elbow. This positioning may create a marked increase in tension and strain on the biceps tendon and bursa.

Other causes include infection, from either an open wound in the shoulder region or a localization of a systemic infection in the bursa.

Signs

Signs of shoulder lameness include:

1. Marked lifting of the head when the limb is being advanced. This results when the horse tries to advance the limb with a minimum of flexion of the shoulder joint.
2. Imperfect flexion of the limb causing the foot to be lifted only slightly off the ground.
3. Shortened cranial phase of the stride.
4. Stumbling caused by insufficient foot clearance and to the short cranial phase of the stride, which causes the toe of the foot to land too soon.
5. Fixation of the scapulohumeral (shoulder) joint, evidenced by restricted movement of the shoulder joint during progression. This is one of the more important signs of shoulder lameness.
6. Indifference to the hardness of the ground. Lameness signs are approximately the same on hard or soft ground if it is level. Soft ground is more likely to impede movement because of the irregular surface.
7. Circumduction (an arcing outward) of the limb in an effort to overcome the difficulty of advancing it.
8. Dropped elbow if the inflammation is severe or if the radial nerve is also injured.

When the horse is in motion, it does not flex the limb properly because of the pain. In acute cases, the limb is usually carried while the horse makes a short jump on the sound limb; it usually will not make any attempt to lift the foot of the affected limb when going forward, but it may use the limb in backing. In less acute cases, observation of the horse during movement shows the fixation of the shoulder joint. When the horse is standing, the foot of the affected limb is placed in back of the normal standing position, and usually rests on the toe. In mild cases, signs similar to the navicular syndrome may occur.

Diagnosis

Diagnosis is based on the signs listed above. Swelling of the bursa at the point of the shoulder is nearly always present, but atrophy of the supraspinatus and other associated muscles should not be confused with bursitis; atrophy of these muscles causes the shoulder joint to appear to be more prominent. A fixation of the scapulohumeral joint is one of the most diagnostic signs of shoulder lameness. This is evident when the horse is in motion.

Direct pressure applied over the point of the shoulder will be painful with acute inflammation of the bursa, but may only cause a mild response in more chronic cases (Fig. 5–137).

A definitive diagnosis can be made with intrasynovial anesthesia (blocking) of this bursa. A sample of synovial fluid can be evaluated is taken to determine if the bursitis is purely inflammatory or a result of infection. X-ray of the shoulder region will rule out other conditions with similar symptoms.

Treatment

Injection of the bursa with antiinflammatories, plus the administration of nonsteroidal antiinflammatory drugs, has proven to be effective treatment. Adequate rest is also required.

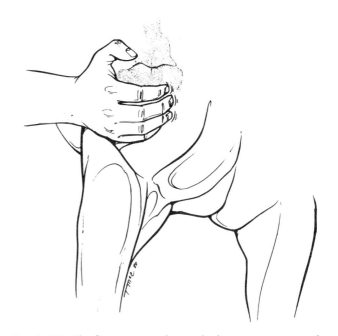

FIG. 5–137. The fingers are used to apply direct pressure over the bicipital bursa region.

When infection is the cause, drainage and flushing of the bursa may be necessary along with high levels of broad-spectrum antibiotics.

Prognosis

The prognosis is guarded to unfavorable. If the condition is chronic when the veterinarian is first called, the prognosis is unfavorable because permanent changes may already have occurred.

Ossification of the Tendon of the Biceps Brachii Muscle

Ossification (a change into bone) of the biceps brachii tendon is rare.

The cause of this disease is unknown, but it would appear that developmental and traumatic conditions involving the shoulder joint may lead to ossification of the biceps tendon.

On gross observation, mild atrophy of the shoulder muscles and, in particular, the biceps brachii muscle may be present in chronic cases. In some, a lowered toe with a longer heel will be evident. At exercise, a moderate lameness is usually observed which is manifested by a reduction in the cranial phase of the stride and a slight reduction in the flexion of the carpus. Even if the condition is bilateral, one limb is usually more affected than the other. Direct deep palpation of the region may result in painful withdrawal. Forcible extension and flexion of the scapulohumeral joint may result in pain and a tendency for the horse to rear. For a definitive diagnosis, x-rays must be taken (Fig. 5–138).

There is no rational treatment available at this time. When shoulder degenerative changes within the shoulder joint result in severe lameness, euthanasia is advised unless the horse can be used for breeding.

The prognosis is poor for long-term athletic function, but good for breeding status.

Inflammation of the Infraspinatus Bursa

The infraspinatus bursa is located between the tendon of the infraspinatus muscle and the caudal eminence of the greater tubercle of the proximal humerus. Inflammation of the bursa is rare.

Severe adduction of the forelimb and/or the possibility of direct trauma to this region is considered to be the cause. Horses cast in lateral recumbency with the lower forelimb entrapped may develop this problem while struggling to free themselves.

The involved forelimb is often held in an abducted position. Adduction of the limb usually elicits a painful response and results in increased signs of lameness on exercise.

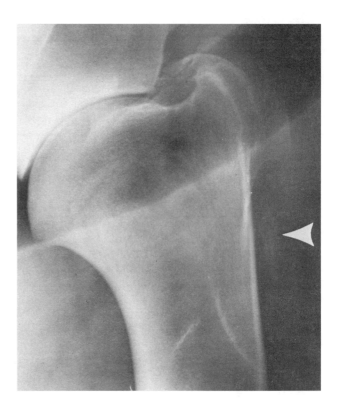

FIG. 5–138. Lateral x-ray of the shoulder of a horse with ossification of the tendon of the biceps brachii muscle (arrow).

In the acute stage, administration of anti-inflammatory agents into the bursa is recommended. With sufficient stall rest (6 weeks or more) and the administration of nonsteroidal antiinflammatory drugs, a good end result can be expected.

In most acute cases, the prognosis should be considered good. Because this condition is so rare, it is difficult to predict outcome.

Osteochondrosis of the Scapulohumeral (Shoulder) Joint

Osteochondrosis (a malfunction in cartilage formation) of the shoulder joint is primarily a disease that affects young, rapidly growing horses. This is not surprising because the primary lesion involves growing epiphyseal cartilage. However, the relationship to rapid growth for this lesion is not as clearly defined as it is for osteochondrosis lesions in the stifle, hock, and cervical (neck) vertebrae, but it seems most likely that it plays a role. Overnutrition imbalanced nutrition, coupled with a genetic predisposition to rapid growth, appears to be a reasonable hypothesis. Presently, osteochondrosis of the shoulder joint is being diagnosed with great frequency in weanlings and yearlings 5 to 10 months of age. When this disease is diagnosed in older horses, the chronic manifestation of secondary degenerative changes within the joint are usually present.

The primary cartilage lesion is usually located at the caudal margin of the humeral head and/or the glenoid cavity (scapula articulation) (Fig. 5–139). This is similar to osteochondritis dissecans (OCD) lesions reported for many other species with the exception that a dissecans (flap or loose body lesion) is not observed. Regardless of the site of the lesion, secondary degenerative change within the shoulder joint is a prominent feature of this disease.

Cause

Osteochondrosis of the humeral head is characterized by disturbance of the normal differentiation of cells in the growing epiphyseal cartilage in the deep layers of the articular cartilage. This in turn causes a failure in the endochondral ossification system, which results in retention of cartilage rather than the formation of bone. As more cartilage is produced, softening of the radial zone in the epiphyseal cartilage occurs. This results in failure of the normal rounded head of the humerus to develop. Eventually the cartilage becomes deformed from a lack of underlying bony support. Secondary degenerative changes within the joint develop because of the abnormal shape of the humeral head and the resultant instability. Osteo-

chondrosis also occurs in the articular surface (glenoid cavity) of the scapula.

Signs

Most cases present with a history of mild to moderate intermittent lameness. Mild atrophy of the muscles associated with the shoulder may also be evident. Horses will often cock (flex) the fetlock of the most severely affected limb. Close observation of the hooves often reveals excessive toe wear and an extra long heel. Exercise usually results in a headnodding lameness characterized by a shortened cranial (extension) phase of the stride. A prominent shoulder lift, reduced carpal flexion, and limb circumduction (outward swing) are present in the most severely affected horses. In a small percentage of cases, swelling of the shoulder joint capsule can be palpated and deep digital palpation causes a painful response. Manipulation in extension and flexion often cause pain and increased signs of lameness on exercise.

Diagnosis

The clinical signs are not specific and occur with many other diseases causing shoulder lameness. In most cases, intrasynovial anesthesia (joint blocking) will lead to a moderate improvement and, in some cases, total relief of signs of lameness will be obtained. Osteochondrosis is likely if bilateral shoulder lameness is present in a weanling or yearling horse.

X-rays are the only means of definitively diagnosing the lesion at this time.

Treatment

Treatment has included rest and confinement for up to 16 months, intraarticular steroids, systemic analgesics, and surgery.

Rest and confinement probably constitute a rational approach for cases with mild to moderate x-ray lesions.

Arthroscopic surgery has been used in a small number of cases, and the results appear encouraging. An important consideration if surgery is contemplated is that many of the signs of degenerative changes within the joint are already present at the time of initial lameness and diagnosis. The more severe these degenerative lesions are, the less successful the surgery will be.

Prognosis

Generally, the prognosis is poor, but depends somewhat on what the horse can be used for and the severity of the osteochondrosis lesion. Horses with mild to moderate lesions can be used for breeding, for pleasure, and in a small percentage of cases, trained for

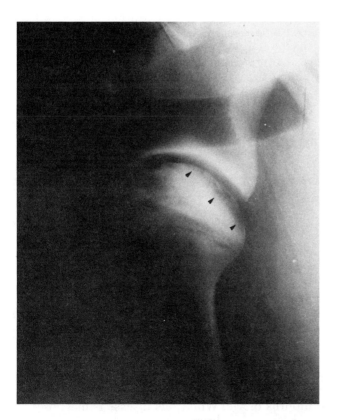

FIG. 5–139. A lateral x-ray of the shoulder joint indicating flattening of the caudal aspect of the humeral head and subchondral lysis (cartilage destruction) (arrows).

racing. Those with severe lesions usually remain lame, but a small percentage may be used for breeding. There is concern regarding the use of these animals for breeding, however, since there may be an associated genetic link for rapid skeletal growth and subsequent development of osteochondrosis. With surgery, an improved outcome can be expected even with severe osteochondrosis lesions.

Arthritis of the Shoulder Joint

Causes

Arthritis of the shoulder joint can have multiple causes, most of which involve traumatic bone changes such as fractures. Fracture of the supraglenoid tuberosity (tuber scapulae) of the scapula and fracture of the lateral tuberosity of the humerus are the most common of these. In these cases, the fractures do not involve large portions of the bone, so the stability of the joint is retained. The irritation caused by these fractures produces an arthritis that causes persistent lameness. In young horses, osteochondritis dissecans or osteochondrosis may cause damage that will remain as chronic osteoarthritis of the shoulder joint.

In foals, an extension of a navel infection may lead to an infectious arthritis. Most commonly, other signs of systemic disease as well as other joints will be involved with the infection.

Trauma is the cause in most cases. Kicks, running into solid objects, and other forms of trauma are nearly always involved.

The course of osteochondrosis is briefly outlined in the Osteochondrosis of the Scapulohumeral Joint section in this chapter. In septic arthritis, the introduction of bacteria usually results from an infected navel (umbilicus). The immune system in young horses may be compromised by insufficient colostrum intake or as a result of primary immune deficiency, a condition seen in Arabian horses. In older horses, penetrating wounds or introduced infections from arthrocentesis (withdrawal of fluid from a joint) may also be considered.

Signs

In general, signs are typical of shoulder lameness, i.e., lifting the head on the affected side when advancing the limb, circumduction (arcing outward) of the limb when advancing it to avoid flexion of the shoulder, and standing with the affected limb so that the foot is behind the opposite forefoot. In some cases, obvious swelling of the shoulder is present. However, in most cases it is difficult to distinguish any difference between the normal and abnormal side. During progression, the horse tends to fix the shoulder joint, resulting in a shortened cranial phase of the stride.

Flexion extension, abduction, and adduction of the limb usually result in painful withdrawal and increased lameness. Careful observation of the shoulder region during movement will reveal the difference in movement in the normal and the affected shoulder.

With infection of the shoulder joint, the horse presents with a nonweight-bearing lameness. Palpation of the shoulder region may elicit pain and increased heat will be felt. In young horses and thin, older horses, a prominent swelling can be felt.

Diagnosis

Because there is often no obvious swelling of the affected side, differential nerve blocks of the distal limb are helpful. When unsoundness still exists after blocking, the shoulder and elbow joints should receive close scrutiny. Whenever possible, an x-ray of the shoulder should be taken. This requires a good x-ray machine. Arthritic changes visible on the x-ray are diagnostic of the condition. Blocking the shoulder joint is also used for diagnosis.

If infection is considered to be the cause of lameness, an arthrocentesis can be performed to retrieve the synovial fluid for analysis.

Treatment

If degenerative changes are already present within the joint, no treatment will be helpful. However, small chip fractures of the lateral tuberosity of the humerus can be removed successfully. Injection of the shoulder joint with a steroid followed by hyaluronic acid (HA) will usually provide temporary relief.

Prognosis

The prognosis is guarded to poor, depending on the cause. If bony changes are present, the prognosis is poor.

Dislocation of the Shoulder Joint

Dislocation of the shoulder joint is a very rare condition leading to a sudden onset of lameness in the horse. The head of the humerus usually dislocates cranially, but in some instances it also dislocates medially.

Causes

This condition may result from the horse pulling and twisting the limb while it is flexed and the foot is held fast. It also has been reported to result from a fall, while the shoulder joint is in the flexed position as might occur during jumping. Whichever the case, this trauma results in the head of the humerus becoming displaced in a cranial or craniomedial position.

Signs

There is usually a history of a sudden severe onset of lameness. The distal limb is frequently adducted (displaced inward) in cases in which the dislocation is cranial, or slightly abducted (displaced outward) in relation to the body if the dislocation is medial. In either case, the limb appears shorter than the opposite side. With cranial displacement, the greater tuberosity and the head of the humerus can be palpated cranial to the glenoid cavity. With medial displacement, the lateral lip of the glenoid cavity can be felt. The limb is usually held in a slightly flexed position and the horse will exhibit a nonweight-bearing lameness at exercise. Affected horses will also violently oppose manipulation of the limb.

Diagnosis

The clinical signs in most cases are diagnostic. If any question should arise, x-rays should be taken after the humeral head is replaced to rule out fractures of the humerus and scapula.

Treatment

The dislocation should be corrected as soon as possible. General anesthesia is required in most cases. In young horses, the affected limb is pulled into extension, and at the same time an assistant pushes or pulls the humeral head back into position. In the mature horse the body is anchored to a fixed object and a tension-creating device is attached to the foot or pastern to apply traction while the operator forces the shoulder back into position. If the humeral head is displaced medially, flexion and adduction of the distal limb are helpful. An audible click will be heard when the humeral head is popped back into place. Assisting the horse during recovery from anesthesia is most important to prevent redislocation of the shoulder.

Prognosis

In most cases, the prognosis is considered good if fractures are not present. It may take anywhere from 4 to 6 weeks before the horse is totally recovered. In situations in which there is no improvement observed within a 2-week period, the prognosis is considered poor for future athletic performance.

Sweeny Paralysis of the Suprascapular Nerve (Atrophy of the Supraspinatus and Infraspinatus Muscles)

The term "sweeny" can apply to any group of atrophied muscles, regardless of location. In popular usage the term generally applies to atrophy (shrinking of tissue) of the supraspinatus and infraspinatus muscles caused by paralysis of the suprascapular nerve.

Causes

Atrophy of muscles results from disuse or loss of nerve supply. In the case of injury to the suprascapular nerve, the cause is usually trauma from a direct blow to the point of the shoulder, or from stretching of the nerve in a sudden backward thrust of the limb, such as during slipping.

Signs

The clinical signs most frequently observed before muscle atrophy occurs is a supporting-limb lameness with rapid outward abduction of the shoulder during full weight bearing (also known as "shoulder pop"). This is best observed as the horse is walked slowly toward the examiner. The outward excursion is easily explained since the supraspinatus and infraspinatus muscles comprise most of the lateral support of the shoulder. Once atrophy begins, the scapular spine becomes more prominent because of the loss of the muscles cranial and caudal to it (Fig. 5–140). Some feel that this outward abduction of the scapula during weight bearing causes intermittent stretching of the suprascapular nerve leading to continued trauma and perpetuation of the paralysis.

Diagnosis

Diagnosis of muscular atrophy is easy, but determining the cause is another matter. Atrophy may result from disuse of the limb as a result of lameness and is not necessarily caused by paralysis of a nerve. The attitude of the limb during motion usually reveals whether lameness is present or whether the condition is actually due to paralysis. Muscular dystrophy (congenital muscle abnormality) can occur and must be differentiated from muscular atrophy.

Treatment

In the past, a variety of unsuccessful treatments have been tried. Surgery involves exposure of the nerve and surgical removal of the surrounding scar tissue. Because the nerve may be intermittently stretched over the cranial border of the scapula during weight bearing, removing a piece of scapula that un-

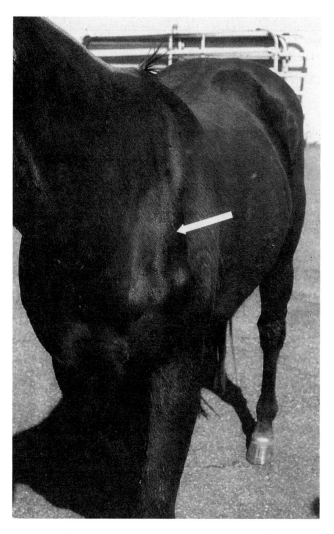

FIG. 5–140. This horse has sweeny. The arrow points to the scapular spine, which has become visible as a result of atrophy of the supraspinatus (cranial) and infraspinatus (caudal) muscles. Note that the lateral tuberosity of the humerus (below the arrow) is also more prominent.

derlies the nerve has been used. This procedure appears to reduce nerve tension and it is thought to further aid in decompression and relieve the potential for intermittent tension of the nerve during full weight bearing and subsequent abduction of the shoulder. Long-term results of these procedures appear promising (Fig. 5–141).

Hand-walking exercise is begun 5 days after surgery and increased according to improvement. The bandage is removed in 4 to 5 days and skin sutures removed in 14 days postoperatively. Six weeks of stall rest with daily hand-walking are recommended. After this, pasture exercise is allowed. After 6 months, active exercise is recommended.

Prognosis

The prognosis is good to guarded. Judgment on the degree of return of nerve function should not be made

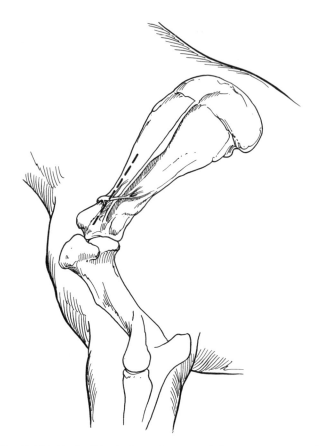

FIG. 5–141. Dashed line indicates location of skin incision centered over the suprascapular nerve and cranial to the scapular spine.

for at least 6 months because a long period is required for regeneration of nerves.

Fractures of the Scapula

Fractures of the scapula are uncommon in horses. The majority of these fractures are simple involving the spine, supraglenoid tubercle (tuber scapulae), neck, and glenoid cavity. However, fragmented fractures of the scapula can also occur. Bone sequestra (piece of dead bone separated from healthy bone) formation is a common finding with displaced fractures of the scapular spine and in cases in which a penetrating wound has resulted in a fragmented fracture of the scapula. Muscle atrophy, from either disuse or damage to the suprascapular nerve, may be seen in more chronic cases. As would be expected, a higher incidence of suprascapular nerve damage occurs with fractures of the neck of the scapula. Damage to the subscapularis nerve and brachial plexus is a rare complication associated with fractures of the scapula. With fractures of the neck of the scapula, the proximal fragment will oftentimes override the distal component in a cranial direction.

Causes

Trauma to the lateral surfaces of the scapula may lead to fracture. It appears that the direction of trauma as well as the force of impact could play a role in the type of fracture that occurs. Fractures of the supraglenoid tuberosity most likely result from forceful traumatic events directed toward the cranial shoulder region. Glancing blows (such as kicks or hitting a fixed object) over the lateral surface could result in fractures of the spine. Penetrating wounds often cause fractures of the spine, and those that penetrate the lateral surface can produce a fragmented fracture of the scapula. More forceful trauma, directed ventral to the spine over the lateral surface, is more likely to result in simple or fragmented fractures of the neck of the scapula and glenoid cavity. A higher incidence of fractured scapulae has been reported in younger horses and polo ponies. Polo ponies are quite susceptible because there is a lot of shoulder contact during performance. In some cases, horses are presented with scapular fractures that do not have a history of trauma. In these, uncoordinated muscle contraction and fatigue may play a role.

Signs

Horses frequently have a history of trauma and signs of lameness ranging from mild to nonweight-bearing. In acute cases with fracture of the spine, horses that exhibit minimal swelling will bear weight and may show only mild lameness during exercise. Direct palpation and close observation of the swelling is the key to diagnosis. For fractures of the supraglenoid tuberosity, the horse will bear weight, but at exercise an obvious shortening of the cranial phase of the stride will be noticed. Deep palpation over this region will lead to a painful withdrawal, and crackling will be felt in acute cases. For a more detailed discussion, refer to the Fractures of the Supraglenoid Tubercle (Tuber Scapulae) section in this chapter. With fractures of the body and neck of the scapula or glenoid cavity, a nonweight-bearing lameness is usually observed with a reluctance to advance the limb when walking. Before extensive swelling occurs, deep palpation may identify a fracture movement, but in most cases, manipulation of the limb in all directions is required to feel the crepitation. In more chronic cases, muscle atrophy and draining tracts from bone sequestration may become apparent.

Diagnosis

The clinical signs locating the lameness problem to the scapula are very important. In the acute case, varying degrees of lameness, localized swelling, and pain on palpation and limb manipulation will be the important features. In the more chronic cases, muscle atrophy, lameness, and draining tracts from bone se-

questra may be important. X-rays of this region are needed for a definitive diagnosis.

Treatment

Bone sequestra resulting from fractures of the scapular spine are treated by surgical removal. In those cases in which sequestra do not form, a bony union can be expected. Transverse fractures of the body and proximal neck of the scapula can be surgically treated with internal fixation in young animals.

Fragmented fractures or fractures of the distal neck of the scapula and those extending into the glenoid fossa are very difficult to treat surgically. Stall rest or slinging of a docile horse may be of help in cases in which there are nonarticular fractures. For treatment of fractures of the supraglenoid tuberosity, refer to the Fractures of the Supraglenoid Tubercle (Tuber Scapulae) section in this chapter.

Prognosis

The prognosis is good for fractures involving the scapular spine and for transverse fractures of the body and proximal neck of the scapula in foals that can be repaired by stable internal fixation. Fractures involving the supraglenoid tuberosity that extend into the joint, distal neck fractures, glenoid fossa fractures, and fragmented fractures all have a poor prognosis for return to function even though bony union may occur after a prolonged rest period.

Fractures of the Supraglenoid Tubercle (Tuber Scapulae)

Fractures of the supraglenoid tubercle (see Chapter 1) are relatively rare. It appears to be a fracture that occurs in horses under one year of age.

Cause

It is postulated that this fracture results from a separation of the physis of the supraglenoid tubercle, since the fracture planes often course along this growth plate. This physis does not close until 10 to 12 months of age.

Signs

In acute cases, an obvious swelling can be localized to the point of the shoulder. At exercise, the cranial phase of the stride is markedly shortened.

Diagnosis

This fracture is one that can be easily missed. First of all, it is an uncommon entity and, secondly, the signs are subtle enough that the swelling or lameness may be attributed to a bruised shoulder. The true extent of the fracture can be realized only with x-rays.

Treatment

At this time, there does not appear to be a successful method of treatment that would return these cases to full function. If left untreated, a fibrous union develops between the supraglenoid tubercle and the scapula which provides an attachment for the biceps brachii muscle not far removed from its original position. However, the displacement is sufficient to mechanically obstruct the full extension of the limb as well as result in secondary degenerative changes in the shoulder joint. Surgical removal of the fractured fragment has proven beneficial in a limited number of cases. After surgery, horses appear more comfortable, and in some cases have been able to perform light work.

Prognosis

The prognosis is poor for future athletic performance and guarded to good for return to pasture soundness.

Rupture of the Serratus Ventralis Muscles

Rupture of the serratus ventralis muscles is a rarely reported condition in horses. These muscles are large, paired, and fan-shaped, and lie in the lateral thorax and cervical (neck) region. The cervical part of each fan-shaped serratus ventralis arises from the last four cervical vertebrae; the thoracic part originates from the first eight or nine ribs. The two parts of the muscle converge to their respective insertions on the proximal cranial and caudal areas on the medial surface of the scapula and the adjacent scapular cartilage. Elastic lamellae from the dorsoscapular ligament penetrate these attachments. The muscles on the opposite side form a support, suspending the thorax between the forelimbs. While the horse is standing, contraction of both muscles elevates the thorax. Contraction of one muscle shifts the weight of the trunk to that side. The neck is also pulled to one side or, if both muscles are contracting, the neck is extended. During locomotion, the cervical part of the serratus ventralis pulls the dorsal border of the scapula craniad; the thoracic part then acts to pull the scapula caudad (see Chapter 1).

When rupture of the serratus ventralis muscle occurs, both left and right paired muscle groups are usually involved.

Causes

Dorsal impact trauma over the withers and neck can lead to rupture of the serratus ventralis muscles. However, it is reasonable to believe that a horse could sustain such an injury from jumping over a high fence or from jumping off an elevated platform.

Signs

Following rupture of these muscles, the thorax drops between the paired scapulae and the dorsal borders of the scapulae assume a position above the thoracic spinous processes (withers). In most instances, the croup will appear higher than the withers. If examined right after the rupture occurs, these horses are in extreme pain.

Diagnosis

The diagnosis is made from the history and clinical signs. X-rays should be taken of the withers region to rule out the possibility of fractures of the dorsal spinous processes.

Treatment

If treatment is attempted, the horse should be placed in a sling support for 30 to 45 days. Nonsteroidal antiinflammatory drugs should be administered if the horse is in acute pain. Even after a prolonged convalescence and after healing has occurred, the withers will be lower than the scapula.

Prognosis

A poor prognosis is given if the serratus ventralis muscle is completely ruptured.

The Tarsus (Hock)

Bone Spavin (Osteoarthritis or Degenerative Joint Disease of the Distal Tarsal Joints)

Bone spavin (true spavin or jack spavin) is an osteoarthritis and periostitis that involves the distal intertarsal, tarsometatarsal, and occasionally the proximal intertarsal joints (Figs. 5–142 and 5–143). The disease usually begins on the dorsomedial surface of these distal joints of the hock, but destructive changes often extend dorsally to involve the dorsal surface of these joints eventually. The early x-ray changes include cyst formation that often involves the adjacent subchondral bone. As the lesion progresses, irregular atrophy of the subchondral bone makes the joint

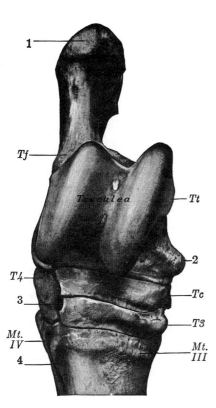

FIG. 5–142. Right hock and proximal part of cannon, dorsal (from front) view. Tt, Tibial tarsal bone; Tf, fibular tarsal; Tc, central tarsal; T3, third tarsal; T4, fourth tarsal; 1, tuber calcis; 2, distal tuberosity of tibial tarsal; 3, vascular canal; 4, groove for great metatarsal artery; Mt. III, cannon bone, Mt. IV, lateral splint bone. The joints most commonly involved with bone spavin are the distal intertarsal joint between the central and third tarsal bones and the tarsometatarsal joint between the third tarsal and third metatarsal bones. Any spavin that involves the proximal intertarsal joint between the tibial tarsal bone and the central tarsal bone has a more unfavorable prognosis. (From Sisson, S., Grossman, J.D.: The skeleton of the horse. *In* Anatomy of Domestic Animals. 4th Ed. Edited by J.D. Grossman. Philadelphia, W.B. Saunders Co., 1953.)

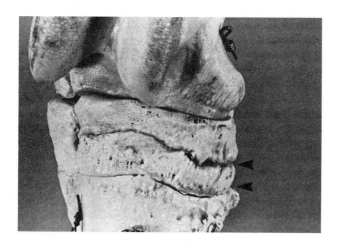

FIG. 5–143. A dried bone specimen from a horse with severe bone spavin involving the distal intertarsal and tarsometatarsal joint spaces (arrows).

spaces appear widened on x-ray examination, and a local periosteal reaction becomes evident. After several months, complete ankylosis (joint fusion) may occur. In other cases, even after prolonged periods of time, only minimal periosteal development will be observed. If ankylosis occurs, the lameness may be abolished.

Degenerative joint disease of the distal joints is considered to be the most common cause of clinical lameness associated with the hock. However, some distinction has been made between clinical entities, and three forms have been described. True spavin (bone spavin or jack spavin) is distinguished from the cunean tendinitis and bursitis (distal tarsitis syndrome observed in harness racing horses). This latter condition is covered on p. 317. Occult spavin or blind spavin has many of the clinical features of bone spavin but lacks x-ray evidence to confirm the diagnosis. However, nuclear scintigraphic studies often show an increased uptake "hot spot" on the radionucleide. Autopsy specimens on these cases indicate ulceration of the articular cartilage and signs of early degenerative joint disease. Some feel that occult and bone spavin should not be considered as separate forms of the disease but rather represent different stages in the development of the same process. Other terms worth mentioning are the blood spavin, bog spavin, and high spavin. Blood spavin is used to indicate a prominent swelling that causes the cranial branch of the medial saphenous vein to distend. Bog spavin is a synovial fluid distention of the joint capsule of the hock. Although bog spavin can occur without bone involvement, it is frequently associated with OCD in young horses. See page 318. High spavin is a bone spavin located more proximally on the hock than a true spavin.

Causes

Bone spavin is observed most frequently in mature horses (3 years and older) that are ridden hard at a gallop (racehorses), horses that jump, and especially western horses used for reining, roping, and cutting. Repeated compression and rotation of the tarsal bones and excessive tension on the attachment of the major dorsal ligaments is thought to be prominent in the development of this disease.

Bone spavin is commonly associated with poor conformation. Sickle hocks and cow hocks predispose a horse to bone spavin. These two malconformations, which often accompany each other, make some cases of bone spavin inheritable. Sickle and cow hocks produce greater stress in the medial aspect of the hock joint. Horses with narrow, thin hocks are more subject to the disease than those with full, well-developed hocks.

So-called "metabolic bone disease" or "developmental orthopedic disease" may be important in the development of bone spavin in the distal tarsal joints of young horses less than 3 years of age. Mineral imbalances, deficiencies, excess protein or protein deficiencies, and endocrine imbalances, have been implicated in defective endochondral ossification (cartilage to bone formation). Several reports have correlated hypothyroidism in foals with collapse of the central and third tarsal bones.

Signs

Horses with bone spavin usually have a lameness history of gradual onset. If the horse is worked hard over several days, the lameness usually worsens, but improves with rest. Racing Thoroughbreds are often not willing to extend (stride out) and exhibit signs of back soreness and forelimb problems. One study of 45 racing Thoroughbreds with bone spavin found that 60% of these horses also had back pain, which was assessed by firm digital pressure. Coexisting forelimb problems included sore front feet and ankles, bucked shins, and knee problems. Interestingly, 85% of the horses in this same study had additions to the hind shoes in the form of heels block or outside stickers. Hunters may start to jump poorly or refuse to jump at all. Reining horses will begin to pivot poorly and stop roughly because of pain. In some cases horses refuse to pivot to the affected side and exhibit their objection by laying their ears back or beginning to buck. Horses that must stop quickly will shift more weight to the least affected limb. This often results in an imbalanced and jerky sliding stop because of the reluctance to firmly plant both hind feet. An affected horse often begins stopping on the forelimbs. The horse may feel stiff or jerky when circled to the affected side.

Pain when the horse flexes the hock joint causes a reduction in the height of the foot flight arc and a shortening of the cranial phase of the stride. The foot lands on the toe and, over time, the toe may become too short and the heel too high. Because of the lower arc of the foot flight, the horse may drag the toe, causing it to wear on its dorsal edge.

Bone spavin lameness tends to be worse when the horse is first used. Horses with mild cases tend to warm out of the lameness after working a short time; in severe cases, exercise may aggravate the lameness. Bone spavin in advanced stages will often cause an enlargement of variable size on the inner aspect of the hock (Fig. 5–144). This enlargement can sometimes be difficult to determine, especially if bilateral spavin is present or if a horse normally has large boxy hocks. When standing, the horse may flex the hock periodically in a spasmodic manner.

Most cases of bone spavin react positively to the hock flexion test. The hock flexion test consists of flexing the hock for 1 to $1\frac{1}{2}$ minutes (Fig. 5–145) and then putting the horse immediately into a trot. A positive reaction to the test is for the horse to take several steps that show more lameness than before the test. In a combined study of 89 race horses (47 from practice, 42 from a referral hospital) with bone spavin, 85% of those examined in the practice and 100% of those examined at the referral hospital showed an in-

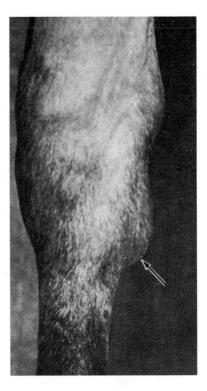

FIG. 5–144. Site of bone spavin of the right hindlimb. The arrow indicates the prominence of new bone growth. (From Veterinary Scope, 7(1):3, 1962; Courtesy of Upjohn Company.)

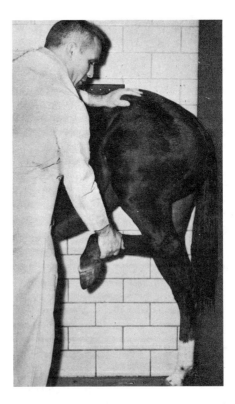

FIG. 5–145. Hock flexion test. The hindlimb should be held in this position for 60 to 90 seconds, and the horse should be observed for increased lameness in the first few steps it takes. Increased lameness is considered to be a positive reaction to the spavin test.

crease in lameness after the hock flexion test. Other conditions, however, may cause this same reaction, especially arthritis in older horses, but in general, the flexion test is considered accurate. It is advisable to conduct the test on both limbs because bilateral bone spavin is common. Gonitis (stifle inflammation) from any cause can produce a reaction to the spavin test. Mild reaction to the spavin test should be viewed with suspicion, and the stifle joint should be carefully examined for problems. The average bone spavin will cause a marked change in the gait, while stifle problems usually causes milder reaction to the test. For this reason, some maintain that the stifle manipulative test should be performed before the spavin test.

As the affected limb is advanced, the sound limb pushes the hips upward so that the affected limb can be advanced with minimum flexion. The tension in the muscles on the sound side may cause the hip on the sound side to look higher, but the unsound hip is pushed higher than it normally would be by this compensatory action. This is commonly called "hiking." This allows the horse to advance the affected limb with minimal flexion (the limb is held rather straight). When viewed from the rear, an asymmetric gluteal rise will be noted. The duration of gluteal use will be shortened on the affected side because the horse is not going through full weight bearing. The foot or shoe may show more wear on the outside because the horse attempts to place most of his weight on the outside of the foot to relieve the pain of the spavin.

Diagnosis

The reduced arc of the foot flight, reduced flexion of the hock, toe wear, and the hock flexion test are used in diagnosis. Infusion of the lower tarsal joints with local anesthetics is helpful in the diagnosis and identifying the joints involved. Lamenesses of the hock and stifle may cause practically identical symptoms. Therefore, careful examination must be given to the stifle as well as to the hock. An enlarged head of the medial splint bone may produce a swelling that looks similar to bone spavin. This can be differentiated by palpation, by its location, and by x-rays. The hocks should be examined carefully both from in front of the horse, comparing the two hocks by observing between the front limbs, and from behind by observing the hocks straight-on and from oblique views. Uneven enlargements are easily detected (see Fig. 5–144), but if the hocks are bilaterally involved, it may be difficult without x-rays to determine if the swelling is normal or not. In most cases, x-rays show that the involvement is on the medial aspect of the proximal end of the cannon bone and on the medial aspect of the third and central tarsal bones, with ankylosis (joint fusion) of the distal intertarsal and/or tarsometatarsal joints (Fig. 5–146). X-rays are essential for accurate diagnosis and prognosis. X-rays also aid in identifying tarsal bone fractures (Fig. 5–147) and cystlike rarefaction (bone becoming less dense) (Fig. 5–148).

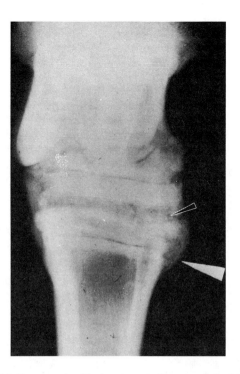

FIG. 5–146. Bone spavin. Black pointer indicates ankylosis (fusion) of the distal intertarsal joint. The white arrow indicates new bone growth on the medial aspects of the third and central tarsal bones. These are typical changes in bone spavin, but the tarsometatarsal joint is not yet fused.

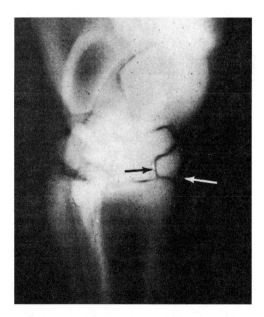

FIG. 5–147. The third tarsal bone is fractured (black arrow) and there is a small chip from this bone dorsally (white arrow). Notice the abnormal shape of the third tarsal bone proximally. This horse showed clinical signs of bone spavin. The periosteal new bone growth on the proximal aspect of the third tarsal bone probably caused the fracture from downward pressure on it by the central tarsal bone. The horse recovered after fusion of the distal intertarsal and tarsometatarsal joints. Surgical intervention should not be used when there is a good possibility of natural repair.

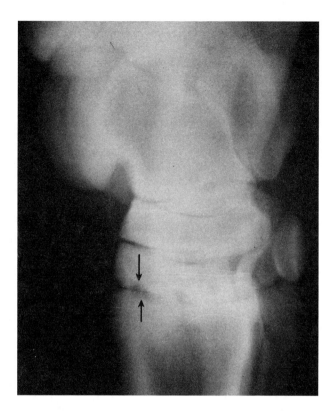

FIG. 5–148. Cystlike bone loss (arrows) located within the tarso-metatarsal joint indicating degenerative joint disease (bone spavin).

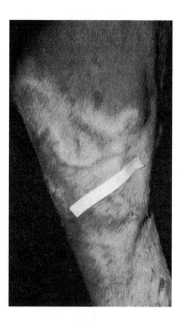

FIG. 5–149. The white tape indicates the course of the cunean tendon where it crosses the medial aspect of the tarsal joint. This is the site of incision for cunean tenectomy.

Treatment

Treatments used include corrective trimming and shoeing, nonsteroidal antiinflammatory drugs at low doses for variable periods, intraarticular (joint) treatment with steroids and hyaluronic acid (HA) and altered exercise programs. Surgical treatments include cunean tenectomy; and surgical arthrodesis. Corrective trimming surrounds balancing the hoof. A flat steel shoe is used and the toe is squared off to ease breakover. The heel may be elevated with pads or wedged shoes to further ease breakover. Low doses of "bute" may be administered for as long as 4 to 6 weeks. Joint injections with a steroid usually provide relief of symptoms, and this is often followed by joint injections of HA 1 to 3 weeks later. Exercise is often reduced to hand walking, initially followed by slow jogging, then gradual increase in exercise over a period of several months. Further joint injection may be required.

Horses that do not respond to conservative approaches are considered for surgery. Cunean tenectomy is removal of a portion of the cunean tendon from the tibialis cranialis muscle (Figs. 5–148 and 5–149). The surgery can be performed with the horse in the standing or recumbent position.

Cunean tenectomy should be considered only as a single procedure if the cunean bursal block gives good relief from lameness. The effectiveness of this surgery

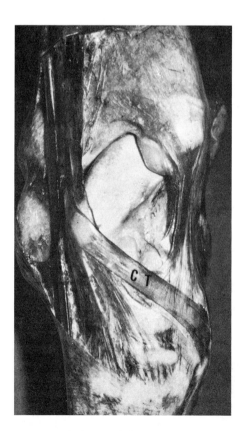

FIG. 5–150. Dorsomedial view of the cunean tendon (CT). Approximately 1 inch of this tendon is removed to treat bone spavin.

appears to depend on the early return to exercise before the scar tissue replacement becomes restrictive.

It is believed that Cunean tenectomy removes a source of pain where the tendon crosses the spavin region; the results of such an operation are variable depending on whether a bursitis of the cunean bursa is present.

Surgical arthrodesis is used to produce satisfactory ankylosis in persistent cases of bone spavin. The distal intertarsal and tarsometatarsal joints are drilled to produce an arthrodesis fusion. Many horses develop osteoarthritis spavin in the second joint even if only one is involved originally. Most commonly, the distal intertarsal joint is involved first, and the tarsometatarsal joint may appear normal on x-ray examination. As little as a year later, change may begin in the tarsometatarsal joint, so both the distal intertarsal and tarsometatarsal joints are surgically arthrodesed as a routine procedure if they are not already ankylosed.

Horses that have bilateral bone spavin can be operated on in both hocks during a single anesthetic period; the horse is rolled over and the procedure repeated.

The horse is rested in close confinement for 30 days and hand-walked only. The skin sutures are removed in 12 to 14 days and bandaging is discontinued after 14 days. Light riding exercise is begun after 30 days and gradually increased. Exercise seems to be important in production of the desired ankylosis.

Some horses take as long as 9 months to 1 year for recovery and complete ankylosis of the involved joints, but most recover in 4 to 5 months. The outlook for recovery is more favorable if only the distal intertarsal and tarsometatarsal joints are involved. If the proximal intertarsal joint is involved, the prognosis is less favorable, but it too should be treated, since this treatment offers the best hope of a complete recovery.

Presently, chemical arthrodesis of the distal tarsal joints is being investigated. Sodium monoiodoacetate (MIA) is the chemical irritant being injected into the distal tarsal joints, and fusion occurs in about 6 months. Unfortunately, only 67% of the horses treated were pain free at the 6-month period. Further investigation on the use of MIA is necessary before it can be recommended for routine use.

Prognosis

Generally, the prognosis for bone spavin is guarded. In those cases that show bony changes in the tarsocrural (tibiotibial) tarsal articulation, the prognosis is unfavorable. A prognosis usually should be withheld until an operation or other methods of therapy are used, especially in those cases showing ankylosis of the intertarsal and/or the tarsometatarsal joints. Complete recovery is expected after surgical arthrodesis in about 80% of the cases where one hock is treated and about 77% of the cases of both hocks are treated surgically. Return to soundness takes anywhere from 8.5 to 12 months. If the proximal intertarsal joint is involved and is surgically treated, about 55% of these horses are expected to become sound. The horse commonly may be slightly lame until warmed up, especially in cold weather.

Although some animals become sound, a predictable decreased height in the foot flight arc is usually present as a mechanical alteration in gait and a firm enlargement associated with the surgical site occurs.

Cunean Tendinitis and Bursitis (Distal Tarsitis Syndrome of Harness Race Horses)

This condition involves inflammation of the cunean tendon, its bursa, and the soft tissues associated with the distal intertarsal and tarsometatarsal joints. It may be the most common cause of hindlimb lameness in harness racing horses. It is thought to be a reversible condition that probably affects the majority of Standardbreds some time during their racing careers. Although it is frequently misdiagnosed as a primary stifle soreness or a partial upward (proximal) fixation of the patella, the stifle may in fact be involved secondarily from protecting the painful hock. Harness horse trainers and veterinarians alike often refer to this condition as jacks, or in some cases, occult or blind spavin because no palpable swelling or pain is present and x-rays usually show no lesion. Although the condition is usually bilateral, it often manifests itself as a single hindlimb lameness that, after injection of a local anesthetic into the joints, will shift to the opposite limb.

The onset of lameness most commonly occurs in the winter and spring as the 2- and 3-year-old Standardbreds are being prepared for summer races. In North America, the average date of onset is usually around March 1, with only a few cases being diagnosed during the racing season.

Causes

The causes appear to be shear stresses that result when the foot impacts the ground at a low angle and again when it pushes off during pacing or trotting. Although the shear stresses are present all the way along the limb, they tend to focus at the tarsus because it is at a 90° angle. These repeated shear stresses result in the inflammation.

Other factors such as improper training and shoeing, abnormal gait, hiking, and accompanying forelimb lameness are thought to play a prominent role in the development of this entity.

Horses that are worked too fast too soon are particularly susceptible. It is speculated that the soft tissues supporting the hock have not developed enough strength to withstand the repeated stress. The average training speed at which this condition develops is at 2 minutes and 30 seconds per mile.

Severe shoeing of the hind feet with calks, grabs, trailers, or bars causes less slippage at impact and takeoff. Thus these shoeing practices all increase the stresses and incidences of this entity. Because some of these shoeing practices are more common in trotters, these horses have a higher incidence of this disease. It may be that many of the interference problems seen in trotters are a result of tarsitis, which often causes the trainer to select even more severe shoeing methods.

Forelimb lameness may result in the horse carrying more weight on its hindlimbs, causing a cunean tarsitis. Pedal osteitis (suspensory ligament desmitis) and flexor tendinitis of the forelimbs are commonly observed. Treatment of the forelimb problem often results in improvement of tarsitis. Additionally, many of these horses exhibit backpain.

Signs

Trainers often report a hindlimb lameness with an insidious onset that is believed to involve the stifle, back, or trochanteric bursa. Although these regions are often painful, the inflammation is probably secondary to a painful hock. At exercise, the horse will frequently carry its hind quarters to the opposite side of the jog cart from the lame limb; it may be difficult to drive, preferring to hold its head to the side of the lameness, and it may begin to interfere and be unable to train as fast. A frustrating feature of this is that most horses look normal when trotted on a lead.

Manipulative tests are important to decide which limb is involved and which joints should be blocked. A lameness with similar signs is gonitis, inflammation of the stifle. Horses with tarsitis usually take only a few lame steps after the flexion test. Those with gonitis are more apparently lame for longer periods of time.

Diagnosis

Intrasynovial anesthesia (joint blocking) of the cunean bursae will usually bring about improvement in the lameness and gait 20 minutes after the injection. A further improvement can be expected within 30 minutes after the injection (see Chapter 3). Interestingly, joint blocking of the tarsometatarsal joint and distal intertarsal joints often results in improvement of the lameness. This is thought to result from blocking of the soft tissues surrounding these joints. If there is improvement from these blocks, it is a good indication that joint injection of a corticosteroid will also be beneficial.

X-rays are usually normal, but in approximately 20% of the cases mild changes may be observed as indicated by spurring and exostosis on the dorsal surface of the central and third tarsal bones.

Treatment

Generally, a combination of therapeutic techniques is used, and the choice depends on the stage of the horse's career and the plans of the owner or trainer. Because the majority of Standardbreds with distal tarsitis have coexisting problems such as sore feet, back pain, and/or suspensory ligament desmitis, these conditions must be treated also for a successful outcome.

The young horse just beginning its racing career is shod with flat quarter-toe shoes behind. In addition, if the feet are misshapen with a steep angle to the medial quarter and with a lateral quarter flare, the shoes should be set full to the inside.

Eliminating fast work for a few weeks will decrease the inflammation, and slow workouts at longer distances (6 to 7 miles) at 4 minute miles will strengthen the soft tissues. Phenylbutazone is recommended to decrease the inflammation. Young horses that do not respond to this treatment should be reexamined.

The experienced competitor with distal tarsitis invariably has coexisting problems which must be discovered and treated. Balancing the feet and the application of flat square-toed shoes is most important. Corticosteroids are injected into the distal intertarsal and tarsometatarsal joints. These injections have a maximum effect in about 4 days. Following this hyaluronic acid can be injected into these joints in 10–14 days. Phenylbutazone is often used to further reduce inflammation, and a rest period of 1 to 2 days with hand walking is usually afforded after the joint injection. Return to training is dictated by the degree of improvement.

Although cunean tendonectomy is a popular treatment for cunean tendon bursitis and some relief in lameness is usually observed, its rationale has been questioned since the removal of these structures further reduces the resistance to shear forces. In fact, no significant difference in racing performance was observed between operated and unoperated horses.

Prognosis

Giving an accurate prognosis is difficult because these conditions appear to be a result of training and management problems. If the trainer will go along with rest periods, reconditioning periods, and altering shoeing methods, a good result can be expected.

Bog Spavin (Idiopathic Synovitis, Tibiotarsal Effusion)

Bog spavin is a descriptive term for chronic distention of the tibiotarsal joint capsule of the hock, causing a swelling of the dorsomedial aspect of the hock joint. Although there are many causes, the distention is due to an acute or chronic low grade synovitis (inflammation of the synovial membrane of a joint).

Causes

Faulty Conformation. A horse that is too straight in the hock joint (when viewed from the side) sickle-hocked or cowhocked is predisposed to bog spavin. If a horse with faulty hock conformation is not affected by bogs as a young horse, it may develop them after training begins.

Trauma. Sprain injury to the hock joint as a result of quick stops, quick turning or other traumas, will cause bog spavin due to injury of the joint capsule or tarsal ligaments.

Other stresses such as lameness in another limb, heavy training, and/or poor shoeing could also be involved in some instances.

Osteochondrosis. Unilateral bog spavin can be caused by chip fractures in the tarsus or osteochondritis dissecans (OCD) lesions associated with the distal tibia and the tibial tarsal bone. Chronic zinc intoxication has been associated with osteochondrosis lesions within the tibiotarsal joint.

Mineral or Vitamin Imbalance. Although deficiencies of calcium, phosphorus, vitamin A or vitamin D, alone or in any combination, have been implicated as causing the problem, there is no scientific evidence for this. Chronic zinc intoxication and copper deficiency have also been implicated in tibiotarsal effusion (fluid distention).

Bog spavin causes a blemish that is serious when due to conformational causes. Once synovial fluid distention of the joint occurs, the condition can be self-perpetuating because of the resultant increase in the intercellular spaces between synovial cells and the dilution of hyaluronic acid by the excess fluid. However, many yearlings show bog spavin in one or both hocks that disappears as they get older. Lameness is seldom present with bog spavin unless it is due to trauma or osteochondritis dissecans.

The synovial fluid changes are usually subtle but are commensurate with a low-grade synovitis.

Signs

Bog spavin has three characteristic fluctuating swellings, the largest of which is located at the dorsomedial aspect of the hock joint (Fig. 5–151). Two smaller swellings occasionally occur on either side of the surface of the hock joint at the junction of the tibial tarsal and fibular tarsal bones. These swellings are lower than the swellings of thoroughpin. When pressure is exerted on any one of these swellings, the other enlargements will show an increase in size and an increase of tension of the joint capsule if held. If the joint distention is severe, a mechanical alteration in the gait (decreased hock flexion and a decreased cranial phase of the stride) may be noted during exercise, but no heat will be felt on palpation. Painful lameness with traumatic bog spavin may result in heat, pain, and swelling over the hock joint. No bone changes will be evident in uncomplicated bog spavin, either

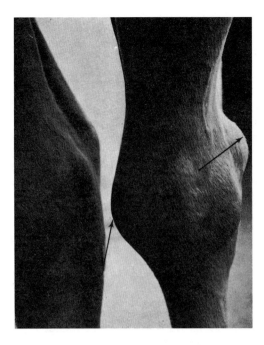

FIG. 5–151. Bog spavin. Arrows illustrate the swellings that occur in typical bog spavin. The dorsomedial swelling is the largest. The swellings at the plantar aspect of the hock on the medial and lateral sides vary in size.

on palpation or on x-rays. A hock flexion test may or may not increase lameness.

Diagnosis

Signs of bog spavin are diagnostic; the only variation is in the size of the three swellings. In most cases, the dorsomedial swelling is the largest, but in some cases the two plantar swellings are more prominent. These three regions are spots where the joint capsule is least inhibited by surrounding tendons, ligaments and retinacula. The lateral swellings must be differentiated from thoroughpin, which occurs at the level of the point of the hock. The most important factor in diagnosis is to determine the cause. X-ray examination is absolutely necessary to rule out chip fractures and osteochondrosis as a cause.

Treatment

Treatment is limited to bog spavins caused by trauma, osteochondrosis, and possibly nutritional deficiencies. Bog spavins associated with conformational defects are difficult to treat because the cause cannot be eliminated. When trauma is the cause of bog spavin, in weanlings and yearlings, usually both hocks are involved, and the problem often disappears as they get older. However, in all cases, an x-ray should be taken to rule out OCD or fracture. For the mature working horse, removal of the primary cause, pressure-wrapping the hock region for 2 to 4 days, and the oral administration of "bute" will often take care of the problem. Again, x-rays should be taken to rule out bony problems and problems associated with tearing of collateral ligaments.

In persistent cases of bog spavin without x-ray evidence of chip fractures or OCD, the blemish can be treated by joint drainage followed by injection of a corticosteroid into the joint. Following the injection of corticosteroids will be a significant reduction in synovial fluid production. In some cases, the joint may be injected with hyaluronic acid (HA) 3 to 4 weeks after the injection of the corticosteroid. Counterpressure by bandaging, following injection, is also recommended. Best results with counterpressure are obtained when elastic bandages are used. The horse should be rested approximately 3 weeks.

A progesterone derivative (Depo-Provera) administered intra-articularly has also been used successfully in some cases of bog spavin. The use of joint drainage followed by the injection of orgotein (Palosein) has also been used. However, Palosein can cause a severe temporary chemical synovitis. Use of a pure fluid form of the drug eliminates the problem.

An alternative treatment is the use of radiation for synovectomy. Six hundred rads applied for 2 to 3 treatments 2 to 3 days apart will affect the synovectomy. This can be done only if the facilities are available.

The recommended treatment for bog spavin caused by chip fracture or OCD is the removal of the fragment and a scraping of the affected cartilage. The arthroscope has proven to be an excellent tool for the treatment of some hock lesions.

Although no specific nutritional abnormalities have been identified the nutritional status of an individual horse should be ascertained as normal when bog spavin without a known cause is encountered.

Tibiotarsal effusion caused by chronic intoxication with zinc appears to respond to removal of the horse from the source of zinc and feeding of a balanced ration, supplemented with 60 g of calcium carbonate per day.

Prognosis

The prognosis for the elimination of bog spavin is guarded because none of the treatments are 100% successful.

Blood Spavin

Blood spavin has no true definition. It usually applies only to an enlarged saphenous vein crossing a bog spavin. It will not be discussed here.

Occult Spavin (Blind Spavin)

Occult spavin is a disease that originates within the hock and causes typical spavin lameness but shows no palpable or x-ray changes.

Cause

It is presumed that trauma is the cause. Most cases of this type of spavin lameness are presumed to be due to lesions within the joint. This damage is usually in the form of ulceration of the articular cartilages. Other pathologic changes may occur, however, such as injury to the small interosseous ligaments that bind the tarsal bones. These changes are not sufficient to be evident on x-ray examination. Inflammation of the cunean tendon and bursa has also been implicated.

Signs

The signs of this disease are those of typical bone spavin lameness, with the exception of physical changes. The cranial phase of the stride is shortened because of the lowered arc of the foot flight resulting from incomplete hock flexion. The same type of rolling action of the hips occurs as in bone spavin. The horse tends to drag the toe of the hoof wall, or of the shoe, and it will wear excessively. The horse responds positively to the hock flexion test and shows all of the symptoms of spavin lameness. Changes indicating bone spavin may become evident later on x-rays.

Diagnosis

Gonitis (inflammation of the stifle) must be differentiated from occult spavin. The use of the intrasynovial anesthesia (joint blocking) of the lower tarsal joints is helpful in localizing the lameness to the hock. X-rays should be studied to detect early changes of bone spavin. Nuclear scintigraphy is also helpful in the diagnosis.

Treatment

Horses that respond favorably to joint blocking generally respond to the intra-articular injection of corticosteriods followed by hyaluronic acid injection in 3 to 4 weeks. Hoof care is also important. The hooves should be balanced and flat steel shoes with a square toe used. In some cases, heel wedges may be helpful. Surgical arthrodesis may be considered in cases where signs of arthritis of the distal tarsal joint become apparent.

Prognosis

The prognosis may be guarded to unfavorable.

Osteochondritis Dissecans (OCD) of the Tibiotarsal Joint

Horses with OCD of the hock may initially be thought to have bog spavin. These animals are frequently not lame but are brought in for veterinary examination prior to being put into training. Osteochondritis dissecans lesions in the tibiotarsal joint are frequently confused with traumatically induced fracture.

Cause

Refer to the Osteochondrosis section in Chapter 4 for details.

Signs

Unlike horses with traumatic fracture of the tibiotarsal joint, those with OCD do not have a history of trauma, but an obvious swelling of the joint is evident. At exercise, a range from no lameness to mild lameness is usual, and severe lameness is not associated with this condition. A hock flexion test may increase the lameness slightly. Palpation of the tibiotarsal joint capsule indicates effusion (fluid distention) without painful swelling.

Diagnosis

An x-ray examination is indicated for all young horses thought to have bog spavin.

Treatment

If the free body is present as an incidental finding on x-ray examination, surgery is probably not indicated. However, a common clinical presentation is bog spavin without lameness. Because of the lack of lameness, surgical removal has been questioned. But cases have been encountered in which horses became lame after they were put into training. The usefulness of surgery was substantiated when the racing performance of operated and nonoperated Standardbreds was compared. Horses that were operated on performed significantly better. Horses that have a mild lameness, tibiotarsal effusion, and OCD lesions should be operated on. These loose bodies can be quite large due to continued cartilage growth after detachment from the parent bone. With few exceptions the use of the arthroscope is recommended.

Prognosis

Surgery appears to improve the prognosis for future use.

Slab Fractures of the Central and Third Tarsal Bones

Slab fractures of the central and third tarsal bones are uncommon.

Causes

The distal tarsal bones are subjected to axial compression, torsional forces, and tensile forces during exercise. Their main function is to absorb concussion and to neutralize these twisting forces. When these bones are subjected to the even greater stress of racing speeds, fracture can occur. Asynchronous movement of these tarsal bones that may be caused by ligament damage or rapid changes in lead may result in the fracture. In most cases, these fractures occur in racehorses working at racing speeds.

Signs

The diagnosis of central and third tarsal bone fractures can be difficult, especially when swelling is minimal and a nondisplaced slab fracture exists. However, if the fracture fragments are fragmented, a nonweightbearing lameness can be expected. Typically, fractures of the third tarsal bones do not exhibit external swelling even though they are often displaced dorsally. Because there is a communication between the proximal intertarsal joint and the tibiotarsal joint, tibiotarsal joint effusion (fluid distention) is usually seen with slab fractures of the central tarsal bone. On palpation, heat can be felt and pain leading to discomfort when pressure is applied to the dorsolateral aspect of the distal row of tarsal bones. A marked reaction to the hock flexion test is usually observed. Intrasynovial anesthesia (joint blocking) of the tibiotarsal joint and proximal and distal intertarsal joints can be helpful in locating the fractures. The retrieval of bloody synovial fluid indicates a fracture.

Diagnosis

X-ray examination is required for a definitive diagnosis (Fig. 5–152). X-ray evidence of degenerative joint disease will be present with tarsal bone fractures of long duration. If the fracture is not visible on x-rays, nuclear scintigraphy can be helpful in identifying the site of involvement. Positive bone scans may precede x-ray findings by 2 to 3 weeks.

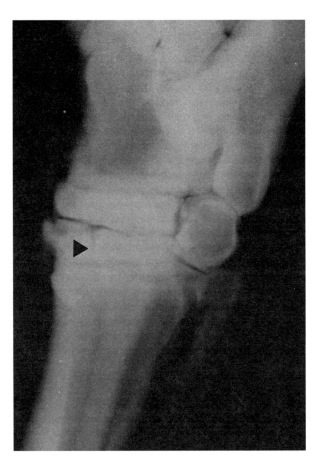

FIG. 5–152. An example of a slab fracture of the third tarsal bone. Arrow points to the fracture line.

Treatment

Although only a small number of cases have been reported, lag screw fixation of displaced fractures appears to be the preferred treatment and provides the best chance for the horse to return to performance. Generally, conservative therapy and surgical removal have proven unrewarding because most horses develop severe degenerative joint disease. However, in one report on three cases of slab fractures (one displaced and two nondisplaced) of the distal tarsal bones which were treated conservatively (prolonged rest and intra-articular hyaluronic acid), all three horses returned to their intended use. The horse with the displaced fracture returned to racing, had 14 starts, and improved his racing times as a 2- and 3-year-old.

Most fragmented fractures are not readily amenable to lag screw fixation and therefore are treated conservatively if breeding status is applicable.

Prognosis

Although some promising results have been obtained with lag screw fixation of these fractures, the prognosis is still considered poor for return to racing performance. Realistically, too few cases have been treated by lag screws to draw a firm conclusion as to the expected outcome. If they are left untreated, nonunions and osteoarthritis can be expected. Mares treated conservatively are usually sound enough for breeding.

Interarticular Fractures in the Tibiotarsal Joint

Interarticular (between two joints or two joint surfaces) fractures are not as common in the hock as they are in the knee and fetlock. They are also frequently confused with osteochondritis dissecans lesions. Fractures can involve any of the bones within this joint. Fragmented fractures occur only rarely.

Causes

Severe stress on the hock joint is undoubtedly the cause of most fractures. However, osteochondritis dissecans may be responsible for some.

Accidents leading to tarsal fractures include being kicked by another horse, racing injury, falls while racing or jumping, and motor vehicle accidents.

Signs and Diagnosis

Grossly, the tibiotarsal joint appears distended with interarticular fractures. Unlike the tibiotarsal joint affected with osteochondritis dissecans, an obvious painful lameness, often with an acute onset, will be reported. On palpation, a painful distended joint is apparent in the acute phase; arthrocentesis (withdrawal of joint fluid) will reveal a bloody synovial fluid. The spavin (hock flexion) test will be positive.

The x-ray examination will usually provide the definitive diagnosis (Fig. 5–153).

Treatment

Depending on the site of the lesion, surgery may be needed to remove the bony fragment. A large fragment near the distal aspect of the bone may be anchored in place with a bone screw in some cases.

Chip fractures are removed through an arthrotomy of the tibiotarsal joint (see Osteochondritis Dissecans of the Tarsocrural (Tibiotarsal) Joint section in this chapter) or with the arthroscope. Impressive results have been observed with conservative treatment of certain fractures. Severely fragmented fractures involving the fragmented tibiotarsal articulation probably warrant euthanasia.

Prognosis

Although the long-term prognosis for traumatic fracture within the tibiotarsal joint has been considered poor, realistically, the prognosis depends largely on the nature of the original injury, its location, and selected treatment. Fractures of the distal tibial malleoli appear to have a good prognosis for return to performance if treated conservatively. Chip fractures involving the nonweight-bearing portion of the tibial tarsal bone also have a good prognosis after surgical removal. Removal of chip fractures of the tibial tarsal bone involving the weight-bearing surfaces carries a guarded prognosis for return to full function. However, this depends somewhat on the size of the fragment, its location, and the duration until treatment. Fragmented fractures of the tibial tarsal bone have a poor prognosis, and euthanasia should be advised.

Fractures of the Fibular Tarsal Bone (Calcaneus)

Fractures of the fibular tarsal bone (calcaneus or "point of the hock") are relatively uncommon. They can be simple chip fractures involving the plantar surface, extend completely through the growth plate in foals, or extend through the body in mature horses. Chip fractures involving the plantar surface can be easily missed on clinical exam. In some cases, however, they go on to form sequestra (a piece of dead bone separated from healthy bone). Physeal fractures and fractures through the body of the bone are often open and are not difficult to diagnose because of the obvious loss of flexor support.

Cause

In most cases, these fractures occur from an external blow, either from the horse being kicked by another horse or the horse kicking a solid object.

Signs and Diagnosis

Chip fractures may be difficult to diagnose on physical examination unless an obvious swelling is present or a draining tract associated with sequestration is observed. On the other hand, fractures through the body or epiphysis are easily diagnosed because there is an obvious loss of function of the gastrocnemius (gaskin) muscle, and the horse will assume a dropped-hock appearance.

The definitive diagnosis is made on x-ray examination (Fig. 5–154).

Treatment

Surgical removal of the chip fractures of the fibular tarsal bone may not be necessary unless they enter the tibiotarsal joint or become sequestered and are accessible to surgical removal.

Although fractures through the main portion of the bone can be difficult to reduce and stabilize, they have been treated successfully with bone plates using the

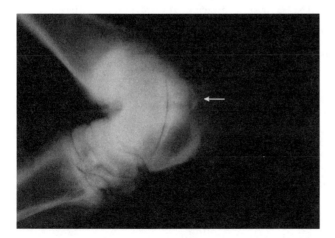

FIG. 5–153. This horse showed obvious lameness that had been present for 1 month. The physical examination pointed to tarsocrural joint effusion. Mild lameness was observed during exercise. X-ray examination identified two chip fractures off the plantar surface of the tibial tarsal bone (arrow).

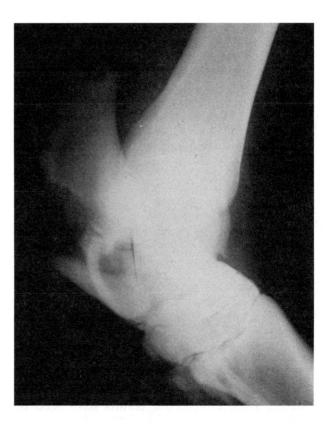

FIG. 5–154. A lateral x-ray of the hock identifying a closed oblique fragmented fracture of the fibular tarsal bone.

tension-band principle, with the additional support of a full-limb cast. Conservative approaches using casting alone have not proven rewarding. There is no rational therapy for the severely fragmented fracture of the fibular tarsal bone, and euthanasia should be advised.

Prognosis

The prognosis for chip fracture of the hock is considered good to guarded depending on its location (intraarticular versus extraarticular), the size of the fragment, and whether it has become a sequestrum. The prognosis for fractures of the growth plate and through the body is considered poor for return to full function.

Dislocations of the Tarsal Joints

Dislocations of the tibiotarsal joint, proximal and distal intertarsal joints, and tarso-metatarsal joint are infrequently encountered in horses. Although fractures of any of the tarsal bones may accompany this injury, if the tarsocrural joint is relatively free of damage, the injury can be treated successfully.

Causes

A severe wrenching or twisting action that may occur from a sudden slip or fall is thought to be involved. Kicks from other horses and entrapment in fixed objects such as fences or cattle guards have also been implicated.

Signs and Diagnosis

Signs are usually quite obvious, because an affected animal will exhibit a non weight-bearing limb deformity associated with the tarsal joints. Crackling may be felt on palpation if the fracture is present. The extent of damage must be verified with x-rays. Dislocations of the tibiotarsal joint is the most severe and, in this instance, the tibia is usually displaced distally and cranially, making it difficult or impossible to realign.

Treatment

Realignment and immobilization with a good-fitting full-limb cast will suffice in most cases of partial dislocations, complete dislocations, and simple fractures without great instability (Fig. 5–155).

If dislocation is associated with fragmented fracture of the tarsal bones or excessive instability is present, a combination of internal fixation and casting is most appropriate (Fig. 5–156, *A* and *B*). In most cases, some

form of internal fixation is advisable. In some cases, tarsocrural joint luxations cannot be reduced.

Prognosis

The prognosis is reasonably good for simple dislocation of the distal tarsal joints without fracture; however, the prognosis worsens from this point if fracture is present. Accompanying fracture within the tibiotarsal joint indicates a poor prognosis. Because tibiotarsal joint dislocations are so difficult to realign, a poor prognosis is given.

Curb

Curb is an enlargement of the plantar aspect of the fibular tarsal bone due to inflammation (desmitis) and thickening of the plantar ligament.

Causes

Predisposing conditions include sickle hocks (sometimes called curby hocks) and cow hocks. Such abnormal conformation imposes additional stress to the plantar ligament and thus tends to produce curb. Inciting causes include violent exertion, trauma from kicking walls or tailgates in trailers, and violent attempts to extend the hock. These causes can produce curb in hocks of normal conformation.

Occasionally a foal is born in which curb appears soon after birth as a result of faulty conformation of the hocks. This faulty conformation may be a result of defective endochondral ossification and partial or complete collapse of the central and third tarsal bones. This set of circumstances has been seen with hypothyroidism in young foals. Associated with this "curby" appearance may be enlarged thyroid glands, a dry coat of hair, and loose flabby appearing muscles. X-rays are definitely indicated for this diagnosis (Fig. 5–157 *A*, *B*, and *C*).

Signs

Curb is indicated by an enlargement on the plantar surface of the fibular tarsal bone (Fig. 5–158). If the condition is in the acute phase, there will be signs of inflammation and lameness. The horse will stand with the heel elevated when the limb is at rest, and heat and swelling can be palpated in the region. Swelling usually does not diminish with exercise, and exercise may actually increase lameness in acute curb. In a severe case, in which trauma has been the exciting cause, periostitis on the plantar aspect of the fibular tarsal bone may result in new bone growth. In chronic cases, tissues surrounding the region often become infiltrated with scar tissue, and a permanent blemish

FIG. 5–155. Ankylosis (joint fusion) of the lower hock joints resulting from complete ligamentous rupture of the tarsometatarsal joint. The limb was immobilized in a plaster cast from the stifle down to and including the hoof.

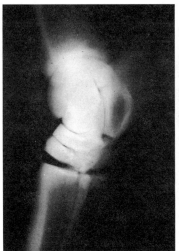
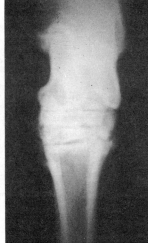
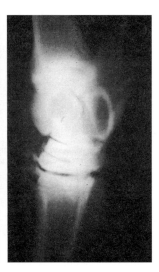

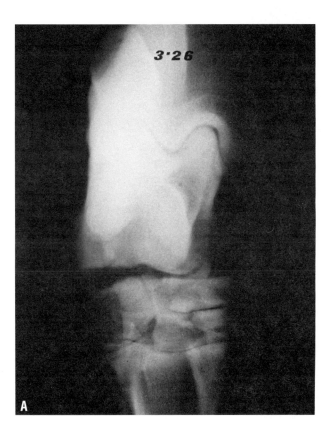
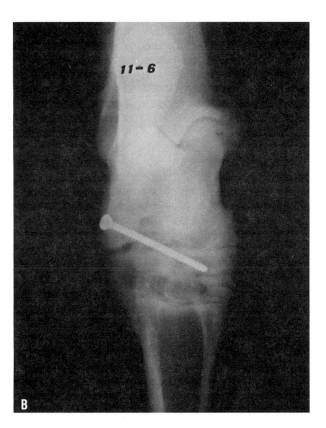

FIG. 5–156. *A,* A dorsal plantar x-ray of a hock illustrating partial dislocation at the proximal intertarsal joint. *B,* This partial dislocation was successfully treated with one bone screw and a cast. Seven-month follow-up indicated good healing. (Courtesy of Dr. C.W. McIlwraith.)

results. Lameness may not be present even though a considerable blemish is evident. Occasionally, the proximal end of the lateral splint bone is large and causes false curb. Careful examination will reveal that the swelling in this region is lateral to the plantar ligament and not on the ligament itself. This finding can be confirmed by x-ray examination if necessary. Ultrasound examination may also be useful.

Treatment

In the early stages of curb, when acute inflammation is still present, cold therapy with ice water packs is most important. Ice is applied 3 to 4 times a day for 20 to 30 minutes. The limb is wrapped between treatments to reduce swelling. Topical application of DMSO may also be used, and administration of a non-

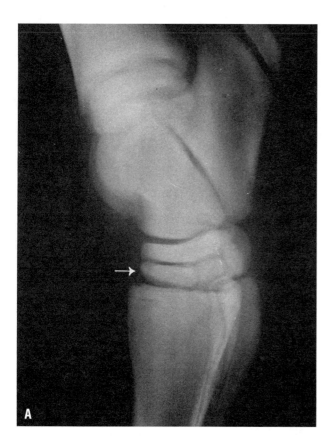

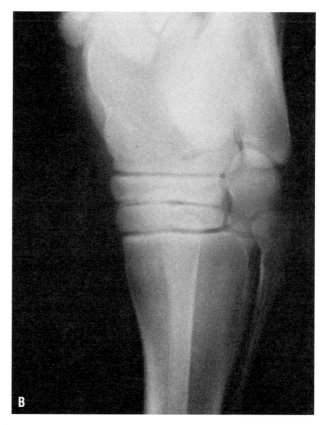

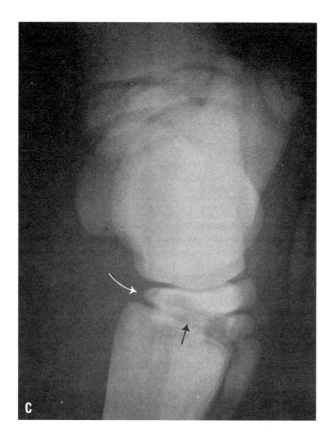

FIG. 5–157. *A*, A lateral x-ray of the tarsus of a 2-week-old foal that has wedging of the third tarsal bone (arrow). On visual observation, the foal appeared to have a "curby" appearance of the plantar surface of the hock region. Treatment consisted of placing this limb in a sleeve cast for 2 weeks. *B*, Follow-up x-rays indicated improvement in the condition. *C*, An oblique x-ray illustrating collapse of the third tarsal bone (black arrow) and wedging of the central tarsal bone (white arrow).

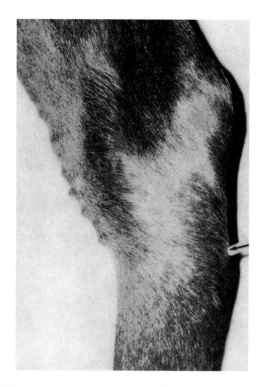

FIG. 5–158. The arrow indicates the swelling caused by inflammation of the plantar ligament, typical of curb. In severe cases, the swelling may extend proximally to the tuber calcis.

steroidal anti-inflammatory drug is also indicated. Cold therapy is continued for 48 hours. Following this, alternating heat and cold treatments can be beneficial. Periligamentous injection of hyaluronic acid may also be used. Rest periods up to several months may be required. Blistering and firing are still done in some regions of the country.

Prognosis

If the horse has good conformation, the prognosis is favorable, providing that the initial acute inflammation is controlled. Poor conformation, however, serves as a continuing cause, and the prognosis is unfavorable. In most cases, some permanent blemish will remain after recovery, even though most horses will be serviceably sound if conformation is good.

Dislocation of the Superficial Digital Flexor Tendon off the Calcaneal Tuber (Luxation of the Superficial Digital Flexor)

Dislocation of the superficial digital flexor tendon off the calcaneal tuber is seen occasionally in horses. The dislocation occurs when one of the attachments of the superficial digital flexor tendon to the calcaneal tuber ruptures. Because of the severe swelling over the point of the hock, a misdiagnosis of capped hock is easily made. However, once the swelling decreases, dislocation can be detected as a slippage of the superficial digital flexor off the point of the hock. Usually the superficial digital flexor dislocates laterally, although medial dislocation has been reported. Initially, affected horses appear quite lame shortly after the injury, but with time the painful response diminishes and a partial loss of complete control of the hindlimb becomes apparent.

Causes

Trauma leading to rupture of either the lateral or medial attachment of the superficial digital flexor to the calcaneal tuber is the cause. It appears that rupture usually occurs about the middle portion of the attachment (between the superficial digital flexor and the calcaneal tuber) possibly indicating a weak point. Medial dislocation has also been associated with a fragmented fracture of the calcaneal tuber.

Signs and Diagnosis

Shortly after the injury, the point of the hock is quite swollen, making it easy to misdiagnose it as a capped hock. As the swelling reduces, the dislocation can be more easily detected (Fig. 5–159). In the acute stage, obvious lameness is present, but with time the horse will appear to have less control of its limb and a periodic displacement of the superficial digital flexor tendon will occur. The displacement is best seen from the rear. While the horse is standing, the superficial flexor can be replaced into its normal position. However, when the horse is walked, the flexor tendon will redisplace and "pop" off the point of the back quite readily. A spavin (hock flexion) test for $1\frac{1}{2}$ minutes usually exacerbates the lameness, although this diminishes with time. On palpation, the dislocation and relocation of the superficial digital flexor tendon can be detected.

Although the diagnosis can be made by clinical signs alone, x-ray will need to be taken to rule out possible fracture. Ultrasound examination is also used to document the injury of the superficial flexor tendon.

Treatment

Surgical repair of the torn tarsal attachment of the superficial digital flexor tendon is recommended. Suturing with either synthetic mesh or screws to stabilize the superficial flexor tendon in its normal position over the point of the hock has been successful.

After surgery, the limb should be immobilized with a cast for at least 30 to 45 days. After this, the limb is supported in a Robert-Jones bandage followed by lesser amounts of support for 30 days. Hand-walking exercise can be begun 7 days after the cast is removed and continued for the next 60 days. Free exercise is begun in a confined area about 4 months postoperatively. In one case in which two screws were used to stabilize the superficial digital flexor tendon, a heavy cotton wrap was used in the immediate postoperative period.

Prognosis

Realistically, too few cases have been treated surgically with long-term followup to make an objective prognosis of the outcome.

Thoroughpin

Refer to the Tenosynovitis section in Chapter 4.

Rupture of the Peroneus Tertius

The peroneus tertius is a strong tendon that lies between the long digital extensor and the tibialis crani-

alis muscle of the rear limb. It is an important part of the reciprocal apparatus, mechanically flexing the hock when the stifle joint is flexed. When this muscle is ruptured, the stifle flexes, but the hock does not.

Causes

Rupture of the peroneus tertius is usually caused by overextension of the hock joint. This may occur if the limb is entrapped and the horse struggles violently to free it. Rupture may also occur during the exertion of a fast start, when tremendous power is transferred to the limb, causing overextension. It can also occur after a full-limb cast is applied to the hindlimb.

Signs

Signs of rupture of the peroneus tertius are well defined. The stifle joint flexes as the limb advances and the hock joint is carried forward with very little flexion. That portion of the limb below the hock tends to hang limp, giving the appearance of being fractured as it is carried forward. When the foot is put down, the horse has no trouble bearing weight and shows little pain. As the horse walks, however, it will be noted that there is a dimpling in the tendon of Achilles. If the limb is lifted from the ground, one can easily produce a dimpling in the tendon of Achilles by extending the hock (Fig. 5–160). It will be noted that the hock can be extended without extending the stifle; this cannot be done in the normal limb.

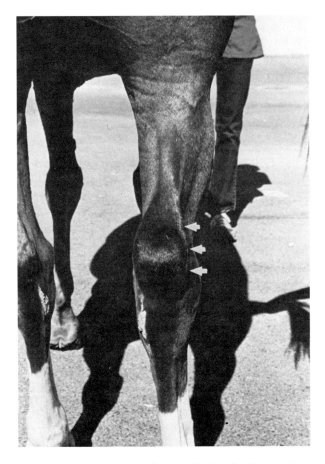

FIG. 5–159. Arrows point to the lateral edge of a dislocated superficial digital flexor tendon. This horse sustained the injury 4 weeks previously.

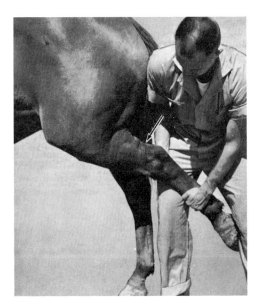

FIG. 5–160. Rupture of the peroneus tertius. The arrow indicates a dimpling in the Achilles tendon when the limb is extended. Note that the hock is extended, but the stifle is flexed; this cannot be done in a normal limb.

Diagnosis

The diagnosis is easily made by the symptoms described above.

Treatment

Complete rest appears to be the best treatment. The horse should be placed in a box stall and kept quiet for at least 4 to 6 weeks. Then limited exercise should be given for the next 2 months. Most cases will heal and show normal limb action and, if properly conditioned, most horses can return to normal work. Surgical intervention is not recommended. Hand-leading is advisable when exercise is first begun. This will help control the horse and prevent reinjury.

Prognosis

The prognosis is guarded to favorable. When the horse is properly rested by box-stall confinement, healing usually occurs. If healing is not evident at the end of 4 to 6 weeks, the prognosis is unfavorable, as the tendon may not unite. Final appraisal cannot be made for at least 3 months after the injury.

Rupture of the Achilles Tendon

Rupture of the Achilles tendon includes the tendons of the gastrocnemius (gaskin) muscle and the superficial flexor of the hindlimb. It is rare for both of these structures to rupture, but when they do, it is a very serious lameness.

Cause

Trauma producing severe stress to these two tendons or lacerated wounds is the most common causes of rupture.

Signs

Signs of Achilles tendon rupture are characteristic. The hock of the affected limb is dropped to the ground or very near to it. The angle of hock deflection is greater than that in rupture of the gastrocnemius tendon alone. The horse has great difficulty in advancing the limb at all and is helpless, especially if both Achilles tendons are ruptured. The limb or limbs cannot support weight.

Treatment

Treatment using a full-limb cast including the hoof and extending it as high on the limb as possible is recommended. This is usually up to the stifle joint. The horse must then be placed in a sling and kept in the cast and sling for 6 to 10 weeks. If the horse will not tolerate these methods of treatment, euthanasia is usually required.

Prognosis

The prognosis is always unfavorable, and only an occasional case recovers (Fig. 5–161A).

Rupture of the Gastrocnemius Tendon

Rupture of the gastrocnemius tendon may occur in one or both hindlimbs. It is rare for both the superficial flexor tendon and the gastrocnemius tendon (Achilles tendon) to be ruptured at the same time. The gastrocnemius tendon apparently ruptures before the superficial flexor tendon.

Cause

Trauma is the cause in all cases. In some cases, the horse is found with the condition in one or both limbs, but the cause is not known. Rupture of this tendon can result from strenuous efforts at stopping or from any other exertion in which great stress is applied to the hock in an attempt to extend it.

Signs

Signs of gastrocnemius tendon rupture are characteristic. The hock or hocks of the affected limb(s) are dropped so that there is an excessive angle to the hock joint (Fig. 5–161B). If the condition is bilateral, the horse appears to be squatting and cannot straighten the hindlimbs. The limb(s) can be advanced and the horse can walk, but at no time do the hock joints assume a normal angle. If the entire tendon of Achilles is ruptured, the limb cannot support weight.

Treatment

Because of the persistent flexion of the hocks, the muscle ends are unable to make contact, making recovery difficult. Placing the horse in a full limb cast and slinging it so that tension on the gastrocnemius tendon and superficial flexor tendon is eased may be beneficial if used for prolonged periods.

Prognosis

The prognosis is unfavorable because of problems inherent with immobilization of the hindlimb.

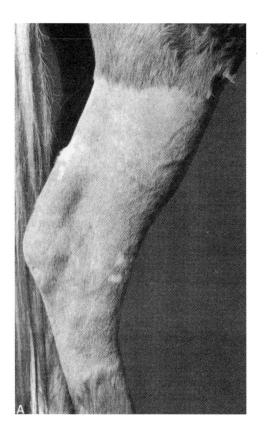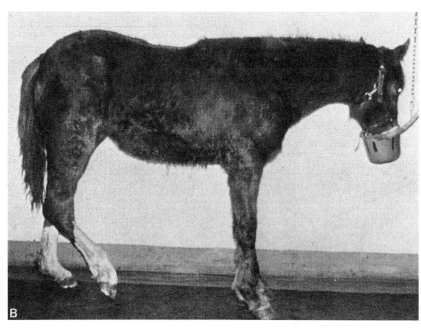

FIG. 5–161. *A,* Healed rupture of the Achilles tendon. Note the enlargement of the healed tendon. Treatment consisted of 6 weeks of limb immobilization in a cast from the stifle down to and including the hoof. (Courtesy of Dr. J.T. Ingram.) *B,* Rupture of the gastrocnemius muscle. Notice the extended stifle joint with flexion of the hock joint.

Stringhalt

Stringhalt is an involuntary flexion of the hock during progression and may affect one or both hindlimbs.

In North America, the disease is usually seen as an isolated occurrence, and although improvement occurs with rest, spontaneous recovery is not observed. Reports from New Zealand and Australia indicate that outbreaks of a stringhalt-like syndrome have been observed. The outbreaks occur in late summer and autumn and are associated with drier than normal summer months.

Causes

The true causes is unknown, although the condition has been blamed on nervous diseases, degeneration of the sciatic and/or peroneal nerves, affections of the spinal cord, toxic factors, and articular lesions within the hock and stifle joints.

Signs

Signs of the disease are quite variable. Some horses show a very mild flexion of the hock during walking, whereas others show a marked jerking of the foot toward the abdomen. The dorsal surface of the fetlock may actually hit the abdominal wall in severe cases. Some horses show these signs at each step, while in others it is spasmodic. In nearly all cases, the signs are exaggerated when the horse is turning or backing. It is usually most noticeable after the horse has rested, but the signs may be intermittent and may disappear for variable periods of time. Any breed may be affected, and mild cases may not hinder the horse in use. Cold weather may cause an increase in signs, and usually there is a tendency toward decreased intensity of signs during warm weather. Most horses affected have a nervous disposition, which may play a part in the cause. The character of the lameness can be confused with intermittent upward fixation of the patella. In some cases blocking the small tarsal joints may eliminate the clinical signs of the lameness.

Diagnosis

The lameness is easily diagnosed, but in some cases signs may be absent at the time of examination. The condition is sometimes confused with fibrotic myopathy, in which the foot is jerked suddenly downward and backward before being put to the ground, and with intermittent upward fixation of the patella, which resembles stringhalt more closely. In stringhalt, there is no locking and releasing of the patella, and the patella cannot be locked when forced upward and outward on the trochlea of the femur. X-rays of the back region should be taken if joint blocks of the region eliminated the lameness.

Treatment

The treatment is surgical for isolated cases and consists of removal of the portion of the tendon of the lateral digital extensor that crosses the lateral surface of the hock joint. Surgical correction can be performed in a standing position, or preferably in lateral recumbency on a surgical table.

The incisions are kept bandaged for 10 days. Most cases show an almost immediate improvement, with complete recovery within 2 to 3 weeks. Other cases may take several months for any great improvement to occur, and still others may never show complete recovery. In cases that recur after several months or a year, an additional portion of the lateral digital extensor muscle may be removed.

Most horses suffering from the stringhalt-like syndrome occurring during outbreaks recover spontaneously without treatment once they are removed from pasture. Recovery can often be prolonged, from several weeks to 12 months.

Prognosis

The prognosis is guarded to favorable. Nearly all isolated cases show some improvement after surgery, but the degree of improvement is not predictable beforehand.

The prognosis appears to be favorable for horses suffering from a stringhalt-like syndrome since spontaneous recovery occurs in most cases.

Shivering

Shivering is characterized by involuntary muscular movements of the limbs and tail. The hindlimbs and the tail are usually affected, but sometimes the forelimbs may be involved.

Causes

The cause of shivering is unknown. Some suggest that it is a nervous or neuromuscular disorder subsequent to influenza, strangles, or other systemic diseases.

Signs

In mild cases, the signs may be difficult to detect because they occur at irregular intervals, but in most cases they are characteristic. They are usually evident when an attempt is made to back the affected horse. As the horse attempts to back, he jerks a hind foot from the ground and holds it in a flexed position abducted from the body. The limb shakes violently, while the tail is elevated and quivers. After a short time, the quivering ceases and the limb and tail return to a normal position. The symptoms usually recur if attempts are again made to force the horse to back. In some horses, the signs are most evident when the horse is turned or forced to step over an object or when his foot is raised from the ground by hand. The eyelids and ears may flicker, and the lips may be drawn backward.

If a forelimb is involved, the limb will be raised and abducted with the carpus flexed. The muscles above the elbow joint will quiver until signs disappear.

Treatment

No efficient method of treatment is known.

Prognosis

The prognosis is unfavorable because the signs usually tend to increase in severity over time. Horses with mild symptoms may be used for work in some cases.

The Tibia

Fractures

Fractures of the tibia are varied and occur with about the same frequency as other proximal limb fractures in horses. Although the complete oblique and spiral fractures are the most common types, fractures of the proximal and distal physis do occur in foals, especially between 1 to 6 months of age. Incomplete (stress) fractures of the tibia can present a diagnostic challenge and can be difficult to treat. Avulsion (separation) fractures of the tibial tuberosity have also been described. Midshaft oblique fractures and spiral fractures can be fragmented to varying degrees, and are frequently open because of the severe overriding of the sharp fragments.

Causes

The causes of tibial fractures are multiple, although external trauma (e.g., kicking) or abnormal stresses are frequently implicated. Fractures caused by torsion combined with bending and axial compressions have been described. Fractures have resulted from falls during a race and have also occurred spontaneously. Incomplete fractures have probably been preceded by a stress fracture resulting from repeated cyclic stress during racing. Growth plate fractures frequently occur during halter breaking. Avulsion fractures of the tibial tuberosity have resulted from an external blow from a polo stick or from kick injury.

Signs

Complete fracture of the tibia is characterized by inability to bear weight on the affected limb and marked soft tissue swelling and crackling associated with the gaskin (crus). Craniomedial overriding of the proximal fragment in relation to the distal segment frequently results in an open fracture. Fractures of the proximal and distal growth plates usually produce a lateral deviation of the limb distal to the fracture (Figs. 5–162A and B and 5–163A). Their configuration can be determined only with radiographs.

Incomplete fractures of the tibia are most frequently seen in race horses, and can be difficult to diagnose. Some clinical features that may cue the examiner to this include: 1) A history of marked lameness with acute onset, 2) pain on palpation localized to the proximal gaskin, and 3) the delayed appearance of soft tissue swelling over the distal component of the fracture. Avulsion fractures of the tibial tuberosity are seen with an acute painful lameness associated with a prominent swelling and pain and a crackling feeling on palpation of the tibial tuberosity.

Diagnosis

Except for incomplete fracture of the tibia, diagnosis of these fractures presents very little challenge. However, x-rays are definitely necessary if surgical treatment is contemplated. Incomplete stress fractures of the tibia may require nuclear scintigraphic evaluation to make the diagnosis in early cases. However, after 2 to 3 weeks, a hairline fracture and proliferation of bone adjacent to the fracture may become apparent on x-rays.

Treatment

Fractures of the proximal two thirds of the tibia in horses are difficult to immobilize for transport and for treatment because the stifle cannot be incorporated in the cast except in young foals. In fact, if a cast is applied, it usually exacerbates the problem because the increased weight of the cast distal to the fracture acts like a pendulum and the fracture becomes the fulcrum. Fractures of the distal third of the tibia can be stabilized somewhat through the application of a full-limb cast placed as high as possible to incorporate the stifle, or in combination with a Thomas splint. This is more effective for young foals than it is for adults.

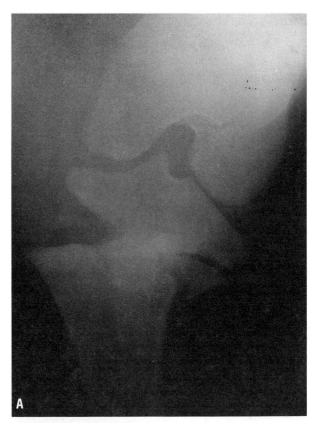

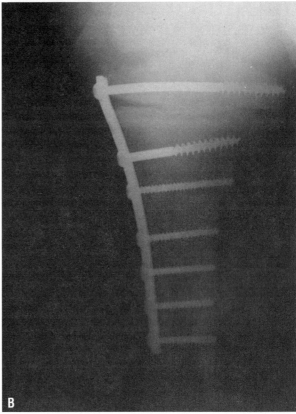

FIG. 5–162. *A*, A fracture of the proximal tibial physis. *B*, A single bone plate placed on the medial side of the tibia was used as treatment. (Courtesy of Dr. C.W. McIlwraith.)

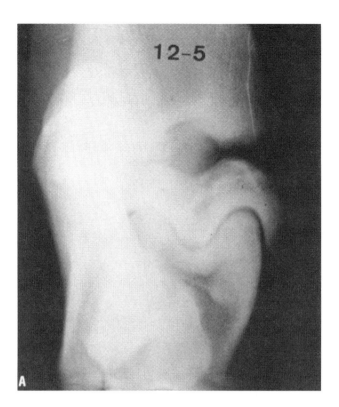
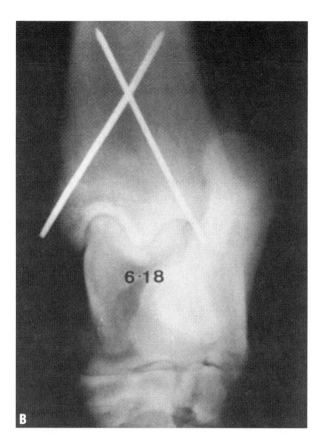

FIG. 5-163. *A*, Cranial caudal x-ray of a fracture of the distal tibial physis. *B*, After realignment, two pins and a full-limb cast were used to treat this fracture.

Generally, if the fracture is open, time should be taken to clip and antiseptically prepare the area for sterile bandage application before transport. Antibiotics should also be administered.

Realignment and treatment of complete midshaft spiral oblique fractures is difficult in the mature horse and still very challenging in the foal. If realignment is not a great concern, the combined application of a cast and Thomas splint in conjunction with slinging has proven successful.

Internal fixation with compression plates has also been successful, particularly in foals. Half-pin and transfixation pinning have also been used successfully in a limited number of cases in foals. It is doubtful that the application is useful in adult horses.

Nondisplaced fractures of the proximal growth plate in young foals can be handled conservatively by stall confinement. Displaced proximal growth plate fractures have been handled successfully with pins or a single boneplate.

Incomplete spiral and oblique fractures of the tibia can be treated by internal fixation using intrafragmentary compression or by the use of casts and Thomas splints. Stress fractures are generally best treated by strict stall confinement for periods up to 3 months.

Fractures through the distal growth plate or transverse distal tibial fractures can be treated by casting alone in foals. The cast should be placed as high as possible to incorporate the stifle if possible. Displaced growth plate fractures in yearlings can be treated successfully with cruciate pinning (Fig. 5-163B).

Euthanasia is advised for adult horses that have sustained severely fragmented fractures except in exceptional circumstances.

Prognosis

The prognosis for a fractured tibia in an adult is poor. The prognosis is guarded to poor in foals and depends totally on the type of fracture sustained, its duration, and the treatment selected. Even with the successful application of internal fixation, the prognosis should be delayed until the healing process is well advanced.

Traction Apophysitis of the Tibial Tuberosity

This condition is reported to affect horses. It is definitely known to occur in dogs and man; in man, the disease is known as Osgood-Schlatter disease. However, it appears that the diagnosis has been abused, because many of the so-called pathologic changes of the tibial tuberosity that appear on x-rays are normal for young horses.

Causes

Trauma to the tibial tuberosity resulting from tension on the patellar ligaments attaching to the tibial tuberosity caused by training of young horses has been blamed for the condition. However, it is also possible that so-called "separation" of the tibial tuberosity may occur from partial upward fixation of the patella. Apophysitis is found in horses up to 3 years of age.

Signs

The signs of this condition are vague. They include mild swelling, tenderness, and pain over the tibial tuberosity following strenuous exercise. The horse will trot in a "dog fashion" because of the short stride of the affected hindlimb. If the lesion is bilateral, the stride will be shorter in both hindlimbs and the toe may be "dubbed off" as a result of the low arc of the foot in flight. Flexion of the affected hindlimb or limbs will exacerbate the lameness. Also, some horses have signs of lumbar kyphosis (hump in their backs).

Diagnosis

The diagnosis is based mainly on x-ray examination. X-rays should be taken of both hindlimbs for comparison.

Treatment

Stall rest or confinement in a small paddock for 3 months is essential. Rest is important because exertion may cause complete avulsion of the tibial tuberosity; however, this is unlikely, because it is rare to find avulsion of this process, even in cases of severe trauma.

Prognosis

The prognosis is good to guarded. The horse should be returned to work on the basis of the findings on the radiographs.

Avulsion Fracture of the Tibial Tuberosity

Avulsion fracture of the tibial tuberosity is uncommon. The tuberosity is a traction epiphysis and serves as a site for insertion of the quadriceps muscle group. The physis underlying the tibial tuberosity is com-

posed of a modified fibrocartilage to counteract the tension stresses of the quadriceps muscles. In horses, it is partially ossified at birth and fuses to the proximal tibial epiphysis during the second year of life. Complete x-ray union occurs between 36 and 42 months of age. Trauma from kicks, stepping in holes, and falling has been documented. The resultant tension on the tibial tuberosity by the quadriceps muscles causes the fractured tuberosity to avulse (separate). Lameness can range from moderate to nonweight-bearing. There may be obvious swelling at the site of the fracture and crepitation (crackling of bone) and pain may be appreciated on palpation. Limb flexion is also painful. The diagnosis is made on x-rays. Bone plates and screws and wires used as a tension band have been used to successfully treat these fractures. The prognosis is guarded to poor and depends on the number of fracture fragments, duration of injury, and whether or not the stifle joint is involved. Generally, the greater number of bone fragments, the longer duration, and if the stifle joint is involved, the poorer the prognosis.

Fracture of the Fibula (Discontinuous Fibula)

Extensive x-ray studies have revealed that what often appears to be a fracture of the fibula is merely a defect in the union of the proximal and distal segments of the bone (Fig. 5–164). This defect in union of the bone can be demonstrated in a high percentage of horses. When x-rays are taken of the opposite fibula, it is usually found that the defect is present there too. Fracture of the fibula can occur as a result of a direct trauma but it probably does not cause the lameness.

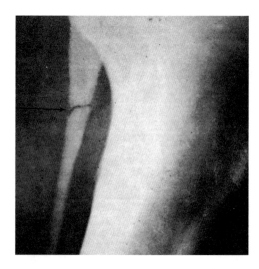

FIG. 5–164. "Fracture" of the fibula. The arrow indicates a normal fibrous junction in the bone, which is frequently found in normal horses.

Fibrotic and Ossifying Myopathy

Fibrotic and ossifying myopathy (muscle disorder) most commonly occur in the hindlimbs of horses. They result from injuries to the hamstrings: the semitendinosus, semimembranosus, and biceps femoris muscles (Fig. 5–165). The fibrotic (abnormal fibrous tissue formation) lesion in the semitendinosus muscle is most important because adhesions form between this muscle and the semimembranosus and biceps femoris muscles. These adhesions limit the action of the semitendinosus muscle, causing an abnormal gait. This lameness most often occurs in Quarter Horses because of the type of work they perform. Ossifying (a change into bone) myopathy in the hindlimb, which also results from previous injury to these muscles, is assumed to be an ossification of a fibrotic myopathy lesion. The signs of lameness are the same as with fibrotic myopathy because the adhesions extending from the bony lesion to the adjacent muscles cause a similar restriction of the limb. Ossifying myopathy has also been observed in the forelimb.

A congenital form of fibrotic myopathy-type syndrome has been identified. Horses are born with an alteration in their gait, characteristic of fibrotic myopathy of the hindlimb. On palpation, a tightening of the semitendinosus muscle is detected but no firm thickening of the muscle typical of fibrotic myopathy is palpated. Because no fibrous thickening of the muscle is present, congenital restrictive myopathy may be a more appropriate description of this entity.

Causes

Trauma is thought to be the cause of fibrotic and ossifying myopathy. Ossifying myopathy is a complication of the fibrotic lesion that also results from trauma. Involved muscles may be injured during sliding stops in rodeo work, or in other ways, such as resisting a scotch hobble or catching a foot in a halter, or from intramuscular injections. The problem is usually unilateral. In some cases, the exact cause of the injury is not known, since clinical signs may not be present during the myositis (muscle inflammation) stage. When the injury heals and adhesions form between the involved muscles, these adhesions cause lameness.

The cause of the congenital form is unknown.

Signs

The signs are caused by adhesions between the semitendinosus muscle and the semimembranosus muscle medially, and between the semitendinosus and the biceps femoris muscle laterally (Fig. 5–165). These adhesions partially inhibit the normal action of the muscles. In the cranial phase of the stride, the foot of the affected hindlimb is suddenly pulled caudally 3 to 5 inches just before contacting the ground (Fig. 5–166). Usually the lameness is most noticeable when the horse walks. The cranial phase of the stride is shortened, and consequently the caudal phase is lengthened. This abnormal gait, which is easily identified, may result from either fibrotic or ossifying myopathy. Because the lameness is mechanical and is not

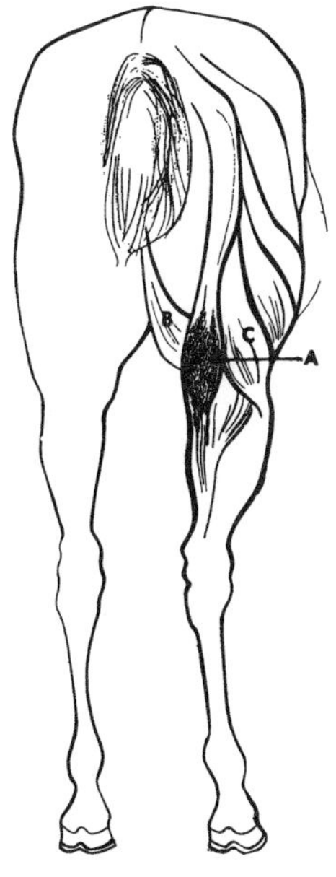

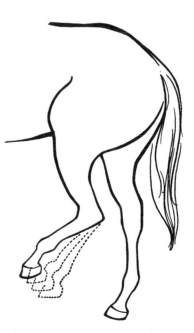

FIG. 5–165. Muscles involved in fibrotic myopathy. *A,* Fibrotic myopathy region in semitendinosus muscle. *B,* Semimembranosus muscle. *C,* Biceps femoris muscle.

FIG. 5–166. Typical action of a hindlimb affected by fibrotic or ossifying myopathy of the semitendinosus muscle. The foot jerks backward 3 to 5 inches just before it is put on the ground.

initiated by pain, it is not altered by any manipulative test. An area of firmness can be palpated over the affected muscles on the caudal surface of the affected limb at the level of the stifle joint and immediately above it (Fig. 5–167).

Diagnosis

The diagnosis is based on the altered gait and on palpation of a hardened area on the caudal surface of the limb at the level of the stifle joint. In making the diagnosis, stringhalt should also be considered. In stringhalt, the limb is pulled toward the abdomen, whereas fibrotic myopathy the foot is pulled toward the ground in a caudal direction just before the foot contacts the ground. In fibrotic myopathy the limb is limited in the cranial phase of the stride by adhesions and by lack of elasticity in the affected area of the muscle belly, causing the limb to be pulled caudally before the full length of stride is reached. Ultrasound examination may be helpful in some cases to define the degree of muscle involvement.

Treatment

Although surgical removal of a 4-inch portion of the semitendinosus tendon and muscle at the level of the stifle joint has been used to treat the traumatically induced fibrotic myopathy. A preferred approach that is less traumatic to perform is a semitendinosus tenotomy.

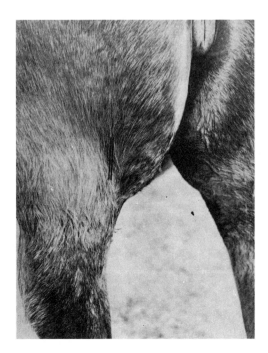

FIG. 5–167. The double lines indicate the region most commonly involved with fibrotic or ossifying myopathy.

Prognosis

With partial myectomy (removal of a portion of a muscle) and semitendinosus tenotomy, some relief will be evident in all cases. After healing, some cases develop characteristic but less pronounced signs, although limb function will be nearly normal and signs will not be noticeable except in the walk. Occasionally, it takes 3 to 7 days for the maximum benefits of surgical correction to become evident.

One report cites a 50% frequency of complications after the partial myectomy of the semitendinosus (e.g., wound dehiscence, disfigurement, scar formation and recurrence of lameness).

The prognosis for tenotomy (removal of a portion of a tendon) of the tendinosus insertion of the semitendinosus muscle appears to be at least equivalent to the myectomy procedure.

Disruption of the Caudal Component of the Reciprocal Apparatus

This is an uncommon problem that results from disruption of the proximal attachments of the gastrocnemius and or superficial digital flexor muscles to the femur. Partial or complete disruption of the reciprocal apparatus can occur, depending on the number of proximal attachments that are lost. Avulsion (separation) fracture of the attachments may also be seen.

Causes

Trauma from falling and slipping may cause this condition. It has also been observed to occur spontaneously during exercise.

Signs and Diagnosis

Proximal swelling is seen on the proximal lateral tibial region and varying degrees of hock flexion with extension of the stifle will be observed depending on the number of proximal attachments that are lost. Ultrasound examination can be helpful in defining the degree of damage, and x-rays are needed to confirm if any avulsion (separation) fracture exists.

Treatment

Stall confinement for 90 days and possibly external support (splinting) in the most severe cases appears to be the approach of choice. Attempts to suture would be futile because the muscle has no muscle power.

Prognosis

On the basis of a limited number of cases, a grave prognosis is given with complete disruption and a guarded prognosis is given for partial disruption of the caudal component of the reciprocal apparatus.

The Stifle

Lamenesses of the Stifle Joint (Gonitis)

Because the stifle joint is the largest and most complex joint in the horse, it is not surprising that injury to it represents an important cause of hindlimb lameness. Briefly, this joint consists of two separate articulations (femoropatellar and femorotibial) and three synovial compartments (femoropatellar, lateral femorotibial, and medial femorotibial) (Fig. 5–168A). The medial femorotibial and femoropatellar joint spaces frequently communicate (65% of cases), and occasionally the lateral femorotibial and femoropatellar joint pouches do as well (17.5% of cases). Fibrocartilaginous menisci (crescent-shaped structures) are interposed between the articulations of the lateral and medial femoral condyles and the proximal tibia. Cruciate ligaments positioned cranial and caudal within this joint stabilize it in a cranial and caudal direction, whereas lateral and medial femorotibial collateral ligaments provide support laterally and medially (Fig. 5–168B). Because of its complex makeup, damage to one region within the stifle joint frequently results in involvement of other structures, which makes the diagnosis and treatment difficult.

As with any joint, injuries to the stifle can be separated into soft tissue and bony lesions. Both often present clinically with a generalized swelling in the stifle region that is referred to as gonitis. The term gonitis is vague, meaning inflammation of the stifle joint. The term does not really constitute a diagnosis; it merely describes a general region of involvement. It is generally accepted that soft tissue injury is more common than bony involvement.

Causes

The stifle joint is subject to numerous forms of insult including trauma, infection, congenital malformation, defective development (osteochondrosis), vascular disturbances, and degenerative processes. The following are conditions of the joint that may cause gonitis.

Partial or Complete Upward Fixation of the Patella. This can cause gonitis and may produce articular cartilage changes of the patella. Irritation causes thickening of the synovium, and roughening of the patella and medial trochlea of the femur may occur.

Sprain or Rupture of the Medial or Lateral Collateral Ligaments. Any form of sprain from mild to sprain fracture will produce gonitis. The medial collateral ligament is the one most commonly ruptured. Rupture causes complete incapacitation because of resulting instability and osteoarthritic changes. Damage to the medial meniscus will eventually occur, either when the medial collateral ligament is torn or from the instability of the femorotibial joint.

Injury to the Cranial or Caudal Cruciate Ligaments. Sprain of these ligaments may occur to any degree. Sprain fracture also occurs (Fig. 5–169). If the ligament is sprained but not ruptured or a partial sprain fracture occurs, diagnosis is difficult. X-rays may reveal separation of the tibial spine (see Fig. 5–169). The cranial cruciate ligament is the one most commonly ruptured and may be damaged along with the medial collateral ligament. Damage to the medial meniscus can occur, either when the cranial cruciate ligament is damaged or from the resulting instability of the femorotibial joint.

Injury to the Menisci. Meniscal injuries occur in the horse but are difficult to diagnose. The medial meniscus is the one most commonly damaged. Persistent effusion (fluid distention) of the joint and chronic lameness can result (Fig. 5–170).

Injuries to the Joint Capsule. The joint capsule may be injured and the fibrous portion partially torn from its attachment. This type of injury is rare.

Severe Trauma to the Joint. This may produce an injury such as a fractured trochlea of the femur or fracture of the patella. This is also a rare type of injury.

Although fractures can involve the proximal tibia, the femur and the patella, fractures of the trochlear ridges of the femur appear to be the most common. Usually direct trauma is the cause and is accompanied by fairly obvious swelling and lameness. However, if a history of trauma is not given, and some days have passed since the injury, this may be difficult to differentiate from osteochondrosis.

Chondromalacia (Degeneration of Articular Cartilage) of the Patella. Although it is believed that partial and complete upward fixation of the patella may cause damage to the articular surface of the patella that results in chondromalacia, this has not been clarified completely.

Osteochondral Fragmentation of the Distal Patella. This condition has been observed following medial patellar desmotomy. On x-rays, bony fragmentation, spurring, and subchondral lysis (bone loss) at the distal aspect of the patella have been observed.

Infectious Arthritis. Infectious arthritis may result from septicemia, especially in foals. On x-ray, the epiphysial subchondral bone often appears lytic (exhibiting bone loss).

Osteochondritis Dissecans and Subchondral Bone Cysts. Osteochondritis dissecans that affects the trochlear ridges, primarily the lateral one, and subchondral bone cysts affecting primarily the medial condyle of the femur, are relatively common causes of gonitis in young horses under 3 years of age (see Chapter 4, Osteochondrosis). Subchondral bone cysts of the proximal tibia and a typical osteochondritis of the tibial spine have also been observed.

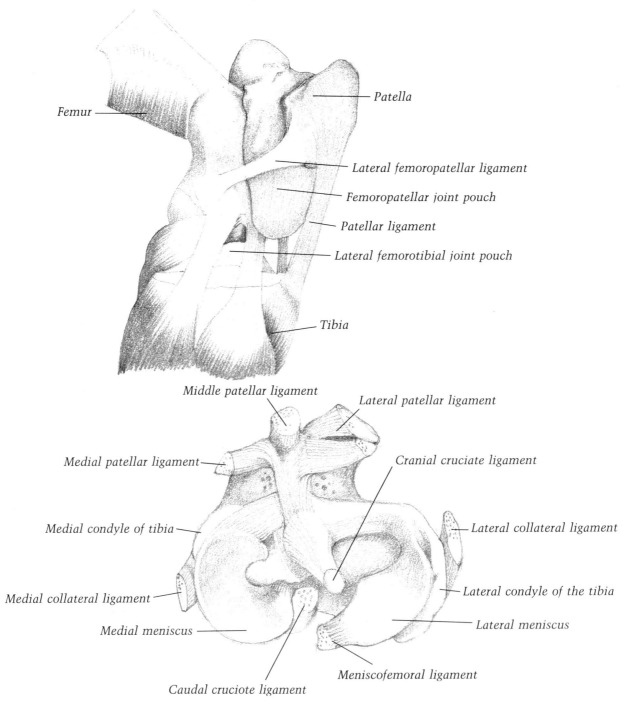

Femur

Patella

Lateral femoropatellar ligament

Femoropatellar joint pouch

Patellar ligament

Lateral femorotibial joint pouch

Tibia

Middle patellar ligament

Lateral patellar ligament

Medial patellar ligament

Cranial cruciate ligament

Medial condyle of tibia

Lateral collateral ligament

Medial collateral ligament

Lateral condyle of the tibia

Medial meniscus

Lateral meniscus

Caudal cruciote ligament

Meniscofemoral ligament

FIG. 5–168. *A,* Lateral view of stifle illustrating the femoropatellar joint pouch, the lateral femorotibial pouch, and various ligaments. (From Sisson, S., Grossman, J.D.: Anatomy of Domestic Animals. 5th Ed. Philadelphia, W.B. Saunders, 1975.) *B,* Top view of the right tibia illustrating the menisci and the various ligaments. (After Sisson, S., Grossman, J.D.: Anatomy of Domestic Animals. 5th Ed. Philadelphia, W.B. Saunders, 1975.)

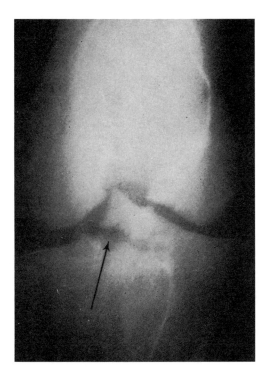

FIG. 5–169. Fracture of the tibial spine associated with rupture of the cranial cruciate ligament (sprain-fracture). Fracture of this spine usually does not accompany rupture of the cruciate ligaments.

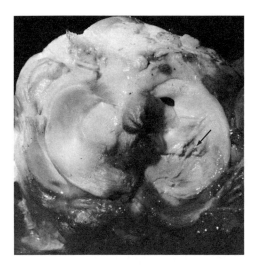

FIG. 5–170. Wrinkling and tearing of the medial meniscus (arrow). This type of injury can occur with or without tearing of the ligaments of the stifle. When upward fixation of the patella and ligamentous injury can be ruled out, tearing of the medial meniscus should be considered in chronic gonitis.

Osteoarthritis. Osteoarthritis of the stifle joint is usually observed in older horses. Prolonged instability from sprain trauma to the collateral ligaments or cruciate ligaments, chip fractures, fractures, chronic synovitis capsulitis, osteochondritis dissecans, and subchondral bone cysts can result in this type of change.

Epiphysitis. Epiphysitis of the distal femoral physis or proximal tibial physis is a rare cause of mild lameness associated with the stifle.

Miscellaneous Causes. Miscellaneous soft tissue injuries to the quadriceps femoris muscle, patellar ligaments, and other surrounding muscles can produce signs of gonitis. Dislocations of the patella should also be included in this category.

From the above, it can be seen that lameness associated with the stifle joint can be complex. Any one or any combination of the above structures may be injured. Several types of arthritis may affect the stifle joint, including serous arthritis, osteoarthritis, and septic arthritis. Navel ill of foals is the most common cause of septic arthritis.

Signs

On gross observation, distention of the stifle joint (gonitis) may be seen when the horse is viewed from the side (Fig. 5–171). With long-standing stifle involvement, atrophy of the gluteal muscles on the affected side may also be apparent. Wearing of the toes is also a common finding (Fig. 5–172).

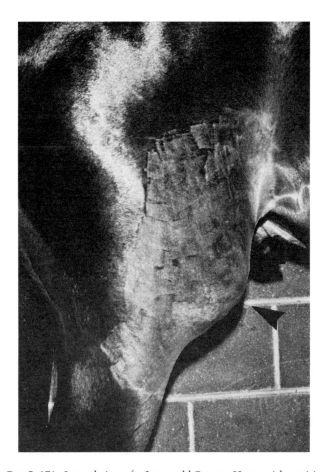

FIG. 5–171. Lateral view of a 3-year-old Quarter Horse with gonitis (arrow).

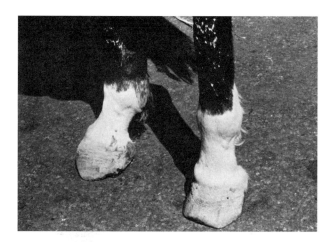

FIG. 5–172. This horse has bilateral chronic swelling of its femoropatellar joint capsules. Note the excessive toe wear.

The degree of lameness varies according to the severity of the injury. Involvement of the menisci and the cruciate or collateral ligaments usually produces severe lameness. Complete or incomplete upward fixation of the patella can also produce gonitis, but signs of lameness are less acute. If the patella partially or completely locks, irritation of the synovial structures occurs, and chronic distention of the joint capsule and persistent lameness eventually result.

Generally, the cranial phase of the stride is shortened and the foot is carried closer to the ground. A toe drag is frequently heard when the horse advances the limb at a trot, and the toe wear is obvious in chronic cases. When the horse is viewed from the rear, asymmetry in the gluteal rise while trotting will be noted. Although the hip on the affected side usually elevates more than its opposite member, the duration of gluteal use is shorter. This is frequently referred to as the "hip hike."

On palpation, distention and thickening of the femoropatellar joint capsule can be felt between the patellar ligaments. To gain a full appreciation for the degree of distention, a comparison should be made with the opposite limb. In a well-behaved animal, this can be done at the same time while standing behind the horse. In others, it will have to be done individually. It is difficult to palpate distention of either the lateral or medial femorotibial joint, but when these joints are distended, the proximal tibia just cranial to the collateral ligament becomes less distinct.

Diagnosis

Diagnosis of stifle joint involvement is made by careful observation of the gait, palpation of the joint, and elimination of other types of lameness.

The patella is forced proximally and laterally in an attempt to lock the medial patellar ligament over the medial trochlea. Horses that are in a lot of pain will frequently attempt to kick. Pulling the horse by the tail or pushing the horse to the side of the examiner will help assist in this maneuver. If the patellar ligaments catch and the horse is unable to flex the limb when it walks off, upward (proximal) fixation of the patella is a problem. On the other hand, if crepitation and pain are elicited with manipulation and a tendency to catch the patella with increased lameness for the first few steps, partial upward fixation of the patella should be suspected (see Upward Fixation of the Patella section in this chapter).

A flexion test of the hindlimb that flexes the hock and stifle, and to some extent the hip, often causes increased signs of lameness, but usually less severe than those observed with hock problems. With serious damage to the articular surfaces, ligaments or menisci, profound lameness may result.

A cruciate ligament test should be run to identify sprain trauma or cruciate rupture. The simplest way to do this is for the examiner to place the palm of his hand on the proximal end of the tibia, and while the other hand is used to pull the tail toward the examiner, the tibia is forced caudally and pressure is released cranially. Crackling, pain, and laxity when the joint comes forward indicate a rupture of the cranial cruciate. Pain and crackling, with laxity when the tibia is forced caudally indicates a rupture of the caudal cruciate ligament (Fig. 3–40). In both cases, horses present with severe lameness.

The collateral ligaments are examined for sprain trauma and rupture by abducting and adducting the limb. The medial collateral ligament is easily checked by placing the shoulder on the lateral side of the stifle and pulling the distal part of the hindlimb away from the horse (Fig. 3–41). With sprain trauma, increased pain will be perceived as well as increased lameness. Ultrasound examination can be helpful in diagnosing the degree of sprain injury. With rupture, the horse is in severe pain and may fall over in an attempt to get away from the examiner. Although the distal limb is adducted to identify problems with the lateral collateral ligament, it is rarely involved.

Intrasynovial anesthesia (joint blocking) of the stifle joint can be helpful.

A complete series of good quality x-rays are needed to evaluate the stifle joint.

Arthroscopy can be used for direct visualization of the intraarticular structures of the stifle joint. Relatively good visualization of the synovial membrane, articular surfaces, menisci, and intraarticular ligaments can be made. Additionally, arthroscopy not only facilitates biopsy but tissue removal for diagnostic examination also provides a means of photographic documentation of pathologic changes within the joint.

Treatment

The treatment obviously depends on the cause of the stifle problem. For recommended treatments of upward fixation of the patella, patellar fracture, osteochondritis dissecans, subchondral bone cysts, or fracture, refer to those sections in this chapter.

If the gonitis is believed to be caused by sprain and injury to the joint capsule or ligamentous attachments without rupture, absolute rest should be enforced for a long period. Confinement should consist of a minimum of 45 days in the box stall and then a minimum of 2 months in a small paddock; in some cases, 3 months in a box stall may be necessary. Nonsteroidal anti-inflammatory drugs are a logical choice and are administered according to response.

If there is a rupture of one of the collateral or cruciate ligaments of the joint, or damage to the medial meniscus, stall confinement for prolonged periods followed by gradual increase in exercise may return the horse to breeding soundness. One case of successful surgical repair of a complete rupture of the medical collateral ligament has been documented. If there is complete rupture of more than one ligament, euthanasia for humane reasons is justified. and chronic lameness will result. If x-ray examination indicates osteoarthritic changes associated with fractures within the joint, the prospects for treatment are also unfavorable (see Fig. 5–169). In septic (infectious) arthritis of the stifle joint, the joints can be treated with intraarticular lavage (flushing) after antibiotic sensitivity of the organism has been determined. Broad-spectrum antibiotics should also be given.

Prognosis

If the gonitis is caused by upward fixation of the patella or mild sprain trauma to the ligaments, the prognosis is favorable, as long as cartilage changes are not extensive. For the other causes, the prognosis is guarded to unfavorable. Horses do not return to a sound condition if x-ray changes of osteoarthritis can be demonstrated.

Upward Fixation of the Patella

Upward fixation of the patella occurs on the medial trochlea of the femur between the middle and medial patellar ligaments (Fig. 5–173). The fixation of the patella on the medial trochlea of the femur prevents flexion of the affected hindlimb. It is sometimes called a dislocation, although this is a misnomer. The fixation can be either intermittent or complete.

Causes

There may be a hereditary predisposition to upward fixation of the patella brought about by conformation. A horse having a steep angle between the femur and tibia, or so-called "straight hindlimb," with what appears to be a long tibia, may be predisposed to the condition. Some cases of upward fixation can be the result of trauma incurred when the limb was overextended. Debility and poor conditioning also can be predisposing factors. Horses with poor muscling (e.g., young or unconditioned) through the stifle are also predisposed. Upward fixation has also been observed in horses abruptly taken out of training and confined to a stall. Apparently, the rapid loss of muscle and ligament tone allows a greater range of movement of the patella, and fixation can occur. This is usually relieved shortly after the horse is put back into exercise. Once upward fixation occurs, the ligaments may be stretched, so recurrence is common. The condition may be present in only one hindlimb, but careful examination often reveals susceptibility in both hindlimbs. Shetland ponies are probably most often affected in this manner.

Although all these conditions may predispose a horse to intermittent or complete upward fixation, the underlying cause may be a disorder of the neuromuscular mechanism that normally releases one patella from its resting position. For example, spasms of the medial thigh muscles (sartorius and gracilis) that insert on the medial patellar ligament may prevent the patella from being released during flexion.

Signs

In acute upward fixation of the patella, the hindlimb is locked in extension (Fig. 5–174). The stifle and hock cannot flex, but the fetlock can. The condition may temporarily relieve itself only to lock again in a few steps, or it may remain locked for several hours or even days. In some cases there is only a "catching" of the patella as the horse walks and the limb never truly locks in extension. This "catching" of the patella is most noticeable when the horse is turned in a short circle toward the affected hindlimb. This intermittent upward fixation of the patella can cause the lameness to be confused with stringhalt, and careful physical examination is required.

Another helpful diagnostic aid is to walk the horse up and down a slope. Because horses with intermittent upward fixation of the patella are reluctant to fully extend the stifle when they walk uphill, they assume a slightly crouched position and are reluctant to allow the stifles to be thrust caudally. As they descend the slope, a jerky gait will be noted as the result of incomplete extension of the stifle. If the stifle does go into full extension, a catch leading to a toe drag will occur in some cases.

Upon palpation, when the limb is locked in extension, the ligaments of the patella are tense and the patella is locked above the medial portion of the trochlea of the femur (see Fig. 5–173). When the horse is forced to move forward with the limb locked, it drags the front of the hoof on the ground. In some cases, a snapping sound may be heard when the patella is released from the trochlea.

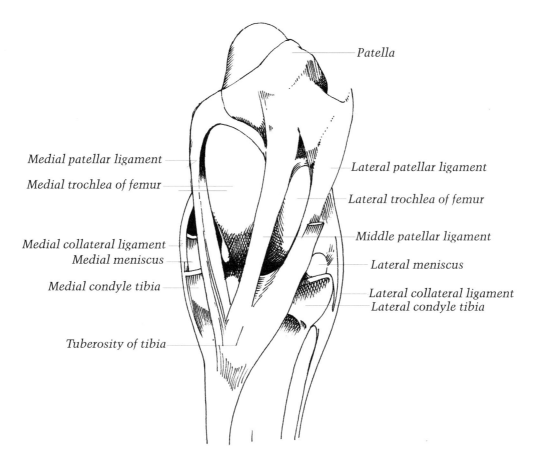

FIG. 5–173. Cranial view of the stifle joint illustrating the patella, three patellar ligaments, and the trochlea. (After Sisson, S., Grossman, J.D.: Anatomy of Domestic Animals. 5th Ed. Philadelphia, W.B. Saunders, 1975.)

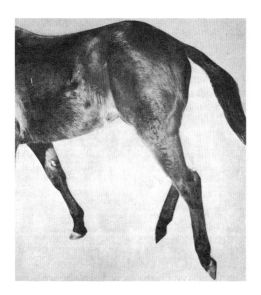

FIG. 5–174. Upward fixation of the patella. The limb is locked in extension as the horse attempts to pull the limb forward. Note that the left fetlock, pastern, and coffin joints are flexed while the stifle and hock joints are locked in extension.

Diagnosis

The signs are typical and, if the limb is locked, the diagnosis is simple. In cases in which a partial locking or complete locking is observed, the veterinarian might force the patella upward and outward. If the limb can be locked in extension for one or more steps, it is predisposed to upward fixation of the patella. In some cases, this condition is chronic, causing an inflammation of the stifle joint. The inflammation in the joint may remain even though upward fixation is corrected. The joint capsule will be checked for distention by palpating between the lateral and middle patellar ligaments and between the middle and medial patellar ligaments. Excess fluid or thickening of the joint capsule indicates that gonitis is present.

When intermittent upward fixation of the patella is present, confusion with stringhalt sometimes exists. In this case, careful observation of the gait and stifle joint will reveal whether the patella is "catching."

The condition is commonly bilateral, although it may be worse in one limb. In some vague cases, it will be noted that the horse tends to drag the toe when advancing the limb. The flight of the foot has a low arc, and there is a short cranial phase to the stride. In such a case, the patella may be locked in upward fixation with the hand. X-rays of the stifle in horses under 3 years of age will eliminate the possibility of concurrent osteochondritis dissecans and subchondral bone cysts.

Treatment

The treatment is varied and depends on the severity of the condition. In intermittent upward fixation of the patella, all efforts are made to treat the condition conservatively. This includes training to improve muscle tone and possibly to reduce muscle spasms. Exercise in soft sand arenas should be avoided. Although there are no good follow-up studies, injection of the patellar ligaments with irritants can be used. Medial patellar ligament desmotomy (surgical severance) is used only as a last resort. On the other hand, medial patellar ligament desmotomy may be the first choice in treatment when the patella cannot be "unlocked" (permanent upward fixation).

When desmotomy is performed, no riding or training should occur for approximately 12 weeks so that full accommodation to the loss of the ligament can occur before stress is imposed on the joint. Both limbs may be done at the same time if necessary. If surgical correction is carried out before gonitis or damage to the articular cartilage of the patella becomes evident, the method of treatment affords a high rate of recovery.

Prognosis

The prognosis is generally favorable for both conditions (intermittent and persistent upward fixation). However, even after prolonged rest periods, fragmentation of the distal patella may occur after desmotomy of the medial patellar ligament. If fragmentation does occur, arthroscopic surgery will be needed.

Chondromalacia of the Patella

Chondromalacia of the patella has been defined as a degeneration of the articular cartilage of the patella that may result from an inflammatory disease of the stifle joint or from a combination of inflammation and pressure exerted upon it from a partial or complete upward fixation of the patella. However, there is little clinical evidence to support this diagnosis as a singular entity at this time. The cause is felt to be repeated trauma from a malaligned patella. With this information, it is tempting to extrapolate the disease to the horse with so-called "loose" patellas. However, there are no reports on the clinical incidence of the disease, and the lesions are also seen on the articular surfaces

of clinically normal horses. It is possible that these lesions also represent a form of osteochondrosis.

Tumoral Calcinosis (Calcinosis Circumscripta)

Refer to Chapter 4, Tumoral Calcinosis.

Osteochondrosis of the Stifle

Refer to Chapter 4, Osteochondrosis.

Patellar Dislocations

Although patellar dislocations exist, they are considered a rare entity. The condition is usually congenital, being recognized shortly after birth. Varying gait abnormalities will alert one to the problem. Lateral, medial, unilateral, and bilateral dislocations have been described, but the unilateral, lateral dislocations is by far the most common. The dislocation can range from a mild intermittent partial dislocation to a complete dislocation that is difficult to replace manually.

Causes

Trauma is thought to be the cause. The condition can also occur in association with defective development of the lateral trochlear ridge caused by osteochondritis dissecans.

Signs

Signs vary according to the position and degree of displacement of the patella. Complete displacement of the patella usually results in an inability to extend the stifle. When complete dislocation of both patellas occurs, the horse is often unable to stand and assumes a rather classic crouched position. Persistent lateral partial dislocation of the patella appears much like upward fixation of the patella. The limb is held in extension, causing it to be placed caudolaterally. When the limb is advanced, an awkward swinging gait with typical toe dragging occurs. Horses exhibiting intermittent unilateral partial dislocation of the patella with spontaneous relocation often move fairly normally, only to suddenly lose their extensor support when the patella displaces. Because some of these animals have a fairly normal gait, the condition is often missed until serious degenerative changes within the joint have occurred.

On palpation, varying degrees of patellar displacement and joint capsule distention will be detected. Although complete dislocations can be difficult to replace, the intermittent partial dislocations are usually not.

Diagnosis

X-rays should be taken to confirm the diagnosis, identify the amount of degenerative changes occurring within the joint, and determine the degree of displacement.

Treatment

Relocation and stabilization of the patella in its proper axial alignment within the trochlear groove are achieved by a relaxing incision on the side toward which the patella is luxated and a tightening of the loose side (away from the patella).

Prognosis

The prognosis is considered guarded in all cases and becomes poor if the condition is bilateral and degenerative joint disease is present. The potential genetic characteristics of the congenital form should be considered.

Fracture of the Patella

Fracture of the patella is rare in horses and may be related to size, somewhat protected location, and great range of motion. Direct trauma to the patella usually results in the bone being pushed away rather than fractured. When fractures do occur, they are usually associated with severe soft tissue trauma involving the ligaments and the capsule of the stifle joint. Both transverse (horizontal) and longitudinal fractures occur.

Causes

Direct trauma to the patella while the stifle joint is semiflexed may be the most likely cause. In this position, the patella becomes fixed against the trochlea, and its mobility is reduced. Kicks from other horses and running into solid objects have also been documented. Patella fractures have also been documented after slipping or falling.

Signs and Diagnosis

Horses present with an acute onset of lameness and a significant painful swelling associated with the cranial aspect of the stifle. On palpation, pain and sometimes a crackling feeling will be noted. Flexion of the stifle joint exacerbates the lameness and the painful

response. X-rays are required to document the nature of the fracture (Fig. 5–175).

Treatment

Prolonged stall rest may be useful for nondisplaced fractures. Rest periods from 3 to 5 months are required. Partial patellectomy (surgical removal) of fracture fragments that are too small for internal fixation has proven beneficial. Most of these fragments can be removed with the arthroscope. Internal fixation should be considered for large displaced and comminuted (many fragments) fractures. Successful treatment of transverse and longitudinally placed fractures of the patella has been documented. Of the two, the longitudinal fracture is easier to realign and stabilize, and there is less chance of having it displace after surgery. Transverse fractures, on the other hand, are more difficult to treat successfully because of the tendency of the proximal segment to become displaced proximally by the pull of the quadriceps femoris muscles. In either case, failure to achieve good anatomic realignment can result in degenerative changes within the stifle joint.

Prognosis

The prognosis depends on the combined evaluation of the patellar fracture and the soft tissue injury. Conservative treatment is usually less than satisfactory unless the fracture is nonarticular or a nondisplaced articular fracture exists. The prognosis for articular fractures or osteochondral fragments that are surgically excised appears good. In one case series, 10 of 14 cases in which partial patellectomy was used for the removal of intra-articular fractures of the medial patella returned to full athletic function. Internal fixation provides the most ideal set of circumstances for a favorable outcome for displaced fractures.

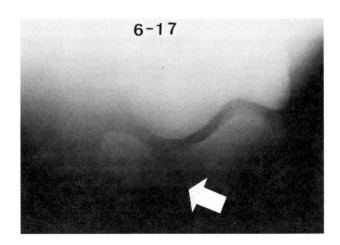

FIG. 5–175. A skyline x-ray view of the stifle joint indicating a fracture of the patella (arrow).

The Femur

Fractures

Fractures of the femur are relatively common in horses. In foals, fractures often involve the proximal and distal growth plate. Adults, on the other hand, usually sustain fragmented fractures of the femoral shaft. Femoral shaft fractures are usually severely displaced, making it difficult to realign the fracture at surgery.

Causes

Young foals frequently sustain femoral fractures during the initial handling and often during halter breaking. Occasionally, the mare steps on the foal, causing this type of injury, or the foal becomes entrapped under a fence. In mature horses, considerable force is required to fracture the femur.

Signs

Horses with femoral fractures frequently have a history of severe trauma leading to a nonweight-bearing lameness. When viewed from the side, the affected limb may appear slightly shortened with the hock held higher than the opposite hindlimb and a dimpling of the musculature overlying the fracture may be observed (Fig. 5–176). In some, obvious swelling may be present. During movement, a nonweight-bearing lameness will be noted. On palpation, excessive movement of the distal limb will be detected. In younger horses, swelling can be observed in association with the fracture site and a crackling feel may be apparent. Generally, there is swelling (e.g., hematoma) associated with these fractures. Because of bone

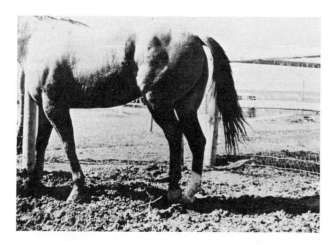

FIG. 5–176. A horse with a fractured femur. Notice that the left hindlimb is shorter than the right. The point of the hock is held higher and the musculature overlying the femur is dimpled.

displacement, the patella often feels loose and can be manipulated easily in a lateral and medial direction.

Proximal growth plate fractures in young horses can be difficult to diagnose. Frequently these foals can bear weight, and because of the fracture location, swelling is not readily apparent in acute cases. Fractures of the distal growth plate are usually easy to diagnose because of the displacement and swelling associated with the stifle region.

Diagnosis

Although the clinical signs are informative, except for the proximal growth plate fractures, x-rays are important to make a definitive diagnosis and pinpoint the exact location of the fracture.

Treatment

Treatment of femoral shaft fractures depends on the age of the animal and the type and location of the fracture. Generally, euthanasia should be performed for adults and yearlings that have sustained femoral shaft fractures unless exceptional circumstances exist. Although attempts at treatment can be made, they are usually futile. Occasionally, femoral fractures in growing horses heal with stall confinement alone. Of course, bone displacement and a subsequent shortening of the limb and permanent lameness may exist. Stall confinement alone is rarely sufficient for the adult horse.

In young foals sustaining femoral shaft fractures, pinning has been used successfully. However, this technique is most useful in very young, sedate foals (Fig. 5–177 *A* and *B*).

Compression plating is probably the treatment of choice for very young foals that have sustained femoral shaft fractures. It is the only method that ensures good stability of the fracture during the healing process.

Although distal growth plate fractures are difficult to treat, pins or screws can be considered. Fractures of the proximal femoral growth plate have been treated successfully by pinning, cancellous bone screws, and the use of the dynamic hip screw system. Repair of displaced fractures requires surgical realignment.

Prognosis

The prognosis for fracture of the femur depends largely on the age of the horse, the location and type of fracture, and its intended use. A much better prognosis can be expected in young animals with simple oblique midshaft fractures that are stabilized by internal fixation. Both proximal and distal growth plate fractures have a guarded prognosis for return to normal function. Surgical removal of the femoral head may be considered as a salvage procedure for breeding.

Generally, femoral fractures in the yearling and mature horse carry a very poor prognosis for a successful outcome.

Femoral Nerve Paralysis (Crural Paralysis)

Paralysis of the femoral nerve affects the quadriceps femoris group of muscles. This muscle group is composed of the rectus femoris muscle, the vastus lateralis muscle, the vastus medialis muscle, and the vastus intermedius muscle. This large muscular mass covers the front and sides of the femur and inserts onto the patella.

Causes

Femoral nerve paralysis may arise from trauma or from unknown causes, and may be associated with azoturia ("tying up"). Injury to the nerve may occur from overstretching of the limb during exertion, kicking, slipping, or tying horse in a recumbent position.

Signs

The horse will not be able to bear weight on the affected limb. In standing position, all joints of the affected limb are flexed as a result of this condition. The horse has difficulty advancing the limb, but can do so because the hock can be sufficiently flexed to pull the limb forward. During movement, the horse will not be able to bear weight on the limb, so compensation must be made in the gait. After the condition has been present for some time, atrophy of the quadriceps muscles occurs, causing these muscles to lose their normal softness and become more like tendinous structures.

Diagnosis

The signs listed above are characteristic and are used for diagnosis. Electromyography of the quadriceps femoris muscles five days after the first signs of femoral nerve paralysis will provide a definitive diagnosis.

Treatment

No treatment is known. If the condition is caused by injury of the femoral nerve, the animal should be stalled for a long time. Nonsteroidal antiinflammatory drugs are administered. The muscles should be massaged whenever possible and, if some function returns, exercise should be used to minimize atrophy. If the cause is azoturia, exercise is an important part of

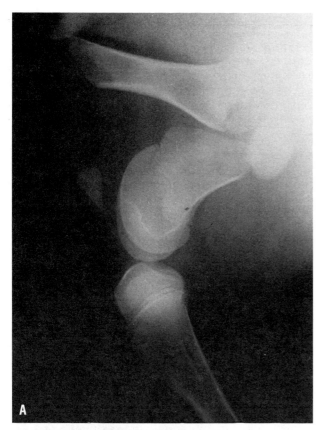

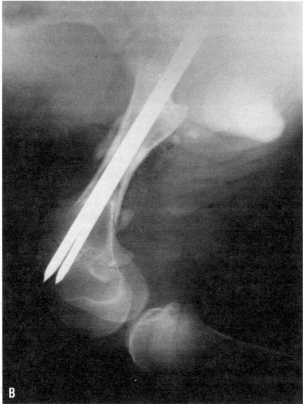

FIG. 5–177. *A*, An example of a closed oblique fracture of the distal third of the femur in a young foal. *B*, This fracture was successfully repaired with large Steinmann pins.

the treatment. Injections of selenium/vitamin E combinations and thiamine are recommended.

Prognosis

The prognosis is guarded to unfavorable if the cause is azoturia. At least 30 days are required for function to return completely. If damage to the femoral nerve is the cause, a year may be required before the outcome is known. Electromyographic examination will document improvement over time.

Trochanteric Bursitis (Whorlbone Lameness)

This lameness, most common in Standardbreds, is an inflammation of the bursa beneath the tendon of the middle gluteus muscle as it passes over the greater trochanter of the femur.

Causes

Lameness is caused by bruising as a result of the horse falling on the affected side, by straining the tendon during racing or training, or by a direct kick on the trochanter. It has also been found following an attack of distemper. In most cases, bone spavin also exists in the affected hind limb, and hock lameness produces the bursitis.

Trochanteric bursitis also occurs in horses racing on small tracks, where the turns are close together, and in horses working on their hindlimbs that are frequently exercised in soft, deep arenas. Short heels, long toes in the hindfeet seem to predispose to this lameness.

Signs and Diagnosis

Pain may be evident when pressure is applied over the great trochanter. At rest, the limb may remain flexed; as the horse moves, weight is placed on the inside of the foot so that the inside wall of the foot wears more than the outside wall. This can be best seen when observing the horse from behind; the foot is carried inward and the horse sets the foot down on a line between the forelimbs. The horse tends to travel in "dog fashion" because the hindquarters move toward the sound side because the stride of the affected limb is shorter than that of the sound side. After the condition has been present for some time, atrophy of the gluteal muscles occurs. In cases where the cause has been a severe trauma, such as a direct kick, the cartilage or the bone of the trochanter may be fractured, causing persistent lameness.

Treatment

Injection of the bursa with anti-inflammatory agents is apparently the most effective method of treatment. Other treatments consist of injections of irritants into or around the bursa. Phenylbutazone given orally may also relieve pain. When the cartilage or bone has been damaged with fracture or periostitis, treatment is difficult. Surgery or injection of irritants may be indicated.

Prognosis

The prognosis is guarded to unfavorable. If the horse responds to therapy within 4 to 6 weeks, he may again become sound. However, if the injury is more severe, the lameness may remain indefinitely or may recur when the horse is put back into training.

The Coxofemoral (Hip) Joint

Rupture of the Round Ligament of the Coxofemoral Joint

The hip joint of the horse has several ligaments to help hold it together. The largest and strongest is the round ligament between the head of the femur and the acetabulum. Occasionally, stresses occur that cause rupture the round ligament, but do not produce hip dislocation. In this case, the head of the femur has a greater range of motion than is normal, causing degenerative changes in the joint.

Cause

Trauma is the cause of round ligament rupture. The same stresses that cause dislocation of the hip joint can cause rupture without actual dislocation.

Signs

Signs of round ligament rupture are very similar to those of dislocation. The notable exception is that the limbs are of the same length. The signs that characterize round ligament rupture are the toe-out, stifle-out, and hock-in appearance of the affected hindlimb. This same appearance is also present in luxation of the hip joint, but the limbs are uneven in length (Fig. 5–178). Comparison of the limbs will show that they are equal in length when the ligament is ruptured and dislocation has not occurred. Some cases may require x-ray examination.

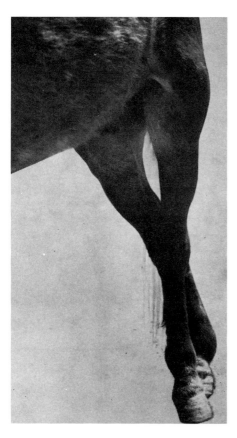

FIG. 5–178. Rupture of the round ligament of the coxofemoral joint. The stifle-out, toe-out, hock-in attitude of the limb typifies rupture of the round ligament. This same limb attitude is also present when the joint has luxated. When the round ligament ruptures, but the joint does not luxate, the limbs are the same length.

Diagnosis

Diagnosis is based on the signs of stifle-out, toe-out, and hock-in appearance with equal length of the limbs. If the condition is of long standing, an x-ray will show severe degenerative osteoarthritic changes. Otherwise, the abnormal position of the femoral head in the acetabulum can be identified. Nuclear medicine studies can also document the injury.

Treatment

There is no effective treatment.

Prognosis

The prognosis is unfavorable because the increased range of motion of the femoral head usually causes severe degenerative joint disease.

Coxofemoral Luxation (Dislocation of the Hip Joint)

Although dislocation of the hip joint of horses is not common, when it does occur, young horses and ponies are most frequently affected. In horses, the ilium tends to fracture before dislocation of the hip occurs.

Causes

In most cases, trauma is the cause. Violent overextension and falling on the point of the stifle with the femur in a vertical position occasionally produces fracture and/or luxation of the hip joint. A tethered horse that catches its foot in a rope may dislocate the hip in the struggle to free itself. The hip may also be dislocated if the horse fights a sideline or as a result of some other such trauma. The acetabulum is deep and the head of the femur is large, so a great trauma would be necessary to dislocate this joint.

Because of the deep acetabulum in the horse, fractures of the dorsal rim occur frequently with dislocation. Also, abnormalities of the hip joint associated with absence or tearing of the ligament of the head of the femur (round ligament) or the accessory ligament can predispose to dislocations with or without associated trauma. Hip dislocations are often complicated by upward patellar fixation.

Signs

The horse, which has both an accessory and a round ligament of the hip joint, must suffer a tear of the round ligament for the hip to dislocate. The femur is usually displaced upward and forward (craniodorsally) when the hip luxates (Fig. 5–179). Signs that usually accompany dislocation are limited cranial stride because of a pronounced shortening of the limb, and more prominence of the greater trochanter of the femur. Soft-tissue swelling may make this prominence difficult to determine in early stages. Crackling of the joint, as a result of the femur rubbing on the shaft of the ilium, may cause one to think the pelvis is fractured. The limb appears to dangle somewhat because of shortening. The toe and stifle turn outward and the hock inward (see Fig. 5–178).

Treatment

In horses that have not fractured the dorsal rim of the acetabulum, the dislocation can be realigned while the horse is under general anesthesia by direct traction and manipulation if good muscle relaxation is obtained. A surgical approach can be used in cases that cannot be realigned with closed manipulation.

If the head of the femur remains in place for approximately 3 months, the muscles will usually keep it in place.

If the dorsal rim of the acetabulum is fractured in association with hip dislocation, simple realignment of the femur is futile. In young animals surgical removal of the femoral head and neck and dorsal rim of the fractured acetabulum should be considered and will aid in the development of a pseudoarthrosis.

Prognosis

The prognosis is guarded to unfavorable. Horses may return to complete soundness after the head of the femur is replaced, but this is the exception and not the rule. Some horses, however, can be made sound enough for breeding purposes. If the animal is valuable, surgical correction is advisable and should be done; otherwise, euthanasia may be necessary.

The Pelvis

Aorto-iliac Thrombosis

Thrombus (an obstructing clot) formation in the caudal aorta, iliac arteries, or femoral artery as the re-sult of damage by Strongylus vulgaris (strongyles) occasionally causes an exercise-induced hindlimb lameness in horses. Such thrombi cause lameness of the hindlimb as a result of circulatory interference (Fig. 5–180). Aorto-iliac thrombosis has also been associated with ejaculatory failure in stallions.

Causes

It is thought that the thrombi are caused by larval forms of Strongylus vulgaris. However, other causes have been suggested.

Signs

Signs vary with the size of the thrombus and the amount of occlusion (blockage) of the blood vessel. Signs also vary in the time of their appearance after exercise. If the thrombus is small and the occlusion of the vessel is not great, the horse may be exercised vigorously before lameness occurs; however, in most cases the lameness occurs shortly after exercise begins and so may be confused with azoturia. While the horse is at rest, the blood supply to the muscles may be adequate to prevent lameness, but some horses will be lame even when walking.

When lameness appears, profuse sweating, pain, and anxiety occur if the horse is forced to continue the exercise. The affected limb will be cooler than the opposite member, and pulsation of the femoral artery will be less than that in the opposite limb, unless both limbs are involved. An outstanding characteristic of this lameness is its intermittent character; it appears with exercise and disappears with rest. If the thrombosis is bilateral in the aorta, the horse may have difficulty in supporting his hindquarters.

The veins on the affected limb will be more or less collapsed, while the veins on the normal limb will stand out. Another sign that may be present in a uni-

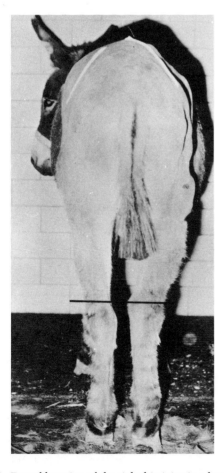

FIG. 5–179. Dorsal luxation of the right hip joint in a burro. Notice the shortening of the right hindlimb, as shown by the point of the right hock being higher than the point of the left hock.

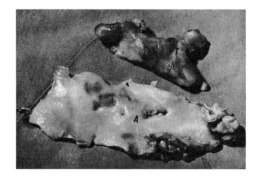

FIG. 5–180. Portion of aorta (A) and its enclosed thrombus (T). The bifurcation of the thrombus on the right shows how it had occluded not only the aorta but the iliac division. The horse afflicted with this thrombus was able to move only a few steps before incoordination and pain began. The condition was diagnosed by rectal examination, which revealed very weak pulsation in the iliac arteries.

lateral affliction is that the affected limb will not sweat, while the opposite normal limb does.

Ejaculatory failure may also be seen in breeding stallions.

Diagnosis

The diagnosis can be made on the basis of clinical signs and by rectal examination of the aorta and the iliac arteries. Ultrasonic evaluation of the terminal portion of the aorta and the aortic quadrifurcation (four branches of the iliac arteries) is useful in obtaining a definitive diagnosis, especially in horses with equivocal findings on rectal palpation.

Treatment

Treatments have included plasma volume expanders, aggressive worming programs with Ivermectic, phenylbutazone, and controlled exercise to induce collateral circulation. None of these treatments have shown consistent benefit, and some cases remain static or worsen, requiring euthanasia.

In the absence of treatment, the vessels may in time be able to establish collateral circulation that will overcome the effects of the thrombus. However, some horses become progressively worse, and euthanasia is necessary.

Prognosis

The prognosis is always guarded, and unfavorable if there is bilateral involvement or if the horse seems to be getting progressively worse.

Fractures of the Pelvis

Fractures of the pelvis in horses are uncommon. The reported incidence ranges from 0.9% of all lameness to 4.4% of all hindlimb lameness, and the prevalence of pelvic fractures is greater in females under 4 years of age. They are most commonly found in the wing and shaft of the ilium, but fractures of the tuber coxae, symphysis pubis, obturator foramen, acetabulum, and ischium also occur. (Fig. 5–181).

Clinically, horses often have a history of a fall or an accident while being hauled, with an acute onset of severe unilateral hindlimb lameness. The diagnosis may be difficult without x-rays or bone scintigraphy. Uncommonly, some horses may bleed to death as a result of sharp fracture fragments lacerating the internal iliac arteries in the pelvic canal.

Cause

Trauma is the cause in all cases. Horses that slip and fall on their sides may fracture the pelvis. Horses can also fracture the ilium by fighting a sideline or struggling while the hindlimbs are tied in a casting harness. The hip articulation of horses is rarely dislocated because of the strong formation of the hip joint; the ilium or acetabulum usually fractures instead. Acetabular fractures frequently result when the horse slips or "does the splits" (spread-eagles). Occasionally the fractures occur spontaneously while a horse is being ridden or while racing.

Signs

Signs of fracture of the pelvis are variable because of the different sites of fractures (Fig. 5–181). However, a horse will often have a history of trauma or a fall that resulted in a severe (grade III to IV) unilateral lameness with eventual muscle atrophy over the affected site. Shortly after the injury, swelling is noted that gradually distributes to more distal sites (e.g., stifle) because of gravity. The first signs of muscle atrophy are generally seen 2 weeks after the injury and the degree of atrophy is dictated by the severity of the lameness and pelvic injury. Also, bony prominence asymmetry of the tuber coxae, tuber ischii, tuber sacrale, and greater trochanter of the proximal femur may be seen or felt on palpation. In some cases, the fractured pieces of bone become sequestra (separated pieces) and must be removed surgically.

If the fracture occurs through the symphysis pubis or the obturator foramen, the horse often appears to be lame in both hindlimbs, walking with a hesitating gait that is short in the cranial phase of the stride. Also, swelling of the vulva or vagina from edema and hemorrhage may be observed in fillies or mares.

With the exception of fracture of the tuber coxae, if the fracture is acute (less than 48 hours), limb manipulation on the affected side will cause pain and a crackling may be felt or heard. As time passes, these signs will be reduced.

In one study of the eight horses examined within 36 hours of injury, only four (50%) had evidence of crackling with limb manipulation. Rectal examination is done to feel for asymmetry and crackling of bone when the horse is moved. In one study, only 4 of 9 horses with pelvic fractures had some abnormality.

Diagnosis

The diagnosis may be made on the basis of physical signs and examination by rectal palpation. A vaginal examination should be performed on mares, for this can be most helpful in identifying fractures of the pubis and ischium.

A definitive diagnosis usually requires x-rays or bone scintigraphy. General anesthesia and dorsal re-

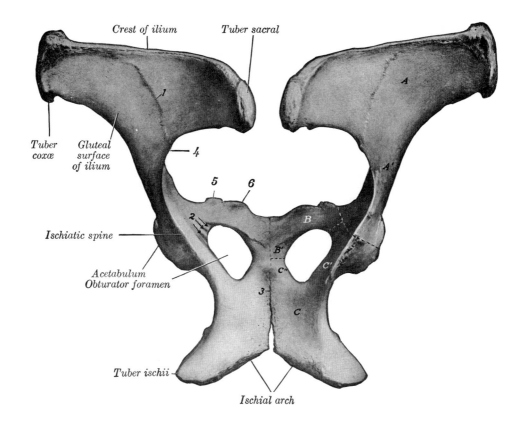

FIG. 5–181. Dorsal view of the pelvis. The dotted line indicates primitive separation of three bones, which are potential fracture sites. A, wing of ilium; A', shaft of ilium; B, acetabular branch of pubis; B', symphyseal branch of pubis; C, body of ischium; C', acetabular branch (or shaft of ischium); C″, symphyseal branch of ischium; 1, gluteal line; 2, grooves for obturator nerve and vessels; 3, symphysis pelvis; 4, greater sciatic notch; 5, iliopectineal eminence; 6, pubic tubercle. (From Sisson, S.: Anatomy of Domestic Animals (Grossman, J.D., ed.). 4th Ed. Philadelphia, W.B. Saunders Co., 1953.)

cumbency are required for a good x-ray examination. Although this approach has been perceived to be risky, with a good chance of worsening the fracture during recovery from anesthesia, it has not proven to be the case in two large studies. However, this approach is not necessary if the diagnosis can be made on physical examination. Bone scintigraphy can be done in the standing horse, and increased uptake "hot spots" will be observed at the fracture site.

Treatment

At present, no surgical methods have been devised for correcting fractures of the pelvis in horses. The best treatment appears to be to place the horse in a box stall and limit its movement for at least 3 months and provide analgesia as needed. Healing of the pelvis, however, sometimes does not take place until a year after the original injury. If the horse is valued highly by the owner, it should not be euthanized until a year has passed, provided that the horse is not suffering great pain. Surgical removal of a bone fragment from a fracture of the tuber coxae or tuber ischii will be necessary if the fragments become sequestra.

Prognosis

The prognosis is guarded in all cases. In one case study, 7 (64%) of 11 cases recovered and 4 (36%) of the 11 horses were sound. In another case series, 46 (60%) of 77 cases had a favorable outcome and 23 (30%) of the 77 horses returned to performance. Approximately 50% of the horses with acetabular fractures were able to return to performance.

Sacroiliac Joint Syndrome (Dislocation) (Strain Dysfunction)

The sacroiliac joint in the horse is a diarthrosis (consisting of two joints) formed between the articular surfaces of the sacrum and the ilium (Figs. 5–182 to 5–184). The surfaces are not smooth in adult horses, but are marked by reciprocal prominences and depressions covered by a thin layer of cartilage. The joint cavity is only a cleft and is often crossed by fibrous bands. The joint capsule is very close-fitting and is attached around the margins of the articular surfaces. The joint is reinforced by strong ligaments. Movement in the joint is not observed in adult horses, with

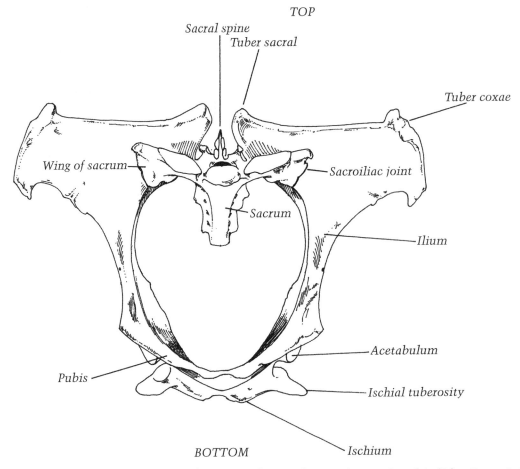

FIG. 5–182. Cranial view of the pelvis illustrating the sacroiliac joints and various bones making up the pelvis. (After Sisson, S., Grossman, J.D.: Anatomy of Domestic Animals. 5th Ed., Philadelphia, W.B. Saunders, 1975.)

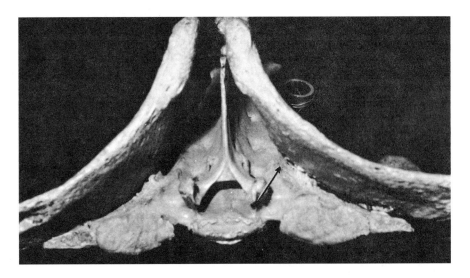

FIG. 5–183. Skeletal model of the sacroiliac joint. Arrow points between the sacrum and ilium. (From Adams, O.R.: Subluxation of the sacroiliac joint in horses. Proc. AAEP, 1969, p. 191.)

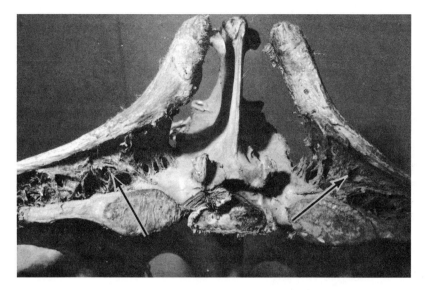

FIG. 5–184. Skeletal model of sacroiliac joint. Arrows point to dried and separated ventral sacroiliac ligament. (From Adams, O.R.: Subluxation of the sacroiliac joint in horses. Proc. AAEP, 1969, p. 191.)

stability, not mobility, being desirable. Because the sacroiliac joint is not meant to be mobile, stresses that produce tearing of these supporting ligaments may produce instability and partial dislocation. Once the continuity of the joint is disturbed, there may be chronic pain resulting from the partial displacement and instability.

Causes

Falls, slipping, and any other trauma that causes twisting or high stress to the sacroiliac joint resulting in acute damage to the ligaments and subsequent instability can cause the lameness. It may also result from repeated trauma rather than a single event. Trotters that turn in one direction on tracks with poorly banked turns appear to be more susceptible to this injury. Others that are at high risk are horses that work primarily at gaits other than a gallop (draft, carriage, and endurance horses and Standard bred racehorses). For whatever reason, tall horses of large body size appeared to be more susceptible.

Signs

The clinical signs are highly variable. Usually stiffness mild pain, and lack of impulsion in the hindquarters are seen. In the acute phase pain may be produced when pressure is put on the tuber coxae to cause rotation of the pelvis and move the sacroiliac joint. There often is some surrounding muscular pain, caused by spasm of the surrounding muscles in their attempt to reestablish the rigidity of the sacroiliac joint. Hindlimb flexion and manipulation may cause pain, but this is variable. Rectal examination with

pressure applied to the region may also cause pain. The condition is most often chronic, and the tuber sacrale may become prominent, either unilaterally or bilaterally, depending on whether one or both sides are involved (Figs. 5–185 and 5–186). The prominence of one or both of the tuber sacral (hunter's bumps) of one or both sacroiliac joints may be due to a partial dislocation of the sacroiliac joint or result from bone malformation and or muscle atrophy. Generally, during this phase, the horse has a history of poor performance; there will be varying degrees of muscle atrophy of the hind quarters, and on palpation, rectal examination, and flexion tests. No pain will be elicited. A lack of flexibility will be observed when downward pressure is applied to the tuber coxae.

The lameness may be unilateral or bilateral or shifting from one side to the other, depending on whether one or both sides are involved. The common complaint in hunter-jumper horses is that the horse is stiff and refuses to jump, or does a poor job of it.

In the harness racehorse, the clinical signs are most clearly seen at the trotting and pacing gaits and rarely seen at the walk. It is best to observe the horse after a fast workout. Characteristic signs include the affected pelvic limb's staying on the ground too long and then suddenly being jerked forward. Normally, the hind feet impact the ground before the forefeet; however, with sacroiliac syndrome, the forefeet hit first because of protraction delayed of the hindlimb. A hiking or jerking motion of the hip is commonly observed early on when the horse is exercised in circles. Later, hiking occurs when the horse is trotted in a straight line.

When the horse is walking, movement of one or both tuber sacral may be noticeable. In inactive cases, nonmovable displacement (hunter's bumps) will be present unilaterally or bilaterally.

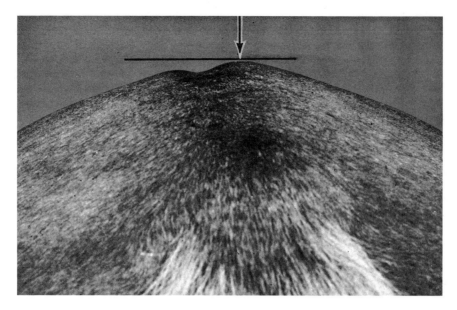

FIG. 5–185. Arrow points to upward displacement of tuber sacral ("hunter's bump"). The view is over the rump of the horse, looking forward. This area may move when the horse is walking and may show unilateral or bilateral displacement in subluxation of the sacroiliac joint.

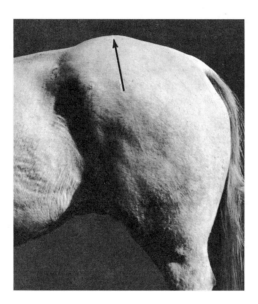

FIG. 5–186. Side view showing location of tuber sacral (arrow). This point should be closely observed when a horse walks for signs of movement and, in old cases, for signs of unilateral or bilateral displacement. (From Adams, O.R.: Subluxation of the sacroiliac joint in horses. Proc. AAEP, 1969, pp. 191–207.)

Diagnosis

In some cases of sacroiliac partial dislocation, there may be slight motion of one or both tuber sacral during walking, and close observation should be made at this point. Whenever there is unevenness or excessive prominence (hunter's bumps) of the tuber sacral, one should consider that at least at one time there had been movement and partial dislocation of this joint (see Fig. 5–185). Unfortunately, due to its protected ("hidden") location, joint blocking of the sacroiliac joint cannot be done.

Although x-ray studies require special equipment, they can be informative. Slight rotation of the pelvis or sacrum can be identified along with widening of the sacroiliac joint space, and in some, degenerative changes can be observed. Nuclear scintigraphy may also be helpful in localizing the problem to this site.

Treatment

In the acute phase, because some ligamentous attachments are injured, time must be allowed for healing to occur. This means rest, preferably in a box stall for at least 30 to 45 days. The ligamentous attachments must be allowed to rejoin and, if injury has been severe, the cartilaginous junction may be damaged enough to cause bony fusion of the joint. Repeated injury may produce a chronic, persistent lameness. In the chronic phase, intermittent use of nonsteroid anti-inflammatory drugs (e.g., bute) and controlled exercise to build up the muscles in the hindquarters and back may be helpful. Generally, however, a mild lameness will persist and a lower line of performance is to be expected.

Prognosis

The prognosis is always guarded. Even with healing of the acute injury, horses cannot return to their previous level of performance. Residual stiffness and lack of impulsion in the hindlimbs are common complaints. In a retrospection study in Standardbred trotters with this problem, a significant reduction in performance level was found.

The Thoracolumbar Spine

Associated Back Problems

There is little doubt that back problems associated with the thoracolumbar spine are an important cause of altered performance in horses. A higher incidence of thoracolumbar problems has been noted in competitive jumpers (show and eventing), dressage horses, and reining horses.

Although a wide range of problems can affect the thoracolumbar spine, they can be separated into three major categories: 1) Congenital deformities of the spine, 2) soft tissue injury, and 3) bony problems associated with the vertebra. Congenital deformities of the thoracolumbar spine include abnormalities in the curvature (scoliosis or lordosis), and vertebral fusion (synostosis). Soft tissue problems include sprained muscles, strained ligaments, disc disease (very rare), and skin lesions from sitfast (saddle sores or protrusion of the vertebrae) and warbles underneath the saddle area. Bone damage includes ossifying spondylosis, spondylosis deformans, overriding of the dorsal spinous processes (Kissing Spines) arthrosis (joint degeneration) of the articular processes, and fractures of the dorsal spinous processes, articular processes, neural arch, and vertebral bodies. (Fig. 5–187). Fractures that frequently result in myelopathy (spinal cord disease) will be covered in The Wobbler Syndrome section in this chapter.

Although there is an acute awareness on the part of the veterinarian as well as the horse owner that back problems exist, and the back is frequently examined as a site of lameness, it is still difficult to obtain a definitive diagnosis. The diagnosis is difficult because

of the variable clinical picture, variable temperament of the horse, the inability to directly palpate and manipulate the thoracolumbar vertebrae, and the expensive equipment required to radiograph this region. To add to the confusion, sensitive skin (thin-skinned) horses and "cold-backed" horses persistently resent palpation of the back, which may be incorrectly interpreted as a back problem. "Cold-backed" horses that show a persistent hypersensitivity over the back and dip and stiffen the back when the rider first mounts it, rarely have radiographic changes. After the initial stiffness is gone, no effect in performance is noted. The question of whether the reaction resulted from pain or guarding because of previous injury, or simply the horse's temperament, is unknown.

Causes

Although there are many causes of back injury (direct trauma, poor-fitting saddles, improper seating of the rider, twisting and wrenching of the spine), there appears to be a correlation between the horse's conformation, sex, use, and breed as to the type of injury that is sustained.

Generally, horses that are short-backed with limited flexibility are more prone to vertebral lesions, whereas horses with long flexible backs are affected more frequently with muscular and ligament strain. Mares are more frequently affected with ossifying spondylosis, and overriding of the dorsal spinous processes is more frequently observed in geldings. Where sacroiliac strain is most prevalent in horses jumping at speeds (hunters, hurdlers, steeple chasers, point-to-pointers), bone damage to the thoracolumbar spine is more frequent in competitive jumpers. Musculoligamentous strain occurs with about equal frequency no matter what type of jumping is involved. Thoroughbred racehorses are more frequently affected with soft tissue injury than with lesions to the vertebrae. Also bone damage to the thoracolumbar spine is most likely to be centered around the midpoint of the back, while soft tissue injury is more frequently just caudal to the withers and over the loin.

It is suggested that spondylosis deformans results from excessive dorsiflexion (hollowing) that occurs when the horse's back muscles fatigue. This, in turn, leads to tearing of the ventral and ventrolateral aspects of the anulus fibrosis, compressing the intervertebral joint, and eventually leading to impingement of the dorsal spinous processes (Kissing Spines). In the most advanced cases, fusion occurs between the intervertebral joints.

Signs

Horses with chronic thoracolumbar problems frequently have a history of loss of performance indicated by stiffness, inability to stride out, lack of enthusiasm for work, lack of fluidity and timing when

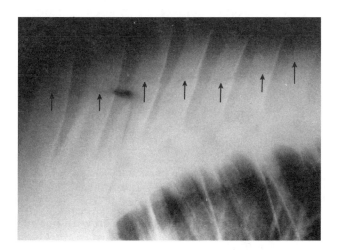

FIG. 5–187. A lateral x-ray of the withers of a horse indicating fracture of the dorsal spinous processes of T4 through T10 (arrows).

jumping, and a loss of "suppleness" in the back. Horses that have sustained recent acute trauma to the vertebral column exhibit rather precise signs of back pain. Horses with severe thoracolumbar pain may have difficulty in straddling to urinate and defecate, or may exhibit a reluctance to lie down or roll on their backs. In some cases, horses resent having their hindlimbs picked up, making it difficult for the farrier to shoe the horse. In those with fracture, stiffness, malalignment of the vertebral column, and a neurologic deficiency may be a part of the history.

On visual examination, the horse should be viewed from the side to observe for the dorsoventral curvature (lordosis or kyphosis, hollowing or arching) of the spine, and the alignment of the summits of the dorsal spinous processes. An elevation or swelling may indicate trauma to the soft tissue or dorsal spinous processes from the saddle if it is located over the withers, or from a fall if located in the caudal, thoracic, or lumbar region. Atrophy of the dorsal musculature should also be noted. The sacroiliac region is usually best viewed from behind while the horse is standing square on all four limbs. The typical signs of hunter's bumps should be noted (refer to sacroiliac subluxation). The lateral curvature of the thoracolumbar spine is best appreciated from above while the animal is standing square on all four limbs and the head and neck are held straight. Abnormal curvature of the thoracolumbar spine may indicate vertebral injury, malformation, or muscle spasms (spastic scoliosis) (Fig. 5–188).

On palpation, sensitive (thin-skinned) horses or "cold-backed" horses frequently withdraw rapidly when palpated over the thoracolumbar spine. This is often misconstrued as a sign of back soreness emanating from the spine or musculoligament support structures when, in fact, it is more likely a sign of skin sensitivity. The open hand with fingers extended should be used to evaluate back pain. Hands are gently run along the dorsal musculature from the withers to the base of the tail, and the pressure is increased after each passage. A positive sign of back pain is elicited when the horse cringes and the muscle firmness (spasm) is evidenced over the site of the lesion. The muscle response of the horse is one of guarding to prevent movement of the affected region. Some horses exhibit a more dramatic response and grunt, kick, or rear when pressure is applied. In any case, this sign should be repeatable and the intensity should not decrease with subsequent palpation. The dorsal spinous processes are palpated, and they should be evenly spaced, axially (centrally) aligned, and about the same height except for the elevations associated with the withers and the depression associated with the lumbosacral junction. Dorsiflexion (hollowing) of the back is checked by forcefully pinching the longissimus muscles on both sides of the dorsal spinous process. Reluctance to hollow the back can indicate a problem. Lateral flexion of the back is assessed by running a ballpoint pen down from the longissimus dorsi muscle to the lateral thoracic area. This is done on both sides. Horses with back problems often exhibit

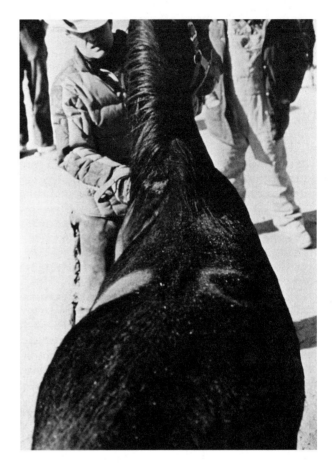

FIG. 5–188. An example of right lateral curvature of the thoracolumbar spine that may indicate injury to the vertebrae, malformation of the vertebrae, or muscle spasms.

less expressive (reduced) lateral flexion and guard against it by splinting (tensing) the musculature. Ventroflexion (humping) of the back is checked by running a ballpoint pen over each croup. Again, reluctance to flex is often indicative of a problem. Usually the most affected side shows the least amount of movement. A rectal examination might be performed to evaluate the sublumbar muscles. Although rectal examinations are rarely informative for thoracolumbar problems, they can be beneficial in identifying problems associated with the sacroiliac and sacrococcygeal regions.

At exercise, a stiffness of the back may be evident, particularly when the horse is turned sharply to one side or the other. A shortening of the stride with decreased hock flexion and a tendency to drag the toes may also be evident. Signs like these make it difficult to make a distinction between hock and stifle lameness. If the pain is quite severe, horses may exhibit a wide straddling hindlimb gait. On backing, the horse may be reluctant at first to raise its head. When moving backward, it may do so in a rather awkwardly flexed position.

Longeing the horse at a trot for 10 to 15 minutes is often helpful. Before exercise, a blood sample might be taken to obtain baseline data on serum muscle enzymes. Exaggerated contraction of the longissimus dorsi muscle may be evident. Some horses may elevate their heads higher than normal and will be reluctant to stride-out or change leads. Although this is not definitive for back pains, some horses swish their tails incessantly. After exercise, another blood sample is taken immediately and 18 to 24 hours later. Active muscle damage is identified by a 2- to 5-fold increase in muscle enzymes as compared to resting levels.

Diagnosis

Because many of the signs associated with thoracolumbar pain are nonspecific, other conditions need to be ruled out. They include problems associated with the pelvis, stifle, and hock joints primarily, but compressive myelopathy (spinal cord disease), bad-fitting saddles, and temperament problems should also be considered.

X-ray examination of the thoracolumbar spine, although difficult, can be valuable for the identification of vertebral lesions (see Fig. 5–187). However, a negative x-ray examination does not mean the thoracolumbar spine is not involved. Powerful equipment is required to x-ray the horse's vertebral column. Although equipment is now available to examine the thoracolumbar spine in the standing horse, better films are usually obtained while the horse is under general anesthesia (Fig. 5–189).

Nuclear medicine (scintigraphy) can also be helpful in identifying both soft tissue and bone problems associated with the back.

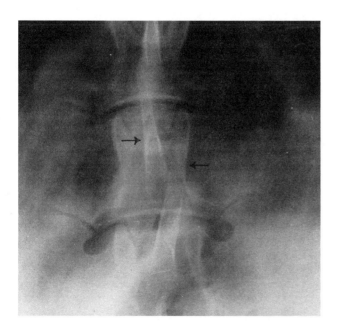

FIG. 5–189. A dorsal ventral x-ray of the lumbar spine. Note two spinous processes (arrows) are displaced to opposite sides, indicating fracture of the spinous processes.

Treatment

A number of conservative treatments are used for thoracolumbar disorders. Some physiotherapeutic techniques available include short-wave diathermy, Faradaic stimulation, thermography, ultrasound, deep massage by cyclotherapy, and pulsing magnetic field. Refer to Chapter 7 for more information about these treatment modalities. Swimming has also been recommended. Manipulative techniques (chiropractic and osteopathic) have also been receiving much attention. All of these treatments have one thing in common, and that is that no control studies have been performed to evaluate their efficacy as a treatment. Anti-inflammatories, long-term parenteral administration of analgesics, and acupuncture have also been used. Several studies have documented the effectiveness of stimulation of acupuncture points with needles, soft lasers, and the injection of saline into acupuncture sites. Treatments are often done weekly, and in one study a mean of 11 treatments was required before the desired effect was realized. Prolonged rest up to 6 months may be beneficial in some cases.

Prognosis

The prognosis depends on the type of injury sustained. A good prognosis can be expected for most cases in which a soft tissue injury involving the support structures has been sustained. The poorest prognosis is expected with spondylosis, in which a high recurrence rate of back pain has been reported. Of course, a very poor prognosis is given for cases sustaining fracture of the vertebral column as well.

Overlapping (Impingement) of Thoracic and/or Lumbar Dorsal Spinous Processes ("Kissing Spines")

Overlapping of the thoracic and/or lumbar spinous processes can result in a lameness from pain caused by pressure on the dorsal spines from enlargement of the proximal ends. The condition occurs most often in young mature Thoroughbreds with short backs that are being used principally for jumping and eventing. The impingement of the spinous process occurs most frequently beneath the saddle region (T12-T17) (Fig. 2–5) but can occur in the caudal withers and cranial lumbar regions.

Causes

The horse may have suffered an injury to the back, although a clear history of this is not always obtained. This injury may be caused by such mishaps as going over backward or falling. Signs may not be evident until 2 to 3 years after the injury.

Probably the most common causes of the condition are the conformation of the vertebral column and the type of work performed. Horses that go through maximum flexion and extension during performance (e.g., during jumping) are most prone to this condition.

Signs and Diagnosis

The onset of signs is often insidious. There is usually a history of increasing stiffness of the back, a reduction in hindlimb impulsion, and a disinclination to work. Loss of muscle mass on either side of the spinous process may be observed.

Changes in behavior and temperament may also be reported. The horse may resent saddling and grooming. Bucking and lying down after saddling may occur. As the cinch is tightened, the horse may groan and exhibit other signs of discomfort. Pressure along the back may cause signs of pain in some cases. Many other variations may result.

Palpation along the back may reveal irregularities in the size of the summits of the spinous processes of the thoracic or lumbar vertebrae. Deep digital palpation is necessary in most cases to reveal these changes. Examination should begin forward at the withers and work backward. One will have to differentiate resentment shown by some horses to this examination from distress resulting from a pathologic condition. Tests of the spine to show loss of flexibility are useful. (Refer to Chapter 3, in the section, Examination of the Back) A horse with overlapping of the spinous processes will show little or no movement from these tests. Direct infiltration of local anesthetics between and around the impinging dorsal spinous processes often eliminates the pain and is helpful in the diagnosis. X-rays of the dorsal processes will greatly aid the diagnosis.

The above signs are by no means specific and may be shown in other types of lameness, especially partial dislocation of the sacroiliac joint. Tying-up syndrome and arthritis of the spine might also cause some similar signs. One must always consider that a horse who discovers that by malingering in some way, such as lying down when saddled, he may end the riding session. Diagnosis is best established with history and with positive changes with manipulation, palpation and x-rays. A positive radiographic examination will show diminished space between, and possibly overlapping of, the affected dorsal spinous processes.

X-ray changes associated with overlapping of the dorsal spinous processes are not always related to clinical signs. Many horses exhibiting x-ray changes performed satisfactorily.

Treatment

Conservative treatment (rest), is the treatment of choice in most cases. Surgery should be relegated for the most severely involved cases.

Surgical treatment will give satisfactory results in most cases, if the diagnosis is accurate. The summit of the affected spinous process is removed. If there is pressure between as many as three spinous processes, removal of the center one will usually relieve the symptoms.

Aftercare consists of 2 to 3 months in a box stall and 1 month of hand-walking before beginning riding. Some cases do not show full benefit for several months.

Prognosis

The prognosis is guarded. Diagnosis is sometimes difficult because of the large x-ray machine required for adequate x-rays, and the fact that not all horses with x-ray signs of overriding of the dorsal spinous processes show clinical signs.

Muscle Problems

Muscle Strain of the Psoas and Longissimus Dorsi Muscles

Strain of the epaxial muscles is undoubtedly a common cause of back injury in horses. This involves primarily the longissimus dorsi muscles, whose main action is to extend (dorsiflex) the back or, if acting singly, to laterally flex the spine. Strain may occur as a result of slipping or falling or result from a poorly coordinated jump or from overuse.

After severe muscular exertion such as racing or other work necessitating fast starts, the longissimus dorsi and psoas major and minor muscles also may develop (muscle inflammation). The pain in the loin region often causes one to think that the horse has "kidney trouble."

Cause

Trauma from muscular strain is the cause. These muscles are very important in the driving action of the hind limbs and are subject to injury. They are also involved in azoturia and the tying-up syndrome, and myositis may be one of the after effects of one of these diseases. Poor fitting saddles and hind limb lameness can also be the cause.

Signs

The horse's back will appear stiff, and in some cases the muscles will appear swollen. He will not exert normal propulsion of the hindlimbs, and will exhibit pain on pressure over the loin, which may cause him to groan and drop the back under hand pressure. Hand pressure on the psoas group of muscles by way of rectal examination may produce pain. The action of the hindlimb is not normal, in that the gait appears to be stiffened in both hindlimbs. The abdomen may be held rigid as though intraabdominal pain were present. Serum muscle enzymes will be elevated in the active stage of myositis.

Diagnosis

Diagnosis is made by the response of the horse to digital pressure over the loin and pressure to the psoas group of muscles on rectal examination. The signs are present for several days, or even weeks, differentiating it from the tying-up syndrome.

Treatment

Proper rest and training procedures are mandatory. The period of rest will vary with the severity of the injury. In most cases, a minimum of 30 to 45 days is required. In addition, injections of vitamin E and selenium may be useful. Sodium bicarbonate in the grain (2 to 4 oz) daily will relieve symptoms in some cases. Some cases will not respond immediately, and others may require 6 weeks for evidence of recovery. Nonsteroidal antiinflammatory drugs are also useful. Additionally DMSO applied topically may be of benefit. Also in some cases injection of the affected muscles with an antiinflammatory may be beneficial. Electromagnetic fields and massage therapy may also be employed. The horse should not be put back in training until all signs of pain have disappeared for 3 weeks after therapy is discontinued.

Prognosis

The prognosis is good to guarded. The possibility of recurrence of injury is real. However, most horses return to full use.

Muscular Dystrophy

Muscular dystrophy (muscle dysfunction and deterioration) has been observed in horses. It differs from simple atrophy in that the muscle completely disappears. The cause of muscular dystrophy is unknown. Complete loss of the muscular tissue is obvious. Signs of lameness have not been observed. Dystrophy leaves a deformity in the limb and a deep grooving where the muscle was. No treatment is known for muscular dystrophy. The prognosis is unfavorable, and if dystrophy should involve muscles in other regions of the body, it could cause lameness and permanent disability.

The Wobbler Syndrome

The wobbler syndrome describes a set of symptoms rather than a specific disease. Commonly, the signs are ataxia (incoordination) and paresis (weakness). An ataxic horse might stand with the hindlimbs spraddled and when moving might move the limbs very widely or have a tendency to cross the limbs and step on its other feet. Weakness is characterized by stumbling, dragging the toes, having difficulty in stepping over obstacles, and being easily pulled or thrown off balance.

The causes of the wobbler syndrome are varied, and the diagnosis, treatment, and prognosis are discussed below under each cause.

Cervical Vertebral Malformation (CVM)

CVM is an abnormality of the cervical (neck) vertebrae that causes pressure on the spinal cord and results in incoordination. Thoroughbred and Quarter Horse males under 4 years are most commonly affected. Diagnosis is made through regular x-rays and positive contrast myelograms and CT scanning to highlight soft tissue damage and the site of spinal cord compression. Treatment includes either fusion surgery or laminectomy (removal of bone and soft tissue compressing the spinal cord). The prognosis is guarded for a return to athletic function.

Equine Protozoal Myeloencephalitis (EPM)

EPM is caused by a parasite that invades the spinal cord and brain stem, causing damage. This condition may begin as an obscure lameness and may be more severe on one side than the other but is often difficult to diagnose. Drug treatment is helpful, but there is a guarded prognosis for complete recovery without relapse unless drug therapy is maintained.

Equine Degenerative Myeloencephalopathy (EDM)

Less common than CVM, EDM is a progressive degeneration of the spinal cord and brain stem that usually begins before 3 years of age. Deficiencies of vitamin E have also been implicated as a cause.

Equine Herpes Virus–1 (EHV)

EHV is a form of the rhinovirus that causes abortion in mares and respiratory disease in young horses. Weakness and incoordination are often preceded by fever, cough, and nasal discharge. Other symptoms include loss of tail tone and bladder control. Sampling of serum and spinal fluid is helpful in diagnosis. Treatment includes drug therapy. Many horses recover from EVH.

Fractures

Traumatic fractures of the cervical vertebrae are most common in foals and weanlings. The symptoms vary greatly. X-rays are essential for diagnosis. Treatment depends on the clinical signs and the nature of the fracture. If the horse is only mildly affected and the fracture is stable, stall confinement with minimal handling is recommended. If the neurologic signs are severe, manipulation and surgery are indicated. The prognosis depends on the severity of the trauma and the time elapsed before treatment.

CHAPTER SIX

Shoeing for Soundness

CHERRY HILL and RICHARD KLIMESH

Shoeing can be preventive, corrective, or therapeutic. *Preventive* trimming and shoeing are characterized by balance, support, and protection. The goals of preventive shoeing are long-term soundness for performance. *Corrective* trimming and shoeing consist of alterations in the hoof to affect stance or stride and in some cases breakover. Properly employed corrective farriery does not *force* a limb into an abnormal position; it *allows* the hoof and limb to attain a desirable configuration, achieve more normal movement, and enhance breakover. *Therapeutic* shoeing is designed to protect or support a damaged hoof or limb or to prevent or encourage a particular movement until healing can take place. Corrective and therapeutic farriery may be helpful in the treatment of some lamenesses but have no beneficial effect in others. Although some lamenesses are not affected by shoeing, preventive shoeing should be a part of every horse's routine hoof care program.

Trimming and Shoeing

Good shoeing is an art and a science. For farriers to do their best work, a proper area should be provided and well-mannered horses presented (Fig. 6–1). There should be a place to tie horses safely at a height above the withers. The area should be well lighted, uncluttered, and level. The floor should be a concrete slab or rubber mat, not a muddy or rocky paddock or a dusty barn aisle full of gravel or potholes. Shade and shelter should be provided for summer as well as for winter work. Adequate light and access to electrical outlets for power tools are essential. It is a horseowner's responsibility to present a farrier with cooperative horses that have been trained to have their limbs handled and their hooves worked on.

Step-by-Step Shoeing Procedure: Before removing the old shoes, the farrier discusses with the trainer or owner any problems or concerns in the way of moving. If the horse is a regular client, the farrier consults notes related to the horse's previous shoeings. Then, if necessary, the horse's movement is evaluated. The owner may be asked to lead the horse at a walk and trot in a straight line so that the farrier can watch (from the front, rear, and side) the manner in which the horse picks up his hooves, moves them, and puts them down.

As the farrier watches a horse move, he is primarily watching how the hoof lands. The hoof should land

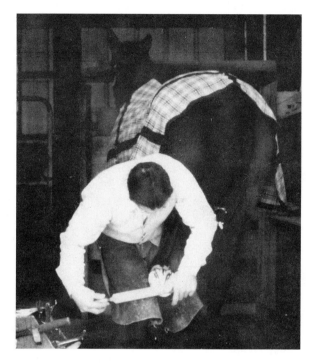

FIG. 6–1. A good work area for shoeing.

flat or slightly heel first but generally not toe first. If the hoof is not landing properly when it is time for a reset, it indicates that the hoof was not correctly shod in the first place, the hoof has grown out of balance since the last shoeing, the horse is compensating for pain, or the horse's conformation is such that the hoof does not land flat. The way a hoof lands differs with each gait and from forelimb to hindlimb. Most horses require shoeing every 5 to 8 weeks partly because the hoof wall at the toe grows faster than that at the heels, which causes the hoof to become imbalanced.

After removing the old shoes, Figures 6–2 to 6–11, each hoof and shoe is examined for clues to the horse's wear patterns. The hoof angle can be determined using a hoof gauge, and the length of the untrimmed hoof can be measured with dividers or a ruler. The balance, shape, and symmetry of the hoof are assessed, noting any tendencies to form flares or dishes. Hoof symmetry is evaluated in relationship to the heel bulbs and the lower limb.

Figures 6–12 to 6–23: Next the sole is pared if necessary, the hoof wall is nipped or rasped, and any

HOW TO REMOVE A SHOE

Necessary tools from left: clinch cutter, hammer, pull-offs, and crease nail puller (Fig. 6–2).

Using the chisel end of the clinch cutter, open the clinches by tapping the spine of the clinch cutter with the hammer (Fig. 6–3).

The clinch is the end of the nail folded over; this is what needs to be opened so that the nails can be pulled through the hoof wall without breaking off large hunks of hoof (Fig. 6–4).

If the shoe is creased, use the crease nail puller to extract each nail individually, allowing the shoe to come off (Fig. 6–5).

Nails with protruding heads can be pulled out using the pull-offs (Fig. 6–6).

If the nails cannot be pulled out individually, remove the shoe with the pull-offs. After the clinches have been opened, grab the shoe heel and pry *toward* the center of the frog. Do the same with the other shoe heel (Fig. 6–7).

When both heels are loose, grab one side of the shoe at the toe and pry toward the center of the frog (Fig. 6–8). Repeat around the shoe until it is removed. *Never* pry toward the outside of the hoof, or you risk ripping big chunks out of the hoof wall. As the nail heads protrude while the shoe is loosened, pull them out with the pull-offs.

Pull any nails that may remain in the hoof (Fig. 6–9).

To protect the hoof until the shoe is replaced, either wrap the hoof edges with tape (Fig. 6–10), or, if the horse has a tender sole, tape a cloth over the bottom of the hoof (Fig. 6–11) or use a protective boot. If the shoes are being pulled to let the horse go barefoot, a qualified farrier should trim the hoof to minimize breakage and ensure balance.

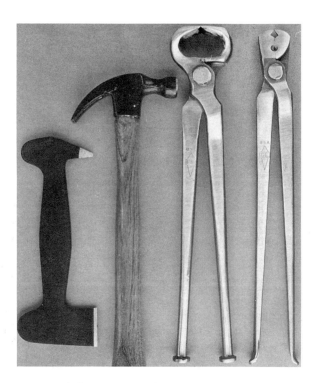

FIG. 6–2. Tools for removing a shoe.

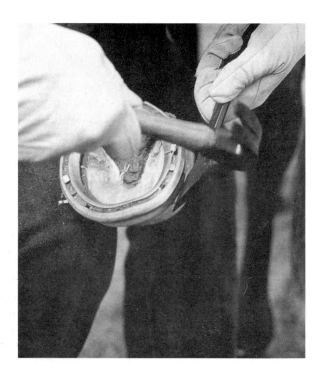

FIG. 6–3. Opening a clinch.

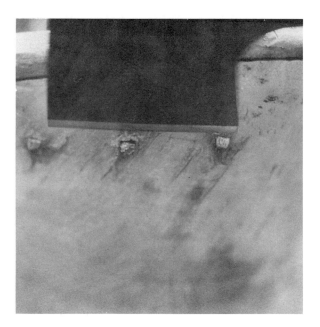

FIG. 6–4. Clinch cutter in position.

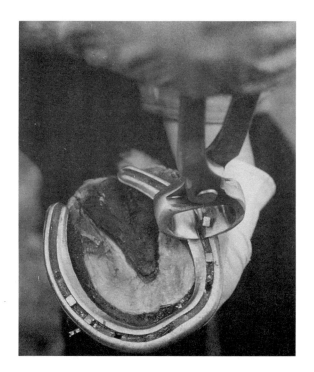

FIG. 6–6. Using pull-offs to remove nails.

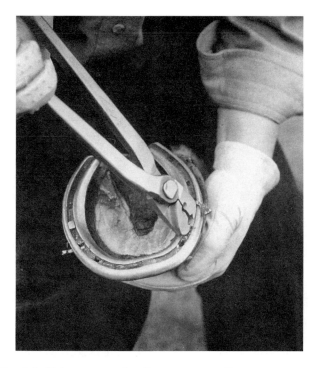

FIG. 6–5. Using crease nail puller to remove nails.

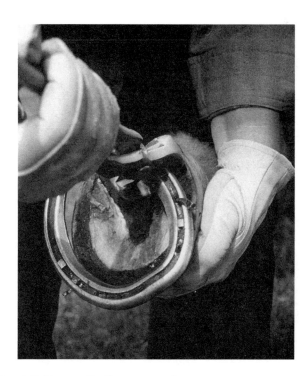

FIG. 6–7. Using pull-offs to remove shoe.

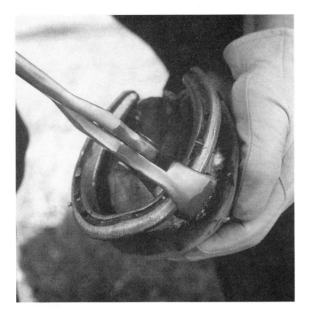

Fig. 6–8. Using pull-offs to remove shoe.

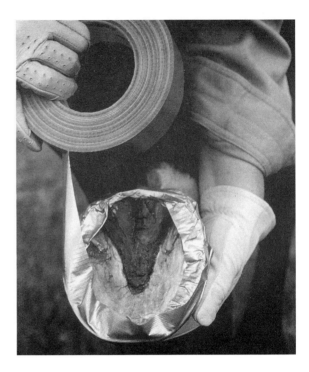

Fig. 6–10. Taping of hoof.

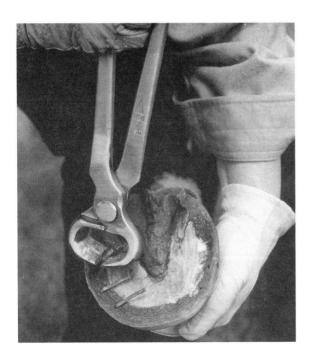

Fig. 6–9. Removing remaining nails.

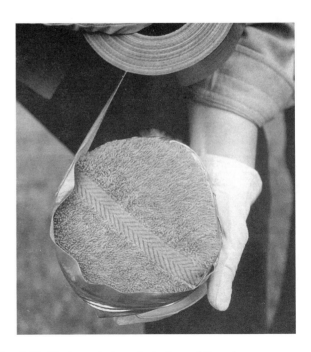

Fig. 6–11. Taping a cloth to the bottom of the sole.

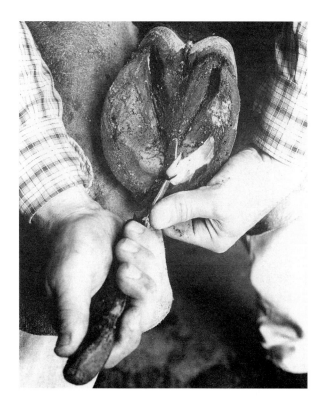

FIG. **6–12.** Trimming the sole.

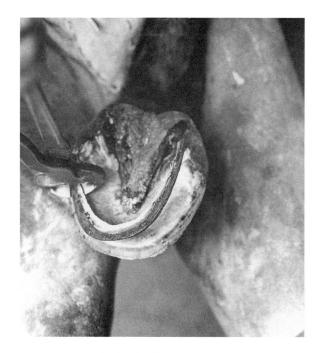

FIG. **6–14.** Nipping the hoof wall.

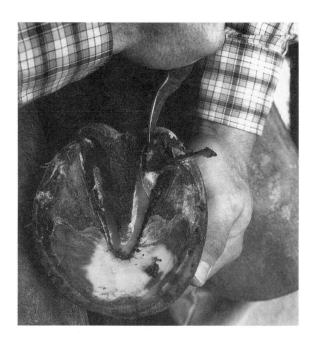

FIG. **6–13.** Trimming the frog.

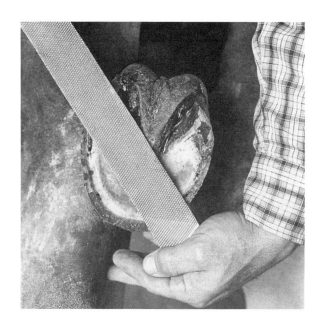

FIG. **6–15.** Rasping the bottom of the hoof.

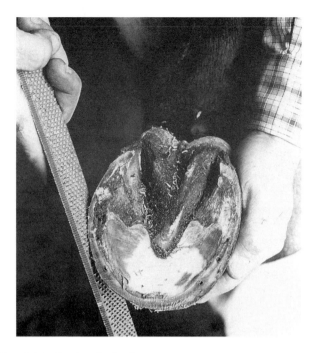

FIG. 6–16. Shaping the hoof.

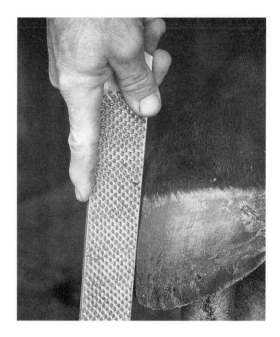

FIG. 6–18. Checking for dish.

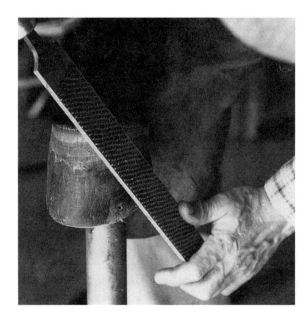

FIG. 6–17. Dressing a flare.

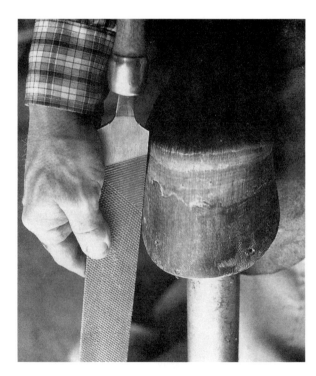

FIG. 6–19. Checking for flare.

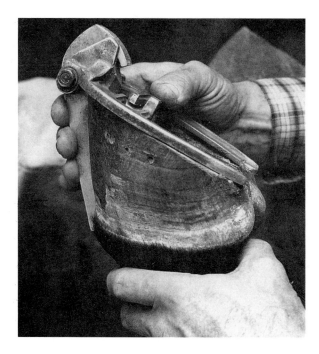

FIG. 6–20. Measuring hoof angle.

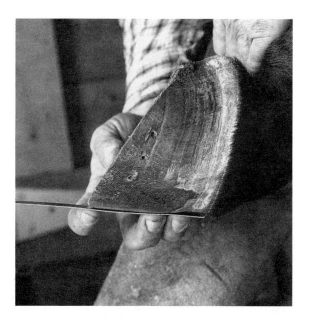

FIG. 6–22. Measuring toe length.

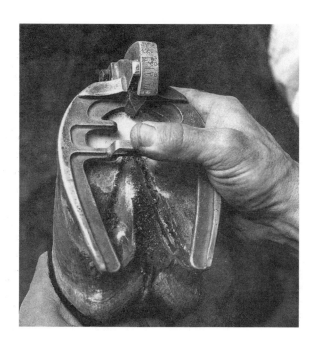

FIG. 6–21. Reading the hoof gauge.

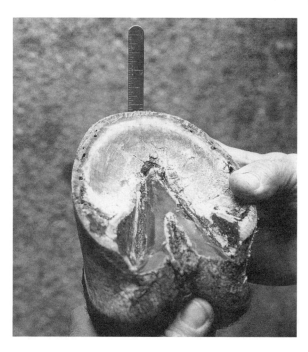

FIG. 6–23. Reading the ruler.

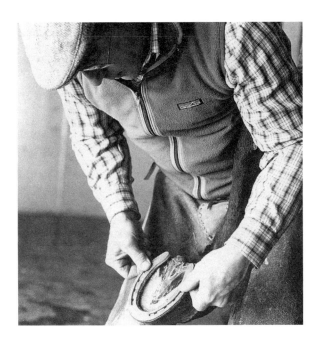

FIG. 6–24. Positioning shoe on hoof.

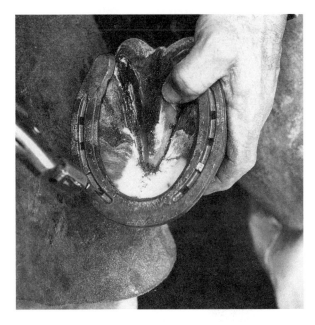

FIG. 6–26. Nailing.

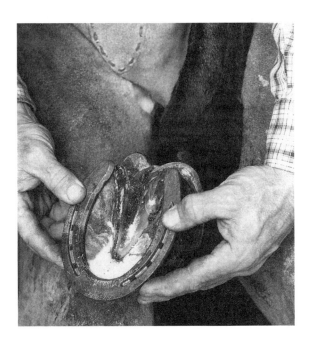

FIG. 6–25. Checking shoe fit.

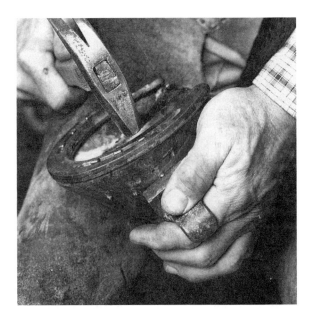

FIG. 6–27. Setting clinches.

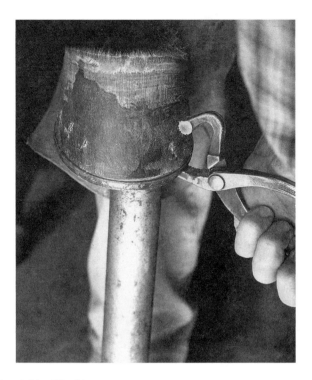

FIG. 6–28. Clinching.

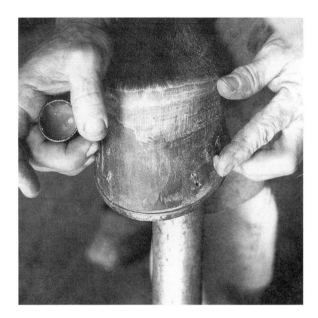

FIG. 6–29. Filling nail holes.

excess frog is trimmed. The outside of the hoof wall is rasped (dressed) if it has flares or dishes. Once trimming is completed, the hoof angle and length are measured, and the levelness of the hoof wall is evaluated. The proper size and type of shoe for the horse are then selected.

Figures 6–24 to 6–28: A good farrier shapes the shoe to fit a prepared hoof, not the other way around. Generally, it is a good sign if, once the farrier has begun shaping the shoe, he does not go back to the hoof with a rasp. When the farrier is satisfied with the shape of the shoe and the way it seats on the hoof wall, he begins nailing. Usually two nails are driven, and the sharp tips are wrung off or bent over and the hoof is set down to see how the shoe is positioned on the hoof. Then the remaining nails are driven and wrung off or bent over. After the nails have been driven, the clinches are set or tightened and filed or cut to a short consistent length. The clinches are then folded flat against the hoof wall and filed smooth.

Figure 6–29: Some farriers apply a hoof sealer to prevent drying out of the hoof, especially if the outer surface of the hoof wall has required rasping. Wax or another substance is used to fill all nail holes. This prevents mud, urine, and water from invading the hoof and causing cracks.

Principles of Preventive Shoeing

Preventive shoeing should be a part of every horse's routine hoof care program. The balance, support, and protection afforded by preventive shoeing contribute to a horse's comfort during movement.

How to Recognize a Good Preventive Shoeing Job

Hoof Preparation

Static versus Dynamic Balance. *Static balance* refers to geometric equilibrium of the hoof at rest (Table 1). Generally, when the ground surface of the hoof is perpendicular to the axis of the limb (when viewed from the front, the medial and lateral walls are equal in length, and the coronet is parallel to the ground), the hoof is in static balance. *Dynamic balance* takes into account the action of the hoof and limb. In its most complete sense, dynamic balance refers to the relationship of all the limbs in motion. For a hoof to be functionally balanced for efficient motion and symmetric strides, the trimming and shoeing must take conformation and other factors into consideration. Achieving dynamic balance, especially when working on a gait abnormality, often involves trial and error. Static balance addresses appearance; dynamic balance focuses on function. The more hoof and limb conformation deviate from standard guidelines, the less likely are static and dynamic trimming techniques to produce similar results.

Toe-Heel Tubule Alignment. The angle of the hoof at the heel should be parallel to the angle at the toe. When the heel angle is 5° less than the toe angle, the hoof is said to have underrun heels (Fig. 6–30). In such a case, the horn tubules at the heel are crushed and collapsed forward and are often more nearly parallel than perpendicular to the ground surface. It is as if the tubules at the heel are "lying down on the job." Rarely

TABLE 6–1. *Shoeing Quality Control Checklist*

Hoof preparation
    Static versus dynamic balance
    Toe-heel tubule alignment
    Dorsal-palmar (plantar) balance
    Medial-lateral balance
    Length
    Levelness
    Sole
    Frog
    Shape
    Symmetry of hoof pairs

Shoe preparation
    Selection
    Fit
    Hoof expansion
    Heel support
    Contact with the wall
    Sole pressure

Nails
    Heads
    Placement
    Pattern
    Clinches

Details

is the heel angle steeper than the toe angle, but it may appear that way if the toe is allowed to grow out with a dish.

Dorsal-Palmar/Plantar (DP) Balance. DP balance refers to the hoof angle (relationship between the dorsal wall of the hoof and the ground) and the alignment of the hoof angle and the pastern angle. Hoof angle is measured at the toe with a hoof protractor (see Fig. 6–20). For years textbooks cited 45 to 50° as "normal" for the front hoof angle and 50 to 55° for a hind hoof angle. But everyday observations by practicing farriers and research indicate that normal front pastern and hoof angles for domestic riding horses range from 53 to 58° and normal hind angles from 55 to 60°, with an occasional normal horse outside of these ranges. (The range of toe angles in wild horses has been reported to be 50 to 60° in the front and 53 to 63° in the hind hoof.)

Each horse has its own "ideal" hoof angle. The angle of the hoof is considered correct when the hoof and pastern are in alignment; that is, the dorsal surface of the hoof is parallel to an imaginary line (axis) passing through the center of the long pastern bone (Figs. 6–31 and 6–32). The goal is actually to align the dorsal surface of the coffin bone with the long pastern bone axis. The hoof wall is used as a guide because, in the normal hoof, the dorsal surfaces of the hoof wall and coffin bone are parallel.

This alignment is best viewed from the side of the horse with the horse standing squarely on a hard, level surface with the cannon bone vertical. It is important to use a line through the center of the long pastern bone for the pastern angle. Using the irregular surface formed by hair and skin at the front of the pastern will result in inaccurate alignment.

Because more lamenesses are associated with low heels (and low hoof angle) than steep heels (and higher hoof angles) and because the hoof angle gets progressively lower during the 6- to 8-week shoeing cycle (because the toe grows faster than the heel), it is usually best for the horse to be shod a little on the steep side.

If the hoof angle is too low in relation to the pastern angle, the center line will be broken back near the vicinity of the coronary band (Fig. 6–33). The lower the hoof angle, the higher the pastern angle and the more broken-back the hoof-pastern axis. Decreasing hoof angle increases the strain on the deep digital flexor tendon.

If the hoof angle is too high in relation to the pastern angle, the line will be broken forward. The higher the hoof angle, the lower the pastern angle and the more broken-forward the hoof-pastern axis. Increasing hoof angle decreases the strain on the deep digital flexor tendon but does not change the strain on the superficial flexor tendon.

Medial-Lateral (ML) Balance. ML balance refers to the relationship between the medial (inside) wall of the hoof and the lateral (outside) wall of the hoof. Determining ML balance is one of the most challenging aspects of farriery and relies as much on art as it does on science. The goal is to trim the hoof in such a way that the ground surface of the hoof is centered beneath the limb. This allows the hoof structure to bear the weight of the limb evenly. Altering the relative lengths of the sides of the hoof shifts the position of the hoof beneath the limb. Lowering the lateral wall tends to position the hoof more toward the midline of the horse, whereas lowering the medial wall tends to position the hoof away from the midline of the horse. But repositioning the limb by trimming may have undesirable consequences.

There are many methods for determining ML balance, none of which works for all horses. Whether a farrier (or veterinarian) chooses a static or dynamic approach and which specific guideline he follows depends on his experience, the age of the horse, the degree of abnormality, the accompanying problems, and the horse's use.

One method of achieving *static* ML balance is to trim the hoof so that the coronet is parallel to level ground (Fig. 6–34). This works with relatively straight limbs. But if a hoof has remodeled over a period of years to accommodate deviations in the limb, this trimming method may put uneven stress on the limb.

A similar method is to trim the hoof so that the plane of the ground surface is perpendicular to the cannon bone. A "T-bar" or similar device can be used to make this determination. This method is also suitable for normally conformed limbs.

Another method is to trim the hoof so that its ground surface is perpendicular to the midline of the horse. This can be checked by picking up the forelimb. With the horse's knee flexed and the cannon lightly resting in the hand, the farrier sites across the ground

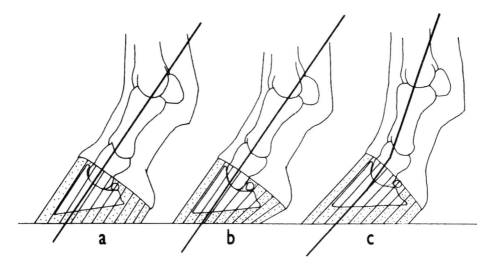

Fig. 6–30. *A*, Normal: tubules parallel from toe to heel. *B*, Underrun heel: tubules not parallel. *C*, Low heels: tubules parallel. (From Hill, C., Klimesh, R., Maximum Hoof Power. New York, Howell Book House, 1994.)

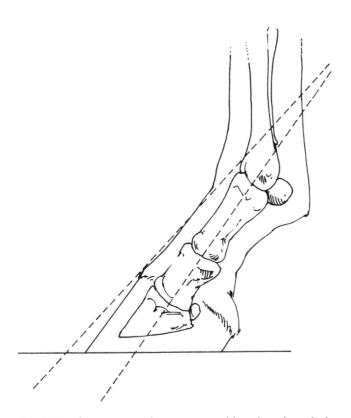

Fig. 6–31. The pastern angle is represented by a line through the center of the long pastern bone, not a line at the dorsal surface of the pastern. (From Hill, C., Klimesh, R.: Maximum Hoof Power. New York, Howell Book House, 1994.)

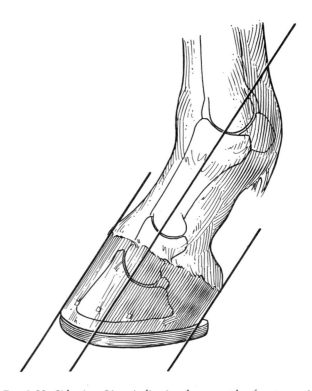

Fig. 6–32. Side view. Lines indicating the correct hoof pastern axis.

surface of the hoof. This approach works well on horses whose limbs deviate from the ideal and often results in *dynamic* ML balance.

It is generally agreed that the hoof is in dynamic balance when the medial and lateral walls strike the ground at the same time. If a hoof is landing on the lateral wall first, that side is assumed to be longer and should be trimmed shorter to allow a flat landing. Shoe wear, however, must be considered before the hoof is trimmed. If a horse *lands* on its lateral toe, it often *loads* on its medial heel. This diagonal imbalance can cause jamming of the coronary band at the medial heel, which can result in sheared heels.

Some horses are conformed so that it is impossible to achieve a flat landing. Overzealous trimming should be avoided because lameness could result from

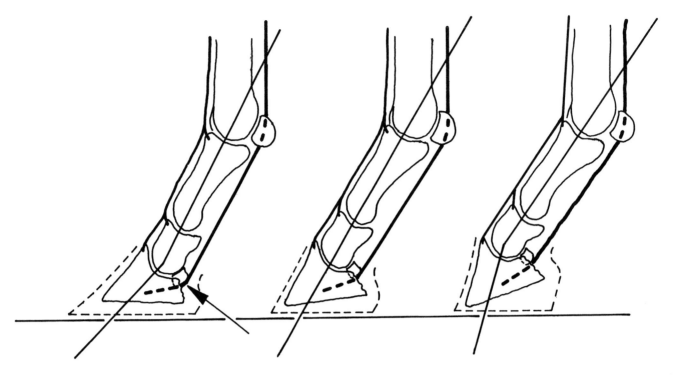

Fig. 6–33. *A*, Broken back axis resulting in excess pressure on the navicular region as indicated by arrow. *B*, Straight axis. (*Note*: it is normal for the bottom of the coffin bone to be 5° to 7° above the horizontal.) *C*, Broken forward axis. (From Hill, C., Klimesh, R.: Maximum Hoof Power. New York, Howell Book House, 1994.)

attempting to make a sound horse's apparently unbalanced hooves conform to an "ideal." It is important to realize that the way the hoof contacts the ground differs with each gait and from fore to rear. A hoof that does not land flat at the walk may land flat at the trot or canter. Landing flat is only one guideline to balance, not a hard and fast rule.

Many hooves, especially hind hooves, cannot be balanced dynamically by trimming the medial and lateral sides to be equal in length. Examining the shoe for wear can help determine a plan for trimming that will result in even wear on both branches of the shoe (Figs 6–35 and 6–36). Usually, if the side of the hoof (shoe) that shows the least amount of shoe wear is trimmed shorter, the subsequent wear on the shoe will be equal. This rule may not apply for a horse that is lame or has an unusual way of going, so it is wise not to rely on just one guideline when attempting something as complex as balancing the equine limb. It is valuable to record the trimming approach and to label and save the used shoes so that changes in the wear pattern can be noted and future trimming adjusted accordingly.

If the hoof wall is worn too short to balance by trimming alone, wedge pads, shims, or custom shoes can be used to achieve balance until the hoof grows.

Length. The length of the hoof is measured at the center of the toe from the point where the soft coronet meets the hard hoof wall (coronary rim) to the ground surface. The toe length determines the length of the lever that the limb must break or pivot over. Long toes

create a longer lever arm, a delayed breakover, and increased pressure on the palmar/plantar portions of the distal limb. Trimming the toe too short, however, can invite bruises.

The appropriate toe length of a freshly trimmed hoof ready for shoeing varies according to the horse's conformation and breed. For example, the toe length of a small Arabian might be 3 inches, that of a Quarter Horse $3\frac{1}{2}$ inches, and that of a Warmblood 4 inches. If a horse is to be barefoot, the hoof is left $\frac{1}{4}$ inch longer than if it is to be shod. The optimum length of the hoof wall is actually dictated by the optimum thickness of the sole.

Levelness. The entire bottom of the hoof wall should be level so that it makes perfect contact with a smooth ground surface or a flat shoe (Fig. 6–37). Any unevenness will cause the hoof to bear weight unevenly. In some cases, a farrier may purposely remove a portion of the hoof wall at the ground surface to "relieve" a crack, flare, or displaced coronet. In most instances, however, the hoof wall should be level.

Sole. The natural sole is slightly cupped from side to side as well as from front to rear. At the time of trimming, the farrier pares the sole to a concave shape but not so thinly as to cause the horse to be sore when he walks on gravel. If the sole is left too thick, however, it can reduce hoof expansion during weight bearing and may inhibit the natural springing action of the hoof capsule, which is an important shock-absorbing function. Also, a thick sole often prevents the farrier from trimming the toe sufficiently to attain DP bal-

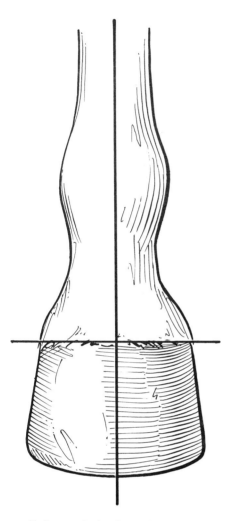

FIG. 6–34. Hoof balance. The hoof is said to be in balance when an imaginary line through the coronet is parallel to the ground surface and perpendicular to a line that bisects the limb axis when viewed from the front.

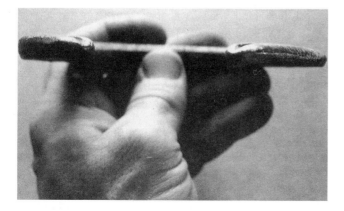

FIG. 6–35. The farrier examines the shoe for wear.

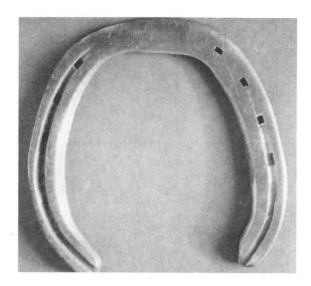

FIG. 6–36. Uneven shoe wear: The right branch has worn the right crease completely away.

ance. The bars should not be weakened by excessive trimming, but long, deformed horn should be removed.

Frog. The frog should be smoothly pared, with no loose or overgrown tissue that could trap dirt and manure and harbor anaerobic thrush organisms. The clefts of the frog at the heels should be trimmed out so that the hoof can self-clean. It is not necessary or desirable for the frog to bear weight when the horse stands on level ground.

Shape. The inside wall is generally steeper than the outside wall. The wall at the toe is usually thicker than at the quarters. The entire hoof wall from the coronary band to the ground should be straight, that is, without dips or bulges. Flares and dishes tend to be self-perpetuating. If there are any dishes (dips in the toe) or flares (dips in the sides of the hoof), the wall should be rasped straight. This encourages the growth of a normal hoof shape.

To evaluate shape, the farrier finds the normal center of the sole, most recently referred to as Duckett's Dot. On the *average riding* horse, Duckett's Dot is located $\frac{3}{8}$ inch back from the tip of the trimmed frog. Once the horse's hoof has been trimmed and shaped, the distance from the dot to the toe should equal that from the dot to the outermost border of the medial wall (Fig. 6–38). The distance from the dot to the lateral wall is usually greater.

Symmetry of Hoof Pairs. Generally, the toe length of a hoof should be equal to that of its mate. Variation in hoof angle, however, often occurs in paired limbs because of individual limb conformation. In some instances, the difference should be minimized through trimming and shoeing, but in many cases the mismatched limbs should be allowed to be different. Dynamic balance will indicate which path the farrier should choose. In some cases, the hooves will be

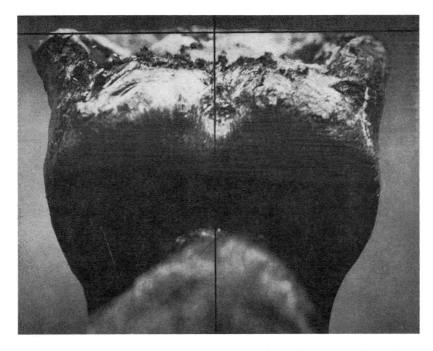

FIG. 6–37. Graphic demonstration of foot level. An imaginary line bisecting the limb longitudinally and a transverse line across the heels should give two 90° angles at their intersection. If the transverse line is tilted either way, the foot is off level.

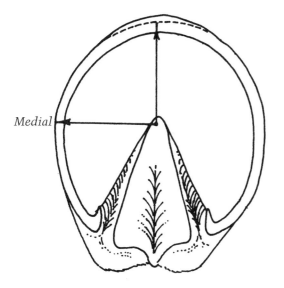

FIG. 6–38. Duckett's Dot. (From Hill, C., Klimesh, R.: Maximum Hoof Power. New York, Howell Book House, 1994.)

trimmed and shod differently so that they move the same.

There is a normal difference in shape and hoof angle between forefeet and hindfeet. Most forefeet are larger, rounder, and wider at the heels and have a flatter sole than the same horse's hindfeet. Hindfeet are commonly one shoe size smaller, are more pointed at the toe, and have a more concave sole and higher hoof angle.

Shoe Preparation

Selection. The size of the shoe should be appropriate for the size of the horse and hoof. The shoe should be strong enough to support the horse's weight but not unnecessarily heavy, or it might negatively affect the horse's stride and agility. The shoes should provide adequate protection, support, and traction. The nail heads are protected from wear by setting them in either a crease or a hole stamped in the shoe (Fig. 6–39).

Hot versus cold shoeing refers to the way the farrier makes, shapes, or applies shoes. Hot shoeing means that the farrier makes the shoes from scratch in a forge, or modifies keg shoes in a forge or fits a hot shoe to the hoof. Cold shoeing means the farrier shapes and applies the shoe without heating it up. Many farriers use a combination of hot and cold shoeing techniques.

Steel, the material most commonly used in making horseshoes, (Fig. 6–40) is a combination of iron and other elements, mainly carbon. Steel is graded by the amount of carbon it contains; the higher the carbon content, the harder the steel. Mild (low carbon) steel is used for horseshoes because it is easily shaped and yet durable enough to last for one or more shoeing periods. A high carbon steel, such as used for springs or tools, would last longer but would be more difficult to shape and would have less traction on hard surfaces. All but the largest sizes of mild steel horseshoes can be shaped while cold to fit the hoof. Large shoes, as for warmbloods and draft horses, must be heated in a forge to be shaped.

Aluminum is also used for horseshoes and it is lighter than steel (Figs. 6–41 to 6–44). Because of this

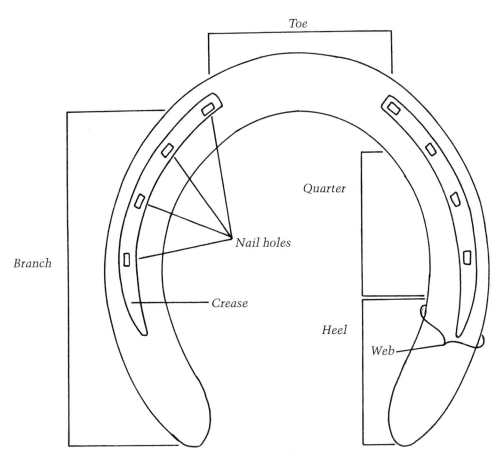

Fig. 6–39. Parts of a shoe. (From Hill, C., Klimesh, R.: Maximum Hoof Power. New York, Howell Book House, 1994.)

weight advantage, aluminum is the material of which most Thoroughbred racing shoes, or "plates" are made. Using aluminum, a shoe can be made wider for support or thicker to alter DP balance without the weight increase associated with a similar steel shoe. Being softer than steel, however, aluminum does not wear as long as steel so many aluminum shoes are equipped with steel inserts at the toes where the most wear occurs. Modern manufacturing processes are producing shoes of aluminum alloys that wear much longer than the earlier aluminum shoes. However, if these shoes are heated for shaping or forming clips, the wear is often greatly reduced.

Because aluminum shoes bend or spring more easily than a steel shoe, they often cannot provide the support that a horse needs. This is especially true with larger horses or with jumpers where there is a great deal of force upon landing and turning.

Another drawback of aluminum horseshoes is that in the presence of moisture, galvanic corrosion occurs between the steel nails and the aluminum. This reaction corrodes the hoof surface of the shoe and affects the hoof itself. Evidence of this corrosion is seen as a pasty white substance between the shoe and hoof when the shoe is removed.

Titanium is a corrosion-resistant element with the strength of steel and the lightness of aluminum. Be-

cause titanium was considered a strategic material until recently, civilian access to and research with titanium have been limited. Testing is under way that may result in a titanium shoe that can be worked like a conventional shoe and that will provide the horse with the best properties of both steel and aluminum.

Attempts have been made for years to develop a successful plastic horseshoe. The main drawback of nail-on plastic shoes is that the inherent flexibility of the material does not provide sufficient support for a horse's hoof. Also, the slippery surface of the plastic encourages the hoof to spread over the edges of the shoe.

Plastic horseshoes that are glued to the hoof wall by means of a cuff or series of tabs are valuable in therapeutic applications. They are used when the wall is too damaged or weak to hold nails securely and on foal hooves that are too thin-walled to nail safely. Because the application of glue-on shoes is relatively nontraumatic, they can be used on laminitic horses and other horses in extreme pain.

Several types of horseshoes are available that combine a core of steel or aluminum with an outer shell of plastic or rubber. These shoes give more support to the hoof than plastic alone, and many can be shaped like a conventional steel shoe. The supposed advantage of these shoes is their ability to absorb shock.

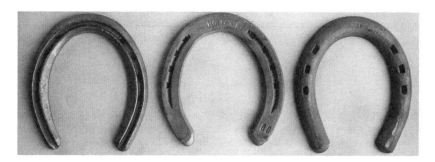

FIG. 6–40. *From left*: rim shoe, plain shoe, half round shoe.

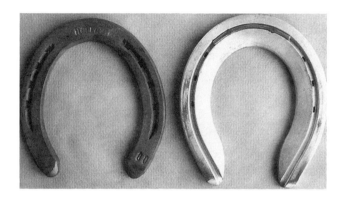

FIG. 6–41. *From left*: plain steel shoe, wide web aluminum shoe.

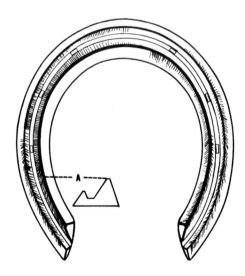

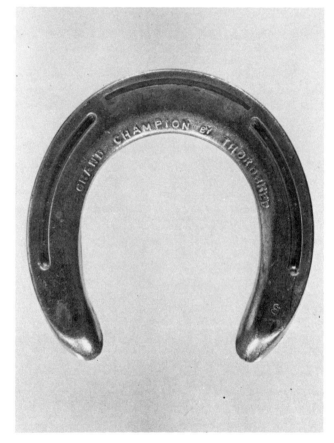

FIG. 6–43. Top view of an aluminum wedge shoe.

FIG. 6–42. Ground surface view of a polo shoe. The low outside rim facilitates breakover in any direction. Inset shows a cross section of the web with A the inside rim.

There is a scarcity of independent research, however, concerning the effectiveness of shock-absorbing hoof wear and of the effects of shock on the equine limb.

Horseshoes are either individually hand-forged by the farrier or mass-produced in a factory. At one time, factory-made shoes were transported in wooden kegs, and therefore the term "keg shoe" refers to a ready-made commercial shoe. When keg shoes were lacking in both quality and variety, it was worth the farrier's time to hand-forge the shoes he used. Today keg shoes are available in many shapes, materials, thicknesses, widths, and qualities. Many top farriers seldom find it necessary to make a shoe from bar stock; others enjoy the forge work so much that they hand-make all the shoes they apply.

It is common for farriers, however, to modify keg shoes to suit particular purposes. The most common

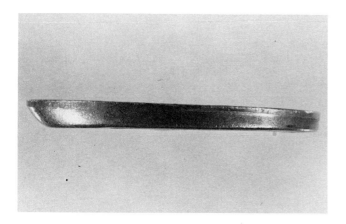

FIG. 6–44. Side view of an aluminum wedge shoe. Note the toe of the shoe (*right*) is thinner than the heels.

modifications are repositioning the nail holes, adding a bar, altering the shape of the toe (rolled, rocker, square), altering the heel shape and length (trailers, extended heels, spooned heels), and forging or attaching clips.

Fit. A shoe should follow the natural shape of the properly prepared hoof, being neither too wide nor too narrow, too short nor too long. When it is viewed from above with the foot on the ground, from $\frac{1}{16}$ to $\frac{1}{8}$ inch of the edge of the properly fitted shoe should be visible from the quarters back to the heels (Fig. 6–45). This indicates that the shoe has adequate allowance for heel growth and expansion.

Hoof Expansion. A shoe is fitted full to accommodate heel movement and normal increase in hoof width during the 5 to 8-week shoeing period. With each step, as the horse's weight descends on the foot, it causes movement (expansion) at the heels (Fig. 6–46). As the weight is lifted, before breakover, the heels return (contract) to their original position. These events are evidenced by the grooves worn in the hoof surface of the shoe.

Because the hoof is cone-shaped, as it grows longer, the base of the cone essentially gets wider, while the steel shoe that is nailed to it remains its original size. Therefore, it is necessary to start out with the shoe wider, so that after 3 to 4 weeks, there is still support for the heel area of the hoof, which becomes wider than when the shoe was applied.

Too little expansion room allows the hoof wall to spread over the edge of the shoe as it grows, resulting in lack of support and hoof wall and sole damage (Fig. 6–47). Too much expansion room increases the chance that the horse will step on the shoe or catch it on something. Upright hooves need less expansion room than flatter, spread-out hooves with more sloping walls.

Heel Support. Enough shoe should extend beyond the heels so that the limb is adequately supported. Generally, the heel of the shoe should be below the mid-

line of the cannon bone when the cannon is vertical (Fig. 6–48). Another guide is that the length of the shoe is equal to or greater than twice the toe length of the prepared hoof (Fig. 6–49). "Short-shoeing" (using a shoe that is too small) does not provide ample support, and this can result in fatigue and damage to the horse's limbs as well as underrun heels (Figs. 6–50 and 6–51).

Contact with the Wall. Unless some of the hoof wall is missing because of hoof damage or has been purposely removed to treat a crack or a persistent flare or other abnormality, the shoe should contact the hoof wall completely. The corner of a business card should not fit between the hoof and the shoe at any point around the outside perimeter of the hoof. Hot-fitting a shoe properly (heating the shoe and pressing it onto the prepared hoof) provides a perfect match between shoe and hoof. When a shoe is cold-fitted, the farrier must be skilled with a rasp to be sure that the hoof and shoe meet all the way around.

Sole Pressure. Although the shoe should be in contact with the entire hoof wall, it should not contact more than $\frac{1}{8}$ inch of the sole. If a horse has very flat soles, the inner edge of the hoof surface of its shoes need to be relieved to avoid creating unwanted sole pressure (Figs. 6–52 and 6–53). This is especially important when the horse is shod with wide-web shoes (Fig. 6–54). Sole pressure can disrupt blood flow and lead to lameness, abscesses, and corns.

Nails

Heads. The nail head should seat tightly in the crease or stamped hole and should protrude below the shoe about $\frac{1}{16}$ inch.

Placement. The nail should enter the hoof within the white line. If the nail enters outside the white line, the clinches are likely to be too low, and the shoe may not be secure (Fig. 6–55). If the nail enters inside the white line, sensitive structures may be invaded. The tip of the nail is beveled so that it travels in a curved path in dense horn tissue and exits the hoof wall. If the nail is angled to the center of the hoof or placed inside the white line, the soft tissue there may not provide enough resistance to curve the nail outward, and the nail does not exit the hoof wall. The bevel is on the same side as the pattern on the nail head (Fig. 6–56). The nail is placed with the bevel toward the inside of the hoof so that the nail, when driven, curves away from the bevel. Six to eight nails are used; generally none are placed behind the widest portion of the hoof wall. The heel nail holes on most keg shoes are often located too far rearward, so only six nails are used, leaving the heel nail holes empty.

Pattern. The height of the nail farthest back on the shoe should be approximately one-third the distance from the ground to the coronary band. The nail pattern is affected by the quality of the hoof, the skill of the farrier, and the quality and design of the shoes and

SHOE TYPES

Materials
  Steel
  Aluminum
  Titanium
  Plastic
  Plastic or rubber over a steel or aluminum core

Types

Plain shoe—a flat shoe having a crease (also called a fuller or swedge) on the ground surface of the shoe in the area of the nails' heads (Figs. 6–40 and 6–41).

Stamped shoe—a flat shoe without a crease, but with pockets stamped in the shoe for the nail heads; also called a punched shoe.

Rim shoe—a shoe with a crease around the entire ground surface for traction and for recessing the nail heads (Fig. 6–40).

Training plate—a light, thin steel shoe.

Polo shoe—a light, thin steel rim shoe with a higher inside rim; stronger than a training plate (Fig. 6–42).

Barrel racing shoe—a light, thin steel rim shoe with a higher outside rim.

Toed and heeled—steel shoe having a bar protruding across the ground surface of the toe and a square protrusion called a calk at each heel to provide traction in soft footing.

Half round—shoe with stamped nail holes that is flat on the hoof surface and round on the ground surface (Fig. 6–40).

Racing plate—a very light, thin aluminum shoe, usually with a steel wear insert at the toe, available in a wide variety of styles.

Wedge shoe (swelled heel)—steel or aluminum shoe thicker at the heels than at the toe (Figs. 6–43 and 6–44).

Wide web shoe—shoe formed from wider steel (Fig. 6–41).

Sizes

There is no standard among horse shoe companies regarding shoe sizes. A shoe that has a 14-inch circumference (from heel to heel) could be one of eight different sizes (ranging from #1 to #12), depending on the company that makes it. The Farrier Industry Association has developed a chart that categorizes most available steel, aluminum, and plastic horse shoes according to their circumference from heel to heel (See Resource Guide at the end of the chapter).

nails being used. Ideally the nail pattern should form a straight line (Fig. 6–57), and the two toe nails should be at equal heights when viewed from the front.

Clinches. The clinches should be "square," that is, only as long as they are wide. Such clinches open easily, allowing the shoe to come off if it gets caught on something. Rectangular clinches are longer than they are wide. Because such clinches usually hold the shoe on securely, if a horse gets the shoe caught on a fence or steps on it, he may rip large portions of his hoof off along with the nails and the shoe. Clinches should be uniform and set flush with the hoof wall. Clinches should not be set into a groove filed in the hoof wall. They should feel smooth to the touch.

Details

The hoof wall should be smooth, never rasped above the clinches unless it is necessary to remove a flare. The edge of the hoof wall as well as the edge of the shoe should be smooth. Old nail holes should be filled with wax (see Resource Guide) or other appropriate substance to prevent moisture, mud, and other contaminants from entering the hoof.

Any exposed edges of the shoe should be rounded (Fig. 6–52) with a rasp or grinder to decrease the chance that the shoe will come off if stepped on. Also, this removes any burrs or steel slivers that may injure a person handling the feet.

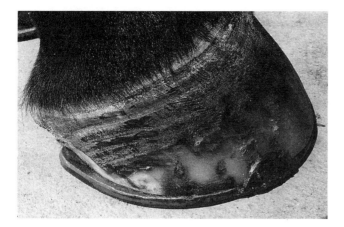

FIG. 6–45. Good shoe fit.

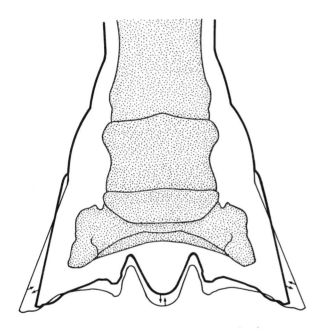

FIG. 6–46. During weight-bearing, the frog and sole are forced downward causing expansion of the hoof wall. During non-weight-bearing, the reverse occurs.

Common Hoof Problems and Treatment

Neglect

Failing to provide regular, competent hoof care is a main cause of problems. Neglect includes allowing the bare hoof to wear too short, or to grow so long that it breaks off, leaving shoes on so long that the hoof grows over the shoe (Fig. 6–47) or grows imbalanced (Figs. 6–58 and 6–59); overfeeding and underfeeding; and failure to examine the hooves regularly for imbedded rocks, nails, and other foreign objects.

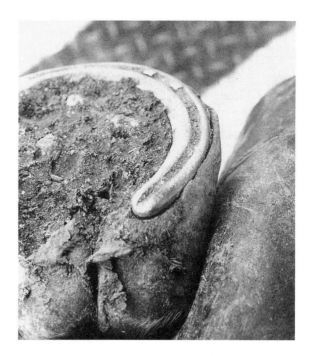

FIG. 6–47. The hoof spread over shoe from quarter to heel. It is way overdue for shoeing.

Hoof Damage

Broken hooves can alter hoof balance and cause lameness (Fig. 6–60). It is not uncommon, however, for flared hooves to break even though the horse remains sound. Similarly, a horse can rip off a shoe and portions of hoof wall and be reshod routinely. When a large section of hoof wall is missing, hoof repair may be necessary. A farrier can use hoof repair materials that have properties similar to hoof horn and will adhere to the hoof wall for months until new growth replaces the damaged area. These materials can be used to build up the low side of a hoof, replace missing sections of wall, or build up thin walls so that a shoe can be nailed on. The prosthetic hoof can be trimmed and shaped like a normal hoof and is strong enough to secure a nail-on shoe (see Resource Guide).

If thc hoof wall is too weak or damaged to secure a shoe using nails or if the horse is in too much pain to allow the driving of nails into the hoof, glue-on shoes are a good alternative. These shoes are available from several sources (see Resource Guide) in many configurations for various applications from foal treatment to racing shoes to founder treatment. One type of glue-on shoe uses a cuff to which a steel or aluminum shoe of choice is riveted and the cuff glued or taped to the hoof. Another type has plastic tabs around the shoe that are glued onto the surface of the hoof wall.

Poor Hoof Quality

Good-quality hoof horn is dry, hard, and tough, not brittle, spongy, or soft. Poor nutrition, faulty metab-

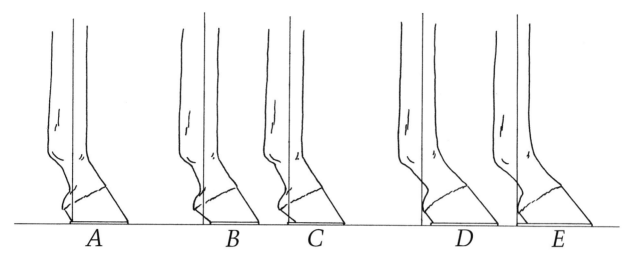

FIG. 6–48. Heel support. *A*, An ideal situation: the hoof is in DP balance, the heels are not underrun, and there is proper heel support. In this case, shoes that extend just slightly behind the heels of the hoof provide adequate support. *B*, Although this hoof is in DP balance, the toe-heel alignment is not parallel, and the heels are underrun. When the shoe is fit to the heels, the hoof is "short shod" and inadequately supported. *C*, The same hoof as in *B* but properly supported with a longer shoe. *D*, This hoof is in DP balance, and the toe-heel alignment is parallel, but the low hoof-pastern angle results in the hoof being too far ahead of the limb. When the shoe is fit to the heels, the hoof is "short shod" and inadequately supported. *E*, The same hoof as in *D* but properly supported with a longer shoe. (From Hill, C., Klimesh, R.: Maximum Hoof Power. New York Howell Book House, 1994.)

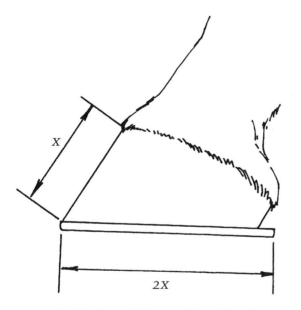

FIG. 6–49. A shoe length guide. (From Hill, C., Klimesh, R.: Maximum Hoof Power. New York, Howell Book House, 1994.)

olism, unhealthy environment, improper management, disease, certain drugs, and trauma are all factors that can affect hoof quality.

In some cases, poor hoof quality is caused by poor nutrition. In others, the problem lies with a horse's inability to synthesize essential nutrients. A horse's ration should provide adequate amounts of the essential amino acid DL-methionine, biotin (a component of the vitamin B complex), and other nutrients. Often, it is necessary to use a supplement to meet a horse's nutritional requirements (see Resource Guide). If nutrition is adequate, poor-quality hooves might be caused by other genetic influences, poor management practices, or both.

Historically, advice for improving hoof quality has ranged from prescribing hoof dressings and packings to standing a horse in the mud around its overflowing water trough. Contrary to what is often believed, many hoofs crack and peel from *too much* moisture or repeated wet-dry episodes rather than not enough moisture. Current recommendations include providing the horse with adequate exercise (which provides moisture internally via the blood) and maintaining the external moisture at a constant, relatively dry level.

In a normal hoof, the outer hoof layer is dense and tough with a moisture content of 15 to 20%. The inner layer averages about 45%. The two layers are joined together by interlocking sheaves of epidermal (insensitive) laminae (from the outer layer) and blood-rich dermal (sensitive) laminae (from the inner layer).

Adequate moisture in the inner layer is provided by blood and lymph vessels in the laminae. Moisture diffuses outward from the moist sensitive laminae toward the dry, hard outer wall. When blood circulates freely to and from the hoof, the dynamic balance of moisture is operating at an optimum level. When there is a lack of exercise or a disease of the hoof such as laminitis or navicular syndrome, an imbalance in the hoof, or an ill-fitting shoe, circulation is interrupted to the point where moisture is no longer provided through the blood flow. A hoof that is too dry is inflexible and an inefficient shock absorber. It also tends to contract and tighten around the sensitive in-

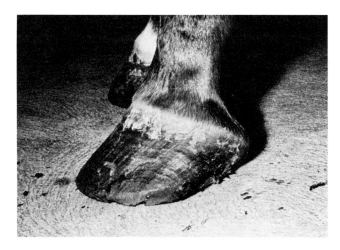

FIG. 6–50. Before trimming and shoeing, a horse with a long toe and underrun heels.

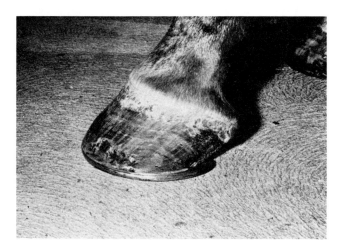

FIG. 6–51. The same hoof as in Fig. 6–50 after trimming and shoeing. The toe is rasped shorter and lowered, and the heels are left higher. The shoe is fit well back on the foot to expand past the heels.

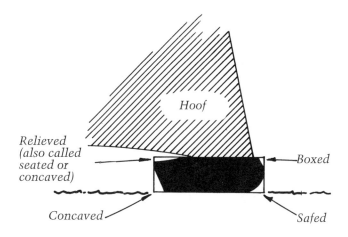

FIG. 6–52. Modifications made to shoe edges. (From Hill, C., Klimesh, R.: Maximum Hoof Power. New York, Howell Book House, 1994.)

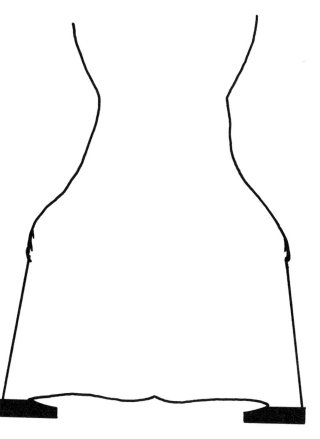

FIG. 6–53. The hoof surface of the shoe is relieved to prevent sole pressure. (From Hill, C., Klimesh, R.: Maximum Hoof Power. New York, Howell Book House, 1994.)

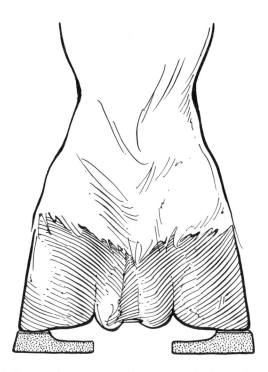

FIG. 6–54. A wide-web shoe with a concaved solar surface. This protects the sole without applying pressure to it.

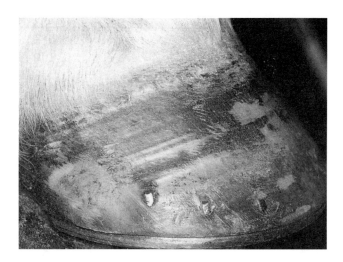

FIG. 6–55. Low clinches.

ner structures. If a horse is getting adequate exercise, the moisture level of the inner layer remains constant.

A hoof that is kept too soft (e.g., when a horse is in a wet environment or hooves are regularly covered with hoof dressing) contains too much moisture in the external hoof wall. The soft wall cannot oppose the pressure from the inner structures of the foot, and the hoof spreads out and flattens. Excess moisture weakens the hoof material; soft, punky hoof walls often peel and separate, resulting in no solid hoof wall to bear the horse's weight or to hold a nailed-on shoe.

Too much moisture can also make a horse's soles soft and susceptible to sole bruises and abscesses. Research has shown that the condition of hooves worsens during hot, humid weather, especially when horses are turned out at night. In such a situation, horses walk around in dew-laden pastures at night and then are either left out where the sun will dry the hooves or are put in a stall where the bedding dries them. Horses that repeatedly walk through mud and then stand in the sun experience a similar decay in hoof quality. In both cases, the hoof is going through a stressful moisture-related expansion/contraction that damages the hoof structures. Mud has the effect of drawing out moisture and oils and tightening pores, much like a poultice. In the process of drying out, the outer layer of the hoof wall will attempt to bend or warp but cannot do so because of the hold the inner layer has on it. Instead, it develops cracks and checks to relieve the stresses from the shearing forces of the opposition of the layers. The cracks may then become packed with more mud and dirt so that they cannot close. The cracks can continue to get larger and spread upward.

Because excess moisture can be so damaging to a hoof, some experts discourage application of any grease or oil to the hoof. Because the hoof has two natural protective layers, dressings may not be able to penetrate the hoof anyway. A waxy covering, the periople, is located at the coronary band and is visible as an inch-wide strip that encircles the top of the hoof. The protective, varnish-like outer layer of the hoof wall, the stratum tectorium, is composed of hard horn. Both coatings retard moisture movement from either direction, from the outside environment into the hoof or from the inner layer of the hoof to the outside.

Hoof dressing is warranted when the bulbs of the heels begin to crack. To restore their pliability, a product containing animal grease, such as lanolin or fish oil, can be applied daily until the desired result has been achieved. A hoof sealer, which penetrates better than a dressing, is often very beneficial in stabilizing hoof moisture content if a horse is in very wet or very dry conditions.

A horse with low-quality hoof horn requires at least a year for new growth from the coronary band to reach the ground. In the meantime, a farrier can try to minimize trauma to the weak hooves by using fewer nails, thinner nails, clips, hand-forged shoes with strategically placed nail holes, acrylics to build up thin walls, or glue-on shoes.

Poor Hoof Shape

The hoof capsule is a very plastic structure that adapts in shape to the stresses that are placed on it. The higher its moisture content, the more plastic it is. Fortunately, many deformed hooves can be reformed by the farrier. Every time the hoof is trimmed, its shape should be evaluated and adjusted to ensure it is growing in the proper manner. When a hoof is being actively reformed, the change in shape during one trimming may be dramatic (Fig. 6–61). Even with "normal" feet, however, with each shoeing the hoof must be shaped and the shoe carefully adjusted. Whether this is done or not is often the difference between a "good" farrier and a "fast" farrier.

Flares in the sidewalls of the hoof can result from an ML imbalance, a genetically or nutritionally weak hoof structure, a too-high moisture content in the hoof, or, most likely, a combination of these factors. A flare on only one side of the hoof is usually caused by ML imbalance. If the hoof wall flares out on both sides, it is usually a combination of hoof conformation and high moisture.

Contracted Heels

Contraction of one or both heels of a hoof can be caused by long toe–low heel (LT-LH) configuration; lack of use of the foot (such as when the limb is injured and non-weight-bearing for a period of time or when the horse's exercise is restricted); or physical restriction of the hoof by horseshoe nails, clips, bandaging, or cast.

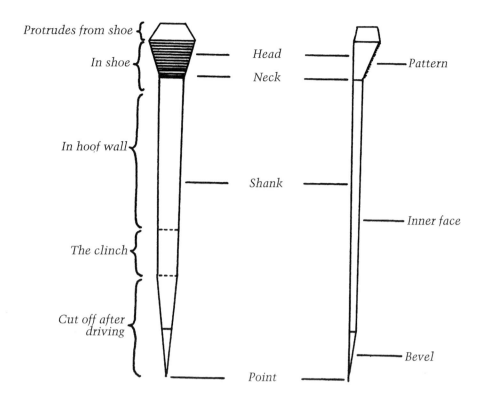

FIG. 6–56. Parts of a nail. (From Hill, C., Klimesh, R.: Maximum Hoof Power. New York, Howell Book House, 1994.)

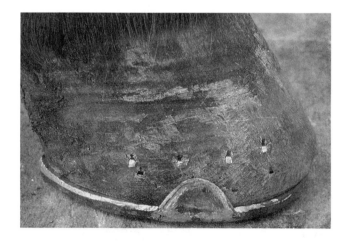

FIG. 6–57. Clinches showing good size, height, and pattern. Note nail holes have not yet been filled. Also note squared toe shoe.

Identification of contracted heels can be made by the following method: The width of the heels $\frac{1}{4}$ inch from the buttresses should equal or exceed the width of the trimmed hoof 1 inch back from the toe (Fig. 6–62). If the heel measurement is less than the toe measurement, the heels are said to be contracted. Some horses, however, have a congenital or adapted hoof shape that fits the definition of contracted heels, but the hoof is balanced by other criteria and the animal is sound. In these cases, it is not advisable to try to spread the heels.

As a hoof deviates toward LT-LH, the hoof elongates from toe to heel, and the heels generally get closer together. When the horse's weight rotates over the long toe in a prolonged breakover, the heels of the hoof are drawn inward. Balancing the hoof and shoeing with a squared toe shoe that provides adequate heel support allows such a hoof to function more normally and encourages the heels to spread.

When a horse lacks exercise, the blood flow in the hoof is decreased, causing a drop in the moisture content of the hoof capsule. In the idle horse, the lack of pressure pushing outward from the descending weight of the horse during movement coupled with an increased inward-curling force from the drying outer hoof wall causes the hoof capsule to contract at the heels. This contraction can compress the sensitive inner structures of the hoof and result in lameness or soreness.

The treatment is to increase the exercise level of the horse and retard the evaporation of internal moisture by application of a hoof sealer (see Resource Guide). In some instances, a shoe with slippered heels (Fig. 6–63) may be applied until the hoof regains its shape. The heel portion of the bearing surface of this shoe is sloped outward to spread the hoof physically as the horse's weight descends. If the horse cannot be exercised, the moisture content of the hoof may need to be increased by wet bandages or by placing the horse in a stall with damp sand or sawdust. Other, more dramatic mechanical devices have been used to spread

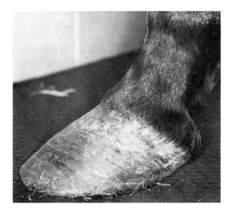

FIG. 6–58. Neglect: Before trimming.

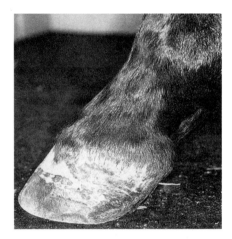

FIG. 6–59. The same hoof as in Fig. 6–58, after trimming.

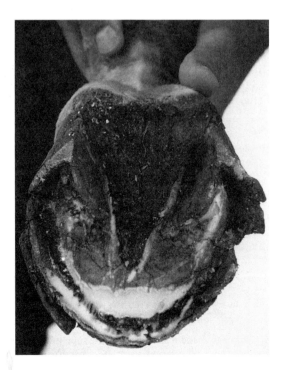

FIG. 6–60. A broken and separated hoof.

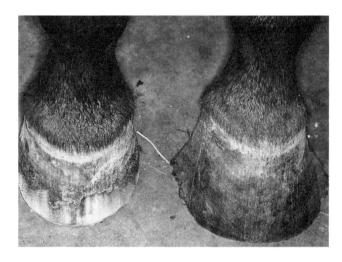

FIG. 6–61. Hoof shape can be altered quite dramatically in one trimming.

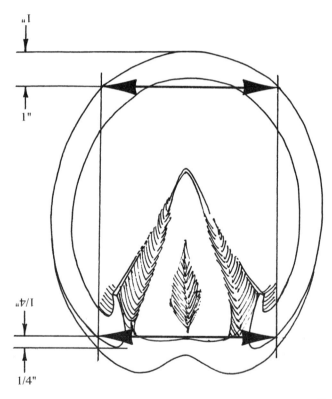

FIG. 6–62. One method of identifying contracted heels. (From Hill, C., Klimesh, R.: Maximum Hoof Power. New York, Howell Book House, 1994.)

the heels of a contracted hoof physically, but these are futile without removing the cause of contraction.

When the hoof must be in a cast or restrictive shoe for a long period to treat an injury, the heels usually contract. A similar contraction may result from consistently nailing on shoes with the nails too far back toward the heels. The last two nail holes on many factory-made shoes are behind the widest part of the hoof. These last two nails should usually be omitted unless they are specifically used to restrict the expansion of a bilaterally flared hoof. In most cases, the hoof will return to normal when the restriction is removed, the hoof is balanced, and the horse resumes regular exercise.

Long Toe–Low Heel (LT-LH) and Underrun Heels

When proper DP hoof balance is not maintained by trimming or shoeing, the hoof attains an abnormal LT-LH configuration, which can result in excess flexor tendon stress and cause heel soreness, cracks, contracted heels, and development of the navicular syndrome.

The LT-LH configuration can occur in several ways. A horse with poor-quality hoof horn is left barefoot; the hooves are not trimmed regularly and grow a long toe; the horse receives poor trimming and shoeing; the horse is overdue for shoeing.

If the heel is trimmed too short, the toe is left too long, and a shoe is placed on the hoof, the hoof angle is fixed at the outset at a too-low angle, and it becomes worse as the hoof grows. Even with a properly balanced hoof, if the shoe is left on too long, the heels will expand over the shoe and the horn at the heels will be crushed while the toe continues to grow longer and is prevented from wear by the shoe.

The LT-LH configuration places excess stress on the flexor tendons and navicular region and can cause underrun heels, an often irreversible condition in which the angle of the hoof horn at the heels is lower than the toe angle by 5° or more.

In trimming a hoof with *low* heels, the toe of the hoof wall is trimmed as short as is practical, tapering off toward the quarters. The heels are taken down only enough to get a good bearing surface of healthy horn, and this can often be accomplished more precisely with the rasp alone, minimizing the risk of trimming them too much.

Underrun heels, however, often should be trimmed short so that the support for the hoof is more rearward.

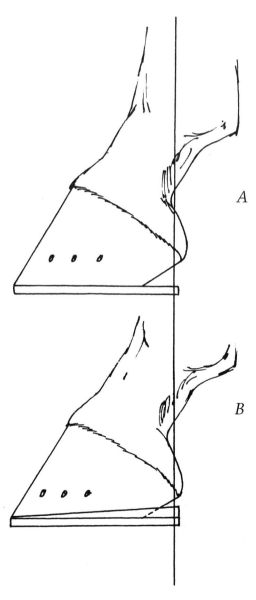

FIG. 6–64. Although *A* and *B* provide adequate support, *B* will more likely correct under-run heels and result in fewer lost shoes. (From Hill, C., Klimesh, R.: Maximum Hoof Power. New York, Howell Book House, 1994.)

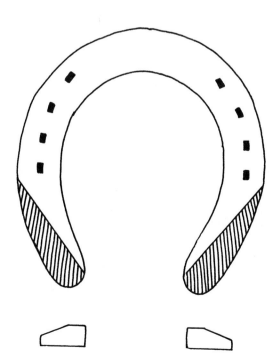

FIG. 6–63. Slipped shoe.

Leaving underrun heels long in an attempt to align the hoof-pastern axis only forces the heels to grow farther forward underneath the limb (Fig. 6–64) and creates an open invitation for lost shoes. After trimming the heels very short, the hoof-pastern axis can be aligned by elevating the heels with wedge-heel shoes or wedge pads (degree pads) (Fig. 6–64). An alternative is to rebuild the heels to a normal length and angle with a prosthetic hoof material (see Resource Guide). The hoof can then be shod in a normal manner.

Navicular Syndrome

Navicular syndrome is a chronic forelimb lameness involving the navicular bone and associated structures. Not all lamenesses associated with the heel area of the hoof, however, should be attributed to navicular syndrome. Factors thought to predispose a horse to navicular problems include poor conformation, improper or irregular shoeing, and stress to the navicular region. A common error that can lead to navicular syndrome is associated with the false economy of stretching the intervals between shoeings. As a hoof grows past its optimum reset time, the toe gets too long and the heel too low, resulting in a broken back axis. Increased pressure between the deep flexor tendon and the navicular bone may cause the heel pain associated with navicular syndrome (see Fig. 6–33).

The egg bar shoe (see egg bar shoe later in this chapter) has proved beneficial in the treatment of the navicular syndrome. It is a noninvasive, inexpensive treatment with virtually no negative side effects or risks. In addition, the egg bar shoe has positive effects on hoof conformation. Some horses show dramatic clinical improvement soon after egg bar shoes are applied as if their call for support was answered. Some underrun hooves, however, have gone past a critical horn tubule angle and have reached the point of no return. Even though these hooves are not likely to show a reversal of the underrun heel condition, the horse may be usable and comfortable working in egg bar shoes or full-support shoes for many years.

Full pads are often prescribed for horses that have navicular syndrome. Hooves with wide open, low heels are sometimes believed to have incurred navicular pain or heel soreness from the direct concussion to the frog and heel region. Full pads used to *protect* this area can actually *transmit* the concussion to the navicular region. A straight bar or full-support shoe might be more effective in providing protection for this type of navicular problem.

Wry Hoof

A wry hoof (diagonal ML imbalance) is a deformation that is usually, but not always, associated with sheared heels. The entire hoof wall, when viewed from the front, appears to sweep off to one side. When a hoof is wry to the inside, the medial wall flares inward and the outer wall curls in underneath the hoof. A wry hoof is caused primarily by a ML imbalance. This imbalance can be the result of improper trimming, from pain in the limb, which causes the horse to land more heavily on one side of the hoof, or from the way in which the hoof is worn as the horse turns in a habitual way in a stall or pen.

To return a wry hoof to a normal configuration, the flare is dressed off (Fig. 6–65A, B) and the hoof is shod with a bar shoe that is centered beneath the limb. This means that the shoe extends beyond the turned under hoof wall by as much as $\frac{1}{4}$ to $\frac{3}{8}$ inch and is shod close to the wall on the flared side.

The remaining hooves should be checked closely for balance because abnormalities affecting the shape of one hoof often affect the other hooves, usually the diagonal limb.

Sheared Heels

ML imbalance can lead to sheared heels and cracks. On a straight limb, lines from the coronet to the ground on the medial and lateral sides of the hoof are the same length, and the coronet forms a smooth line around the top of the hoof. The hoof strikes the ground flat (both sides simultaneously) at a walk.

When one side of the hoof becomes too short through wear or trimming, uneven stress is placed on the entire hoof structure. When a disproportionate amount of weight is borne by one side of the hoof, the entire side of the hoof wall can be dislocated upward, actually shearing the heels between the bulbs (Fig. 6–66). Grasping a heel of a sheared hoof in each hand, one can sometimes move the heels independently. Some horses' hoof structure adapts to this sheared configuration over many years, making a return to normal impossible and in some cases undesirable. If imbalanced during the formative years, a hoof may be permanently fixed into that abnormal balance, which then becomes "normal" for that horse. A recent development of sheared heels, often causing soreness and lameness, can usually be remedied by therapeutic shoeing methods.

If a small area of the hoof wall is allowed to be too long (such as when the shoe does not fit flat on the hoof) or if a small area of the hoof is growing faster, focal pressure is directed up the hoof wall, which can cause a section of the coronet to be displaced upward (and may result in a crack in the hoof wall at that point). A coronet displacement often goes undetected and can be the cause of subtle lameness.

The treatment for sheared heels is to allow the displaced hoof wall to drop down to its original position. The hoof is trimmed in balance as if it were not sheared, and a bar shoe is fit to the hoof. Before the

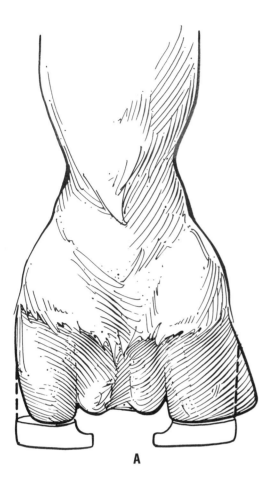

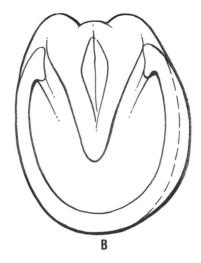

FIG. 6–65. Placement of a shoe on a wry foot. *A*, The shoe is placed where the foot should be. *B*, The dotted line indicates the flared hoof wall that will be rasped off.

bar shoe is applied, the ground surface of the displaced heel is further trimmed ("floated") so that it will not bear on the shoe. There should be a gap of $\frac{1}{4}$ to $\frac{1}{2}$ inch between the shoe and the hoof, tapering to meet at midquarter (Fig. 6–67). Some hooves will remodel in one or two shoeings. Other long-standing cases may never return to normal.

The treatment for a displaced coronet is similar to that for sheared heels. Below the site of the displacement (following the horn tubules to the ground surface), the hoof wall is sculpted out to parallel the bulge at the coronet (Fig. 6–68). This will allow the displaced portion of the hoof wall to descend to the shoe and the coronet to assume its normal position.

This reforming of the hoof is often facilitated (after trimming in the aforementioned manner) by leaving the shoes off of the affected hooves and keeping the horse in a stall with a base of damp sand or a deep layer of dampened coarse sawdust for several days. The hoof will reform (and deform) more readily with a greater moisture content, and this footing will support the entire ground surface of the hoof, allowing the hoof wall to settle down to a normal level. The hooves might also be encouraged in this remodeling by wrapping them with moist bandages and by periodically rasping the ground surface of the hoof at the site of displacement as it settles. For more information, refer to sheared heels and quarters, Chapter 5.

Cracks

Cracks are separations or breaks in the hoof wall. Vertical cracks between the tubules that compose the hoof horn are referred to by their location, such as toe cracks, quarter cracks, and heel cracks. Cracks that originate at the coronet are called *sand cracks* (Fig. 6–69), whereas those that start at the ground surface are called *grass cracks*.

A horizontal crack in the hoof wall is called a *blow-out* (Fig. 6–70). Blow-outs are caused either by an injury to the coronary band or by a blow to the hoof wall. A blow-out usually does not result in lameness and many times goes unnoticed until the farrier spots it. Once they occur, these cracks seldom increase in size horizontally and usually require no treatment. Because the hoof is weaker at this site, however, a blow-out can set the stage for a vertical crack if the hoof is weakened by excess moisture or is not in ML balance.

Cracks do not "heal" back together. The hoof wall must be replaced primarily by new growth from the coronary band just as a damaged fingernail must grow out. This will take from 9 to 12 months. For optimum hoof growth, it is essential that the ration contain nutrients necessary for healthy hoof horn (see Resource Guide).

Sand cracks can result from an injury to the coronet or from an infection in the white line ("gravel") that

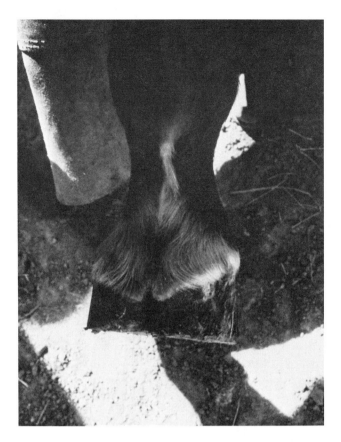

FIG. 6–66. Backview of a horse with sheared heels. Note the medial coronet of the heel and quarter region are higher than the lateral side. The medial hoof wall is also straighter than the lateral side.

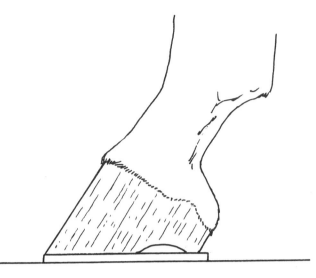

FIG. 6–68. Treating a displaced coronet. (From Hill, C., Klimesh, R.: Maximum Hoof Power. New York, Howell Book House, 1994.)

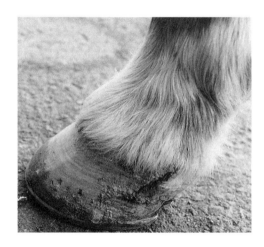

FIG. 6–69. Sand crack.

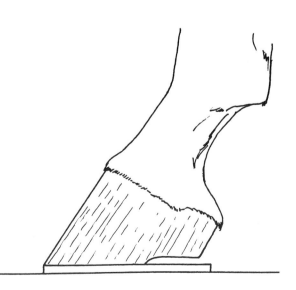

FIG. 6–67. Floating a heel. (From Hill, C., Klimesh, R.: Maximum Hoof Power. New York, Howell Book House, 1994.)

breaks out at the coronet. Sometimes a horse bumps the coronet when loading or unloading from a trailer, or the horse might strike the coronet during fast work or an uncoordinated movement.

A wet environment containing sand or gravel can soften a horse's hooves and allow particles to be forced up into the white line. If infection results, it can travel upward through the laminae and break out at the coronet, possibly causing a crack to form. Cracks often appear at the site of a displaced coronet (Fig. 6–71).

The first step in dealing with sand cracks is to determine the cause and remove it. This, accompanied by a good shoeing, may be all that is necessary to stabilize the hoof as it replaces the damaged horn. Severe cracks can be held immobile by a variety of methods until the hoof grows out. These have included nailing or screwing across the crack; drilling holes on either side and lacing the crack up like a boot; fastening a metal plate across the crack; and patching the crack

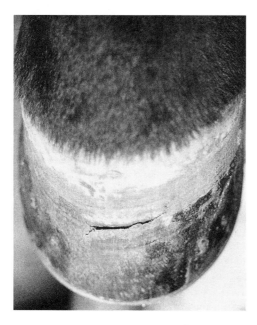

FIG. 6–70. Blow-out crack that has grown down from its initial site near the coronary band.

together with plastic, fiberglass, or other materials (Fig. 6–72).

Today the farrier and veterinarian can choose from several "high-tech" hoof repair materials developed specifically to bond to the hoof wall. Some of these materials mimic the consistency of the hoof wall so that once applied they can be nailed into, trimmed, and rasped along with the hoof wall as it grows down. The prosthetic materials can be used to fill the crack completely or to form a patch across the crack (see Resource Guide).

Before the crack can be stabilized, it must be thoroughly cleansed of dirt, loose hoof horn, and bacteria. If there is any evidence of moist tissue, the crack must be treated by a veterinarian until it is completely dry. Applying any type of patching material over a moist crack would seal in bacteria, providing the perfect environment for an infection to develop or escalate.

Chronic or severe cracks toward the heel of the hoof are sometimes dealt with by removing the section of the hoof wall behind the crack (Fig. 6–71). The hoof is then supported by a full-support shoe until new hoof grows down. A similar but less involved approach is to apply a full-support shoe and "float" the portion of the hoof behind the crack. Floating means to trim that portion of the hoof about $\frac{1}{4}$ inch shorter so that it will not contact the shoe (Fig. 6–71). By eliminating weight-bearing behind the crack, movement of the two halves of the crack is minimized, and the hoof often grows down intact. A horse that is very active or in work, however, is likely to need to have the crack more securely stabilized.

Grass cracks most often appear in unshod hooves that have been allowed to grow too long. Often all that is needed to control these cracks is a good trimming.

More severe cracks may require shoes for several months until new hoof tissue can grow down and replace the cracked horn. To help toe cracks grow out, the hoof angle must be kept up where it belongs and a square-toed shoe applied to minimize the prying effect of breakover.

Surface cracks are tiny fissures that cover varying portions of the hoof wall. They are most often caused by a change in hoof moisture, such as when a horse on wet pasture is put in a stall with dry bedding or when a horse that has been standing in mud then stands in the sun. Surface cracks are remedied by stabilizing the horse's moisture balance, minimizing his exposure to wetness, and using a hoof sealer. Thick hoof dressings may fill the cracks and improve the exterior appearance of a hoof, but a hoof sealer is more beneficial to long-term hoof health (see Resource Guide).

Bruises, Corns, and Abscesses

When the hoof is trimmed, the outer wall should be long enough so that it is the primary weight-bearing structure, not the sole. Pressure on the perimeter of the sole inside the white line can cause pain and can compress the blood vessels beneath the sole. If the wall is trimmed too short, if the sole is very flat, or if a barefoot horse has worn its hooves so short that the soles are flat or protruding below the hoof wall, the sole is likely to be bruised (Fig. 6–73). Horses in muddy pens, whether shod or barefoot, often bruise their soles when the temperature drops and the lumpy mud freezes hard.

Normally the healthy sole has a concave shape like a shallow bowl and is about $\frac{1}{4}$-inch thick on a saddle horse. A properly trimmed sole "gives" or has springiness only under *very heavy* thumb pressure. If the sole gives to *moderate* pressure, it may be too short to protect the inner structures adequately from bruising especially on rocky or frozen ground. A thin-soled horse may lack confidence of movement and be "off." Bruising may develop into an abscess, which can cause varying degrees of lameness. The abscess can even affect the coffin bone in some cases. If a thin sole is the result of recent trimming, the horse, even when shod, may be "ouchy" when walked over gravel or rough ground that contacts the sole. Usually in a week or two, the sole thickens enough for the horse to be comfortable.

Corns are bruises or abscesses that occur inside the buttress where the hoof wall curves to join the bars. This site is actually referred to as the *seat of corn*. Corns are usually caused by pressure from a horseshoe or from a stone wedged between the shoe and the hoof. When the hoof is trimmed, the seat of corn should be pared below the level of the hoof wall to prevent contact with the shoe. If a shoe is left on too long and the hoof overgrows the shoe, the heels often collapse, and pressure is put on the seat of corn resulting in a bruise or abscess. A corn can cause varying degrees of lame-

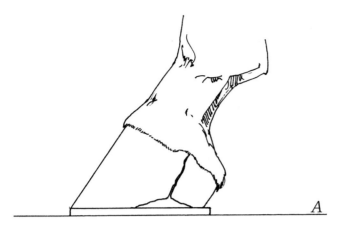

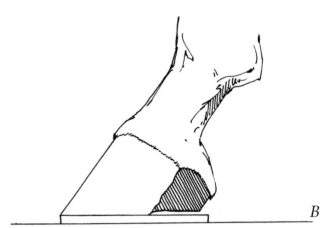

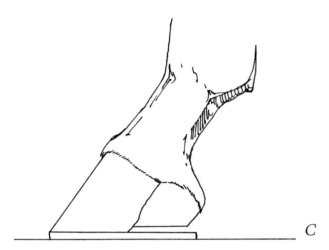

FIG. 6–71. Treating a crack. *A*, Relieving. *B*, Resecting. *C*, Floating. (From Hill, C., Klimesh, R.: Maximum Hoof Power. New York, Howell Book House, 1994.)

ness. Trimming to remove pressure on the corn may be all that is required. If the corn is infected, it is treated as an abscess.

Full pads are often used to protect a bruised sole while it heals. If a pad is applied over a sole bruise that is on the verge of abscess, however, it will tend to fester the abscess quickly. The horse may exhibit great pain a day or so after the pad has been applied necessitating the removal of the pad. Once the abscess has been treated by a veterinarian and has dried out, a pad can be reapplied, if necessary, for protection.

Hot Nail

A horseshoe nail driven into the hoof wall that puts pressure on the sensitive inner structures without actually piercing them is referred to as a close nail (Fig. 6–74). A close nail may cause the horse immediate discomfort or may go unnoticed for many days or until the horse is put into work. Usually the offending nail can be located by the use of a hoof tester or by judi-

cious tapping with a hammer at the location of each nail. Removal of the close nail often returns the horse to soundness because the sensitive structures have not been invaded.

A nail that is driven *into* the sensitive structures of the hoof is called a *hot nail*. A hot nail usually causes the horse to exhibit immediate pain unless the horse is under sedation. If the animal is normally fractious when being shod, the response to a hot nail may go unnoticed. On removing a hot nail, blood is likely to be seen in the nail hole and on the nail itself. The hole should be flushed with an antiseptic such as povidone-iodine (Betadine) and plugged to prevent contamination. A nail should not be placed in the hole. The horse should be current on tetanus vaccination and should be observed for several days for continuing or developing lameness.

If an abscess develops, a veterinarian should be contacted. Usually the shoe is removed, and the hoof is soaked in a hot water Epsom salt solution twice daily for 2 to 3 days. When the veterinarian determines that the infection has cleared, the shoe can be replaced.

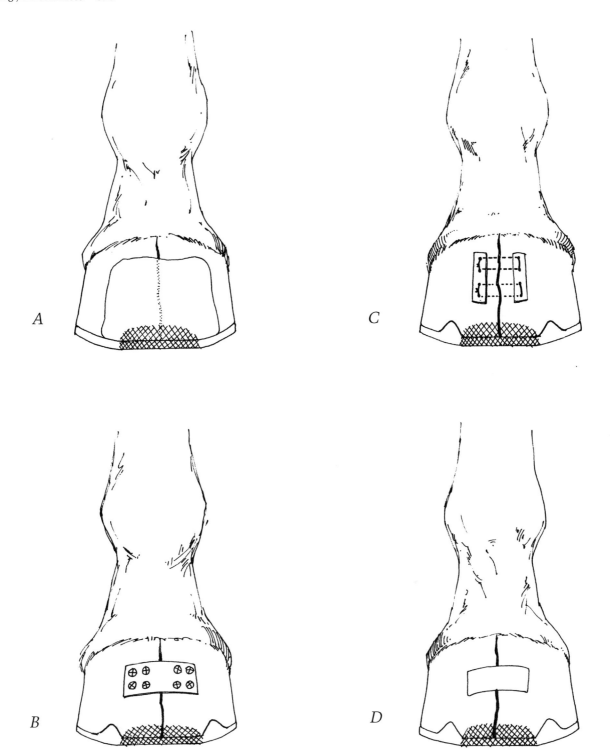

FIG. 6–72. Stabilizing a crack. *A*, Acrylic patch. *B*, Screwed-on plate. *C*, Laced patch. *D*, Glue-on patch. Cross-hatched areas indicate squared toe. (From Hill, C., Klimesh, R.: Maximum Hoof Power. New York, Howell House, 1994.)

Thrush

Thrush is caused by anaerobic bacteria that thrives in the warm, dark recesses of the hoof. The bacteria's foul-smelling black exudate is most commonly found in the clefts of the frog and if left untreated can invade sensitive tissues, especially deep in the central cleft, and cause lameness. Thrush also inhabits separations and cracks in the hoof wall, especially if the horse is in a moist environment. Cleanliness is the best prevention and the first step of any treatment program. Sugardine is effective for treating thrush: A thin paste is made from white sugar and Betadine scrub and spread on the cleaned areas daily until the problem is

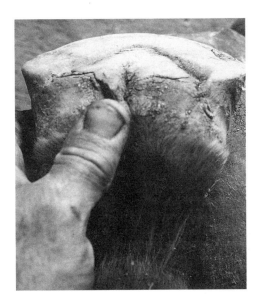

FIG. 6–73. Excess hoof wall wear resulting in sole pressure.

resolved. Commercial preparations for treating thrush are available and are effective in varying degrees. Severe cases of thrush can be treated with the CVP gasket pad (see section on pads later in this chapter).

White Line Disease

When an area of separation occurs in the hoof wall, it provides a moist, dark environment, ideal for the growth of horn-digesting organisms. Soil and manure may be forced up into the interlaminar space as the white line deteriorates. If left unchecked, this situation can progress to white line disease and result in lameness and much expense.

White line disease, sometimes incorrectly called seedy toe, is caused by invasion of the inner horn by bacteria, fungus, or yeast, which results in varying degrees of damage to the structural integrity of the hoof. There seems to be a greater occurrence of the condition in hot, humid climates.

The area of an affected hoof is characteristically filled with a white cheesy material and air pockets that are often packed with debris. The disease starts at ground level and, if not controlled, can work its way up to the coronary band.

An affected horse may show symptoms similar to those of laminitis: lameness, heat, sole tending to be flat, slow horn growth, tenderness when nailing, and pain over the sole when hoof testers are applied. There may be areas of the hoof wall that, when tapped, give a hollow sound. Depending on the extent of the damage, lameness can result from mechanical loss of horn support. In severe cases, the destruction of the laminae may allow a rotation of the coffin bone to occur.

Any separation in the white line should be considered a seed for white line disease. A separation is often found between the heel and the quarter in the white line. The cavity may be $\frac{1}{4}$ inch deep or extend halfway up the hoof wall. The space is usually filled with a white chalky substance or thrush's foul-smelling, tarlike residue. These heel caves can be treated by digging out as much of the decomposed horn as possible and packing the hole using the CVP method (see section on pads later in this chapter). If the hole is deep, the treatment materials may need to be layered. A shoe is applied to protect the packing and to prevent further contamination. The horse should be kept in a dry environment and the shoes reset regularly at which time the packing is replaced. The hoof deterioration can usually be prevented from spreading with this treatment and the hoof grows down solid. If the area of separation is large or extends for a distance along the white line, the aforementioned treatment is used in conjunction with the application of a CVP gasket pad. Treatment of severe cases of white line disease may involve a partial resection of the undermined hoof wall by a veterinarian.

Bowed Tendon

An inflammation of the flexor tendon (usually the superficial flexor tendon of the front limb) is called a bowed tendon. Flexor tendon strain is the main cause of bowed tendon. The strain can be brought about by poor hoof and limb conformation (long, weak pasterns), poor or irregular shoeing (lack of adequate support), muscle fatigue, heavy footing, a misstep, and work at speed.

Even if a hoof is trimmed to a proper hoof angle, if the shoe that is applied is too short and does not provide adequate tendon support, problems may result. As a hoof grows longer, the attached shoe migrates forward on the hoof so that the heels of the shoe end up farther forward than they started. If the shoe is fit flush with the heels at the start, in 6 weeks, the shoe will not even cover the hoof at the heels, let alone support it. If a horse is in heavy work, a good form of insurance against bowed tendons would be extended heels or egg bar shoes. For more information, refer to tendinitis, Chapter 4.

Arthritis

Arthritis is a general term for joint inflammation. The chain of events leading to arthritis can be complex and interrelated. The initial cause may be hard use, a fall, a blow to the joint, poor conformation, inadequate conditioning, or inadequate farrier care. Affected joints often show pain on flexion, and a decreased range of motion may be observed. Treatment aims at relieving pain and preventing further damage. In some cases, farrier adjustments are necessary to help alleviate arthritic pain. Balancing the hoof and removing traction devices are the most common ad-

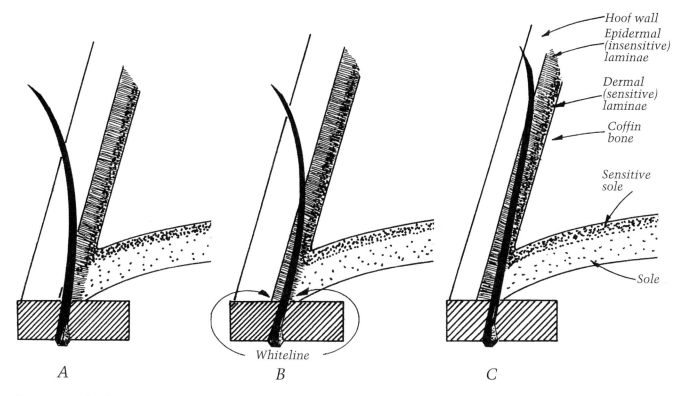

Labels on figure: Hoof wall; Epidermal (insensitive) laminae; Dermal (sensitive) laminae; Coffin bone; Sensitive sole; Sole; Whiteline

A *B* *C*

FIG. 6–74. Nail path. *A*, Good nail. *B*, Close nail. *C*, Hot nail. (From Hill, C., Klimesh, R.: Maximum Hoof Power. New York, Howell Book House, 1994.)

justments. Using a plain or wide web shoe will allow the horse to slide as it lands. Using a shock-absorbing pad may give the horse some relief. Horses with bone spavin may get relief from wedge heels or wedge pads with a squared or rocker toe shoe. See Chapter 4.

Coffin Bone Fracture

Horses turning at speed (barrel racing, roping, jumping) sometimes fracture a coffin bone (Fig. 6–75). Depending on the location and severity of the fracture, it is possible that treatment can restore the horse to its previous level of performance. The Klimesh Contiguous Clip Shoe may be helpful in this regard. The shoe effectively immobilizes the hoof capsule and the coffin bone inside. Depending on the configuration of the hoof and the management of the horse's environment, it may be necessary to use a full pad or a metal plate to prevent trauma to the coffin bone through the bottom of the hoof. See contiguous clip shoe later in this chapter. For more information on coffin bone fracture, refer to Chapter 5.

Laminitis

Laminitis results in an acute inflammation and damage of the basement membrane attachments be-

tween the dermal (sensitive) and epidermal (insensitive) laminae in the hoof that can be caused by a wide variety of factors, including overeating of grain or pasture, trauma, and foaling complications. The chronic form of the condition is often referred to as founder. It is likely that a number of horses experience mild laminitis and recover without it ever being recognized. Other horses that experience mild laminitis may or may not be diagnosed as such by the veterinarian and may recover and return to normal work with or without (or despite) treatment.

Horses that suffer significant hoof damage from laminitis, resulting in weeks or months of unsoundness, are unlikely ever to return to their previous level of performance. Some of these horses can become sound enough for light turn out. Mares so affected, however, may not be able to bear the additional weight of a pregnancy without refoundering.

Successful treatment of laminitis involves a cooperative effort from the horse owner, veterinarian, and farrier. Although an experienced veterinarian and farrier can set the stage for a horse's recovery, the owner's long-term commitment to the treatment program is of paramount importance. Dealing with laminitis can require emotional strength and a considerable investment of time and money. Besides initial emergency care, a horse suffering from severe laminitis will need frequent farrier attention and periodic veterinary care for a year or more. Most horses require daily treatment and specialized management and close supervision for life. Some horses, despite con-

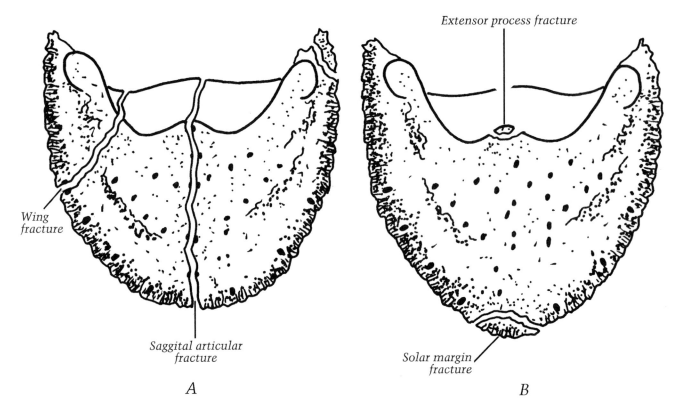

Extensor process fracture

Wing fracture

Saggital articular fracture

Solar margin fracture

A

B

FIG. 6–75. *A* and *B*, Types of coffin bone fractures.

scientious treatment and care, will fail to improve and may worsen. Because laminitis is the second leading cause (next to colic) of equine death, prevention is essential. The horse's weight should be monitored closely; the horse must not be able to get into the feed room; and the horses that are turned out on pasture must be carefully selected and monitored. For more information, refer to Chapter 5.

Clubfoot

A DP imbalance at the other end of the scale from LT-LH is the clubfoot, which is essentially a short toe–long heel. This type of imbalance may affect a hoof that has been non-weight-bearing for a period of time, because of an injury, for example. In this case, the clubfoot is usually temporary in nature and can be coached back to a normal shape by judicious trimming and proper exercise.

Another type of mild clubfoot is caused by excessive wear of the bare toe from pawing, toe dragging, or poor-quality hoof wall. This type of clubfoot can often be controlled by application of a half-shoe, also called a tip shoe. Usually made from the toe portion of a light shoe like a training plate, the half-shoe protects the toe of the hoof and leaves the heels bare to wear off in a normal fashion. The ends of the half shoe are tapered or set into the hoof so that there is not an abrupt step where the shoe makes the transition to the quarters

of the hoof. If the toe of the hoof is worn back, the toe of the half-shoe can be extended out to the normal point of breakover. A side benefit of the half-shoe is that it cannot be stepped off.

A more serious type of clubfoot is caused by a contraction of the flexor muscle-tendon unit that attaches to the coffin bone. This clubfoot may occur in one or both feet. It most commonly affects the fronts. The reasons for this contracture are not clearly understood, but as the muscle-tendon unit tightens, it pulls the heels of the hoof off the ground and they tend to grow long. The horse's weight is shifted on to the toe, which causes excessive wear and a dishing of the toe.

Trying to lower the heels of this type of clubfoot forcibly is rarely a good idea. In most cases, such an approach makes the clubfoot worse. It is better to support the heels by an elevated shoe or a shoe in conjunction with a wedge pad. If, when the horse is standing squarely, there is $\frac{1}{4}$ inch of space between the heels of the clubfoot and the ground, the amount of elevation should be $\frac{1}{2}$ inch or more. This procedure allows the heels to bear weight, takes some weight off the toe, and lessens the constant strain on the deep flexor muscle-tendon unit. Sometimes this breaks the contraction cycle, allowing the muscle to relax enough so that the hoof can be gradually lowered down over a period of weeks to a more normal angle. In other cases, the horse may never be able to have its heels lowered but may be comfortable and even usable with the elevated heels. Carpal check ligament desmotomy in conjunction with therapeutic shoeing can be rewarding in difficult cases.

Foals with mild to moderate clubfeet, if diagnosed and treated early, have a fair chance to perform unencumbered as adults. Advances in glue-on shoe technology allow corrective shoes to be applied to foals at a few weeks of age. Intravenous treatment with tetracyclines by the veterinarian may be used. It is difficult to predict, however, which foals will respond to treatment. Yearlings that have had extensive corrective trimming and shoeing to correct clubfeet may appear normal, but radiographs may show malformations of the coffin bone. Further treatment using carpal check ligament desmotomy and therapeutic trimming and shoeing may improve this situation and return the horse to performance. For more information regarding flexion deformities, see Chapter 4.

Mismatched Feet

Mismatched feet, or high-low syndrome, usually affects the front feet. One hoof tends toward LT–LH, and the other tends to be clubby. Some farriers report that more than half of the horses they shoe have mismatched feet to some degree.

One approach to dealing with the high-low syndrome is to lower the heels of the steep hoof and elevate the heels of the low hoof so hoof angles match. Where the initial difference between the feet is slight (less than 5°), this method usually works fine and does not affect the horse's performance.

If the difference in toe angles is 5° or greater, however, it is usually better not to force the hooves to be the same angle. Mismatched feet on a sound horse are more "balanced" than matching feet on a lame horse. This is why some farriers shun the use of a hoof gauge as a trimming guide. They believe that it is better to align the hoof and pastern of each foot visually and to evaluate the horse's movement when determining how to trim.

To attain dynamic balance and an even stride, it may be necessary to shoe a horse with two different shoes on the fronts. For example, a horse might wear a squared-toe egg bar on the low hoof and a thicker, full-toed plain shoe on the steep hoof. The egg bar provides support for the low heels and the squared toe helps speed breakover. The thicker shoe on the steep hoof makes up for the extra weight of the egg bar on the low hoof. The lower hoof seems to have more natural "action" anyway, and the steep hoof may need an even heavier shoe to balance the movement. This symmetry of limb movement is more important for horses that are being judged in the ring on the correctness of their gaits. With most horses, however, it is sufficient to concentrate on shoeing to provide necessary support.

When trimming mismatched feet, it is easy to trim the steep hoof too short. For this reason, it is best to trim the low hoof first and then the steep hoof only enough to match the toe lengths. One method of evaluating relative toe lengths is to stand the horse on a flat level surface and view the knees from the front. The bumps on the insides of the knees should usually be the same level. If necessary, a rim pad or wedge pad can be used to elevate the low hoof.

Lost Shoes

Lost shoes are a cause of hoof wall deterioration, either by a sudden loss of hoof wall at the time the shoe is lost or by wear and breaking of the now bare hoof resulting in loss of DP or ML balance. If a horse loses a shoe soon after he is shod, it is likely to be due to the horse stepping on the shoe or getting it caught on something. If a horse loses a shoe later in the shoeing period, it may be due to the wear on the nails or the shoe, which causes looseness. Eighty to 90% of lost shoes are front shoes.

Causes. Lost shoes are due to a variety of hoof-related factors as well as to a horse's overall conformation and way of going, poor riding, and poor management. Not all horses lose shoes. In a study that spanned a 3-year period, one farrier documented that 80% of all lost shoes were attributed to 20% of the horses. Certain horses in that 20% group lost most of the shoes. One client's gelding lost more shoes in 1 year than another client's four horses together lost in more than 10 years. The average shoe loss in this study was 1.33 shoes per horse per year.

Wet Environment. Excessive moisture is a major cause of lost shoes; soft hooves do not hold nails securely. Besides disrupting the moisture balance of the hoof, mud is thought to remove shoes mechanically. Although it is unlikely that mud can actually suck a shoe off, deep mud can interfere with a horse's timing and balance. The mud might slow down one limb, and another one comes unstuck suddenly and lands haphazardly and plucks off a shoe. (*Note*: Other heavy or deep footing, such as sand, snow, or even long grass, can also alter limb movement and result in lost shoes.)

Hoof and Limb Conformation. A horse with an exaggerated angle to its front pasterns, especially one with his limbs set ahead of his body and underrun heels, requires front shoes placed so far back on the hoof (for flexor tendon support) that the shoe could easily be stepped on. Underrun heels, those that angle forward rather than more nearly vertical, can develop in a matter of months by leaving shoes on too long or by using a shoe that is too short. Underrun heels are difficult, if not impossible, to correct; aggressive treatment includes using a shoe with a generous base of support at the heels, which can easily be stepped on. To minimize repeated lost shoes, however, the heel support may be compromised temporarily, but this means that the underrun heel condition has less chance of correcting itself.

The base-narrow, toed-out horse may step off a front shoe with the other front foot. Also, horses can inherit or develop poor-quality hooves. Thin hoof walls and shelly horn make lost shoes much more likely.

Leaving Shoes on Too Long. This is a common cause of lost shoes. When a shoe is left on too long, the hoof overgrows the shoe at the heels and quarters. The small amount of hoof wall left to support the horse's weight often collapses, and the shoe is forced up into the hoof, frequently becoming imbedded in the sole. This deforming of the hoof wall is a cause of underrun heels. The nails are then too long and the loose clinches work on the nail holes making them larger. The loose nails then get sheared off or the shoe rotates on the hoof and gets stepped off. When a shoe is left on too long, the hoof grows out of balance (LT-LH), which can result in a delayed breakover and lost shoes as a result of overreaching.

Good Shoeing. One of the ironies of lost shoes is that the better a horse is shod, the greater the chances might be for the horse to lose a shoe. A farrier's first priority can be to keep a shoe on at all costs, or it can be to shoe the horse for balance, support, and long-term soundness. It is erroneous to think that a good shoeing job consists of a close fit around the entire edge of the hoof with little heel showing and eight heavy nails with long clinches holding the shoe on securely. A shoe that is fit full and fit to support a horse properly has more steel exposed at the quarters and heels, which may be more likely to be stepped on, especially if the horse is not moving properly.

If a horse steps on his shoe or gets it caught in wire, it is better for the shoe to come off cleanly than for the horse to damage his hoof or limb structures because the shoe was on too securely. Therefore, the nails used should be high-quality slim nails with thin shanks. The clinches should be relatively small, about $\frac{1}{8}$ inch square, and smooth, so when a shoe does get caught, the clinches open up easily and slide cleanly through the nail holes in the hoof wall, not taking chunks of hoof wall with them.

If the horse is of the larger breeds or is involved in a sport requiring quick stops or turns, clips can be added to the shoe to reduce shearing force on the nails. If the hoof is soft or weak, clips will help secure the shoe and prevent the nails from breaking out the hoof wall.

Shoes with eight nails and long clinches resist the forces of the struggling horse. The long clinches do not open up easily and can pull large hunks of hoof wall away with them when the horse finally does wrench the shoe off. This not only results in extensive hoof damage, but it may also result in a sprain damage.

Miscellaneous Causes. Miscellaneous causes include alteration in stride owing to the use of traction devices and unusual one-time circumstances, such as the horse who takes a misstep in his pen or stall, the horse who steps on himself while backing out of a trailer, or the horse that steps off another horse's shoe. In certain circumstances, such as with long-distance horses, new shoes and nails wear out and come off before the hoof is ready to be trimmed.

First Aid for a Lost Shoe. Even if a hoof has not been damaged by the act of losing a shoe, the hoof can quickly be chipped or bruised if it is not protected. When a horse has lost a shoe, the hoof should be cleaned thoroughly and either a protective boot or tape should be applied. The horse should be kept in a clean, dry stall until the shoe is replaced. It is a good idea for trail riders to carry a rubber boot on rides. If a hoof is damaged, it can be repaired with prosthetic materials or glue-on shoes until new hoof grows down to replace it.

Spooned-heel shoes on the front hoofs can be helpful for pawing horses and chronic overreachers (Fig. 6–76). The front shoe heels are bent toward the vertical until they almost contact the heel buttresses about midway between the bulb and the ground surface. Great care must be taken in fitting the shoes because the shoe is pulled forward as the hoof grows longer. The spooned heels can cause damage to the heel bulbs if fitted too close.

On horses that need a lot of heel support and tend to overreach, heel shields can be welded around the edge of the shoe heels. These shields prevent the hind shoe from grabbing the edge of the front shoe heel and pulling it off. Again, care must be taken in fitting these shoes so that the normal migration of the shoe forward does not cause the heel shields to contact the heel bulbs.

Horse owners should perform a daily inspection that includes picking out a horse's feet. It is important to recognize normal hoof smell, texture, and sensitivity so that abnormalities can be detected. An owner should be capable of recognizing a bent shoe, a loose clinch, an overgrown hoof wall. All shod horses should be reset on a regular schedule regardless of whether the horse is ridden.

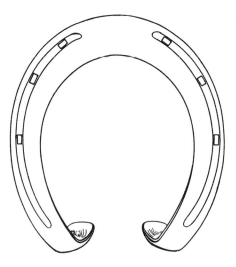

FIG. 6–76. Ground-surface view of spoon shoe. The spoons extend upward and cover the heels of the foot preventing the horse from pulling a shoe if it overreaches.

Stress and Strain Owing to Improper Traction

Sliding plates on reining horses and wide web shoes sometimes provide *inadequate* traction. The result can be strained tendons or sprained ligaments. Traction devices such as toe grabs, heel calks, and borium sometimes provide *too much* traction. The resulting excess torque can lead to strain or sprain and may contribute to a fracture. For more information, see traction later in this chapter.

Limb Deformities

Incorrect "corrective" trimming of young horses can be responsible for acquired limb deformities and resultant lamenesses and gait defects. See foal hoof management later in this chapter.

Corrective and Therapeutic Trimming and Shoeing Techniques

Corrective trimming and shoeing alter the hoof to affect stance or stride including breakover. *Therapeutic* shoeing is an important part of some lameness treatments. Corrective and therapeutic shoeing techniques aim to restore DP balance, ML balance, shape, and hoof integrity as well as provide additional support, protection, and traction, if necessary. In addition, corrective shoeing techniques can sometimes be helpful in resolving movement abnormalities (Fig. 6–77).

The implementation of corrective and therapeutic shoeing techniques should be a team effort between an experienced, skilled farrier, a competent equine veterinarian, and a responsible horse owner.

To Attain Dorsal-Palmar Balance

The most common DP imbalance is LT-LH often accompanied by underrun heels. In trimming a hoof with low heels, the toe of the hoof wall is trimmed as short as is practical, tapering off toward the quarters. The heels are taken down only enough to get a good bearing surface of healthy horn, and this can often be accomplished more precisely with the rasp alone, minimizing the risk of trimming them too much. Trimming underrun heels extends the base of support of the hoof rearward; leaving underrun heels long in an attempt to align the hoof pastern angle only forces the heels to grow further forward underneath the limb (see Fig. 6–48).

Horses that have low heels and a broken back hoof-pastern axis often benefit from the application of *wedge-heel shoes* or *wedge pads* (degree pads) applied between the hoof and a flat shoe. Wedge-heel shoes are thicker in the heel than in the toe (see Figs. 6–64 and 6–44). Wedge pads are thick on one end and taper to very thin at the other end (Fig. 6–78). Depending on how much the heels of the hoof need to be elevated, the farrier can use a single wedge pad of the appropriate thickness or a stack of several.

Wedge pads not only can realign hoof-pastern angles, but also can prevent direct pressure on the navicular region. The thicker wedge pads are often stiff enough across the heels to protect the frog and thus the navicular region from direct ground pressure, provided that there is no undue pressure on the frog from its excess length or from improper hoof packing. Wedge pads are available as full coverage pads or as bar pads, which have an open center thus permitting the sole to respire normally. The open center, however, collects debris that can be difficult to clean out. Horses with bone spavin (arthritis of the distal tarsal joints) may get some relief from wedge heels or wedge pads with a squared or rocker toe shoe.

A less common DP imbalance is that of a short toe/long heel. It is important to determine the cause of the long heel before attempting to lower the hoof to align with the pastern. Damage to the hoof or limb structures can be caused by trimming the heels too much and trying to force the heels down. Short toe/long heel often occurs to a hoof that has been non-weight-bearing for a period of time because of an injury to the limb or can be a result of a flexural deformity (contracted muscle-tendon unit) associated with the deep digital flexor tendon. To prevent the overly long heel horn from deforming, it is helpful to trim the heels down to as near normal length as practical and then elevate the heels using wedge pads or an elevated heel shoe to allow the hoof to bear weight evenly. Although this trimming and shoeing procedure is helpful, the underlying cause must be addressed for a satisfactory outcome. Desmotomy of the carpal check ligament may be required in some cases.

A half-shoe is often used for a short toe–long heel condition that results from toe dragging, pawing, or other causes of excessive toe wear. This shoe can be made from the front half of a training plate that covers the toe and leaves the heels bare. The ends of the half-shoe are tapered or set into the hoof so that there is not an abrupt step where the shoe makes the transition to the heels of the hoof. This shoe protects the toe of the hoof while allowing the heels of the hoof to wear down as they grow.

The half-shoe is often useful in treating mild cases of clubfoot. In this application, the toe of the shoe is extended past the toe of the hoof from $\frac{1}{4}$ to $\frac{1}{2}$ inch to retard breakover and stretch the deep digital flexor muscle-tendon unit.

To Restore Hoof Shape

The flare should be dressed off and that side of the wall should be shortened (lowered). The quarter where the flare was located should be sculpted out with the

SHOEING PRESCRIPTION FORM (FIG. 6–77)

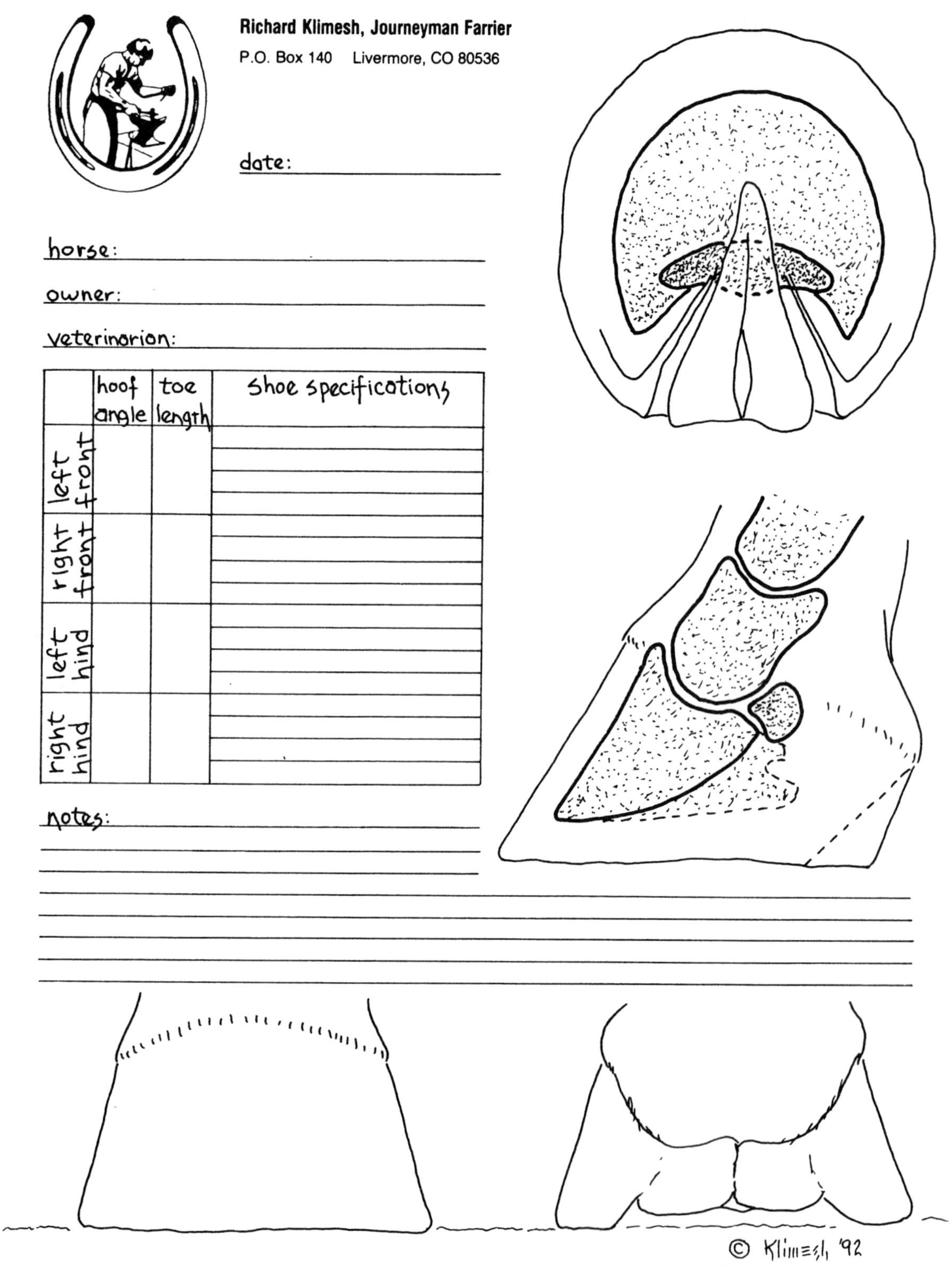

Richard Klimesh, Journeyman Farrier
P.O. Box 140   Livermore, CO 80536

date: _____

horse: _____

owner: _____

veterinarian: _____

	hoof angle	toe length	shoe specifications
left front			
right front			
left hind			
right hind			

notes: _____

© Klimesh '92

FIG. 6–77. Shoeing prescription form.

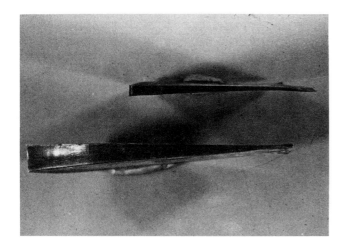

FIG. 6–78. Plastic wedge pads.

rasp so that the hoof at that area bears no weight. This removes the bending forces on the horn tubules and will result in the new hoof horn growing down straighter.

Many horses have "pancake" hooves that tend to spread out and become flat. The treatment for these hooves includes stabilizing their moisture content by keeping them in a dry environment and applying a hoof sealer to minimize the absorption of external moisture. The flares should be dressed off to about half the thickness of the hoof wall and a shoe applied with side clips located across the widest part of the flared hoof (Fig. 6–79). (The shoe should be a bar shoe or an open shoe that is strong enough to withstand the spreading forces of the hoof.) The straighter the hoof wall becomes, the stronger it is. Once the shape of the hoof is restored and the moisture content stabilized, the hoof can often be shod with a regular shoe with no clips.

Often the hoof is not flared symmetrically but distorted across the diagonal of the hoof base, such as a medial toe flare with a lateral heel flare. Along with this, the opposing points (the medial heel and lateral toe) are pulled inward. Trimming the hoof into balance may prevent further distortion of the hoof, but a shoe is usually required to reform the hoof to a more functional symmetric shape. The shoe is applied with clips across the longest diagonal. These clips contain the hoof as it grows down, encouraging expansion across the narrow diagonal, and the result is a more symmetric hoof.

A flare at the front of the hoof wall is called a dish. Most hooves dish to some degree, and as part of the regular trimming process this dish should be dressed so that the hoof wall at the toe is straight from the coronet to the ground. If this is not done, the dish will cause the breakover point of the hoof and the entire base of support to be too far forward. The presence of any dish can easily be seen by laying a straight edge such as a rasp against the hoof wall (see Fig. 6–18).

A dished toe is sometimes the result of a contraction of the muscle-tendon unit at the back of the limb. This contraction exerts constant pull on the coffin bone within the hoof capsule, which causes the hoof wall to bend away from the coffin bone and result in a dish. The treatment is to elevate the angle of the hoof by trimming or by using a wedge pad or shoe. This often lessens the pull on the coffin bone enough to allow the muscle-tendon unit to relax. Then the hoof may be lowered over several trimming periods back to its normal angle. In some cases, a carpal check ligament desmotomy may correct the problem if it persists.

A clubfoot or even just a normally steep hoof might develop a dish if the heels are lowered too much in an attempt to "balance" the foot. These types of hooves are better maintained at a relatively steep angle of 60 to 65°.

As with flares, an increase in hoof moisture allows the hoof wall to dish more easily, so it is best to keep the hooves dry, using a hoof sealer if necessary.

To Provide Additional Support

Extended Heel Shoes

Extended heel shoes are used to lengthen the base of support for the limb. In a properly trimmed hoof, the length of the support base (shoe) should be at least twice the toe length (see Fig. 6–49). In an ideally conformed hoof, the amount of shoe extended past the heel of the hoof is from $\frac{1}{8}$ to $\frac{1}{4}$ inch, enough to allow for the normal forward migration of the shoe over the 5- to 8-week shoeing period. Hooves with varying degrees of underrun heels require more length of shoe to achieve the necessary support.

The shape of extended heel shoes when applied to the front feet usually follows the shape of an egg bar shoe, and in fact, they are called "open egg bars." On the hindfeet, the extended heels can be bent straight back to form a true extended heel shoe or bent out 45° to form bilateral trailers (Fig. 6–80). Bilateral trailers widen as well as lengthen the support base adding stability to the limb. Also, with the shoe heels bent outward (Fig. 6–81), the clefts of the frog clean easier than with an open egg bar shoe, but unfortunately these shoes further prevent the natural rotation that occurs during the impact phase of the stride. The danger of using these shoes on the front is that the trailers are likely to be stepped on. Generally, extended heel shoes are an excellent support shoe and performance enhancer when used on the hindfeet of horses engaged in strenuous athletic activities such as dressage and jumping.

Egg Bar Shoe

A shoe with extended branches that curve inward and connect to each other at the heels is an egg bar

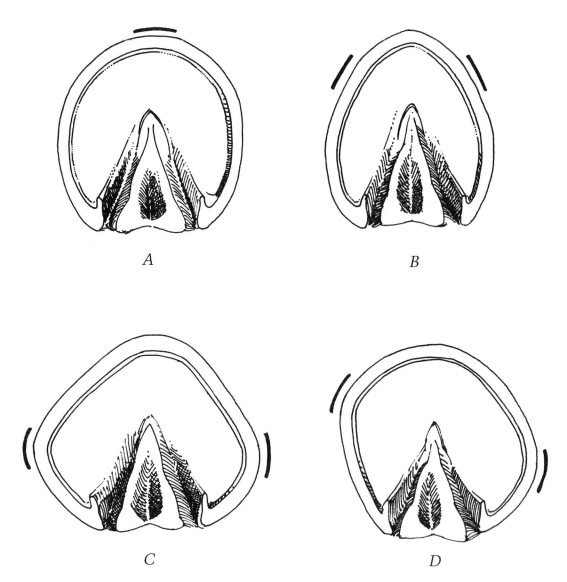

A

B

C

D

Fig. 6–79. Clip positions. *A*, Toe clip. *B*, Forward-placed side clip. *C*, Rearward-placed side clip. *D*, Asymmetric side clips. (From Hill, C., Klimesh, R.: Maximum Hoof Power. New York, Howell Book House, 1994.)

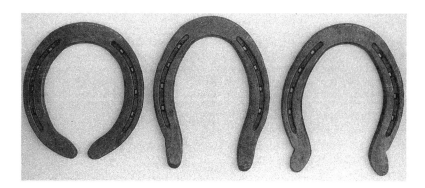

Fig. 6–80. *From left*: open egg bar, extended heels, bilateral trailers.

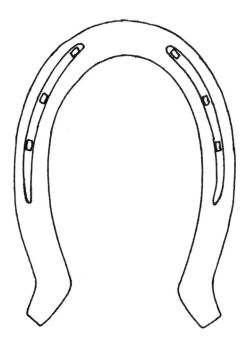

FIG. 6–81. Shoe with trailers.

(Fig. 6–82). Egg bar shoes provide a large, stable base that extends behind the heels. This longer base supports the heels in soft footing, prevents the hoof from rocking back, and takes some stress off the deep digital flexor tendon and the navicular region.

Egg bar shoes can often interrupt the undesirable cycle leading to contracted heels; collapsed, underrun heels; and flat soles. A flat-soled hoof is a "dead hoof," one that lands with a thud; it is not conformed to transmit resilient energy. Such a hoof shod with an egg bar shoe may, over time, begin to develop a more cupped (concave) sole, a desirable configuration that encourages a trampoline-like contraction and expansion resulting in the hoof springing off the ground.

By virtue of the shape of the bar and the extra amount of material in an egg bar shoe, the horse's weight is spread out over a larger area of ground than with a conventional shoe. An egg bar shoe instantly gives a horse a larger base of support. This is particularly important for horses that have a disproportionate relationship between their body weight and the circumference of their hooves (heavy horses, small hooves).

The egg bar shoe is especially beneficial for the Thoroughbred-type hoof with heels that have collapsed forward and inward resulting in an underrun hoof, often with a flat sole. It is equally helpful for the Warmblood-type hoof that often is flared outward on the sides with heels collapsed forward. When factors cause the tubules to begin angling forward, the hoof can quickly get caught in a self-perpetuating chronic condition that is often irreversible.

The weight of a horse with underrun heels or a long toe–low heel axis is concentrated at the back of the hoof or even *behind* the hoof causing excess tendon stress. In soft or deep footing, the larger ground surface of an egg bar "catches" the horse's weight as it descends down the limb, thereby reducing the strain on the deep flexor tendon and relieving some of the tension on the navicular region and the coffin joint. The egg bar extends the base of support and effectively redirects the horse's weight forward toward the center of the hoof. This contributes to the development of a more desirable, upright hoof/pastern axis.

Because the bar of an egg bar is located behind the frog, the heel bulbs are protected. The egg bar shoe not only prevents the heels from sinking down into soft footings, but also protects the bulbs from the destructive trauma of striking the ground.

The hoof must be trimmed properly before an egg bar shoe is applied. If the toe is left long, it will impede breakover and defeat the purpose of the shoe. Modifying the toe of the shoe can ease breakover. The egg bar shoe should be fitted wide from the broadest part of the foot toward the rear. The length of the egg bar shoe depends on the configuration of the hoof. It may be so short as to resemble a straight bar shoe, or it may extend to the back of the heel bulbs forming a true egg shape.

Because the egg bar shoe consists of more material than a standard shoe, the action of the horse may be affected by the additional weight. The hoof may reach a higher arc in its flight, and the knees and hocks may exhibit a greater degree of flexion. During extension, the slight increase in weight at the end of the limb may result in a slight exaggeration of the horse "throwing the foot forward." If this is the case and the action is undesirable, an aluminum egg bar is appropriate.

Depending on the circumstances, the horse wearing bar shoes may require different management. A bar shoe tends to collect and retain bedding, mud, or manure, so the hooves must be cleaned regularly. Horses wearing egg bars should not be turned out in deep or muddy footing.

The egg bar shoe is used in a wide variety of therapeutic applications ranging from sheared heels to chronic suspensory problems. Egg bar shoes are also used on performing show jumper, hunter, dressage, cutting, reining, pleasure, and trail horses. In addition to increasing the useful life of a horse, the egg bar shoe encourages the development of a more correct, functionally sound hoof. Recognition of the value of egg bar shoes has prompted several manufacturers to add both steel and aluminum egg bar shoes to their product lines.

Full-Support Shoes

A full-support shoe is an egg bar shoe with a frog support plate (Fig. 6–83). It is often called a heart bar/egg bar, although this is technically not correct. The plate of the full-support shoe contacts a large portion of the frog, whereas the tip of a true heart bar may

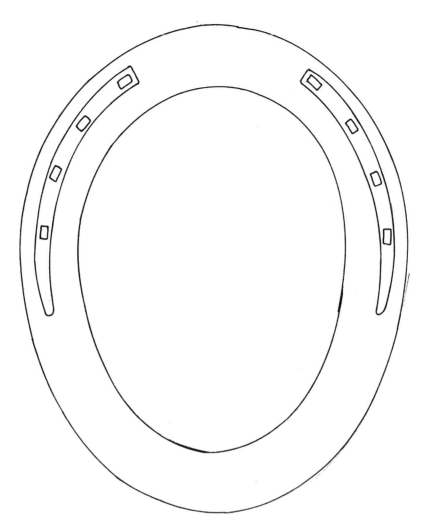

FIG. 6–82. Egg bar shoe. (From Hill, C., Klimesh, R.: Maximum Hoof Power. New York, Howell Book House, 1994.)

only contact a small area of the frog (the size of a dime). Full-support shoes are available commercially or can be made by a qualified farrier. The full-support shoe is used to treat hooves with flat or dropped soles and hooves with weak or underrun heels. A portion of the horse's weight is carried by the frog plate, allowing the heels of the hoof to grow down without being crushed.

This shoe is also useful in the treatment of hooves that have had a portion of the hoof wall removed (as in a heel resection for a crack) or injured (as in a heel avulsion). Contrasted to an egg bar shoe, which is used to support a hoof that has had the heel "floated" to allow a displaced heel to descend to the shoe, the full-support shoe is used when it is desirable to stabilize the hoof capsule while the hoof grows new horn.

A heel resection exposes a portion of the full-support (or egg bar) shoe, and the risk of the horse stepping it off is increased. To prevent the hindfoot from stepping off a front shoe, heel shields or wide clips can be welded around the exposed portion of the front shoe.

A full-support shoe is fitted in the same manner as the egg bar shoe described previously. The frog plate should follow the shape of the frog and support it completely from $\frac{1}{2}$ inch back from the tip of the trimmed frog. When the shoe is set on the prepared hoof, the frog plate should just contact the frog. The frog support plate should not extend beyond the boundaries of the frog, or circulation within the hoof might be impaired. If the frog is recessed below the level of the hoof wall, shims of the appropriate size and shape can be attached to the frog plate to achieve contact.

The configuration of the full-support shoe makes it difficult to keep the sole clean, especially if the horse is in mud, gravel, or dirty bedding. If the hoof wall is of poor quality or the horse is in undesirable footing, a full pad may need to be used with the full-support shoe.

In lieu of a full-support shoe, a full-support pad can be used. This type of pad is available commercially or can be fabricated by an experienced farrier. It might be difficult to fit the pad properly to the frog, however,

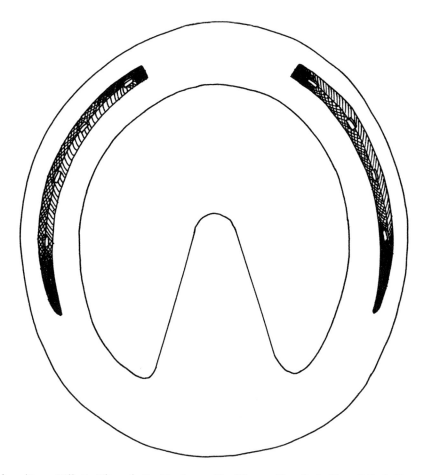

FIG. 6–83. Full-support shoe. (From Hill, C., Klimesh, R.: Maximum Hoof Power. New York, Howell Book House, 1994.)

because the opaque pad surface prevents direct observation of frog contact. To function properly, the ground surface of the pad must be supported beneath the frog either by a frog plate on the shoe or by the addition of a frog-shaped shim (the thickness of the shoe) on the pad itself (Fig. 6–84).

Heart Bar Shoe

This shoe is basically a straight bar shoe with a specialized frog plate (Fig. 6–85). In laminitis cases, the heart bar shoe is used to support the coffin bone via the frog. The rigid heart bar is welded in place and applies a fixed amount of support (see focal versus diffuse later). The adjustable heart bar uses a screw to vary the amount of support provided to the frog. Both types can be used with a full pad if a frog-shaped shim is fixed to the hoof surface of the pad to transfer the support to the frog and to prevent any pressure from being applied to the sole. The location of the tip of support is approximately $\frac{3}{8}$ inch back from the apex of the trimmed frog. Ideally the location is determined from x-ray films by measuring the length of the coffin bone and coming back from the tip of the coffin bone 33% of its length.

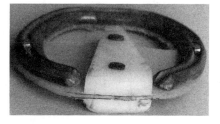

FIG. 6–84. Frog support pad.

There is some debate as to whether the entire frog plate should contact the frog (diffuse support) or just an area at the tip of the plate the size of a dime (focal support). Successes and failures have occurred with both methods. The focal support method requires extremely accurate measurement and placement of the heart bar tip as well as optimum amount of support (pressure). This in not an easy shoe to build and apply correctly and can be misapplied. The diffuse support method is more forgiving in that the amount of support pressure is less critical.

In some laminitis cases, it is necessary to remove portions of the hoof wall, usually at the toe, but sometimes at one or both quarters as well. This resection

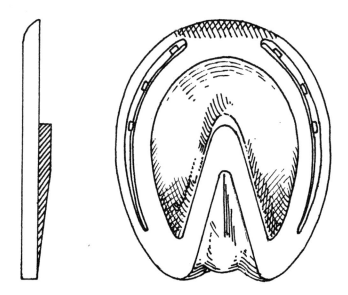

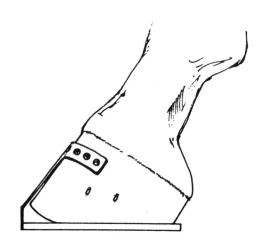

FIG. 6–85. Heart bar shoe.

relieves pressure between the hoof wall and the coffin bone, allows the coffin bone to be reoriented with the hoof capsule, and removes the dead tissue (laminar wedge) that impedes the proper growth of new hoof tissue. If resection is confined to the toe, there is usually sufficient hoof wall remaining to support the attachment of a heart bar shoe by nails or glue. Side clips are often placed just behind the resected area to prevent the weakened wall from spreading and to help secure the shoe to the hoof.

If the hoof wall is too weak or shelly to attach nails and glue-on shoes are not available, the shoe can be secured by using one or more T-bars or goosenecks (Fig. 6–86). The base of the T-bar is welded to the edge of the shoe, and the cross bar is attached to solid horn high up on the hoof wall. When the exposed laminae have dried and cornified sufficiently, a prosthetic hoof material can be used to rebuild the hoof to its normal shape. A shoe can then be attached to the rebuilt hoof by glue or nails.

Other Bar Shoes

A bar can be placed anywhere across the branches of the shoe to protect the hoof from ground contact and trauma. A *straight bar* connects the heels of the shoe and protects the frog (Fig. 6–87). If the frog is prominent or the heels low, the bar can be set away from the frog and is called a *drop bar*. A *cross bar* can go diagonally across the shoe or straight across to protect the sole or the navicular region of the frog. The *V bar* shoe (Fig. 6–88) extends from the heels over the frog to connect to the toe of the shoe. It can be used in conjunction with a frog support pad for a laminitic hoof to protect the tender sole area just ahead of the frog. A wide bar bisecting a *straight bar* shoe is used for the same purpose and is called a *phi bar*. It is im-

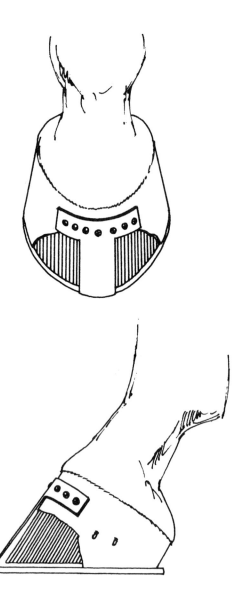

FIG. 6–86. Gooseneck.

portant that, if a pad is used, it is riveted to the central bar in front of the frog to hold the pad away from the sole.

It is imperative that a bar that crosses the hoof does not contact the sole at any point because it could impair circulation within the foot or cause bruises and abscesses. When using a bar to protect the hoof, it is important to keep debris (e.g., bedding, manure, rocks, dirt) from accumulating because this puts pressure on the hoof during weight-bearing and defeats the purpose of the bar. A full pad with careful attention to amount of packing may be helpful (see pads later).

A therapeutic bar shoe that is used to elevate the heel of the hoof significantly is called a Patten shoe (Fig. 6–89). The Patten shoe is used on a convalescing horse in the treatment of lacerated flexor tendons and contractions of the flexor muscle-tendon unit. This shoe can be forged from one piece of steel or fabricated from a standard shoe with the addition of the heel elevation bar either by bolts or by welding. Many variations of this shoe are in use, some of which can be adjusted for elevation while on the horse, but most have to be removed, adjusted, and reset onto the hoof.

Contiguous Clip Shoe

The Klimesh Contiguous Clip Shoe (Fig. 6–90) can be used in treating fractures of the coffin bone. The shoe is made by first fitting a straight bar or egg bar shoe (depending on the hoof configuration) to the trimmed hoof. The shoe should have a deep crease for the nail heads, such as a rim shoe, to facilitate removal of the nails individually at time of reset. It may be advisable to use a rocker or squared toe to minimize the pull of the deep digital flexor tendon on the coffin bone during breakover. The shoe is fit close around the entire perimeter of the hoof wall with no allowance for normal expansion.

A series of tall clips (16-gauge uncoated steel) are welded around the outer perimeter of the shoe. The shoe is nailed to the hoof using four nails, and the clips are bent in with a hammer to within $\frac{1}{16}$ inch of touching the hoof wall.

A hard-setting acrylic (see Resource Guide) is then applied between the clips and the hoof wall. This effectively immobilizes the hoof capsule and the coffin bone inside. Depending on the configuration of the hoof and the management of the horse's environment, it may be advisable to use a full pad or a treatment plate to prevent trauma to the coffin bone through the bottom of the hoof.

The shoe can be easily removed by pulling the four nails with a crease nail puller and gently prying the clips away from the hoof wall with a clinch cutter. The hoof capsule usually has contracted to some degree during the 6-week shoeing period, which facilitates removal of the shoe. At time of reset, the bar of the shoe

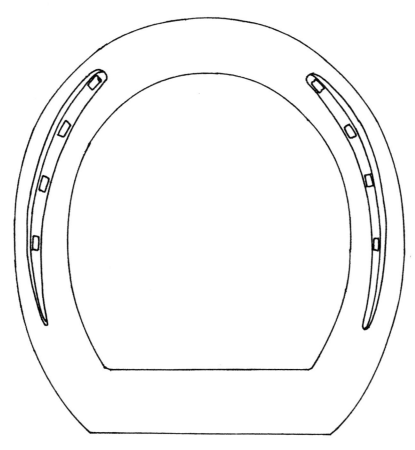

FIG. 6–87. Straight bar shoe. (From Hill, C., Klimesh, R.: Maximum Hoof Power. New York, Howell Book House, 1994.)

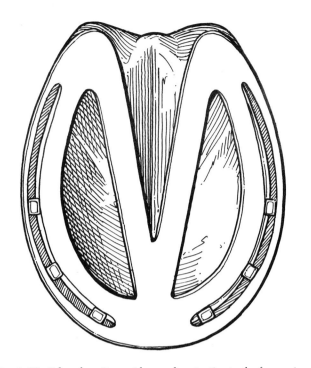

FIG. 6–88. V-bar shoe. It provides good protection to the frog region.

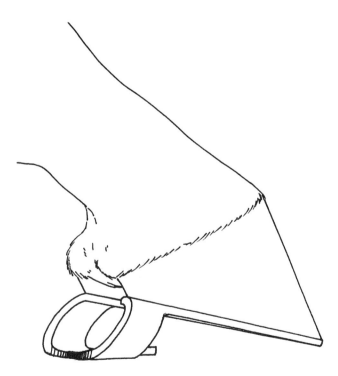

FIG. 6–89. Patten shoe.

may need to be cut and rewelded to accommodate the smaller size of the hoof. When lameness is no longer evident and the x-ray films show satisfactory healing, the hoof can be shod with a bar shoe and two side clips to stabilize the hoof and prevent refracture.

To Provide Protection

Pads

There are four main reasons to use hoof pads: to protect the sole, to reduce concussion, to change the angle of the hoof, and to prevent snowballing. Wedge pads were discussed in the section on balance. The other three functions of pads all relate to protection.

A full pad is a protective material covering the entire bottom of the horse's foot and is installed between the hoof and the shoe with or without hoof packing. Full pads may be made of leather, plastic, and other synthetic materials. Side clips are often used with pads to help maintain the position of the pad and shoe on the hoof and to decrease the stress on the nails.

Horses that have flat or thin soles may benefit from wearing full pads. Even horses that have a normally concave sole, if worked regularly on gravel or rocky terrain, may require full pads to prevent bruising.

Hoof Packing

Opinions differ on whether to pack the space between the pad and the hoof and what materials to use for packing. Although tradition calls for pine tar with oakum, using it has drawbacks. Oakum is a loose, stringy hemp fiber that retains water, breaks down over time, and shifts beneath the pad, often working out between the heels. Another option is silicone, which is either squirted into the sole space from a caulking gun after the shoe and pad are in place or mixed with a catalyst to speed curing and applied to the sole before the shoe and pad are nailed on. There are several drawbacks, however, to using silicone. It tends to concentrate moisture and heat against the sole, and if too large an amount is used, it puts pressure on the sole and prevents the sole from descending as part of its normal shock-absorbing function. Also, silicone allows sand and mud to accumulate between the pad and the sole, causing sole pressure.

Commercial hoof packing preparations are available that can be used with varying degrees of success (see Resource Guide).

CVP Method

A healthy alternative for packing is the Klimesh CVP Gasket Pad. CVP stands for the three main ingredients: copper sulfate powder, venice turpentine, and polypropylene (poly) hoof felt. Poly felt, which does not readily absorb water, was developed specifically as a hoof packing material. The copper sulfate and venice turpentine combine to make a medicated

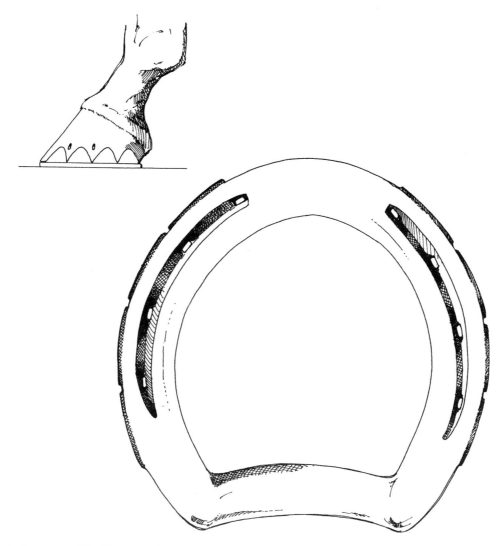

FIG. 6–90. Klimesh Contiguous Clip Shoe.

adhesive that binds the poly felt to the sole forming a gasket between the pad and the hoof. This gasket protects the hoof wall and sole from the invasion of sand, dirt, mud, water, and other foreign matter for the entire 5- to 8-week shoeing period.

The venice turpentine is spread onto either the hoof or the poly felt, and the copper sulfate lightly sprinkled over it, or the two are stirred together to form a light green mixture (approximately 3 T copper sulfate to 1 pint venice turpentine), which is then spread onto the hoof or felt. The copper sulfate migrates into fissures in the hoof wall and sole, preventing the growth of undesirable organisms and eliminating the foul odor often associated with the use of full pads. The CVP packing forms a barrier against the hoof that prevents excess moisture from baths, creeks, or muddy pens from softening the hoof. If *too much* copper sulfate is used, however, the hoof tissues may dry out and become flaky. After the hoof is trimmed and ready for the pad and shoe, the commissures of the frog are filled with appropriately sized pieces of poly felt

lightly coated with the CVP mixture. If the frog is recessed below the level of the hoof, pieces of CVP are placed on the back half of the frog to build up the area between the heels to the level of the trimmed hoof wall. This prevents mud and debris from getting between the pad and the sole.

If the sole has an extreme cup to it, CVP is used to fill the area level with the wall. The packing should not bulge out the center of the pad when it is applied to the hoof. As the horse moves, the CVP packing will be compressed and conform to the contours of the sole and frog. If the horse loses a shoe, often the CVP gasket will remain adhered to the sole, providing sole protection until the pad and shoe can be replaced.

Pad Uses

Full pads are often used to protect a bruised sole while it heals. If a pad is applied over a sole bruise that may abscess, however, it tends to fester the abscess

TYPES OF PADS

Full flat pads—cover the entire sole. They are used primarily to protect the sole and to keep it clean of snow and debris.

Leather pads—conform to the sole, absorb water and eventually deteriorate, and compress between the shoe and the hoof. They do allow the hoof to respire more than plastic pads.

Plastic pads—are available in a variety of thicknesses, hardnesses, colors, and durability that allows many types to be reset. They do not allow the hoof to respire and may or may not conform to sole.

Shock-absorbing pads—are used to reduce concussion and vibration to the hoof and limb structures; however, their effectiveness is debated.

Wedge pads—are used to elevate one portion of the hoof, usually the heels. They are available in full or bar (open) style.

Bubble pads—are full, hard pads with a 2-inch diameter convex (on ground surface of pad) dome near center. Originally designed for antisnowballing, they are also used to relieve pressure over navicular or other sole area. Traction is reduced.

Rim pads—fit between the shoe and the hoof wall; the sole and frog are open. They are used to put more distance between the sole and the ground.

Tube type rim pads—are composed of a small rubber tube that lines the inside rim of the shoe and is held in place by an attached flat, thin portion that lies between the shoe and the hoof; designed to eliminate snowballing.

---

quickly. The horse may exhibit great pain after the pad has been on for a short period, necessitating the removal of the pad. Once the abscess has been treated (see treatment plate) and has dried out, a pad can be applied again, if necessary, for protection.

For many years, full pads were used in the treatment of acutely laminitic horses, with the belief that the pads provided protection for the horse's sore feet. The pressure transferred to the sole by a pad and packing, however, may compromise blood flow and lead to further degeneration of vascular structures within the hoof. In addition, abscesses are common in recently foundered hooves. Often the pain experienced by a foundered horse is thought to be due not only to the inflamed laminae, but also to the pus and gas pockets formed in the sole. Pads may tend to increase the pressure of the abscesses on the sensitive sole and make treatment difficult. A good number of horses with *chronic* founder have found comfort with a hard plastic pad and minimal packing of hoof felt and venice turpentine.

In cases in which injury or surgery results in a partial loss of the hoof wall, a full pad can keep the sole free from debris and decrease the amount of bandaging material needed. Full pads may be prescribed for horses that have navicular syndrome, particularly those cases that are the most painful to hoof testers over the central third of the frog. Hooves with wide-open, low heels are sometimes believed to have incurred navicular syndrome or heel soreness from the direct concussion to the frog and heel area. In some cases, full pads used to *protect* this area actually *transmit* the concussion to the navicular region. A straight

bar or "V" bar shoe might be more effective in providing protection for this type of navicular problem.

Along with the use of full pads comes an interruption in hoof moisture balance. When a full pad covers the sole of a hoof, outward moisture migration via the sole is halted, and the hoof structures can become softened and thereby weakened. In addition, full pads tend to trap moisture from slush, mud, snow, and normal hoof respiration next to the hoof structures, causing deterioration and providing a suitable environment for growth of bacteria, fungus, and yeast (see section on CVP pad). Some believe that horses tend to develop an even thinner and more vulnerable sole from wearing pads full time and therefore become pad dependent. Some horses with weak soles have developed a thick normal sole with the use of full pads and the CVP method.

Traction is decreased with a full flat pad; the cup of the bare sole and the frog are covered; therefore, the grip of the shoe is all that remains. Some full-support pads have an artificial frog built onto the ground surface, which helps compensate for traction loss. The added weight of a pad and packing can exaggerate a horse's action and travel deviations.

There are many pads on the market that claim to protect the horse by reducing concussion. The effectiveness of shock-absorbing pads is largely undocumented and widely debated. A properly shod healthy foot provides all the shock absorption necessary for normal work by transferring the energy of the hoof's impact to the shock-absorbing structures: the hoof wall, the laminae, the frog, the digital cushion, and the blood vessels. If the hoof structures are abnormal or the work is excessive, concussion-reducing pads are sometimes prescribed. Success depends on the type of pad used, the horse's conformation and degree of soundness, the footing, and other management factors.

A wide variety of concussion-reducing pads are available as full pads or rim pads. The material of the pads must have the ability to absorb the force of concussion quickly and release it slowly. With the repeated compression and expansion of the pad may come a permanent compression of the pad material or a sideways shift of the pad or an actual cutting into the pad by the hoof wall. The result may be loose clinches, premature wearing of the nail holes, loose or lost shoes, and possible weakened or split hoof walls.

Snowballing can be stressful to the support structures of a horse's limb whether the horse is standing or moving. The barefoot horse is the best equipped for shedding snow and ice from its hooves, but if shoeing is needed for traction or protection, several antisnowballing pads are available. Full flat pads, full pads with a convex bubble in the center, and tube-type rim pads all work with varying degrees of success depending on installation, hoof shape, and temperature and type of snow.

Some breed and performance associations have rules specifically related to the use of hoof pads at horse competitions. It is the horse owner's and exhibitor's responsibility to know and abide by the pertinent regulations.

Wide-Web Shoes

Wide-web shoes are used to protect the perimeter of the sole and to provide more ground contact and a more stable support for the hoof. These shoes have gained popularity with increase in the population of the larger Warmblood horses. Because of their extra width, these shoes are more resistant to deforming under the weight of a horse. Their increased surface area is thought to dissipate some of the shock of impact.

One drawback to increased ground surface contact is a decrease in traction. When used on performance horses, wide-web shoes often require some sort of traction device (see section or traction). When a wide-web shoe is used on a hoof with a flat sole, it is necessary to relieve or concave the inner hoof surface of the shoe or apply a rim pad between the shoe and the hoof wall to prevent pressure from being applied to the sole (see Fig. 6–54). On some commercial wide-web shoes, the nail holes are placed proportionately farther inward on the web. Care must be taken when applying these shoes to thin-walled hoofs to avoid driving a close or hot nail. This is less of a problem with hand-forged wide-webbed shoes because the farrier can take the wall thickness into account when placing the nail holes.

Treatment Plate

A treatment plate, or hospital plate, is used to protect the sole or frog and also to provide regular access to these areas for inspection and medication. These shoes are extremely useful in treating feet with dropped sole, protruding coffin bones, sole abscesses, and puncture wounds to the sole or frog. Although a hard plastic pad or metal plate can simply be taped to the bottom of the shoe to serve this purpose, if treatment extends over more than a few days, a treatment plate that bolts on to the bottom of the shoe will be much more economical in terms of both time and money. Treatment plates can be custom-made by an experienced farrier and are available commercially. If positive protection is required but access for treatment is not necessary, a steel plate can be permanently welded to cover the center of the shoe and used with CVP packing.

To Alter Gait Defects

Breakover Alterations

Breakover is the phase of the stride between stance and swing (see Chapter 2). It is the moment when the hoof prepares to leave the ground. It starts when the heel lifts and the hoof begins to pivot at the toe and ends when the toe leaves the ground. The deep digital flexor tendon (assisted by the suspensory ligament) is still stretched just before the beginning of breakover to counteract the downward pressure of the weight of the horse's body.

The ideal hoof breaks over near the center of the toe. The location of breakover is different for front and hind hooves. The coffin bone and hoof of a front foot are usually round with sloping hoof walls and wide areas of support on each side of the hoof. This configuration encourages breakover to occur at the center of the toe. For this reason, front shoes usually show the most wear at the toe (Fig. 6–91).

Hind hooves are more pointed and triangular in shape and have straighter walls with less lateral sup-

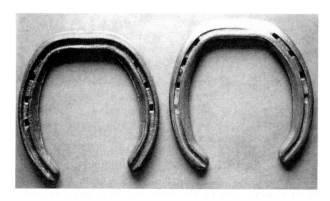

FIG. 6–91. Left: new squared toe shoe. Right: Wear from breakover on a squared toe right front shoe.

port than front hooves. The hindfeet are the horse's means to push, pivot, and change direction, so they perform a wide variety of medial-lateral movements. Also, most horses are conformed and travel in a slightly toed-out configuration in the hind. This allows the hip and stifle to move freely forward (and slightly to the outside) without being hindered by the flank and coupling. Therefore, hind hooves (and shoes) often do not break over at the center of the toe but slightly to the inside of center. Instead of showing wear from breakover at one particular point the way front shoes do, however, hind shoes usually show wear more evenly from sliding as they hit the ground.

The point of breakover should not be *forced* to occur at a point that is unnatural for the individual horse. A hoof can be *encouraged*, however, to break over in a position that contributes to balanced movement. If a horse's hooves are balanced, the horse is most likely breaking over at its ideal spot.

Provided that a horse's hoof is aligned with the pastern, some correlations can be drawn between angles and breakover. Longer or lower pasterns (53° or lower) result in the hoof being on the ground for a longer period of time than those with shorter or more upright (59° or higher) pasterns.

The length and position of the hoof's base of support in relation to the cannon and fetlock determine how much time and effort it takes to breakover. A hoof is in the proper position to support a horse's weight if the bulbs of the heels are approximately underneath the midpoint of the cannon bone (when standing) and the heels of the hoof only slightly ahead of the bulbs (see Fig. 6–48A). Hooves that are small or have underrun heels (and are not shod to counteract this) sink more at the heels during loading and therefore experience more stress, require more effort to lift, and have a delayed breakover.

Dishes or extra length of toe, if not removed, increases tendon stress and delays breakover. If a dish is not rasped to result in a straight hoof wall from the coronary band to the ground, the shoe is likely to be applied ahead of the optimum point of breakover.

Various modifications to standard shoes and several specialized shoes can specifically affect breakover (Fig. 6–92).

Squared toe: The toe of the shoe is squared and set back from the toe of the hoof to facilitate easy breakover. The toe of the hoof is usually rounded with the rasp to prevent chipping. Used on the hindlimbs, squared-toe shoes may help prevent the stepping off of front shoes (Figs. 6–93 and 6–94).

Roller toe: The hoof surface of the shoe is flat. The ground surface of the shoe has a rounded toe much like a naturally worn shoe.

Rocker toe: The entire toe of the shoe is bent upward. This requires that the toe of the hoof be rasped or cut to fit the shoe. The hoof is encouraged to break over specifically at the point of the rocker location.

Roller-motion shoe: Combining the rocker toe with swelled heels results in a roller-motion shoe (Fig. 6–95).

Half-round shoe: The ground surface of the outside and inside edge of the entire shoe are round. A half-round shoe allows a horse to break over more easily in any direction. (see Fig. 6–40).

Forging and Overreaching Solutions

Forging is a gait defect commonly heard when a horse is trotting (Fig. 6–96). It occurs when a hindfoot (or hind shoe) contacts a front foot (or front shoe) on the same side. Overreaching (Fig. 6–97) is a related gait defect with more serious consequences of an injury to the front limb (heel bulb, coronary band, fetlock, or flexor tendon) or a pulled shoe.

Assuming management and training related factors have been evaluated and modified if required (see Chapter 2), shoeing may be able to help eliminate the problem of persistent forging or overreaching. Most corrective shoeing is based on restoring a horse's normal hoof configuration and balance.

There are no absolutes when it comes to corrective shoeing for forging or overreaching. Although most experts agree how to modify the front feet of a horse that forges or overreaches, the opinions are varied for treatment of the hindfeet. Often, just balancing the front hooves and easing their breakover eliminate forging. This balancing is often accomplished by shortening the toe or raising the hoof angle to align the hoof/pastern axis. Breakover can be eased with a modified (squared, rolled, rocker, or roller motion) shoe.

The DP balance of the rear hooves should be evaluated and adjusted, if necessary. In the case of a horse that is relatively equal in width of chest and hindquarter, putting a modified toe shoe, such as a squared toe shoe, on the hindfeet as well might eliminate forging. Why would this work since the breakover of both the fronts and hinds has been made easier? In the case of a horse with a pointed hind hoof, sometimes squaring the front hooves and leaving the hinds pointed would result in a break in the synchronization of the movement of the diagonal pairs of limbs. Squaring the hind toes may smooth out and equalize the movement. And the square toe on the hind replaces the normally pointed hind toe; a pointed toe would tend to hit and perhaps grab a front shoe more easily than a squared toe would. Using half-round shoes on the hinds may also be helpful.

To prevent pulled shoes caused by overreaching, many farriers remove the sharp outer edges of the shoes. Chamfering the outer edge of the hoof surface of the shoe is called "boxing," and rounding the outer edge of the ground surface of the shoe is called "safeing." These procedures make it less likely that a front shoe will be "stepped off" if contacted by a hind shoe.

Trailers have long been touted as an aid to encourage a hoof to stop sooner on landing if the hoof is meeting the ground heel first or flat. If the thinking is based on a larger surface area providing additional drag or friction, it is faulty, as the opposite is true with

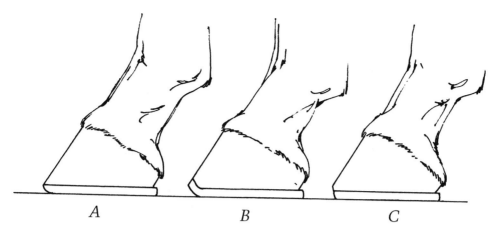

FIG. 6–92. Modified toe shoes. *A*, Rolled toe. *B*, Rocker toe. *C*, Squared toe. (From Hill, C., Klimesh, R.: Maximum Hoof Power. New York, Howell Book House, 1994.)

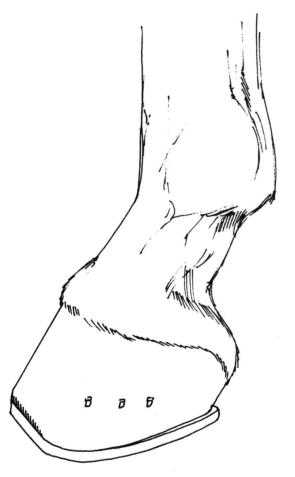

FIG. 6–93. Squared toe shoe. (From Hill, C., Klimesh, R.: Maximum Hoof Power. New York, Howell Book House, 1994.)

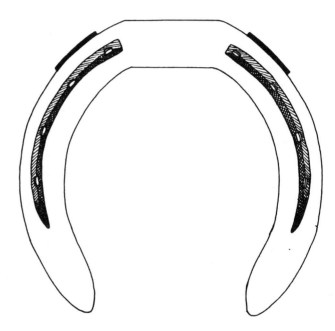

FIG. 6–94. Squared toe shoe with forward placed side clips. (From Hill, C., Klimesh, R.: Maximum Hoof Power. New York, Howell Book House, 1994.)

smooth trailers. A smooth trailer increases the surface area of the shoe and actually provides less traction. A calk or sticker on the trailer would contact the ground sooner and create additional drag, but the trailer just provides a place for the calk to be placed. It is the calk that is doing the stopping, not the trailer. This is where the confusion may have originated.

Even if trailers on the hinds *did* encourage a slightly quicker stop to the hoof's motion as it lands, would it prevent forging or overreaching? According to some slow-motion videos, the answer is no. The moment when contact between the toe of the hind and the front shoe would occur is before the hind shoe (and its smooth trailers) actually touches the ground. Trailers do offer a greater measure of support for the flexor tendons than normal shoes. Exaggerated trailers, however, can be dangerous to people and other horses in the event of a kick. Egg bar shoes are a safer alternative for providing such an extension and support.

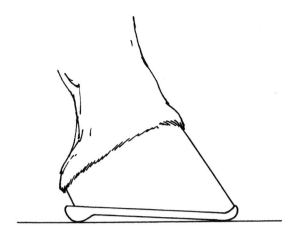

FIG. 6–95. Full roller motion shoe.

Interference Adjustments

Interference refers to a regularly occurring abnormal sideways (axial) limb swing that results in a physical contact with the opposite limb. Why a horse interferes is usually due to a variety of interrelated factors (see Chapter 2), including conformation, soundness, age, conditioning, training, rider proficiency, and farriery. In some cases, finding a solution requires the owner, farrier, and perhaps a veterinarian to work together during a period of trial-and-error.

First, a knowledgeable farrier should examine the horse's shoes for signs of imbalance. Shoe wear, which is related to the hoof landing, loading, and taking off, is valuable information for assessing a foot flight problem. The torque, or twisting force, that the deviating foot experiences and expresses in flight is a direct result of the impact of loading and the release of that force during breakover. If a hoof lands unbalanced, it usually sends the energy upward and forward in an unbalanced fashion, and the flight of the limb or hoof will show a resulting deviation.

Examining the shoe for wear can help determine a plan for trimming that will result in even wear on both branches of the shoe. Signs of unequal shoe wear include a rounding of one area of the shoe, nail heads worn more in one area of the shoe, and a thinning of the shoe in one region. Usually, if the side of the hoof that shows the least amount of shoe wear is trimmed shorter, the subsequent wear on the shoe will be equal. This rule is excepted by a horse that is lame or has an unusual way of going, so it is wise not to rely on just one guideline when attempting something as complex as balancing the equine limb. An examination of the hoof itself can show imbalance, such as in the self-perpetuating condition sheared heels. If one heel is higher than the other, as the horse repeatedly lands with unequal impact, it tends to force the heel even higher.

If the hoof is obviously unbalanced, alternations in trimming and shoeing should come first. Otherwise, conscientious corrections to all riding, conditioning,

and training deficiencies should be made before turning to farriery for additional solutions. Shoeing alterations should be approached conservatively and monitored closely. One of the most serious misconceptions surrounding corrective farriery is the notion that crooked limbs should be made to point forward. Although there can be merit to this in the developing young horse, forcing a foot to conform to an "ideal" on a horse over 1 year of age often results in serious stress to joint alignment and function.

With a toed-out condition, it is not uncommon for the bones from the fetlock to the coffin bone to be aligned in a straight column with even, symmetric joint spaces but with the entire column rotated outward instead of straight forward. If alteration (commonly a lowering of the outside) forces the hoof to point forward, joint spaces on the inside (medial) of the joints become tighter while the joint spaces on the outside (lateral) of the joints become stretched and farther apart. Now there is a problem that if continued can lead to joint inflammation.

When farrier corrections are warranted, they can affect the breakover, flight, landing, or weight-bearing of the hoof. Some interference problems require experimentation over a period of several shoeings before a pattern begins to emerge and the solution materializes. Unfortunately, some horses continue to interfere despite the best management, riding, training, and farrier care.

Breakover

A squared or rocker toe shoe can encourage the breakover to occur off center if desired. Often it is necessary to experiment during several shoeing periods to find the optimum breakover to help an interfering horse. Although it is better to *encourage* breakover to occur at the desired point rather than *prevent* it from occurring at an undesirable point, in some therapeutic instances, toe extensions are used to alter the point of breakover. A toe extension is a metal piece forged or welded to a particular portion of the shoe to inhibit breakover at that point (Fig. 6–98). Toe extensions are used on the inside of a base-narrow toed-out horse to help the horse break over centrally. The extension is added from the center of the toe of the shoe to approximately the second nail hole.

Half round shoes allow breakover in any direction so are inappropriate to use when trying to redirect the breakover but do allow a horse to find its natural breakover point more easily.

Foot Flight

To affect the natural flight of a hoof as little as possible, it is best to use the lightest shoe that still provides adequate support for the hoof. If the foot flight pattern of the front feet needs to be widened, lowering the outside wall, reducing inside flares, and possibly

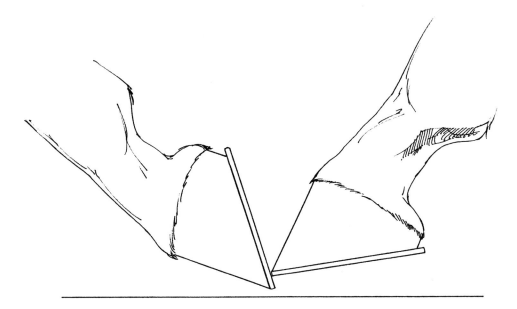

FIG. 6–96. Forging. (From Hill, C., Klimesh, R.: Maximum Hoof Power. New York, Howell Book House, 1994.)

adding a calk on the inside may work. If the foot flight pattern of the hind feet of a cow-hocked horse needs to be widened, lowering the outside wall, adding a trailer on the outside, and adding a calk on the inside may work. If the foot flight pattern of the hindfeet of a base-narrow or bow-legged horse needs to be widened, lowering the inside wall, reducing inside flares, and adding a calk or a trailer on the outside may work. Bear in mind, however, that by lowering one side of a hoof that is in balance to affect foot flight or by using calks on only one branch of a shoe, the limb support structures experience uneven stress and may experience problems worse than interfering.

Undesirable torque in flight is usually due to an imbalanced foot or misaligned limb. Joint rotation, such as seen in the bow-legged or knock-kneed horse, increases as speed or extension within a gait increases. Sometimes the foot flight pattern can be improved by applying the shoes so they are in line with the horse's body regardless of how the hooves point.

Some Standardbred farriers use side-weighted shoes to control knee torque and alter foot flight. These shoes are more appropriate for high-speed or high-action horses than for horses moving at normal gaits. Weight affects front and hind limbs differently. Added weight on a front foot tends to move the limb away from the weighted side. Added weight on a hindfoot tends to pull the limb toward the weighted side.

Landing

Encouraging a hoof to land in a balanced fashion begins with trimming the hoof level and shoeing it to land flat or slightly heel first. If alterations to landing are desired, they are usually accomplished by altering the balance of the hoof. Trailers or calks on one heel of a shoe are sometimes used to turn the hoof on landing, but as previously mentioned calks are considered by many to be dangerous because of the uneven stresses they put on the structures of the limb.

Weight Bearing

Ideally during the loading phase of the stride, the horse's weight is borne over the center of the hoof. If a horse shows a dynamic imbalance in weight-bearing, an attempt to move the hoof under the center of the limb can be made by raising up or lowering the pertinent side of the hoof. Lowering the lateral (outer) wall moves the hoof toward the midline, while lowering the medial (inner) wall often moves the hoof away from the midline. Often a farrier approaches the situation by placing the shoe on the hoof so that the shoe is under the center of the limb although the hoof may be off to one side slightly. In this case, the shoe would fit close on one side of the hoof and extend beyond the hoof on the other side (Fig. 6–99).

To Provide Traction

The barefoot horse (Fig. 6–100) has quite good traction in a variety of situations, especially a horse with a naturally balanced hoof, dense hoof horn, and well-cupped sole. Such a hoof is able to grip most surfaces without hoof damage, and the naturally concave sole sheds mud and slush well. In contrast, the hoof with an LT-LH, brittle or pithy horn and a flat sole has difficulty getting adequate traction. Shod horses often require added traction depending on the season and footing. Horses wearing certain therapeutic shoes may need added traction for security.

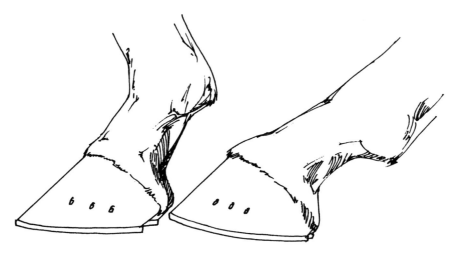

FIG. 6–97. Overreaching: The moment a shoe might be "grabbed" when the front foot is greatly delayed in breakover. (From Hill, C., Klimesh, R.: Maximum Hoof Power. New York, Howell Book House, 1994.)

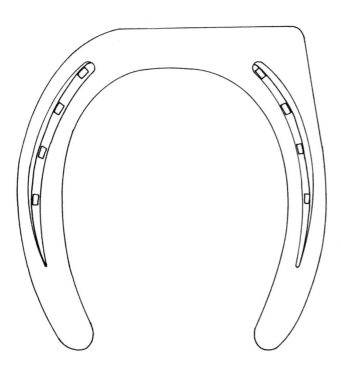

FIG. 6–98. Toe extension shoe.

Traction Principles

Using traction devices unwisely can be dangerous. Adhering to the following principles minimizes risk:

- Determine the activity level of the horse.
- Take into account the normal footing.
- Select the appropriate type of traction device.
- Apply traction devices moderately at first.
- Use traction devices on both feet and on both sides of the shoe to prevent uneven torque.
- Gradually build up the traction to the optimum level.
- Closely monitor the horse for signs of lameness.

- Realize that a small degree of slide on landing is natural and desirable because it dissipates some shock that would otherwise be transmitted to the horse's limb.

It is advisable that clips be used whenever calks, ice nails, or borium is used. Adding traction devices essentially stops the shoe, but the horse's body mass (including the hoof that is attached to the shoe) is still moving forward. Once the nails get loose and movement begins, the hoof wall can split and break. Clips help keep the shoe from shifting and loosening and take much strain off the nails, which can actually shear off.

Usually quarter clips (so called because they are applied at the quarters of the hoof) are used; however, a single toe clip is sometimes used on each front shoe. Quarter clips are applied somewhere between the toe and the quarter on both branches of the shoe.

Traction should be added moderately. The structures of the limb have only a limited capacity to accept torque before something is damaged, no matter how fit the horse is. Torque is the twisting force that occurs when the horse's limb is subjected to opposing forces. Using excess traction or suddenly applying devices unfamiliar to a horse may cause him to exert dangerous stresses on his muscles, tendons, bones, ligaments, and joints.

A hoof (or foot) normally goes through a certain amount of slide and often some degree of rotation as it lands and takes off again. If a horse is deprived of this normal motion (suddenly or excessively), the forces are taken up by the joints, soft tissue support structures, and tendons. Injuries from excessive or inappropriate traction can show up immediately or after long-term use.

A horse needs to become accustomed mentally to his new grab on the ground. He needs to be relaxed enough to devise new ways to balance his body to compensate for the change in traction. Sometimes a

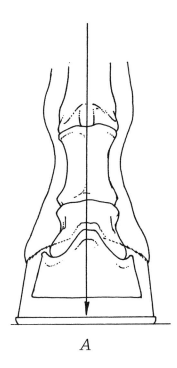
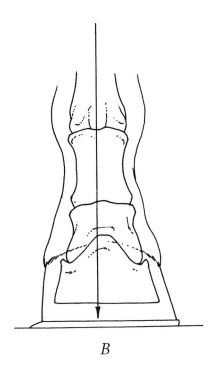

A   *B*

FIG. 6–99. Base of support centered under limb. *A*, Centered hoof. *B*, Offset hoof. (From Hill, C., Klimesh, R.: Maximum Hoof Power. New York, Howell Book House, 1994.)

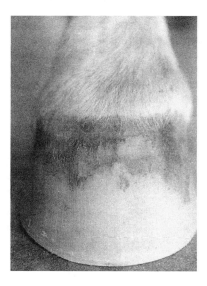

FIG. 6–100. A properly trimmed bare hoof. This also illustrates mild proximal displacement of the coronet.

jumper may be willing to negotiate a tight turn "off balance" if he knows he will not slip and can readily regain his balance with good ground contact. This results in a faster turn but also has the potential for greater trauma to his limbs.

Requiring a horse to work on precarious footing without adequate traction can result in muscle strain (such as in the gluteals and hamstrings) caused by constant slipping. Therefore, optimum traction but no extra is the goal.

Traction should be used bilaterally. Borium spots or smears, ice nails, and calks should always be applied on both sides of a shoe (and on both shoes of a pair of limbs) to prevent uneven torque or twist on landing or take-off. (There are a few instances, however, when the judicious application of only one traction device on a shoe or two different devices on the same shoe might be warranted, such as for correcting a travel defect.) Borium and ice nails are generally used for horses traveling at a slow to moderate speed on slippery footing. Customarily ice nails are applied at the third nail-hole position, at the midpoint of each side of the shoe. This results in the safest grab with minimal torque. Borium is usually added just ahead of both toe nails and just behind each heel nail. Because horses that require calks often are moving at a high rate of speed, the goal is a secure landing, so calks are usually placed behind the heel nail.

The horse should be monitored for signs of lameness and swelling. When a horse realizes that his hooves are going to stick rather than land, slide, and twist, he will be able to adjust his balance and movement accordingly. As traction is increased, it is important to stay within an individual horse's limits of tolerance. The goal is *optimum* traction, not *maximum* traction.

The warning signs of excessive traction are lameness, swelling, heat, a reluctance to work, a shortened stride, and a bad attitude. All of these can indicate that a horse is trying to protect itself. Contrary to what is commonly thought, tendons do not have the ability to stretch more than about 3% of their length without

TYPES OF SHOES AND DEVICES THAT AFFECT TRACTION

Standard keg shoe—plain steel shoes, whether creased or punched for the nail heads, usually provide adequate traction for most situations.

Aluminum—aluminum shoes may have a slightly better grab than steel shoes because aluminum is softer but wears out faster. Wear can be extended by inserting a steel wear plate at the toe or borium to the ground surface. Aluminum racing plates with toe grabs or heel stickers can be used successfully in some situations.

Rim shoes—the nail crease that is on the ground surface of most keg shoes is called the swedge. When swedging extends the entire length of the shoe, it is termed a full-swedged or rim shoe (Fig. 6–101). Lighter variations of the rim shoe are the polo shoe, which is full-swedged with a higher inside rim, and the barrel racing shoe with a higher outside rim. Rim shoes provide added traction because the rims, until they are worn down, grab the ground. Also, the dirt that packs into the swedge provides more traction against the ground than does a flat steel shoe.

Toed and heeled shoes—keg shoes are available with permanent calks forged at the heels or at the toe and heels. In soft footing such as warmer winter conditions, these sink into semifrozen ground or "soft" ice and give good traction. On hard ice or rocks, however, these shoes are not as effective.

Borium—borium (tungsten carbide) or other hard-surfacing materials can be applied to the ground surface of the horse's normal shoe in smears, beads, or points (Fig. 6–102).

Nails—commercial frost or mud nails with ribbed or specially hardened heads can be substituted for regular horseshoe nails to provide added traction. One at each midpoint nail position may be all that is necessary. The treated or pointed heads resist wear and dig into hard ground or ice (Fig. 6–102).

Calks—calks are projections added to the ground surface of the shoe for providing traction. They can be permanent or removable. Threaded studs (removable) have bullet-shaped or blocky heads and range in height from $\frac{11}{16}$ inch for shoe jumpers to $\frac{1}{2}$ inch road calks (Fig. 6–103). Although removable studs offer the advantage of applying the right amount of traction for a particular footing, the sudden change may not allow a horse to adapt to its new traction. Permanent calks are driven or forged into the shoe or brazed or welded onto the shoe (Fig. 6–102). Because of their permanence, a horse can become thoroughly familiar and confident with the new traction, but the amount of traction provided cannot be changed between shoeings to accommodate different footings.

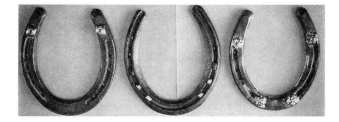

FIG. 6–102. *From left:* studs, ice nails, borium.

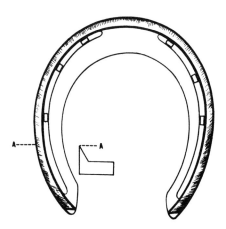

FIG. 6–101. Full-rim shoe. This full rim on the outside edge of the web is used to increase traction, especially among Standardbreds. Inset shows a cross section of the web with rim (A) on the outside.

damage. Exceeding this elastic range can bring about changes to the mechanical characteristics of the tendon fibers and usually results in inflammation (tendinitis). Ligaments have almost no ability to stretch, so when they are wrenched, it usually results in a tear.

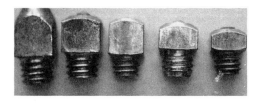

FIG. 6–103. An assortment of screw-in studs.

To Encourage Proper Limb Development in Foals

Foal hoof management should be designed in light of a foal's present configuration and its anticipated adult conformation. A foal should have a veterinary examination the day after birth to determine whether deviations in the foal's limbs are normal or whether they require close observation or treatment. Most angular deformities greater than 15° require immediate veterinary treatment; however, the majority of foals do not fall into this category.

A regular program of farrier care should begin when the foal is about 1 month of age. Overly enthusiastic rasping or radical trimming, however, can do more harm than good with the very young foal. Therefore, it is essential that the farrier and veterinarian confer.

A foal is born with soft feathers of horn on the bottom of its hooves. These wear off by the end of a normal first day. The texture of the hoof itself is cornified yet soft and waxy. It is somewhat that way the first week but gradually hardens to more durable hoof horn. The last bit of neonate (baby) hoof will have grown down to ground level by about 6 months of age. Physeal (growth plate) closure has an important bearing on the timing of corrective treatments.

Many foals born with crooked limbs straighten without any formal treatment, and those that do not can often be corrected with care from a competent veterinarian and farrier and by proper management. For example, many foals are born carpus valgus (knock-kneed); that is, they stand with their knees closer together than their hooves.

Because most newborn foal's chests are very narrow, the front limbs are close together at the chest. The foal, in its attempt to stabilize itself when standing, widens its base of support by increasing the distance between its hooves and allowing the lower limb to rotate outward. This causes the limbs to bend inward at the knees bringing the knees even closer together. The hooves of such foals are sometimes aggressively altered so that the limbs appear cosmetically ideal, but this if often harmful.

Incorrect "Corrective" Trimming

Some age-old corrective trimming principles are no longer employed on foals. One procedure to correct a toed-out horse is to rotate the hoof capsule inward by lowering the outside hoof wall to make it shorter than the inside wall. In addition, a half shoe is applied to the inside wall to rotate the hoof farther inward. This has the effect of moving the limb in under the horse's body and shifting more of the weight to the outside of the limb.

Lowering the outside hoof wall of toed-out foals before 3 months of age, however, can interrupt the normal developmental pattern and result in a varus deformity of the fetlock region (Fig. 6–104). The growth plates of the fetlock region have compen-

sated and remodeled according to the alteration in weight-bearing caused by the trimming. Now the growth plates are no longer in a desirable horizontal configuration.

Impatience to "correct" a normally carpus valgus, fetlock-rotated-out foal by lowering the outside hoof wall can also result in sheared heels and quarters. Such a problem is not likely to occur if the hoof is kept in ML balance and the foal's own development was allowed to correct the carpus valgus condition. Therefore, it is important *not* to lower the outside wall on carpus valgus, fetlock-rotated-out foals under 3 months of age. Squaring the toe of the hoof may help restore ML balance. Because a carpus valgus foal tends to break over medial of the hoof center, squaring the toe encourages a more central breakover.

Knee and Chest Conformation

Depending on chest conformation, a foal is usually somewhat carpus valgus until 6 to 8 months of age. The tighter (more narrow) the chest, the more the face of the knee naturally (and should be allowed to) rotates outward. The fetlocks also face somewhat outward to allow horizontal formation and maintenance of the growth plates. If the fetlocks (and hoof) are forced to face forward by "corrective" trimming, the lowering of the outside of the hoof that causes it to rotate medially may result in the aforementioned sheared fetlock. Such a fetlock joint is no longer hinged perpendicular to the limb. When a foal is improperly "corrected" like this, by the time it matures, it will likely have attained a toed-in stance (Fig. 6–104).

At 8 to 10 months of age, the normal widening of the foal's chest gradually moves the front limbs away from the body allowing the knees to straighten, rotate inward, and be more directly under the body mass in a straight configuration. The fetlocks that have been treated properly also rotate inward and now point straight forward (Figs. 6–105 and 6–106). Those that have been improperly altered may now toe-in with the widening of the chest.

The foal that has a mild-to-moderate valgus (knock-kneed) deformity, if kept level and balanced through the growing months, will stand relatively straight as a yearling because he improves with age and weight gain.

The foal whose entire limb is rotated outward is not so lucky. Little can be done to change this conformational defect of such a foal—one that has a straight limb but a rotational deformity from the elbow down. In many cases, however, if such a foal is kept level and balanced and if the foal develops a sufficient chest, he may become an acceptable athlete, although he may have an odd walk the rest of his life. If this foal is mistakenly diagnosed as having valgus fetlocks and he is inappropriately "corrected" by making the foot face forward, the foal will then have a problem—a toed-in foot with a rotated-out limb. Valgus foals that have the genetics for heavy bodies and wide chests especially should not be treated early or aggressively for their valgus condition, or by the time their chests widen they may have become bow-legged. Questions regarding these problems should be directed to your veterinarian and farrier.

Advances in glue-on shoe technology allow corrective shoes to be applied to foals only a few weeks of age (see Resource Guide).

Regular Farrier Care

Besides assessing a foal's hooves in relation to his limbs when he is standing, a farrier evaluates the foal's hoof wear patterns. In most cases, rasping that is required to balance a hoof should be done conservatively and with close monitoring of the natural wear. By squaring the toe, a hoof can be encouraged to break over at the center. By checking for evenness and symmetry, the farrier can evaluate the natural tendency of the fetlock, pastern, and hoof to align with the cannon. With the foal's front limb flexed at the knee, the farrier lets the extensor surface of the cannon rest in the palm of his hand. The fetlock and hoof are allowed to fall into their normal axis at rest. The farrier can then evaluate the heels for evenness, the relationship of the hoof to the limb, and the symmetry of the frog in relation to the hoof.

Teamwork

A horse's health and soundness are a result of a team effort. The horse owner must take the responsibility for coordinating the efforts of the other team members: the manager, the trainer, the instructor, the rider, the veterinarian, and the farrier.

A horse depends on the team to work well together and make wise decisions. The owner is responsible for providing competent care and management of the horse, which includes feed, housing, exercise, veterinary and farrier care, grooming, and proper training. When any of these duties are entrusted to another person, it is still the owner's responsibility to ensure that things are done correctly.

The veterinarian helps manage a horse's overall health and monitors limb and hoof soundness. A veterinarian should be contacted for advice and treatment related to lameness, wounds, foal hoof management, and nutrition.

The farrier's primary role is to trim and shoe the horse as naturally as possible keeping principles of balance in mind. The farrier's goals should be (1) long-term soundness and (2) optimum performance. In addition, a farrier can assist a veterinarian, to the extent of his or her experience, in the treatment of various hoof and limb problems.

It is important that the veterinarian and farrier have an opportunity to interact. The combination of their knowledge and experience usually benefits the horse.

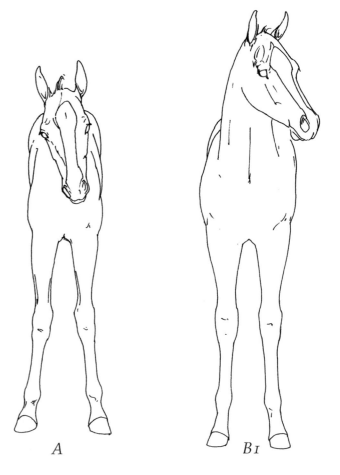

A   *B1*

FIG. 6–104. Correct and incorrect foal trimming. *A*, Suckling foal. *B1*, Weanling allowed to toe-out normally. *C1*, *B1* as yearling now straight. *B2*, Weanling trimmed to stand straight. *C2*, *B2* as yearling now toed-in. (From Hill, C., Klimesh, R.: Maximum Hoof Power. New York, Howell Book House, 1994.)

Whenever a hoof injury involves sensitive tissue (hot nail, puncture, abscess, bleeding crack, coronary wound), it is important that a veterinarian be involved in the treatment. Although the farrier may perform the actual work (paring an abscess, relieving or resecting a crack, treating a hot nail), it should be done under a veterinarian's supervision. Both veterinarians and farriers can provide valuable insights during prepurchase evaluations and for the formulation of management plans.

Farrier Publications

American Farriers Journal, PO Box 624, Brookfield, WI 53008-0624 (official journal of the AFA).

Anvil, PO Box 1810, Georgetown, CA 95634-1810 (practical articles on horseshoeing and blacksmithing).

Hoofcare & Lameness Quarterly Report, PO Box 6600, Gloucester, MA 01930 (practical articles and research on farrier science).

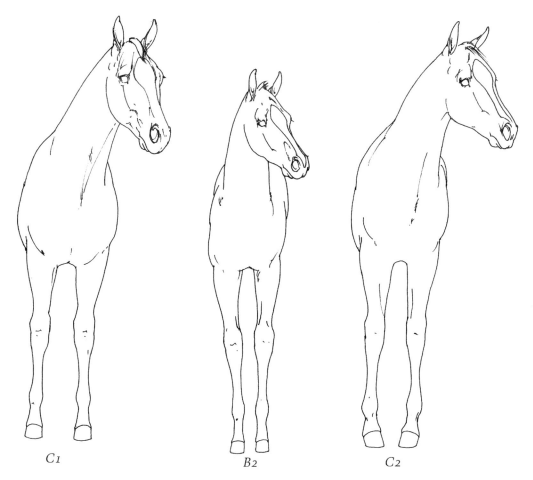

C1   *B2*   *C2*

FIG. 6–104. *Continued*

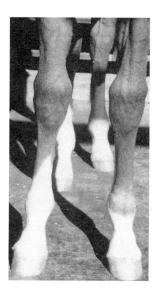

FIG. 6–105. A weanling foal at 4 months.

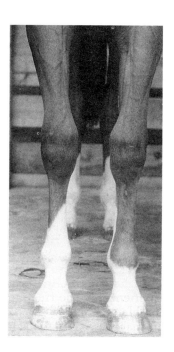

FIG. 6–106. The same horse as in Fig. 6–105 at 10 months.

Farrier Organizations

American Farriers Association, 4059 Iron Works Pike, Lexington, KY 40511; (606) 233-7411.

Brotherhood of Working Farriers Association, 14013 East Highway 136, LaFayette, GA 30728; (706) 397-8047.

Resource Guide

CENTAUR FORGE, LTD., PO Box 340, Burlington, WI 53105; 414-763-9175 (farrier books and tools, shoe size comparison chart, studs, hoof boots, hoof sealer, pads).

CHERRY MOUNTAIN FORGE, PO BOX 140, Livermore, CO 80536 (bulletins: CVP gasket pad, therapeutic shoe construction; Farrier's Formula distributor).

GLU-STRIDER, 1395 Blue Hills Ave., Bloomfield, CT 06002; (203) 242-3650 (glue on-shoes).

HAWTHORNE PRODUCTS, INC., Box 66, RD 2, Dunkirk, IN 47336; (800) 548-5658 (hoof packing).

INNOVATIVE ANIMAL PRODUCTS, GAUTHIER MEDICAL, INC., 6256 34th Ave NW, Rochester, MN 55901; (800) 551-4394 (Equilox, prosthetic hoof repair material).

LIFE DATA LABS, INC., PO Box 490, Cherokee, AL 35616 (800) 624-1873 (manufacturer of Farrier's Formula).

INTERNATIONAL EQUINE PODIATRY, INC., PO Box 507, Versailles, KY 40383; (606) 873-5294 (glue-on shoes).

CHAPTER SEVEN

Methods of Therapy

Physical Therapy

The aim of physical therapy is the restoration of function and promotion of tissue healing by assisting normal physiologic processes. Methods of physical therapy include cold, heat, massage, exercise, light, electricity, manipulation, and mechanical devices. The physiologic response to physical therapy is its effect on the vascular supply; this in turn reproduces similar changes in deeper tissues.

Cold (Cryotherapy)

The application of cold is used in the treatment of acute and hyperacute inflammatory processes. It aids in relief of pain, it reduces inflammation and prevents edema and tissue swelling. There is a decrease in tissue metabolism and possibly some anesthesia. Cold is best combined with compression bandage and rest to limit swelling further. Cold therapy is used during the first 48 hours after trauma has occurred. After this time, it is of less value. It is applied for 20- to 30-minute applications, and at least 1 hour should elapse before it is reapplied. Generally it is applied 3 to 4 times a day.

Cold application can be made by running cold water through a hose on the part or by using a tub or canvas bag to cover the limb. Elaborate whirlpool systems can also be used for hydrotherapy. A word of caution, however, is directed toward this type of treatment for prolonged periods of time. It is not natural for horses to stand in water for 1 to 2 hours a day. The feet become softened and more susceptible to trauma, hoof and sole defects and subsolar abscesses. Moist therapy should not be used if there is an open wound.

Ice cubes in water contained in plastic is helpful in acute noninfectious inflammatory processes. This therapy is most effective in limiting swelling from the acute injury and shortens the recovery period. Swelling is limited by vasoconstriction. If cold is applied too long, there may be a reflex vasodilation, and there is also the possibility of vasodilation after the cold is removed. These are additional reasons for using a compression bandage in conjunction with cold application. Alternating heat and cold are often used on acute noninfectious inflammatory conditions (such as sprain) beginning 48 hours after the injury. Cold is used for injury of muscles, tendons, ligaments, and

joints and for burns. It is particularly effective when it is applied after each workout.

Heat (Thermotherapy)

Heat can be applied as radiant heat, conductive heat, and conversive heat. The physiologic effects of the three methods are basically the same. Radiant heat is applied by infrared light and conductive heat by hot water bottle, electric heating pad, hot fomentations, and poultices. Conversive heat is developed in tissues by resistance to high-frequency electrical energy (diathermy) or sound waves (ultrasound).

Heat is used in an attempt to cause resorption of swelling caused by blood or serum. Heat causes vasodilation, which may increase the number of phagocytes (scavenger cells that can ingest foreign material and bacteria) in the area as well as increase oxygen supply to the part. There is increased metabolism in local cells, increased lymph flow, and a rise in local temperature caused by the vasodilation. Vessel permeability is also increased, and this must be considered when using heat because increased vessel permeability can lead to increased absorption of toxins or occurrence of tissue edema following its use. Heat is usually not used alone but is combined with active or passive action, either manually or by exercise. Heat can spread bacteria and toxic products deeper into surrounding tissues and should not be applied if infection is present. Heat should not be used until infection is under control. Heat is used 48 hours after injury.

Superficial Heat

Some methods of applying heat are designed to cause only superficial inflammation that does not extend far beneath the skin. Hot water poultices, heating pads, a turbulator (whirlpool), and ultraviolet light are used for this purpose. Hot water poultices and a turbulator are application of moist heat, and drugs may be added to facilitate penetration. For this purpose, magnesium sulfate (epsom salts) or mild liniment solutions are commonly used. Magnesium sulfate also acts to draw swelling from the tissue because of the higher osmotic tension in the magnesium sulfate solution. Magnesium sulfate should be added at the rate of approximately 2 cups per gallon of water for this purpose. A turbulator can be used to give passive massage to the part during the application of hot water. A turbulator is a motorized device that agitates the water around the part by pump action. These are expensive and carry some risk of electrical shock. An inexpensive turbulator can be made by reversing a vacuum cleaner hose so that the air blows from the machine instead of sucking air. With the vacuum hose deep in the water that is around the limb, the machine blows air through the hose and turbulates water around the part. Superficial heat of this type is often combined with massage, and following application of heat by one of the aforementioned methods, the part may be massaged using alcohol or other mild rubefacient (causing a reddening of the skin) solutions. These solutions do not have any particular therapeutic value, but they aid the massage and cause a superficial flush. Often the liniment may be credited when improvement was actually the result of the heat and massage.

For deeper penetration, luminous or nonluminous infrared light is used. The luminous type of infrared can be used for frostbite or to aid pointing abscesses. There is a danger of a thermal burn caused by infrared light, and the source should be at least 18 inches away from the part being treated. There is no pain initially, and evidence of thermal burn appears later. It can be applied for 20- to 40-minute applications and repeated at hourly intervals if necessary. The nonluminous type of infrared light heats a metal coil, and this coil radiates the infrared light. This form is usually the best type to use because there is no danger of bulb breakage.

Deep Heat

Diathermy. Diathermy produces a local elevation of temperature within tissues by using high-frequency current or microwave radiation. Diathermy is a relatively impractical therapy for treating horses.

Ultrasound. Ultrasound consists of ultra-high-frequency sound waves produced by the conversion of high-frequency electrical energy waves to sound waves by the crystal in the head of the instrument. A mechanical vibration is produced by the sound waves. This crystal converts electricity to sound, which is measured in watts of output per square centimeter of head surface. The use of ultrasound involves the passage of these high-frequency sound waves (above 20,000 cycles per second) through tissues. The resistance of the tissues to these waves produces heat. This heat penetrates to the bony structures of a joint or limb. Ultrasound is best used for deep heat penetration of muscles (myositis), nerve damage, tendon injury, desmitis, bursitis, and scars in contracted tissue. Other conditions that may respond include splints, spavin, and chronic proliferative (villonodular) synovitis. In some cases, it may be used in combination with corticosteroids. Ultrasound restores function by the relief of pain by the production of heat. It is not of value in bone damage, and if enough is used, bone destruction may occur because of the heat produced.

Ultrasound has also been shown to increase the healing capabilities of tendons treated by percutaneous tendon splitting. Increased vascularization, improvement of the scar tissue formation, and more complete removal of necrotic debris has been noted. Treatment is usually begun 3 days after tendon splitting and continued for at least 18 days.

Ultrasound penetrates deeper (approximately 3 to 5 inches) than diathermy or other forms of heat application described. It also micromassages the tissue. The chassis of the machine should always be grounded to prevent accidental shock to the horse.

Ultrasound should not be used for 48 to 72 hours after injury because it can cause hematoma and seroma if used before this. The duration of application varies between 5 and 10 minutes, and the instrument head should be kept in motion and in contact with the skin. Ultrasound waves do not pass through the air or through hair on the surface of the body. The part should be clipped and shaved, and a coupling agent, such as mineral oil, must be used to establish contact between the instrument head and tissue. High doses of ultrasound cause a rise in tissue heat to as high as 106°F. The temperature rise can cause bone or tissue damage, and care should be taken not to use too high a dosage for too long a time. For this reason, it should not be used directly over the spinal cord region. The instrument head should be kept in motion to prevent heat from accumulating in the tissues. To be most effective, ultrasound should be applied for at least 10 days. After this, alternate-day therapy can be instituted.

Ultrasound is not used over an area of local anesthesia because the horse cannot feel it and thus will not object to levels of heat high enough to cause discomfort. Ultrasound is not used over infected regions because it may encourage the spread of infection. Also, it is not used directly over a surgical site for 14 days after surgery because it may cause the incision to separate. Finally, it is not used over metal implants because the increased heat that is generated may loosen them. Ultrasound is most beneficial when there are no bone changes and when only soft tissues are damaged.

Massage

Massage is used in subacute and chronic swelling and can be combined with the use of liniments, although the main benefit is from massage. The lubrication quality of the liniment usually aids in the massaging. Many liniments receive credit for being good therapeutic agents, when it is actually the massage that reduces edematous (fluid) swelling and aids in relieving pain of an injured tendon or joint. The effect is short-lived, and treatment must be repeated several times a day to be of value. Massage aids in reducing tissue edema (fluid) and also in freeing scar tissue adhesions of the skin to underlying tissues.

Chiropractic Treatment

Chiropractic treatment involves manipulating the vertebrae with gentle force to realign them. It is used primarily for biomechanical problems to remove pain, stiffness, and crookedness. How effective chiropractic treatment is in lameness therapy is not known and cannot be specifically stated until controlled studies are performed and results reported.

Faradic Current

Faradic current is an intermittent alternating electrical current. This electrical current stimulates contraction of muscle and can be varied in intensity and timing so that muscles are contracted and relaxed, thereby preventing atrophy and promoting mobilization of joints. It prevents adhesions and helps disperse inflammatory fluids and hematoma, and because it increases blood flow, it removes the accumulated byproducts from muscle metabolism. This type of therapy is indicated primarily in sprain injury of joints and strain injury of muscles. It probably hastens recovery from this type of injury and helps to alleviate muscular soreness.

Exercise

Depending on the condition, exercise is frequently used to aid in rehabilitation. It is primarily used in subacute and chronic conditions to remove swelling, especially in puncture wounds of the limb, midline incisions, and castrations. Whenever possible, it is combined with massage and the use of liniments. It may also be used to rehabilitate and strengthen the limb after injury to tendon or ligaments. In any case, it must be used with judgment because the horse often tends to overdo it when allowed free access to a corral or pasture. Exercise on a hand lead is usually best when the horse is beginning exercise after surgery for a fractured carpus, sesamoid fracture, and similar conditions. When the initial excitement has worn off, after several days of hand leading, the horse can be turned into a small pen and from there into a pasture as the limb strengthens.

When facilities are available, swimming is an excellent way to rehabilitate and condition the musculature of a horse without concussion to the limbs. Controlled exercise on a hot walker or treadmill or by ponying, however, is used more frequently and is often most practical. Generally, controlled exercise may be begun 2 weeks to a month after surgery and, in most cases, the convalescent period can be shortened considerably by at least 1 to 2 months. If swimming is used, it is not advisable suddenly to work a horse on ground that has only exercised in a pool. Although the muscles are worked, they are not the same as those that develop during running, and the bones may be weaker because they are not subjected to the weight-bearing stresses needed to maintain their strength. It is important, therefore, to gradually incorporate normal workouts gradually into the rehabilitation period.

Surgery

Surgical procedures are performed with the horse either standing or recumbent (lying down) depending on the procedure, the surgeon's preference, and the facilities available. Whether surgery is performed in a large hospital, a small clinic, or in the field, the environment should be as clean and free from bacteria as possible. If surgery is to be performed at a farm, a location that is free of dust, insects, and wind and that has good lighting are chosen.

Standing surgeries are sometimes performed on an outpatient basis; that is, the horse is trailered in to a clinic and taken home on the same day. The horse is first given a sedative or a tranquilizer and then a local anesthetic to desensitize the surgery site. Shortly after the surgery is performed (within 1 to 2 hours), the horse "recovers" from the sedative or tranquilizer and local anesthetic and is ready for transport. Some examples of operations suitable for standing surgery are cryosurgery, medial patellar desmotomy for upward fixation of the knee cap (patella), cunean tenectomy for certain cases of spavin, deep digital flexor tenotomy for persistent laminitis, posterior digital neurectomy, resection of the hoof wall for laminitis, and opening of the sole to allow drainage of an abscess.

Recumbent surgery is performed under general anesthesia. Because of the necessity of presurgical fasting, sterile preparations, and recovery time, recumbent surgery is best suited to equine hospitals that have proper surgical facilities and stabling.

Both standing and recumbent surgeries follow a similar procedure. The surgical site is groomed, clipped closely, shaved, scrubbed with antiseptic soap, and wiped with alcohol. The surgeon also scrubs, wears sterile gloves, and uses sterilized instruments. Meanwhile, the horse has been given a sedative or a tranquilizer as a preanesthetic agent, and when the surgeon is ready, the horse is anesthetized. After the surgery is performed, the horse is then closely monitored during recovery from the anesthesia. Surgical aftercare can include casts, splints, support bandages, or occasionally a sling. Sutures are removed approximately 10 to 14 days after surgery.

Types of Procedures

Joint lavage is a process of using fluids to wash away degradation debris or pus from an infected or damaged joint to restore the lubricating ability of the synovial fluid. Body temperature sterile saline solution (with the possible addition of an antibiotic or dimethyl sulfoxide [DMSO] solution) is injected into the joint and then drained. Joint lavage is most often performed under general anesthesia, although in some cases it can be done while the horse is standing confined in a stock.

Arthrodesis is the ankylosis or fusion of a joint for treatment of bone spavin, ringbone, osseouscysts of the pastern joint, and other types of chronic arthritis (degenerative joint disease). Because movement of these affected joints causes pain, fusion of the joint stops the pain. Arthrodesis is most applicable for low-motion joints. Under general anesthesia, a large portion of the joint cartilage is removed, which ultimately causes the joint to fuse. A method that has worked experimentally, under local anesthesia, involves a substance being injected into the joint that causes cartilage degradation and joint fusion. Unfortunately, this approach results in extreme pain and lameness for prolonged periods before fusion is achieved.

Arthroscopy is a surgery specially suited to chip fractures of the knee, coffin joint, large hock joint, stifle joint, fetlock joint and shoulder joint. It is performed under general anesthesia. A small incision is made to allow the insertion of the arthroscope. Performed properly, there is minimal trauma to soft tissue; therefore, horses can potentially return to work more quickly.

Other Methods of Therapy

Therapeutic Farriery

Corrective trimming and shoeing are an important part of the therapy in many lamenesses. In navicular syndrome, for example, it is often the first treatment initiated to restore balance, provide support, and relieve stress. In traumatic lamenesses, farriery often augments the primary treatment by minimizing stress to and providing stability, support, and protection for the healing limb. Therapeutic farriery is covered in more detail in Chapter 6.

Immobilization

Immobilization is one of the most beneficial and important therapeutic tools for the treatment of musculoskeletal injuries. It simply allows the injured region sufficient time to heal without the risk of reinjury. Confinement within a box stall or a small run for a period of 1 to 6 months is often recommended. The duration of rest is selected from an understanding of the healing characteristics of the injured tissue and how this injury is handled. During confinement, good foot care, parasite control, sanitation, and feeding practices are important. High-quality grass hay or alfalfa should be selected, but the continuation of a high grain ration is discouraged because of the chances of producing an overweight, overactive animal that will place added stress to the injured site. Free choice mineral supplements should be made available at all times. Because horses confined in a stable with a transient population are susceptible to respiratory infections, a regular vaccination program should be maintained.

Cross-tying, running a horse on a wire, and tying the horse to an overhead chain are used to confine the horse's activities further. Of the methods, cross-tying provides the strictest confinement, particularly if the horse is placed in a tie stall that limits it from moving in either direction. It is important, however, to make sure that the horse is not tied so tightly that it cannot reach food or water. Overhead wires or chains allow the horse to move for a limited distance within the stall, but if applied properly they prevent a horse from lying down (Fig. 7–1). Although this type of confinement is useful for a variety of problems, it is most frequently applied when it is undesirable for the horse to pace or lie down. Because horses in these positions become bored, they often develop habits of knocking over their water and feed buckets; therefore, it is best to use attached snap-on feed and water buckets. Young horses less than a year of age do not respond well to this type of confinement initially, but with gentle handling and reduction of grain intake, they usually accept it. Still the horse's disposition must be taken into account because some refuse to accept these measures.

Slings are helpful to stabilize and support a horse that has some difficulty standing on its own if it will accept it. It is of little benefit to the horse that cannot stand on its own once it is stabilized in the upright position. Application of a sling to a horse that cannot stand usually results in further injury or suffocation in some cases. Much to the disbelief of many horse owners, not all horses accept slinging. For some rea-

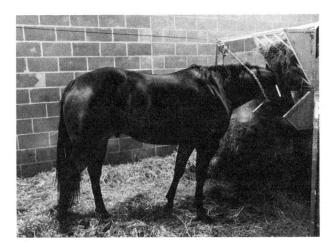

FIG. 7–1. This horse is being run on an overhead wire. The lead rope should be tied short enough to prevent the horse from lying down, but loose enough to allow free movement along the wire's length.

son, the confinement and support frightens them to the point that they will do almost anything to get out of it. Although there are many types of slings available, they all follow a basic design that includes holes for all four limbs and a large belly band that is fixed in place by straps to support the underside of the horse. Chain hoists are attached to the ceiling and are used to elevate the horse. Slinging can be beneficial for horses that are ataxic and, in some cases, when a horse is convalescing from upper limb fracture. Generally, young horses, weanlings to yearlings, do not accept slinging well.

Immobilization of a Part

Immobilization is a beneficial method of therapy for acute inflammatory conditions, but it can be difficult to employ in horses because they may resist the restraint. Immobilization of the part aids in preventing the spread of inflammation and reduces swelling as it reduces movement. It also permits the tissues to heal with minimal scar formation. Immobilization also supports damaged structures, which is especially valuable in the healing of tendons and ligaments. Although immobilization is best done using a cast, compression bandages, cotton bandages, or bandage splints may be of help. Compression bandages should not be used in acute infectious inflammatory conditions until the infection is brought under control. If the infection is not under control, the compression may force the bacteria and associated toxic products deeper into the tissues. Rarely should a compression bandage be left on longer than 3 days without changing. Skin loss from necrosis can occur if this rule is not observed, or the bandage may become so loose that it is no longer effective. Strong liniments should not be used under bandages because they can cause blistering.

Ordinary gauze is extremely inelastic and, when left in place for longer than 24 hours, may cause skin loss. When gauze is used under a compression bandage, it is usually best to use the type known as "Kling" (Johnson & Johnson Co.) or "conforming" gauze, which is much more elastic and does not rigidly oppose the tissue. The same is true of ordinary adhesive tape, and preferably only elastic adhesive tape is used (Elasticon, Johnson & Johnson Co.).

Cotton bandages of varying thicknesses can be used to help stabilize a limb for transport or to provide support after a cast has been removed.

Splints can be used to prevent flexion of a part, to apply tension, and to stabilize a lower limb fracture for transport. Because of the potential complications and additional damage that can result from an improperly applied cotton bandage or splint, these methods of immobilization are best left to an experienced veterinarian.

Casts provide the most stable form of immobilization when applied properly. Generally, a cast is applied while the horse is under general anesthesia. There are certain circumstances, however, in which it is applied in the standing animal.

Application of Counterirritation

Counterirritation is used to stimulate a subacute or chronic inflammatory process to a more acute process in the hope that healing will occur when the acute inflammation subsides. Of the methods available, therapeutic coutery (firing) is the most severe form of counterirritation. It is used most often to treat conditions of the carpus, cannon bone, and fetlock in racehorse. In some cases, it has been used prophylactically (before a problem arises), but there is no evidence to support this approach.

Although counterirritation in the form of sclerosing agents, internal and external blisters, and thermocautery (firing) has been used for many years in the horse, few controlled studies have been performed to assess effectiveness. In inexperienced hands, the use of these methods can add further injury to the horse. For this reason, these techniques are not frequently used.

Rubefacient Products

These produce redness and mild heat by increasing circulation. They are commonly present in various braces and liniments. Many terms are applied to products used for their rubefacient effect. The terms "liniment," "tightener," "brace," and "sweat" are often used. In reality, there is little difference among them.

A *liniment* is any combination of products used for a rubefacient effect. A liniment usually contains one or more of the essential (volatile) oils. Its use on the limbs of a horse can result in considerable edema (fluid swelling) and skin soreness. If the reaction is severe or neglected, scars and denuded areas can result. A horse should not be ridden while skin soreness or edema is present. The blistering effect of a liniment is increased when a bandage is used to cover the area where liniment was applied.

A *tightener* is a term applied to various mixtures that aid in the removal of edema or the fluid in a joint capsule or tendon sheath. The tightener effect comes from the removal of edema or excess synovial fluid so that the tendons and suspensory ligament are more palpable. In most cases, this effect is not due to the drug but to the massage with which the drug is applied and to the compression bandage that is applied over the area after the tightener has been rubbed in.

A *sweat* is a product that causes some moisture accumulation on the skin following its use. Most products including alcohol do this. The skin of a horse can actually exude serum from its surface in the presence of inflammation. A plastic wrapping, oiled silk, or waxed paper is usually applied around the limb after the use of this type of drug mixture. These wrappings themselves can cause the skin to "sweat." In addition to alcohol alone, equal parts of alcohol and glycerin and furacin ointment alone or in combination with DMSO usually 50/50 are also used for this action. Plastic sheeting can be wrapped over the drugs applied and bandaged over to increase the "sweat" effect.

A *brace* is a mixture of substances that is used routinely following workouts. The limbs of the horse are rubbed down before putting on limb wraps each night. In most cases, the massage used in applying the mixture is much more beneficial than the mixture itself, in preventing tendon sheath and joint capsule filling. Massage, plus the compression bandage, would accomplish the same purpose in most cases. Alcohol (ethyl or isopropyl) serves this purpose satisfactorily. Commercial preparations are also popular and can sometimes be used as a "tightener" and a "sweat" as well. Depending on concentrations of various products incorporated in commercial remedies, they may or may not produce a severe irritation when enclosed under a bandage.

Most rubefacient products are not really effective, but the massage and bandaging that go with them probably are. As long as the product does not cause pain to the horse and irritation to the skin, no harm is done. The rubefacient effect is temporary and must be repeated once or twice daily for any beneficial effect at all. A region of muscular soreness or joint soreness that is massaged shows pain relief following application of this type of drug. In just a short time, however, the effect is gone. Plastic sheeting applied to the limb after application of these drugs enhances their effect. It also increases the irritant effect, however, and could damage tissues.

Cryosurgery

Although the use of cryosurgery has received a lot of attention as an effective treatment for tumors, only recently has it been advocated for the treatment of musculoskeletal problems. The technique utilizes extreme cold produced by the application of liquid nitrogen. Cryotherapy has been used for cryogesia (blocking the sensation) of the palmar digital nerves and as a form of freeze firing for bucked shins (dorsal metacarpal disease). It has also been recommended for splints, cunean bursitis, tendinitis, curb, and bowed tendons.

Radiation Therapy

Radiation therapy is another way of producing deep inflammation. It produces an inflammatory reaction that can last for approximately 6 weeks. A minimum of 90 days' rest must be allowed following radiation therapy for best results. Radiation therapy can be applied in a number of ways. The most satisfactory

methods have employed the therapeutic x-ray machine or gamma radiation using cobalt-60 needles.

The following conditions may be treated with radiation therapy: chronic traumatic arthritis and osteoarthritis of the carpal joints, chronic traumatic arthritis and osteoarthritis of the fetlock joint, periosteal new bone growth of the carpal bones, and other conditions in which a deep prolonged inflammatory reaction would be beneficial.

X-Irradiation

The delivery of high-quality x-rays to a specific site is possible, but sophisticated equipment is required to filter the soft x-rays out. Unfortunately, a major drawback to this approach is the cost of equipment to safely deliver the x-rays. Radiation works by causing an irritation that increases the blood supply sufficiently to repair the problem.

Acupuncture

It has been stated that acupuncture prompts the body to heal itself by stimulating acupuncture points with needles, pressure, heat, injections, or implants. Acupuncture is most commonly used to treat sore backs but is used on a variety of other problems as well. How effective acupuncture is in the treatment of lameness is not known and cannot be specifically stated until controlled studies are performed and results reported.

Laser Therapy

Light Amplification by Stimulation Emission of Radiation (LASER) therapy is a recently introduced therapy that stimulates acupuncture points. When the electromagnetic waves are focused as a concentrated beam on a small spot, they can cut through living tissue. At low intensities and wider focus, "cold" or "soft" laser beams can be used to stimulate wound healing by modifying biochemical tissue responses and to suppress pain through the acupuncture release of endorphins. It has been recommended for the treatment of tendon and ligament injuries, arthritis, reduction of inflammation and scar tissue formation, enhancement of wound healing, and for the treatment of burns. As with acupuncture, the use of laser therapy remains an art, and until critical investigative studies prove its value, its widespread use will be limited.

Electrotherapy

Electrotherapy has generated some interest for fracture-repair enhancement. Treatments of delayed unions and nonunions, splints, buck shins, tendinitis, degenerative joint disease, and desmitis in the horse have been reported. What all these treatments have in common is a modification of local tissues such that an environment more conducive to healing occurs.

Electrostimulation (ES)

Direct ES at low amperage (5 to 20 microamp) has been shown to be beneficial in the treatment of delayed unions and nonunions. Because ES requires implants, however, the resulting complications make it an impractical therapy at this time.

Pulsing Electromagnetic Fields (PEM)

The application of PEM is totally noninvasive and has proven to be beneficial in the treatment of nonunions, failed arthrodesis, and congenital pseudoarthrosis in humans.

Reportedly, PEM mimics the normal physiologic responses in bone metabolism, and theoretically the biologic response of bone can be altered by adjustment of wave patterns and pulse rates. Much work, however, is needed to define specifically the influences of wave forms on biologic system responses. Studies representing individual testimonials, although important, in some cases may only serve to delay the basic research that is required to prove the benefit and worth of the pulsing electromagnetic fields.

To date, no research has been done that clearly identified a benefit from this treatment in the horse.

Magnetic Therapy (MT)

Although in use for many years, MT has only recently been subjected to critical investigation. This therapy has been reported to be effective in the treatment of various orthopedic disorders, but only a few controlled studies have been performed. Its major effect, when very low frequencies are used, is to increase the blood supply and the oxygen tension to the treated region. Additionally, there appears to be an ion exchange within the cells and the intracellular spaces that is beneficial, and it appears that local enzymes are affected as well. Even though there have been many testimonials to its benefit, more critical studies are needed before it can be recommended.

TENS and EMS Therapies

Transcutaneous Electrical Nerve Stimulation (TENS) therapy consists of an electrode-containing pad that passes low-voltage electric impulses to the nervous system. The theory is that repeated nonpainful stimulation of sensory nerve fibers breaks the pain cycle by overriding the pain sensation to the brain owing to the "overload" on the nerve tracts and the release of serotonin, a pain-blocking chemical. TENS therapy may be helpful for relief of chronic pain of arthritis in some cases.

Electrical Muscle Stimulation (EMS) uses high-voltage electrical current to create passive muscle contractions. The main application is to "exercise" atrophied muscles or those of a limb that is healing and cannot bear weight. Passive muscle contractions increase circulation, remove waste products, decrease edema, and thereby facilitate healing.

Poultices

These agents work through high osmotic tension to draw fluid from a part toward the surface. Poultices tend to limit infectious or noninfectious inflammatory processes. In some cases, they are applied over puncture wounds. Some of these agents are not applied directly to the skin, for they might cause excessive moistening of the skin. A bandage is placed over the poultice, and it is usually left in position for 12 to 48 hours. A poultice may be reapplied at intervals several times. Covering the poultice with plastic sheeting increases its efficiency.

There are commercially available medicated gauze bandages that serve as support bandages as well as poultice bandages.

Use of Anti-Inflammatory Agents

Anti-inflammatory agents are separated into steroidal and nonsteroidal agents.

Steroidal Anti-inflammatories

Steroidal anti-inflammatories are widely used in the treatment of numerous musculoskeletal problems, and although their adverse effects are well documented, their use has allowed many horses to return to useful competition.

Steroids enter the cell and combine with the cell nucleus to produce new proteins. These newly developed proteins reduce the cell metabolism, which gives rise to the pharmacologic effects. Because intracellular (into the cell) transfer of the corticoids is required, it usually takes several hours for this pharmacologic effect to be realized.

Steroids are renowned for their ability to suppress the immune response and thus make the animal more susceptible to infection. This is a particularly important consideration when these products are used for prolonged periods of time.

Prolonged steroid use is characterized by muscle wasting, suppression of growth in younger animals, altered bone metabolism that leads to osteoporosis, suppression of the immune status, and suppression of the adrenal cortex. The last-mentioned situation is important for animals that are taken off prolonged steroid therapy abruptly because they may suffer from acute Addison's crisis. Other systemic effects of corticosteroids worth mentioning are their effect on the vascular system and the mineralocorticoid effect. These effects plus the suppression of the adrenal cortex have been implicated in the predisposition to laminitis.

Intra-Articular Injection. Intra-articular corticosteroid therapy is commonly used in equine practice today to reduce the inflammation and pain in degenerative and traumatic arthritis. It has permitted many horses to complete their training and compete successfully. Studies have shown, however, that frequent use of some corticosteroids reduces the production of hyaluronic acid and important cartilage constituents while increasing osteophyte formation in joints. This made the articular surface less resilient and more vulnerable to mechanical trauma.

Contrary to this, one controlled study showed the injection of betamethazone (one of the corticosteroids) in the carpal joints is not detrimental when fractures are present and when the horse is worked.

Generally, no joint should be injected with a corticosteroid without a prior x-ray examination. Intra-articular injections of corticosteroids permit a horse to use a joint that has extensive pathologic changes, thereby causing further degenerative changes.

The site of anti-inflammatory action of corticosteroids, following intra-articular injection, appears to be the synovial membrane. These drugs cause a suppression of inflammation that allows recovery of cellular function. Synovial fluid volume is reduced, and its viscosity improves.

Adequate rest should accompany the use of corticosteroids, for they merely decrease inflammation while healing occurs. Too often, the corticosteroids are used to mask symptoms, and the horse is allowed to damage the part further.

The interval between injections depends on the severity of the condition and the degree of response to the previous injection. Some severe inflammatory conditions should be injected every 2 to 3 weeks, whereas less severely affected regions respond with less frequent injections. After the injection of a corticoid into a joint or tendon sheath, the region should be wrapped to establish counterpressure and to promote absorption of excess fluid.

Some products cause joint swelling after administration (synovial flare). This postinjection flare may cause heat, pain, and swelling that may last for a few hours to several days. The reaction is thought to be a crystal-induced synovitis from the crystalline suspension that was injected. This swelling usually disappears in 24 to 72 hours, and the effect of the drug can then be determined.

Besides the postinjection flare, the following adverse reactions to intra-articular steroids have been recognized: (1) Metaplastic bone formations are due to inadvertent injection of long-acting steroids into peri-articular soft tissues. These bony deposits develop over several months and may result in eventual lameness. (2) Septic arthritis is one of the most serious consequences to intrasynovial injections of corticosteroids. The organisms can infect the joint either by direct introduction from the injection or through the bloodstream. In either case, steroids administered intrasynovially or systemically decrease the number of organisms needed to cause a clinical infection. (3) Steroid arthropathy, which may be caused by the repeated injection of steroids, is characterized by a change in cartilage metabolism and an accelerated rate of joint destruction and x-ray evidence of advanced degenerative joint disease. The incidence of this can be markedly reduced by allowing the horse sufficient time to rest after the steroid injection and to use the treatment only when bone changes within the joint are not evident. (4) A predisposition to fragmented fractures of the carpus occurs in the horse worked while under the influence of corticosteroids.

Corticosteroid Therapy for Tendon Injuries. Tenosynovitis (windpuffs) and tendinitis (bowed tendon) of the superficial digital flexor and deep digital flexor tendons and desmitis of the suspensory ligament used to be treated by intralesional injections of steroids. Because of the relatively consistent development of calcification at the injection sites, however, this approach is no longer advocated. Corticosteroids injected into the tendon sheath as a treatment for tenosynovitis is still used and recommended.

Nonsteroidal Anti-inflammatory Drugs

Nonsteroidal anti-inflammatory drugs (NSAIDs) are a group of drugs with a diverse chemical structure that possess similar biologic action. All NSAIDs have a similar mode of action, accounting for both their therapeutic and their toxic effects. They inhibit prostaglandin synthesis and the formation of inflammatory products. This action is responsible for the anti-inflammatory, antipyretic (fever-reducing) and analgesic (pain-reducing) effects. Because the NSAIDs do not have an effect on the preformed prostaglandins, there is a lag time after administration before they exert a therapeutic effect. Although phenylbutazone and flunixin have a relatively short half-life (4.5 hours and 1.6 hours), their clinical effect may last for more than 24 hours after a single dose or as long as 3 days after a final course of treatment.

Despite the low toxicity of NSAIDs, they have been associated with gastrointestinal ulcers and kidney core necrosis.

Phenylbutazone (Butazolidin). Phenylbutazone ("bute") is the most widely used NSAID in equine practice. It is frequently used for the treatment of many problems leading to lameness, including problems with the feet, joints, bones, tendons, and muscles. The well-known analgesic, anti-inflammatory, and antipyretic effects in horses makes it an effective drug for the treatment of a number of injuries. Butazolidin is used intravenously and orally as tablets, powder, or paste.

A controlled study found that essentially 100% of orally administered phenylbutazone paste or powder is absorbed if it is administered before a meal and that a greater variability with decreased levels was found when phenylbutazone was given after the meal. No work has been done, however, to indicate what effect this treatment recommendation might have on the toxicity of this product. Although more expensive, the paste form is easier to administer, and one is more assured that the horse is receiving the correct amount of drug. Alternatively, tablets can be given with either a balling gun or crushed and put with molasses, or a powder form can be given. A greater toxicity was identified in foals when phenylbutazone was administered crushed and suspended in molasses versus when it was given with a balling gun. It is proposed that the molasses increased the contact time of phenylbutazone with the mucosa of the mouth and the gastrointestinal tract, thus increasing its toxic effect.

It is obvious from these studies, despite the evidence that phenylbutazone is well tolerated at recommended to low dosage levels in healthy horses, that its toxic effects are real and must be looked for. Variables such as drug interreaction, breed differences, preexisting disease, age, and overdoses of drug owing to error in weight estimation or frequency of administration may render the horse susceptible to toxicity even at recommended doses.

Ketoprofen. Ketoprofen is a relatively new NSAID approved for horses in 1990. It is recommended for alleviation of pain and inflammation associated with musculoskeletal problems, and it has been shown to be effective as an antiendotoxic drug for treatment of colic. Of the commonly used NSAIDs (Phenylbutazone and Banimine), it has been shown to have the least toxic side effects.

Meclofenamic acid [N-(2,6-dichloro-m-tolyl) anthranilic acid]. A study was done on this drug by four investigators in which it was used for a variety of lamenesses. The drug was given orally. There was no toxic effect, and the researchers believed that there was improvement in a significant number of cases. Other research showed it to be effective for relief of pain in pedal osteitis and laminitis and ineffective in osteoarthritis. Another study identified a negative side effect with a mean decrease of 18% in plasma protein concentration in ponies receiving the recommended doses of meclofenamic acid for 10 days.

Flunixin Meglumine (Banamine). Banamine, a nicotinic acid derivative, is a potent NSAID that is well absorbed and distributed to the body's tissues after intramuscular and intravenous administration. It appears to be a more potent drug than phenylbutazone because 0.5 mg of flunixin megluamine has the equivalent anti-inflammatory effect in a 450-kg horse as 2 g of phenylbutazone.

Flunixin meglumine is reported to be 100% bioavailable after intravenous injection and about 80% bioavailable if it is taken orally. Peak levels are present after 3 minutes when given intravenously and after 30 minutes when given orally. It is unique among the NSAIDs in that it appears to be effective at relatively low plasma concentrations. Even though its plasma half-life is short, about 1.6 hours, it produces a pharmacologic effect of up to 30 hours after a single administration and can be detected in urine for 15 days after treatment.

Although Banamine is frequently used in place of phenylbutazone for treatment of various musculoskeletal problems, it is also effective in the treatment of colic and has proven to be an effective antiendotoxic drug.

Naproxen (Equiproxen). Naproxen is a NSAID especially recommended for the relief of pain and inflammation from myositis and other soft tissue injuries. Although naproxen administered daily decreased the incidence of musculoskeletal diseases in horses during training and racing as compared with controls, it is not thought to be that effective for the treatment of joint disease in horses. Naproxen appears to have a reasonable margin of safety in the horse. Toxicity was not apparent when the drug was administered orally or intravenously at three times the recommended dosage for 42 days. One investigator reported that administration of recommended dosages for 14 days followed by two times this amount for 7 more days did alter plasma protein concentration.

Salicylates (Aspirin). Salicylates, although potent anti-inflammatory agents, have a short plasma half-life in herbivores and for that reason are not often used. They are cyclo-oxygenase inhibitors and follow the typical pharmacokinetics of inhibiting prostaglandins. Aspirin also has an antithiombrogenic activity (reduces clot formation) that makes it a valuable drug in the treatment of laminitis.

Thiosalicylate (Thiolate), a close relative of aspirin, is available in injectable form for horses. It has a longer half-life than aspirin, and for that reason it may be more effective.

Other Anti-inflammatory Drugs

Orgotein (Palosein). This is a metalloprotein isolated from bovine liver. It contains copper and zinc and when administered parenterally is said to be distributed rapidly throughout the body. Clinical tests sponsored by the manufacturer claimed good results in a wide variety of bone, joint, and soft tissue problems.

Orgotein is a superoxide dismutase (SOD) that exerts its anti-inflammatory effect by reducing the superoxide ion radical that is released from cells in inflamed tissues and from white blood cells. SOD is found naturally as an intracellular enzyme that acts to reduce the superoxide ion effect within the cell. Superoxide ions are produced in large amounts by the liver, red blood cells, and macrophage and neutrophil. Within an inflamed joint, these potent superoxide radicals have the capability of degrading cartilage proteoglycans, collagen, and hyaluronic acid. The efficacy of SOD is related to its ability to inhibit the breakdown of the neutrophil and release of the lysozyme, yet it does not interfere with the neutrophil's phagocytic capabilities. Orgotein also scavenges the extracellular superoxide ion, which decreases the potential for further damage.

SOD does not have an antipyretic effect, it is not immunosuppressive, it does not enhance sepsis or interreact with other drugs, and it has no known side effects, even with repeated use. It does have a direct anti-inflammatory effect, and its usefulness in the treatment of arthritic entities when it is administered either systemically or intra-articularly has been documented in the horse.

Dimethyl Sulfoxide (DMSO). DMSO is a solvent and mixes with many other common solvents and with water. It is extremely hygroscopic (moisture absorbing), absorbing 70% of its weight from air under the right temperature and humidity conditions. This hygroscopic property makes sealing the bottle after use mandatory. Its penetration of the skin reaches a maximum when it is mixed with 10% water. If stored with a loose cap, it will absorb water to become rapidly diluted.

DMSO has its greatest use in reducing acute swelling of noninfectious origin. Seromas, hematomas, and edema from trauma, when the skin is not broken, respond to application of this product. It is not to be used on raw wound surfaces.

DMSO apparently can carry drugs through the skin, and various claims have been made for remedies utilizing this quality. The molecular size of the product, however, determines whether it will penetrate or not. DMSO carries irritating drugs into tissue, and one should be cautious before using it on an area to which any type of blistering material containing iodine, turpentine, camphor, or similar substances has been applied previously because it may cause severe reaction owing to deep penetration by these agents. Corticosteroids have been mixed with DMSO so that they are carried to deeper tissues.

Research reports the successful use of DMSO in the treatment of degenerative joint disease in the horse. It has also proved beneficial as a lavage solution for the treatment of septic arthritis or septic tenosynovitis.

Frequently the topical application of DMSO causes a transient irritation in the skin that may cause the horse to bite at the region treated.

This drug has been most effective in the treatment of acute swelling, particularly of the lower limb. The gel form is easily applied either alone or under a bandage or in combination with furacin to make a sweat. The addition of corticosteroids to increase the anti-inflammatory effect can also be used. It can be applied topically, usually two to three times a day, in areas that are not to be rebandaged. Another problem associated with DMSO therapy is hair loss that may leave the horse more susceptible to superficial infection. These effects can be reduced somewhat by combining DMSO with furacin in a 50–50 mixture. It is impor-

tant to obtain proper instructions for applying the drug from the veterinarian.

Adverse reactions documented in humans include minor rashes, increased sensitivity to antibiotics, headaches, dizziness, and generalized dermatitis. The latter three have been reported infrequently. An oyster-like breath is common after contact with DMSO. Minor rashes that occur are often preceded by blisters at the site of application. Because antibiotics can penetrate the skin when applied in combination with DMSO, antibiotic sensitivity may develop in persons applying these drugs. The use of gloves is advocated in all cases when applying the drug; even then it is not uncommon, for those that appear to be susceptible, to have an oyster-like taste in their mouth. Particular caution should be taken by women who are childbearing.

Hyaluronic Acid (HA). HA is a natural constituent of synovial fluid used in treating synovitis/capsulitis problems. Although HA may prevent inflammatory enzymes from degrading cartilage, it does not repair existing cartilage damage. HA also has anti-inflammatory properties. Depending on the severity of the arthritis, the joint's synovial fluid breaks down into a thin, ineffective lubricant that can be enhanced by the high viscosity (thickness) of HA. First 1 to 2 ml of synovial fluid are drained from the joint, then sodium hyaluronate (the acid salt of hyaluronic acid) is injected directly into the joint (intra-articularly). Intravenous administration of HA has also been proven to be beneficial.

Selection criteria for horses appropriate for HA treatment include those that responded positively to joint block, show no bony changes on x-rays, and have no associated joint or ligament problems. In appropriate cases, 80 to 90% of the horses treated with HA experience a beneficial effect. Although a positive response may occur within a few days, the maximum response does not usually appear until 2 weeks after the injection. The effect may last for several months, and there are no side effects. The most beneficial effects have been seen with synovitis and capsulitis in the knee and fetlock joints. After injection, the horse is hand-walked for 5 days and not returned to work for 2 weeks. The use of HA in conjunction with corticosteroids shows an advantage over corticosteroids alone. HA is available in several viscosities; the higher the molecular weight, the more effective and the more expensive.

Polysulfated Glycosaminoglycan (PSGAG). PSGAG (commercially available as Adequan) also occurs naturally in synovial fluid and is partially responsible for the resiliency of cartilage. Treatment of an arthritic joint with PSGAG not only improves the viscosity of the synovial fluid, but also arrests or delays further cartilage damage (chondroprotection) in chronic or recurrent arthritis. It does this by inhibiting the enzymes of inflammation that break down proteoglycans, the substances enmeshed within a collagen framework that give cartilage its compressive stiffness. PSGAG diffuses into the articular cartilage and binds to the collagen molecules, acting as replacement glycosaminoglycans. It is appropriate for treatment of synovitis and capsulitis and may have more far-reaching effects. Although PSGAG is largely chondroprotective in nature, it may also have restorative properties. PSGAG promotes HA synthesis and may be able to replace glycosaminoglycans lost from the cartilage.

More frequent injections may be necessary with PSGAG than with HA, and the beneficial effects from PSGAG treatment may not show up for several weeks. In addition to its intra-articular use, however, it has been used orally and intramuscularly. The latter two methods have the added benefit of treating more than one joint at the same time.

Index

Page numbers in *italics* indicate figures; those followed by "t" indicate tables.